THE Healthcare Quality Book

FOURTH EDITION

THE Healthcare Quality Book

Vision, Strategy, and Tools

David B. Nash • Maulik S. Joshi •
Elizabeth R. Ransom • Scott B. Ransom • Editors

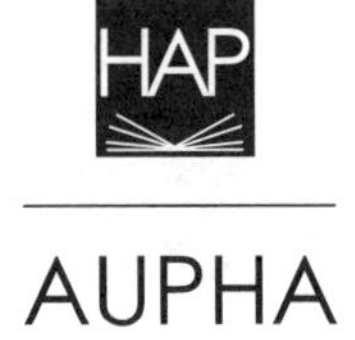

Health Administration Press, Chicago, Illinois
Association of University Programs in Health Administration, Washington, DC

Your board, staff, or clients may also benefit from this book's insight. For more information on quantity discounts, contact the Health Administration Press Marketing Manager at (312) 424-9450.

23 22 21 5 4 3 2

Library of Congress Cataloging-in-Publication Data

Names: Nash, David B., editor. | Joshi, Maulik, editor. | Ransom, Elizabeth R., editor. | Ransom, Scott B., editor.

Title: The healthcare quality book : vision, strategy, and tools / David B. Nash, Maulik S. Joshi, Elizabeth R. Ransom, and Scott B. Ransom, editors.

Description: Fourth edition. | Chicago, Illinois ; Association of University Programs in Health Administration : Washington, DC : Health Administration Press, [2019] | Includes bibliographical references and index. | Identifiers: LCCN 2018060062 (print) | LCCN 2019000071 (ebook) | ISBN 9781640550544 (eBook 13) | ISBN 9781640550551 (Xml) | ISBN 9781640550568 (Epub) | ISBN 9781640550575 (Mobi) | ISBN 9781640550537 (print)

Subjects: LCSH: Medical care—United States—Quality control. | Health services administration—United States—Quality control. | Total quality management—United States.

Classification: LCC RA399.A3 (ebook) | LCC RA399.A3 H433 2019 (print) | DDC 362.1068—dc23

LC record available at https://lccn.loc.gov/2018060062

The paper used in this publication meets the minimum requirements of American National Standard for Information Sciences—Permanence of Paper for Printed Library Materials, ANSI Z39.48-1984. ∞™

Acquisitions editor: Jennette McClain; Project manager: Michael Noren; Cover designer: James Slate; Layout: Cepheus Edmondson

Found an error or a typo? We want to know! Please email it to hapbooks@ache.org, mentioning the book's title and putting "Book Error" in the subject line.

Health Administration Press
A division of the Foundation of the American College of Healthcare Executives
300 S. Riverside Plaza, Suite 1900
Chicago, IL 60606-6698
(312) 424-2800

Association of University Programs in Health Administration
1730 M Street, NW
Suite 407
Washington, DC 20036
(202) 763-7283

BRIEF CONTENTS

Foreword xvii
Brent C. James
Preface xix
David B. Nash, Maulik S. Joshi, Elizabeth R. Ransom, and Scott B. Ransom

Part I The Foundation of Healthcare Quality
Maulik S. Joshi

Chapter 1. Overview of Healthcare Quality 5
Rebecca C. Jaffe, Alexis Wickersham, and Bracken Babula

Chapter 2. History and the Quality Landscape 49
Norbert Goldfield

Chapter 3. Variation in Medical Practice and Implications for Quality 75
David J. Ballard, Briget da Graca, David Nicewander, and Brett D. Stauffer

Part II Tools, Measures, and Their Applications
Elizabeth R. Ransom

Chapter 4. Data Collection 107
John Byrnes

Chapter 5. Statistical Tools for Quality Improvement 127
Davis Balestracci

Chapter 6. Physician Profiling and Provider Registries 171
Bettina Berman and Richard Jacoby

Chapter 7. Health Information Technology in Healthcare Quality and Safety: Prevention, Identification, and Action 189
Sue S. Feldman, Scott E. Buchalter, and Leslie W. Hayes

Chapter 8. Simulation in Healthcare Quality and Safety 213
Hyunjoo Lee and Dimitrios Papanagnou

Part III Culture and Leadership
David B. Nash

Chapter 9. The Patient Experience..233
Deirdre E. Mylod and Thomas H. Lee

Chapter 10. Safety Science and High Reliability Organizing..............253
Craig Clapper

Chapter 11. Education for Healthcare Quality and Safety..................279
David Mayer and Anne J. Gunderson

Chapter 12. Creating Alignment: Quality Measures and Leadership..301
Michael D. Pugh

Chapter 13. Governance for Quality 329
Kathryn C. Peisert

Part IV Emerging Trends
Scott B. Ransom

Chapter 14. Ambulatory Quality and Safety 363
Lawrence Ward and Rhea E. Powell

Chapter 15. The Role of the National Committee for Quality Assurance...389
Michael S. Barr and Frank Micciche

Chapter 16. Value-Based Insurance Design 415
A. Mark Fendrick, Susan Lynne Oesterle, Marianthi N. Hatzigeorgiou, and Margaret F. Shope

Chapter 17. Value-Based Purchasing: The Increasing Importance of Quality Considerations in Funding the Healthcare System 439
Neil Goldfarb

Chapter 18. Medication Use Quality..457
Mel L. Nelson, Matthew K. Pickering, Hannah M. Fish, and Laura Cranston

Chapter 19. Population Health Safety and Quality 475
Keith Kosel

Index..501
About the Editors..547
About the Contributors..551

DETAILED CONTENTS

Foreword xvii
Brent C. James
Preface xix
David B. Nash, Maulik S. Joshi, Elizabeth R. Ransom, and Scott B. Ransom

Part I The Foundation of Healthcare Quality
Maulik S. Joshi

Chapter 1. Overview of Healthcare Quality 5
Rebecca C. Jaffe, Alexis Wickersham, and Bracken Babula
The Growing Focus on Quality 5
Frameworks and Stakeholders 9
Measurement 14
Quality Improvement Models 17
Quality Improvement Tools 22
Conclusion 33
Case Study: Mr. Roberts and the US Healthcare System 33
Case Study: Stopping Catheter-Related Bloodstream Line Infections at the Johns Hopkins University Medical Center and Hospitals Across the United States 38
Study Questions 43
References 44

Chapter 2. History and the Quality Landscape 49
Norbert Goldfield
Introduction 49
Quality Measurement and Management Prior to 1965 50
Medicare, Medicaid, and Subsequent Developments 53
New Outcomes Metrics and the Future of Quality Measurement and Management 63
Conclusion 65
Notes 66

Study Questions 66
References 67

Chapter 3. Variation in Medical Practice and Implications for Quality 75
David J. Ballard, Briget da Graca, David Nicewander, and Brett D. Stauffer
Variation in Medical Practice 75
Analyzing Variation 82
Using Variation Data to Drive Healthcare Quality Initiatives 87
Conclusion 94
Study Questions 95
References 95

Part II Tools, Measures, and Their Applications
Elizabeth R. Ransom

Chapter 4. Data Collection 107
John Byrnes
Considerations in Data Collection 107
Sources of Data 113
Conclusion: Returning to the Case Example 123
Notes 124
Study Questions 125
Acknowledgments 125
Additional Resources 125
References 126

Chapter 5. Statistical Tools for Quality Improvement 127
Davis Balestracci
Introduction 127
Process-Oriented Thinking: The Context for Improvement Statistics 128
Variation: The Framework of This Chapter 130
Plotting Data over Time: The Run Chart 132
Common Causes Versus Special Causes of Variation 134
The Control Chart: A Very Powerful Tool 139
Analysis: The I-Chart Is Your "Swiss Army Knife" 147
An Important Expansion of the Concepts of "Perfectly Designed," Common Cause, and Special Cause 150

Summary 162
Study Questions 164
Additional Resources 164
References 169

Chapter 6. Physician Profiling and Provider Registries 171
Bettina Berman and Richard Jacoby
Background and Terminology 171
The Physician's Role in Improving Quality 174
Use of Physician Profiling and Provider Registries in Healthcare Organizations 176
Examples of Profiles and Scorecards 177
Benchmarking 180
The Measurement and Implementation Process 181
Keys to Success 183
Challenges 183
Physician Profiling and Provider Registries in a Changing Healthcare Landscape 185
Study Questions 186
References 186

Chapter 7. Health Information Technology in Healthcare Quality and Safety: Prevention, Identification, and Action 189
Sue S. Feldman, Scott E. Buchalter, and Leslie W. Hayes
Introduction 189
Health IT in Healthcare Quality and Safety 190
What Does the Literature Say About Health IT Use in Healthcare Quality and Safety? 191
Improving Care Delivery Through Health IT: Case Studies 195
Case Study 1: Prevention 195
Case Study 2: Identification 198
Case Study 3: Action 202
Conclusion 205
References 210

Chapter 8. Simulation in Healthcare Quality and Safety 213
Hyunjoo Lee and Dimitrios Papanagnou
Introduction to Simulation 213
Applying Educational Frameworks to Patient Safety Simulations 218

Simulation in the Patient Safety Landscape 221
Conclusion....................226
Study Questions....................226
References....................227

Part III Culture and Leadership
David B. Nash

Chapter 9. The Patient Experience....................233
Deirdre E. Mylod and Thomas H. Lee
The Patient Experience Emerges....................233
Concerns About Patient Experience Data....................236
Improving Patient Experience Measurement and Reporting....................241
Using Patient Experience Data to Improve....................245
Study Questions....................249
References....................250

Chapter 10. Safety Science and High Reliability Organizing....................253
Craig Clapper
Safety and Reliability....................253
History of the Modern Safety Movement....................256
Reliability as an Emergent Property....................260
Descriptive Theories of High Reliability Organizations..262
Why Should We Care?....................265
Creating Safety and High Reliability in Practice....................266
Important Topics in Safety and High Reliability....................271
Sustaining Cultures of Safety and High Reliability....................276
Study Questions....................276
References....................277

Chapter 11. Education for Healthcare Quality and Safety....................279
David Mayer and Anne J. Gunderson
Introduction....................279
Early Curricular Work in Clinical Quality and Patient Safety....................281
Current Curricular Work in Clinical Quality and Patient Safety....................286
Conclusion....................298
Study Questions....................298
References....................299

Chapter 12. Creating Alignment: Quality Measures and Leadership 301
Michael D. Pugh
Introduction 301
Quality Measures and Metrics 301
Quality Assurance, Quality Control, and Quality Improvement 305
Leadership, Measurement, and Improvement 308
Case Study: Board-Adopted Quality Aims 318
Conclusion 324
Notes 325
Study Questions 326
References 326

Chapter 13. Governance for Quality 329
Kathryn C. Peisert
Background: Why Is Quality the Board's Responsibility? 329
What Are the Board's Quality Oversight Duties? 340
The Board-Level Quality Committee 350
Building a Culture of Quality and Safety 352
Conclusion 356
Notes 356
Study Questions 357
References 357

Part IV Emerging Trends
Scott B. Ransom

Chapter 14. Ambulatory Quality and Safety 363
Lawrence Ward and Rhea E. Powell
The Ambulatory Care Setting 363
Ambulatory Quality Improvement 364
Ambulatory Safety 371
Future Challenges and Keys to Success 374
Conclusion 376
Case Study: A Private Practice in the Pennsylvania Chronic Care Initiative 377
Case Study: Comprehensive Primary Care Plus 379
Case Study: A New Pay-for-Performance Contract 380

Case Study: Referral Follow-Up and Ambulatory Safety 382
Study Questions 382
References 383

Chapter 15. The Role of the National Committee for Quality Assurance 389
Michael S. Barr and Frank Micciche
Healthcare Quality: A Novel Concept 389
Development of the National Committee for Quality Assurance 390
NCQA Adds Practice-Level Focus 393
2009–2017: A New Era of Health Reform 400
Quality Measurement: Assessing Healthcare Performance Across the United States 404
Conclusion 408
Study Questions 409
References 409

Chapter 16. Value-Based Insurance Design 415
A. Mark Fendrick, Susan Lynne Oesterle, Marianthi N. Hatzigeorgiou, and Margaret F. Shope
Introduction 415
Key Concepts in the Shift from Volume to Value 416
Putting Innovation into Action 419
The Future of V-BID 429
Conclusion 433
Study Questions 433
Case Study: Implementation of Connecticut's Health Enhancement Plan 433
References 435

Chapter 17. Value-Based Purchasing: The Increasing Importance of Quality Considerations in Funding the Healthcare System 439
Neil Goldfarb
Introduction and Definitions 439
Overview of Value-Based Purchasing Strategies 440
Public Purchaser Value-Based Purchasing: CMS and Medicare 447
Employers as Value-Based Purchasers 449

Driving Toward a Value-Based Marketplace 453
Study Questions 453
References 454

Chapter 18. Medication Use Quality 457
Mel L. Nelson, Matthew K. Pickering, Hannah M. Fish, and Laura Cranston
Introduction 457
The Shift from Volume to Value in Healthcare 457
Medication Use Expert: The Pharmacist 463
Emerging Trends: Pharmacist Engagement in a Value-Based Healthcare System 467
Conclusion 470
Study Question 470
Interactive Exercise 470
References 471

Chapter 19. Population Health Safety and Quality 475
Keith Kosel
Overview: Where We Stand Today 475
Safety and Quality in Various Populations 478
What Should Safety and Quality Look Like in a Community? 480
Who Should Be Responsible for Population Safety and Quality? 487
Case Study: Hearts Beat Back: The Heart of New Ulm Project 491
Case Study: Boston Community Asthma Initiative 492
The Role of Measurement in Driving Population Health Safety and Quality 492
Going Forward 495
Conclusion 497
Study Questions 497
References 497

Index 501
About the Editors 547
About the Contributors 551

FOREWORD

The modern quality movement has been building for nearly half a century. Wennberg's classic study documenting massive geographic variation in healthcare appeared in 1973. In 1987, researchers established that the amount of clinical variation within a single hospital was larger than the variation among geographic regions. By the mid-1990s, Deming's position that higher quality nearly always reduces operating costs was proving correct. In late 1999, the Institute of Medicine released the *To Err Is Human* report, which launched patient safety as a critical quality focus. Its 2001 successor, *Crossing the Quality Chasm*, reflected the voice of the healing professions calling for fundamental reform of healthcare delivery systems. Literally thousands of successful clinical projects, across a wide range of organizations and settings, have given further support for Deming's premise: The path to financial stability runs through clinical excellence.

But all these years later, has anything really changed? Variation still runs rampant in care delivery services, and patients still suffer unacceptable rates of care-associated injuries and deaths. Costs continue to rise, making essential healthcare services ever less accessible. Why?

Quality improvement theory contains two major parts. The first is data-based problem solving—a set of methods and tools that help identify operational problems, find focused areas for high-leverage change, and then demonstrably fix those problems through measured experimentation. The vast majority of healthcare quality training and most organizational quality initiatives rely on data-based problem solving. However, despite its manifest effectiveness, data-based problem solving innately builds around a series of projects. Clinical researchers sometimes note that "multiple anecdotes do not constitute evidence," and the same is true in quality: Multiple projects do not constitute health system reform.

The second part of quality improvement is what Deming called a "system of production"—the idea that a masterful enterprise will organize literally everything around value-added frontline work processes. This approach starts with key process analysis, a tool that prioritizes the processes that define any organization, and it builds true transparency, embedding data systems that align to key processes. Management structure follows the process structure. A "system of production" is bottom-up healthcare reform. A number of examples—Allina

Health in Minnesota, Mission Health in North Carolina, and Bellin Health in Michigan, to name a few—have shown that these principles can work just as well in care delivery as they do in other industries.

The volume you hold in your hands is about creating a system that supports quality. It outlines the major, essential components, and it shows how to fit those components together. Properly used, it can serve as an operations manual for healthcare reform, laying a foundation upon which you can build a new future. It holds the keys to a care delivery system that delivers

All the right care, but
Only the right care;
Without defect or injury;
At the lowest necessary cost;
Under the full knowledge and control of the patient; while
Learning from every case.

Read it, then go forth and conquer.

Brent C. James, MD, MStat
Salt Lake City, Utah

PREFACE

Transformation, *disruptive innovation*, *redesign*, *reform*—these popular terms all accurately characterize the state of our current healthcare system and its evolution. The changes we are witnessing today are accelerating at a rate that early pioneers in medicine could not have envisioned. All healthcare organizations are facing the challenges of change as they embark on their individual journeys to provide better care, better service, and better overall health for everyone they serve. All organizations are on a different path and have a different destination. However, they all have one commonality: *Quality* is the road map. Improving healthcare quality is the essential strategy to survive and thrive in the future. The difference between organizations that are good and those that are great is determined by leadership, and leaders who are masters of quality improvement are the difference makers.

This textbook provides a framework, strategies, and practical tactics to help all healthcare leaders to learn, teach, and lead improvement efforts. This fourth edition has been updated significantly from the previous editions, but once again it has an all-star list of contributors with incredible expertise and breadth of experience. Like the healthcare field itself, this edition has been improved, reimagined, and redesigned. Organized into four sections, the book focuses on the foundation of healthcare quality (part I); tools, measures, and their applications (part II); culture and leadership (part III); and emerging trends (part IV). Individually, and in aggregate, this book is designed to be both an instructional guide and a conversation starter among all students of healthcare quality—that is, all current and future healthcare professionals.

Part I contains three chapters that together provide a foundation for healthcare quality. In chapter 1, Rebecca C. Jaffe, Alexis Wickersham, and Bracken Babula provide an overview of major reports and concepts, Donabedian's classic structure-process-outcome framework, and methods and tools for quality improvement. The history and the landscape of quality in healthcare are beautifully narrated by Norbert Goldfield in chapter 2. In chapter 3, David J. Ballard and colleagues examine one of the most pervasive and significant issues in healthcare quality—clinical variation. They explain the concept, distinguish between warranted and unwarranted variation, and discuss quality improvement tools that can help manage and reduce unwarranted variation in medical practice.

Part II of the book builds on the foundation and speaks in-depth to tools, measures, and their applications in the pursuit of quality. John Byrnes, in chapter 4, articulates how data are the foundation of quality and patient safety and how the effective and efficient collection of data is critical to all strategic endeavors to improve quality. Davis Balestracci, in chapter 5, reveals how to apply the appropriate statistical analyses to make the information meaningful. In chapter 6, Bettina Berman and Richard Jacoby expertly apply data to the physician and provider registry domain as another tool for leveraging information for improvement. Information technology (IT) is an engine that uses data as fuel and, in chapter 7, Sue S. Feldman, Scott E. Buchalter, and Leslie W. Hayes describe how organizations use healthcare IT in a three-part cycle of prevention, identification, and action with data and information. Chapter 8 rounds out part II's focus on applications of data, information, measures, and tools, as Hyunjoo Lee and Dimitrios Papanagnou provide an overview of how simulation, as they say, "can be used to improve healthcare quality and safety by highlighting its intrinsic ability to expose, inform, and improve behaviors that are critical for effective communication and teamwork."

Whereas part II provides a comprehensive view of the measures, tools, and technologies that are needed to improve quality and safety in healthcare moving forward, part III focuses on what is arguably the key to everything—leadership and culture. To begin this section, Deirdre E. Mylod and Thomas H. Lee, in chapter 9, summarize important aspects of patient satisfaction—a key marker of a patient-centered field. In chapter 10, Craig Clapper, a national expert and teacher in high reliability, reinforces the goals of zero preventable harm and 100 percent appropriate care as cornerstones of a high reliability culture.

In chapter 11, David Mayer and Anne J. Gunderson trace the history of the education movement by outlining key milestone papers and symposia, signaling that there are still significant gaps in the teaching of education for healthcare quality. Chapter 12, by Michael D. Pugh, exquisitely details the why and how of dashboards and scorecards as critical leadership system tools for improvement and accountability. The final chapter in this section, chapter 13 by Kathryn C. Peisert, describes the fiduciary responsibility of the board of directors and delineates its central role in the quality and safety debate. Ultimately, the board bears the responsibility for *everything* in the healthcare organization, including quality and safety.

The textbook concludes with part IV—a compilation of chapters that discuss many of the emerging trends in today's fast-paced healthcare environment. Lawrence Ward and Rhea E. Powell, in chapter 14, consider the multitude of approaches to improving quality and safety in the ambulatory setting, providing contemporary insights for driving improvements in the delivery of care in primary care and specialty provider offices, ambulatory surgery centers, urgent care centers, retail clinics, freestanding emergency departments, and work-based clinics. In chapter 15, Michael S. Barr and Frank Micciche provide an overview of the National Committee for Quality Assurance (NCQA), from its initial role in helping employers and health plans develop quality standards to its present-day work in creating systems to measure those standards, including the Healthcare Effectiveness Data and Information Set (HEDIS) measures, health plan accreditation guidelines, the patient-centered medical home model, and various recognition programs.

In chapter 16, A. Mark Fendrick and colleagues present the fundamentals of value-based insurance design, another trend that impacts all healthcare stakeholders. Neil Goldfarb then shows us in chapter 17 how purchasers select and pay for healthcare services with a greater focus on value. Mel L. Nelson and her colleagues in chapter 18 provide a pharmacy perspective on achieving greater quality and lower cost through effective medication use. Finally, in chapter 19 by Keith Kosel, we review current thinking on population health quality and safety.

Throughout the world, healthcare is changing dramatically. However, that dramatic change will lead to significant advances in patient safety and quality of life only when organizations and healthcare leaders effectively implement quality improvement solutions to our complex problems.

As editors, we use this book extensively, whether for teaching in our courses, as reference material, or for research. The most important use is for leading change within our organizations. We greatly appreciate all the feedback we have received thus far to improve the textbook so that we can all be better leaders and healthcare providers.

Please contact us at doctormaulikjoshi@yahoo.com with your feedback on this edition. Your teaching, learning, and leadership are what will ultimately transform healthcare.

David B. Nash
Maulik S. Joshi
Elizabeth R. Ransom
Scott B. Ransom

Instructor Resources

This book's Instructor Resources include teaching aids for each chapter, including PowerPoint summaries, answers to the end-of-chapter study questions, and a test bank.

For the most up-to-date information about this book and its Instructor Resources, go to ache.org/HAP and search for the book's order code (2382).

This book's Instructor Resources are available to instructors who adopt this book for use in their course. For access information, please email hapbooks@ache.org.

PART

I

THE FOUNDATION OF HEALTHCARE QUALITY

Maulik S. Joshi

Quality is the focal point in the transformation of the healthcare system. A fundamental change in the way care is delivered and financed requires addressing every facet of quality, including

- understanding the gaps and variation from best practices in care and service;
- leveraging data, tools, and information technology to lead quality improvement;
- creating a culture of service excellence, safety, high reliability, and value;
- leading and governing toward population health; and
- engaging with all key stakeholders, such as accrediting bodies, policy makers, payers, purchasers, providers, and consumers.

The three chapters that make up this section of the book provide an overview of quality, trace the history of the quality movement in healthcare, and address the issue of variation in the quality of clinical care. Together, the chapters provide a foundation for leading the healthcare transformation.

Rebecca C. Jaffe and colleagues begin in chapter 1 by providing an overview of major reports and concepts that form the quality foundation. Two Institute of Medicine (IOM) reports—*To Err is Human* (2000) and *Crossing the Quality Chasm* (2001)—are truly landmark documents that articulate major deficiencies in the United States healthcare system and define a strategic road map for a future state of improved quality. The reports highlight the severity of medical errors, estimated to account for up to 98,000 deaths and $29 billion per year, and provide a critical classification scheme for understanding quality defects. The categories are underuse (not doing what evidence calls for), misuse (not appropriately executing best practices), and overuse (doing more than is appropriate). The IOM reports also introduce a game-changing framework for defining six aims of quality: It should be safe, timely, effective, efficient, equitable, and patient centered. Finally, the reports note that, for improvement to be lasting, it must happen at four nested levels—at the level of the patient, the team, the organization, and the environment.

Chapter 1 also discusses the work of Avedis Donabedian, who noted that all evaluations of quality of care could be viewed in terms of one of three measures—structure, process, or outcome. Evaluation based on structure considers characteristics of the people or setting, such as accreditation or physician board certification, that serve as structural quality measures. Assessment of process quality involves measures such as the percentage of diabetic patients receiving a blood sugar test in the previous 12 months, or the percentage of eligible women receiving mammograms. Outcomes, such as mortality rates and self-reported health status, are the ultimate quality measures.

The remaining content in chapter 1 focuses on the methods and tools necessary to achieve the goal of improved quality. Many approaches to quality improvement are available, and all are worth considering. The methods and tools have a variety of names and titles (e.g., the Plan-Do-Study-Act cycle, Six Sigma, Lean), but their success is fundamentally dependent on the culture and capability for executing improvement. Essential to all are the steps of identifying the problem(s), setting measurable aims for improvement, testing interventions, studying data to assess the impact of the interventions, and repeating the cycle of testing and learning. Chapter 1 ends with a discussion of what quality is all about—providing the best care and service to the patient. The concluding case studies highlight opportunities to improve systems of care so that future patients don't have to face the same problems that have plagued the healthcare field to date.

In chapter 2, Norbert Goldfield describes the history and landscape of quality, introducing us to healthcare quality pioneers such as Walter Shewhart, William Deming, and J. M. Juran. Goldfield places a particular emphasis on Ernest A. Codman, who studied results, or what we now call outcomes. The chapter continues with a discussion of Medicare and Medicaid, which serves as a launchpad for addressing important elements of quality—case mix, risk adjustment, claims and medical records, and, ultimately, payment for quality. Malpractice, consumerism, and the politics of healthcare quality represent both challenges and opportunities for the future of quality improvement. Goldfield's calls to action apply the learnings from the past to accelerate better quality data and measurement, better quality management, and the implementation of change in the "small-*p*" politics of healthcare.

In chapter 3, David J. Ballard and colleagues examine one of the most pervasive and vexing issues in healthcare quality—clinical variation. Although variation in medical practice has been studied for nearly a century, John Wennberg and colleagues brought it to the forefront with the development of the

Dartmouth Atlas of Health Care, which accentuated the differences in rates of utilization for many medical procedures in the United States. The color-coded *Dartmouth Atlas* maps reveal the often-stark differences between counties, even those adjacent to each other, in terms of the rates of procedures. Ballard and colleagues note the tenets of warranted variation, which is based on patient preferences and related factors, and unwarranted variation, which cannot be explained by patient preference or evidence-based medicine. The effects of unwarranted variation are well documented and include inefficient care, excessive costs, and disparities in outcomes. The chapter authors emphasize that the goal is not to merely understand the nature of variation but to implement strategies to reduce unwarranted variation. Building on chapters 1 and 2, chapter 3 notes that positive change requires identifying variation in practice, distinguishing warranted from unwarranted variation, and implementing quality improvement tools to manage and reduce unwarranted variation.

The foundation of quality requires us to acknowledge history's lessons to create a better future. Today's challenges are not completely new; many healthcare pioneers studied the early dimensions of quality measurement and management long ago. Sentinel reports and studies over the last two decades have called attention to major gaps in quality, as well as strategies and tools to get quality to where we want it to be. Even with all of this knowledge and evidence in hand, however, we are still confronted by the ubiquitous variation in quality of care. Looking to the future, we must address this variation to ensure that the right care is provided to the right patients at the right time and place.

CHAPTER

1

OVERVIEW OF HEALTHCARE QUALITY

Rebecca C. Jaffe, Alexis Wickersham, and Bracken Babula

The Growing Focus on Quality

The quality of the US healthcare system is not what it could be. Around the end of the twentieth century and the start of the twenty-first, a number of reports presented strong evidence of widespread quality deficiencies and highlighted a need for substantial change to ensure high-quality care for all patients. Among the major reports driving the imperative for quality improvement were the following:

- "The Urgent Need to Improve Health Care Quality" by the Institute of Medicine (IOM) National Roundtable on Health Care Quality (Chassin and Galvin 1998)
- IOM's *To Err Is Human: Building a Safer Health System* (Kohn, Corrigan, and Donaldson 2000)
- IOM's *Crossing the Quality Chasm: A New Health System for the 21st Century* (IOM 2001)
- The *National Healthcare Quality Report*, published annually by the Agency for Healthcare Research and Quality (AHRQ) since 2003
- The National Academies of Sciences, Engineering, and Medicine's *Improving Diagnosis in Health Care* (National Academies 2015)

Years after these reports were first published, they continue to make a tremendous, vital statement. They call for action, drawing attention to gaps in care and identifying opportunities to significantly improve the quality of healthcare in the United States.

"The Urgent Need to Improve Health Care Quality"

Published in 1998, the IOM's National Roundtable report "The Urgent Need to Improve Health Care Quality" included two notable contributions to the quality movement. The first was an assessment of the current state of quality (Chassin and Galvin 1998, 1000): "Serious and widespread quality problems exist throughout American medicine. These problems . . . occur in small and large communities alike, in all parts of the country, and with approximately equal frequency in managed care and fee-for-service systems of care. Very large numbers of Americans are harmed." The second contribution was the categorization of quality defects into three broad categories: underuse, overuse, and misuse. This classification scheme has become a common nosology for quality defects and can be summarized as follows:

- Underuse occurs when scientifically sound practices are not used as often as they should be. For example, only 72 percent of women between the ages of 50 and 74 reported having a mammogram within the past two years (White et al. 2015). In other words, nearly one in four women does not receive treatment consistent with evidence-based guidelines.
- Overuse occurs when treatments and practices are used to a greater extent than evidence deems appropriate. Examples of overuse include imaging studies for diagnosis of acute low-back pain and the prescription of antibiotics for acute bronchitis.
- Misuse occurs when clinical care processes are not executed properly—for example, when the wrong drug is prescribed or the correct drug is prescribed but incorrectly administered.

To Err Is Human: Building a Safer Health System

Although the healthcare community had been cognizant of its quality challenges for years, the 2000 publication of the IOM's *To Err Is Human* exposed the severity and prevalence of these problems in a way that captured the attention of a large variety of key stakeholders for the first time. The executive summary of *To Err Is Human* begins with the following headlines (Kohn, Corrigan, and Donaldson 2000, 1–2):

> The knowledgeable health reporter for the *Boston Globe*, Betsy Lehman, died from an overdose during chemotherapy. . . .
>
> Ben Kolb was eight years old when he died during "minor" surgery due to a drug mix-up. . . .
>
> [A]t least 44,000 Americans die each year as a result of medical errors. . . . [T]he number may be as high as 98,000. . . .
>
> Total national costs . . . of preventable adverse events . . . are estimated to be between $17 billion and $29 billion, of which health care costs represent over one-half.

Although many people had spoken about improving healthcare in the past, this report focused on patient harm and medical errors in an unprecedented way, presenting them as perhaps the most urgent forms of quality defects. *To Err Is Human* framed the problem in a manner that was accessible to the public, and it clearly demonstrated that the status quo was unacceptable. For the first time, patient safety became a unifying cause for policy makers, regulators, providers, and consumers.

Crossing the Quality Chasm: A New Health System for the 21st Century

In March 2001, soon after the release of *To Err Is Human*, the IOM released *Crossing the Quality Chasm*, a more comprehensive report that offered a new framework for a redesigned US healthcare system. *Crossing the Quality Chasm* provides a blueprint for the future that classifies and unifies the components of quality through six aims for improvement. These aims, also viewed as six dimensions of quality, provide healthcare professionals and policy makers with simple rules for redesigning healthcare. They can be known by the acronym STEEEP (Berwick 2002):

1. *Safe:* Harm should not come to patients as a result of their interactions with the medical system.
2. *Timely:* Patients should experience no waits or delays when receiving care and service.
3. *Effective:* The science and evidence behind healthcare should be applied and serve as standards in the delivery of care.
4. *Efficient:* Care and service should be cost-effective, and waste should be removed from the system.
5. *Equitable:* Unequal treatment should be a fact of the past; disparities in care should be eradicated.
6. *Patient-centered:* The system of care should revolve around the patient, respect patient preferences, and put the patient in control.

Improving the quality of healthcare in the STEEEP focus areas requires change to occur at four different levels, as shown in exhibit 1.1. Level A is the patient's experience. Level B is the microsystem where care is delivered by small provider teams. Level C is the organizational level—the macrosystem or aggregation of microsystems and supporting functions. Level D is the external environment, which includes payment mechanisms, policy, and regulatory factors. The environment affects how organizations operate, operations affect the microsystems housed within organizations, and microsystems affect the patient. "True north" lies at level A, in the experience of patients, their loved ones, and the communities in which they live (Berwick 2002).

National Healthcare Quality Report

Mandated by the US Congress to focus on "national trends in the quality of healthcare provided to the American people" (42 U.S.C. 299b-2(b)(2)), the

EXHIBIT 1.1
The Four Levels of the Healthcare System

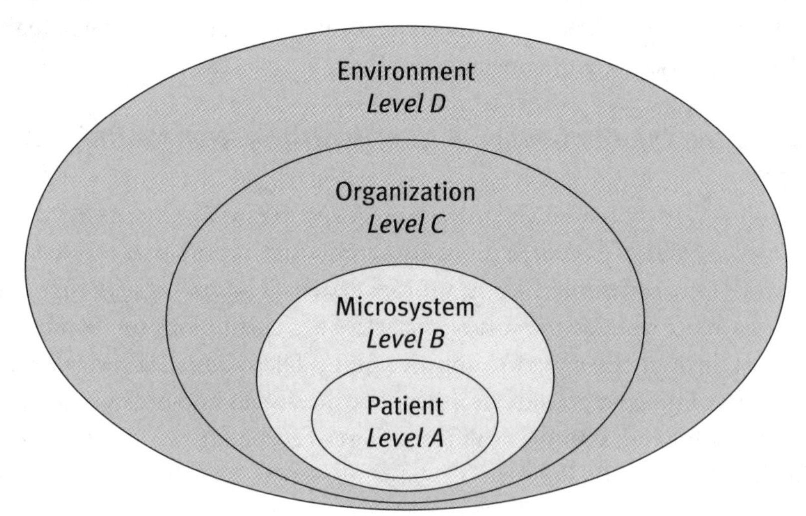

Source: Ferlie and Shortell (2001). Used with permission.

AHRQ's annual *National Healthcare Quality Report* highlights progress and identifies opportunities for improvement. Recognizing that the alleviation of healthcare disparities is integral to achieving quality goals, Congress further mandated that a second report, the *National Healthcare Disparities Report,* focus on "prevailing disparities in health care delivery as it relates to racial factors and socioeconomic factors in priority populations" (42 U.S.C. 299a-1(a)(6)). AHRQ's priority populations include women, children, people with disabilities, low-income individuals, and the elderly. The combined reports are fundamental to ensuring that improvement efforts simultaneously advance quality in general and work toward eliminating inequitable gaps in care.

These reports use national quality measures to track the state of healthcare and address three questions:

1. What is the status of healthcare quality and disparities in the United States?
2. How have healthcare quality and disparities changed over time?
3. Where is the need to improve healthcare quality and reduce disparities greatest?

In its *2016 National Healthcare Quality and Disparities Report*, the AHRQ (2016) notes several improvements, including improved access to healthcare, better care coordination, and improvement in patient-centered care. Despite these improvements, many challenges and disparities remain with regard to insurance status, income, ethnicity, and race.

Improving Diagnosis in Health Care

The National Academies of Sciences, Engineering, and Medicine's (2015) report on *Improving Diagnosis in Health Care* claims that most people will experience at least one diagnostic error—defined as either a missed or delayed diagnosis—in their lifetime. Diagnostic errors are thought to account for up to 17 percent of hospital-related adverse events. Likewise, up to 5 percent of patients in outpatient settings may experience a diagnostic error.

Previous reports had steered clear of discussing diagnostic error, perhaps fearing that the topic assigns blame to clinicians on a personal level. This report, however, proposes an organizational structure for the diagnostic process, allowing for analysis of where healthcare may be failing and what might be done about it. The National Academies recommend that healthcare organizations involve patients and families in the diagnosis process, develop health information technologies to support the diagnostic process, establish a culture that embraces change implementation, and promote research opportunities on diagnostic errors (National Academies 2015).

How Far Has Healthcare Come?

More than 15 years after the prevalence of medical errors was brought to light in *To Err Is Human*, healthcare in the United States has seen a call to arms for the improvement of quality and safety. But has anything really changed? A 2016 analysis published by the *British Medical Journal* suggests not. The article, titled "Medical Error—The Third Leading Cause of Death in the US," delivers a shocking realization of the scope of medical error in healthcare today. Using death certificate records along with national hospital admission data, Makary and Daniel (2016) conclude that, if medical errors are tracked as diseases are, they account for more than 250,000 deaths annually in the United States—outranked only by heart disease and cancer.

To Err Is Human and *Crossing the Quality Chasm* were catalysts for change in healthcare, and they led to increased recognition and reporting of medical error and improved accountability measures set by governing bodies. Nonetheless, more work needs to be done to shrink the quality gap in US healthcare. The remainder of this chapter will focus on frameworks for quality improvement, providing a deeper dive into the STEEEP goals and examining stakeholder needs, measurement concepts, and useful models and tools.

Frameworks and Stakeholders

The six STEEEP aims (Berwick 2002), as presented in *Crossing the Quality Chasm,* provide a valuable framework that can be used to describe quality at any of the four levels of the healthcare system. The various stakeholders involved in healthcare—including clinicians, patients, health insurers, administrators, and the general public—attach different levels of importance to particular aims and define *quality of care* differently as a result (Bodenheimer and Grumbach 2009; Harteloh 2004).

The STEEEP Framework

Safety

Safety refers to the technical performance of care, but it also includes other aspects of the STEEEP framework. Technical performance can be assessed based on the success with which current scientific medical knowledge and technology are applied in a given situation. Assessments of technical performance typically focus on the accuracy of diagnoses, the appropriateness of therapies, the skill with which procedures and other medical interventions are performed, and the absence of accidental injuries (Donabedian 1988b, 1980).

Timeliness

Timeliness refers to the speed with which patients are able to receive care or services. It inherently relates to access to care, or the "degree to which individuals and groups are able to obtain needed services" (IOM 1993, 4). Poor access leads to delays in diagnosis and treatment. Timeliness can also manifest as the patient experience of wait times—either the wait for an appointment or the wait in the medical facility. Timeliness is often a balance between quality of care and speed of care.

Effectiveness

Effectiveness refers to standards of care and how well they are implemented. Perceptions of the effectiveness of healthcare have evolved over the years to increasingly emphasize value. The cost-effectiveness of a given healthcare intervention is determined by comparing the potential for benefit, typically measured in terms of improvement in individual health status, with the intervention's cost (Drummond et al. 2005; Gold et al. 1996). As the amount spent on healthcare services grows, each unit of expenditure ultimately yields ever-smaller benefits until no further benefit accrues from additional expenditures on care (Donabedian, Wheeler, and Wyszewianski 1982).

Efficiency

Efficiency refers to how well resources are used to achieve a given result. Efficiency improves whenever fewer resources are used to produce an output. Because inefficient care uses more resources than necessary, it is wasteful care, and care that involves waste is deficient—and therefore of lower quality—no matter how good it may be in other respects. "Wasteful care is either directly harmful to health or is harmful by displacing more useful care" (Donabedian 1988b, 1745).

Equity

Findings that the amount, type, or quality of healthcare provided can relate systematically to an individual's characteristics—particularly race and ethnicity—rather than to the individual's need for care or healthcare preferences have heightened concern about *equity* in health services delivery (IOM 2002; Wyszewianski and Donabedian 1981). Many decades ago, Lee and Jones (1933, 10) asserted that "good medical care implies the application of all the necessary services of modern, scientific medicine to the needs of all the people. . . . No matter what the perfection of technique in the treatment of one individual case, medicine does not fulfill its function adequately until the same perfection is within the reach of all individuals."

Patient Centeredness

The concept of patient centeredness, originally formulated by Gerteis and colleagues (1993), is characterized in *Crossing the Quality Chasm* as encompassing "qualities of compassion, empathy, and responsiveness to the needs, values, and expressed preferences of the individual patient" and rooted in the idea that "health care should cure when possible, but always help to relieve suffering" (IOM 2001, 50). The report states that the goal of patient centeredness is "to modify the care to respond to the person, not the person to the care" (IOM 2001, 51).

Stakeholders

Virtually everyone can agree on the value of the STEEEP attributes of quality, but clinicians, patients, payers, managers, and society at large attach varying levels of importance to each attribute and thus define *quality of care* differently from one another.

Clinicians

Clinicians tend to perceive the quality of care foremost in terms of technical performance. Their concerns focus on aspects highlighted in IOM's (1990, 4) often-quoted definition: "Quality of care is the degree to which health services for individuals and populations increase the likelihood of desired health outcomes and are consistent with current professional knowledge."

Reference to "current professional knowledge" draws attention to the changing nature of what constitutes good clinical care. Because medical knowledge advances rapidly, clinicians strongly believe that assessing care provided in 2010 on the basis of knowledge acquired in 2013 is neither meaningful nor appropriate. Similarly, "likelihood of desired health outcomes" aligns with clinicians' widely held view that, no matter how good their technical performance is, predictions about the ultimate outcome of care can be expressed only as a probability, given the presence of influences beyond clinicians' control, such as a patient's inherent physiological resilience.

As healthcare has evolved, standards for clinicians have moved beyond technical performance and professional knowledge. Clinicians today are increasingly asked to ensure that their care is patient centered and offered in a way that demonstrates value and efficiency.

Patients

Patients care deeply about technical performance, but it may actually play a relatively small role in shaping their view of healthcare quality. To the dismay of clinicians, patients often see technical performance strictly in terms of the outcomes of care; if the patient does not improve, the physician's technical competence is called into question (Muir Gray 2009). Additionally, patients may not have access to accurate information regarding a clinician's technical skill. Given the difficulty of obtaining and interpreting performance data, patients may make decisions about their care based on their assessment of the attributes they are most readily able to evaluate—chiefly patient centeredness, amenities, and reputation (Cleary and McNeil 1988; Sofaer and Firminger 2005).

As health policy changes, patients, much like clinicians, are becoming more likely to consider cost as part of the quality equation. From the patients' vantage point, cost-effectiveness calculations are highly complex and depend greatly on the details of their insurance coverage. A patient who does not have to pay the full price of medical care may have a very different view of the value of the treatment, compared to a patient who incurs a higher percentage of the cost.

Payers

Third-party payers—health insurance companies, government programs such as Medicare, and others who pay on behalf of patients—tend to assess the quality of care on the basis of costs. Because payers typically manage a finite pool of resources, they tend to be concerned about cost-effectiveness and efficiency.

Though payer restrictions on care have commonly been considered antithetical to the provision of high-quality care, this opinion is slowly changing. Increasing costs, without concomitant improvements in overall quality, have led to more clinicians and patients focusing on the value of care and therefore accepting some limitations. Clinicians continue to be duty bound to do everything possible to help individual patients, including advocating for high-cost interventions even if those interventions have only a small positive probability of benefiting the patient (Donabedian 1988a; Strech et al. 2009). Third-party payers—especially governmental units that must make multiple trade-offs when allocating money—are more apt to view the spending of large sums for diminishing returns as a misuse of finite resources. The public, meanwhile, has shown a growing unwillingness to pay higher insurance premiums or taxes needed to provide populations with the full measure of care that is available.

Administrators

The chief concern of administrative leaders responsible for the operations of hospitals, clinics, and other healthcare delivery organizations is the quality of the nonclinical aspects of care over which they have the most control— primarily, amenities and access to care. Administrators' perspective on quality, therefore, can differ from that of clinicians and patients with respect to efficiency, cost-effectiveness, and equity. Because administrators are responsible for ensuring that resources are spent where they will do the most good, efficiency and cost-effectiveness are of central concern, as is the equitable distribution of resources.

Society/Public/Consumers

At a collective, or societal, level, the definition of *quality of care* reflects concerns about efficiency and cost-effectiveness similar to those of governmental third-party payers and managers, and much for the same reasons. In addition, technical aspects of quality loom large at the collective level, where many believe care can be assessed and safeguarded more effectively than it can be at the level of individuals. Similarly, equity and access to care are important to societal-level concepts of quality, given that society is seen as being responsible for ensuring access to care for everyone, particularly disenfranchised groups.

Are the Five Stakeholders Irreconcilable?

Different though they may seem, stakeholders—clinicians, patients, payers, administrators, and the public—have a great deal in common. Although each emphasizes the attributes differently, none of the other attributes is typically excluded. Strong disagreements do arise, however, among the five parties' definitions, even outside the realm of cost-effectiveness. Conflicts typically emerge when one party holds that a particular practitioner or clinic is a high-quality provider by virtue of having high ratings on a single aspect of care—for example, patient centeredness. Those objecting to this conclusion point out that, just because a practice rates highly in that one area, it does not necessarily rate equally highly in other areas, such as technical performance, amenities, or efficiency, for instance (Wyszewianski 1988). Clinicians who relate well to their patients, and thus score highly on patient centeredness, nevertheless may have failed to keep up with medical advances and, as a result, provide care that is deficient in technical terms. As with this example, an aspect of quality that a given party overlooks is seldom in direct conflict with that party's own overall concept of quality.

Measurement

Just as frameworks and stakeholders are useful for advancing one's understanding of quality of care, so is measurement, particularly with respect to quality improvement initiatives.

Structure, Process, and Outcome

As Avedis Donabedian first noted in 1966, all evaluations of the quality of care can be classified in terms of one of three measures: structure, process, or outcome.

Structure

In the context of measuring the quality of care, *structure* refers to characteristics of the individuals who provide care and of the settings where care is delivered. These characteristics include the education, training, and certification of professionals who provide care and the adequacy of the facility's staffing, equipment, and overall organization.

Evaluations of quality based on structural elements assume that well-qualified people working in well-appointed and well-organized settings provide high-quality care. However, although good structure makes good quality more likely, it does not guarantee it (Donabedian 2003). Licensing and accrediting bodies have relied heavily on structural measures of quality because the measures are relatively stable, and thus easier to capture, and because they reliably identify providers or practices lacking the means to deliver high-quality care.

Process

Process—the series of events that takes place during the delivery of care—can also be a basis for evaluating the quality of care. The quality of the process can vary on three aspects: (1) appropriateness—whether the right actions were taken, (2) skill—the proficiency with which actions were carried out, and (3) the timeliness of the care.

Ordering the correct diagnostic procedure for a patient is an example of an appropriate action. However, to fully evaluate the process in which this particular action is embedded, we also need to know how promptly the procedure was ordered and how skillfully it was carried out. Similarly, successful completion of a surgical operation and a good recovery are not enough evidence to conclude that the process of care was of high quality; they only indicate that the procedure was performed skillfully. For the entire process of care to be judged as high quality, one also must ascertain that the operation was indicated (i.e., appropriate) for the patient and that it was carried out in time. Finally, as is the case for structural measures, the use of process measures for assessing the quality of care rests on a key assumption—that if the right things are done and are done right, good results (i.e., good outcomes of care) are more likely to be achieved.

Outcome

Outcome measures capture whether healthcare goals were achieved. Because the goals of care can be defined broadly, outcome measures may include the costs of care as well as patients' satisfaction with their care (Iezzoni 2013). In formulations that stress the technical aspects of care, however, outcomes typically involve indicators of health status, such as whether a patient's pain subsided or condition cleared up, or whether the patient regained full function (Donabedian 1980).

Clinicians tend to have an ambivalent view of outcome measures. Clinicians are aware that many factors that determine clinical outcomes—including genetic and environmental factors—are not under their control. At best, they control the process, and a good process only increases the likelihood of good outcomes; it does not guarantee them. Some patients do not improve in spite of the best treatment that medicine can offer, whereas other patients regain full health even though they receive inappropriate or potentially harmful care. Despite this complexity, clinicians view improved outcomes as the ultimate goal of quality initiatives. Clinicians are unlikely to value the effort involved in fixing a process-oriented gap in care if it is unlikely to ultimately result in an improvement in outcomes.

Which Is Best?

Of structure, process, and outcome, which is the best measure of the quality of care? The answer is that none of them is inherently better and that the appropriateness of each measure depends on the circumstances (Donabedian 2003). However, this answer often does not satisfy people who are inclined to believe that outcome measures are superior to the others. After all, they reason, the outcome addresses the ultimate purpose, the bottom line, of all caregiving: Was the condition cured? Did the patient improve?

As previously noted, however, a good outcome may occur even when the care (i.e., process) is clearly deficient. The reverse is also possible: Even when the care is excellent, the outcomes might not be as good because of factors outside clinicians' control, such as a patient's frailty. To assess outcomes meaningfully across providers, one must account for such factors by performing complicated risk adjustment calculations (Goode at al. 2011; Iezzoni 2013).

What a particular outcome ultimately denotes about the quality of care crucially depends on whether the outcome can be attributed to the care provided. In other words, one has to examine the link between the outcome and the antecedent structure and process measures to determine whether the care was appropriate and provided skillfully. Structures and processes are essential but not sufficient for a good outcome.

Metrics and Benchmarks

To assess quality using structure, process, or outcome measures, one needs to establish metrics and benchmarks to know what constitutes a good structure, a good process, and a good outcome.

Metrics are specific variables that form the basis for assessing quality. Benchmarks quantitatively express the level the variable must reach to satisfy preexisting expectations about quality. Exhibit 1.2 provides examples of metrics and benchmarks for structure, process, and outcome measures in healthcare.

The way healthcare metrics and benchmarks are derived is changing. Before the 1970s, quality-of-care evaluations relied on consensus among groups of clinicians selected for their clinical knowledge, experience, and reputation (Donabedian 1982). In the 1970s, however, the importance of scientific literature to the evaluation of healthcare quality gained new visibility through the work of Cochrane (1973), Williamson (1977), and others. At about the same time, Brook and colleagues (1977) at RAND began using systematic reviews and evaluations of scientific literature as the basis for defining criteria and standards for quality. The evidence-based medicine movement of the 1990s, which advocated medical practice guided by the best evidence about efficacy, reinforced the focus on the literature and stressed consideration of the soundness of study design and validity (Evidence-Based Medicine Working Group 1992; Straus et al. 2005). As a result, derivation of metrics and benchmarks has come to revolve more around the strength and validity of scientific evidence than around the unaided consensus of experts (Eddy 2005, 1996).

The main insight that can be drawn from a deeper understanding of concepts related to the measurement of healthcare quality is that the type of measure used—structure, process, or outcome—matters less than the measure's

EXHIBIT 1.2 Examples of Metrics and Benchmarks for Structure, Process, and Outcome Measures in Healthcare

Type of Measure	Focus of Assessment	Metric	Benchmark
Structure	Nurse staffing in nursing homes	Hours of nursing care per resident day	At least four hours of nursing care per resident day
Process	Patients undergoing surgical repair of hip fracture	Percentage of patients who receive prophylactic antibiotics on the day of surgery	100 percent receive antibiotic on the day of surgery
Outcome	Hospitalized patients	Rate of falls per 1,000 patient days	Fewer than five falls per 1,000 patient days

relationship to the others. Structural measures are only as good and useful as the strength of their link to desired processes and outcomes. Similarly, process and outcome measures must relate to each other in measurable and reproducible ways—as demonstrated by efficacy studies—to be truly valid measures of quality.

Quality Improvement Models

A number of systems exist to guide the process of quality improvement. At their core, all of these systems are approaches to complex problem solving. Just as the scientific method guides research inquiry in the lab, and just as the diagnostic process guides clinical reasoning, quality improvement models structure the approach to system improvement. All of the models discussed in this section were initially developed for industries outside of healthcare. Their adoption in and adaptation to the field of healthcare quality improvement demonstrate the field's willingness to learn from the success of others, as well as the relative youth of the quality movement in the healthcare arena. Although these models have different names, they have certain core commonalities. Most share the following basic format:

1. Identify the problem
2. Measure current performance
3. Perform a cause analysis
4. Develop and implement an improvement strategy
5. Measure the effect of the intervention
6. Modify, maintain, or spread the intervention

"Form follows function," a concept rooted in the field of architecture, stresses the importance of understanding what you are trying to accomplish before you determine how you are going to do it. Applied to healthcare quality, the phrase highlights the need to understand the purpose behind the effort—the goal—at the individual, departmental, and organizational levels before deciding what improvement process or approach to adopt. The following approaches, though not an exhaustive list, are the ones most commonly applied:

- The Plan-Do-Study-Act (PDSA) cycle
- The model for improvement
- Lean, or the Toyota Production System
- Six Sigma
- Human-centered design

The Plan-Do-Study-Act Cycle

Walter A. Shewhart (1891–1967) developed the PDSA cycle during the 1920s, and the cycle was further described by W. Edwards Deming (1900–1993), who is often regarded as the "father" of quality. Deming (2000b), a statistics professor and physicist by trade, stressed the importance of practicing continuous improvement and thinking of manufacturing as a system. As part of his "system of profound knowledge," Deming (2000a) promoted the idea that about 15 percent of poor quality was because of workers and 85 percent was because of improper management, systems, and processes. In most, but not all, contexts, the stages of this model are plan, do, study, and act. Some may replace the "study" with "check," making the cycle PDCA. Nevertheless, the principles remain the same. In practical terms, the stages of the PDSA cycle can be broken down as follows.

Plan

- Understand the problem and the underlying causes for a gap in quality.
- Establish an objective. What are you trying to accomplish? By how much do you aim to improve, and by when?
- Ask questions and make predictions. What do you think will happen?
- Plan to carry out the cycle. Who will perform the functions? What steps will be performed?
- When will the plan be implemented and completed? Where will the plan/work take place?

Do

- Educate and train staff.
- Carry out the plan (e.g., try out the change on a small scale).
- Document problems and unexpected observations.
- Begin analysis of the data.

Study

- Assess the effect of the change, and determine the level of success achieved, relative to the goal/objective.
- Compare the results with your predictions. Did you meet your aim for improvement? Did anything get worse?
- Summarize the lessons learned.
- Determine what changes need to be made and what actions will be taken next.

Act

- Act on what you have learned.
- Determine whether the plan should be repeated with modification, or whether a new plan should be created.

- Make necessary changes.
- Identify remaining gaps in the process or performance.
- Carry out additional PDSA cycles until the goal/objective is met.

Model for Improvement

Tom Nolan and Lloyd Provost, cofounders of Associates in Process Improvement (API), developed a simple model for improvement based on Deming's PDSA cycle. As shown in exhibit 1.3, the model uses three fundamental questions as a basis for improvement: (1) What are we trying to accomplish? (2) How will we know that a change is an improvement? (3) What change can we make that will result in improvement?

Setting measurable aims is essential for any quality improvement effort. The effort required to bring about improvement may vary depending on the problem's complexity, whether the focus is on a new or an old design, or the number of people involved in the process (Langley et al. 1996). The Institute for Healthcare Improvement (IHI) has adopted the API approach as its organizing improvement model.

Lean, or the Toyota Production System

The Massachusetts Institute of Technology first used the term *Lean* in 1987 to describe product development and production methods that, when compared with traditional mass production processes, produce more products with fewer

EXHIBIT 1.3
API Model for Improvement

Model for Improvement

- What are we trying to accomplish?
- How will we know that a change is an improvement?
- What change can we make that will result in improvement?

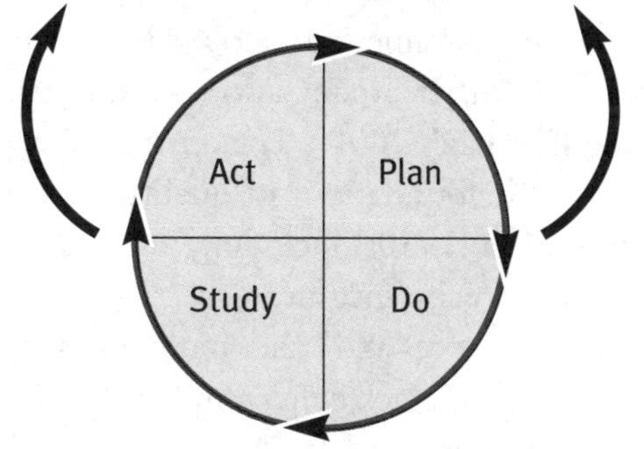

Source: Langley et al. (1996). Used with permission.

defects in a shorter time. Lean thinking, or Lean manufacturing, grew out of the work of Taiichi Ohno (1912–1990), who began developing the concepts as early as 1948 at Toyota Motor Corporation in Japan. As a result, it is also known as the Toyota Production System (TPS).

The goal of Lean is to develop a way to specify the meaning of value, to align steps/processes in the best sequence, to conduct activities without interruption whenever someone requests them, and to perform the activities more effectively (Womack and Jones 2003). Lean focuses on the removal of *muda*, or waste, which is defined as anything that is not needed to produce an item or service. Ohno identified seven types of waste: (1) overproduction, (2) waiting, (3) unnecessary transport, (4) overprocessing, (5) excess inventory, (6) unnecessary movement, and (7) defects. Lean also emphasizes the concept of continuous (one-piece) flow production. In contrast to a batch-and-queue process, continuous flow creates a standardized process in which products are constructed through a single, continuous system one at a time, ultimately producing less waste, greater efficiency, and higher output.

Lean methodology places the needs of the customer first by following five steps:

1. Define *value* as determined by the customer, based on the provider's ability to deliver the right product or service at an appropriate price.
2. Identify the value stream—the set of specific actions required to bring a product or service from concept to completion.
3. Make value-added steps flow from beginning to end.
4. Let the customer *pull* the product from the supplier; do not *push* products.
5. Pursue perfection of the process.

When waste is removed and flow is improved, quality improvement results. The simplification of processes reduces variation, reduces inventory, and increases the uniformity of outputs (Heim 1999).

Six Sigma

Six Sigma is a system for improvement developed by Hewlett-Packard, Motorola, General Electric, and other organizations during the 1980s and 1990s (Pande, Neuman, and Cavanagh 2000). The central concepts of Six Sigma are not new; they build on the foundations of quality improvement established from the 1920s through the 1950s, including Shewhart's research on variation and his emphasis on precise measurement. Six Sigma creates clear roles and responsibilities for executives and other individuals, who may achieve the ranks of champion, green belt, black belt, or master black belt as they develop through higher levels of training and expertise.

With Six Sigma, the aim is to reduce variation and eliminate defects in key business processes. It aims for a rate of no more than 3.4 defects per million opportunities. By using a set of statistical tools to understand the fluctuation of a process, managers can predict the expected outcome of that process. If the outcome is not satisfactory, management can use associated tools to learn more about the elements influencing the process. The primary theory of Six Sigma is that a focus on reducing variation leads to a more uniform process output. Secondary effects include less waste, less throughput time, and less inventory (Heim 1999).

The Six Sigma improvement model consists of five steps that together form the acronym DMAIC:

1. *Define.* Identify the customers and their problems. Determine the key characteristics that are important to the customer, along with the processes that support those key characteristics.
2. *Measure.* Categorize key characteristics, verify measurement systems, and collect data.
3. *Analyze.* Convert raw data into information that provides insights into the process. These insights include identifying the fundamental and most important causes of defects or problems.
4. *Improve.* Develop solutions to the problem, and make changes to the process. Measure process changes, and judge whether the changes are beneficial, or whether another set of changes is necessary.
5. *Control.* If the process is performing at a desired and predictable level, monitor the process to ensure that no unexpected changes occur.

Human-Centered Design

Quality improvement initiatives are increasingly incorporating design concepts as part of an effort to restore the central role of patients and frontline healthcare providers in the improvement process. Existing improvement models emerged primarily out of the manufacturing industry, where reduction in defects, speed of production, and reduction of waste are the primary concerns. Design methods, on the other hand, originate from such industries as architecture, product development, and fashion. Priorities in these fields extend beyond those of manufacturing and include such concerns as customer satisfaction, functional performance, and creativity. When applied to the healthcare setting, human-centered design can encompass a broad array of concepts and practices, including human factors engineering (HFE) and the process of co-creating devices, spaces, and processes with patients or end users. This approach might involve, for instance, purposefully forming a team of industrial designers, patients, and occupational therapists to design a new type of prosthetic device for amputees, or bringing together designers, medical professionals, patients, and family members to create a better waiting room experience (Guinn 2017).

The steps of the design process are as follows:

1. *Empathize.* Thoroughly understand the motivations, needs, and concerns of the client or user.
2. *Define.* Translate the perspectives gained from interviewing and observing the end user into clear design challenges and goals.
3. *Ideate.* Generate a broad array of potential solutions, with minimal self-editing or concern for real or imagined limitations.
4. *Narrow.* Identify the most promising solutions, usually through the application of specific criteria.
5. *Prototype.* Create tangible products representing the potential future solutions, with the goal of communicating back to the end user and further exploring/refining ideas.
6. *Test.* Share prototypes and gather feedback, working toward a final solution.

Two key elements of the design process are empathy building and prototyping. Empathy is key to realizing the promise of patient/person centeredness in the improvement of healthcare services. The depth to which designers aim to understand their users is pivotal to the creation of superior products and services. Prototyping exists in other improvement models, but usually in the form of small-scale implementation of a solution in the actual environment. At its extreme, prototyping may take the form of a pilot, but more frequently it is a lower-fidelity expression of a final product, such as a physical model, storyboard, or simulation. Like the PDSA cycle, application of the design process is cyclical and continues until the goal is met.

Quality Improvement Tools

Understanding the difference between quality improvement models and quality improvement tools is difficult. A quality model is akin to the process of designing and then constructing a house. The tools are the materials and activities that take the design from an abstract concept to a physical structure. An architect does not simply walk onto a building site with an idea in her head. Instead, she creates blueprints that communicate the building plan. The blueprint is a tool that makes the design process visible. Similarly, contractors use physical tools, such as hammers and saws, as well as organizing tools, such as checklists and work schedules, to ensure that the house is built correctly. Similarly, in quality improvement, different tools have different functions and are used at distinct stages. They are not interchangeable, just as you could not substitute a hammer for a saw. We can observe people using the tools of the system, but the system or model itself (e.g., Six Sigma, Lean) is invisible and cannot be observed.

Quality improvement tools can be organized into seven categories, following a framework developed by the American Society for Quality (ASQ) (Tague 2004):

1. Cause analysis
2. Evaluation and decision making
3. Process analysis
4. Data collection and analysis
5. Idea creation
6. Project planning and implementation
7. Knowledge transfer and spread techniques

This section is not intended to be a comprehensive reference on quality tools and techniques; rather, it aims to highlight some of the more widely used tools in each category.

Cause Analysis

Once a gap in quality has been identified, the next step is usually to figure out why actual performance is lagging behind optimal performance or benchmarks. This process is known as *cause analysis*. Skillful cause analysis allows improvement teams to link their solutions and interventions with the underlying reasons for the gaps in care they are working to fix.

Five Whys

The "five whys" exercise is a basic method for drilling down through the symptoms of a process or design failure to identify the root cause. Easy to understand and to perform, it involves simply asking "why?" five times. Users of this technique will quickly identify the more proximal conditions contributing to a quality gap, instead of assuming that the obvious surface conditions are the most important. The benefit of this approach is that it forces users to look beyond their first answer. Any time a breach in protocol is assumed to be the reason for a bad outcome, one must dig deeper, asking why the protocol was not followed, until a root cause is identified. The key to successful use of this technique is not to stop the analysis too early, thus misidentifying the root cause.

Cause-and-Effect/Fishbone Diagram

Most complex problems have multiple root causes, which can be missed using five whys, because that tool encourages one path to be followed at the exclusion of others. Cause-and-effect diagrams, also referred to as *Ishikawa* or *fishbone diagrams*, help to broaden the search for possible root causes. In a fishbone diagram, the problem (effect) is stated in a box on the right side of the chart, and likely causes of the problem are listed around major category headings to the left, resembling the bones of a fish (ASQ 2014). Possible category headings, as shown in exhibit 1.4, include *Technology*, *Team*, *Individual*, *Organization/ Management*, *Protocols*, and *Environment*.

Evaluation and Decision Making

Deciding exactly where in a system to intervene to bring about change often involves a more quantitative approach to cause analysis. Visualizing data can help to identify correlations and patterns to help guide decisions.

Scatter Diagram

Scatter diagrams, also known as *scatter plots* or *x-y graphs*, enable users to identify whether a correlation exists between two variables or sets of numerical data. As shown in exhibit 1.5, when a high correlation exists between the two elements, the data will display as a tight line or curve; when the elements have little correlation, the data will display as a more scattered or "shotgun" distribution. Although correlation does not imply causation, targeting a variable that is highly correlated with the outcome of interest may be more likely to improve performance.

EXHIBIT 1.4
Schematic of a Fishbone Diagram Used in Cause Analysis

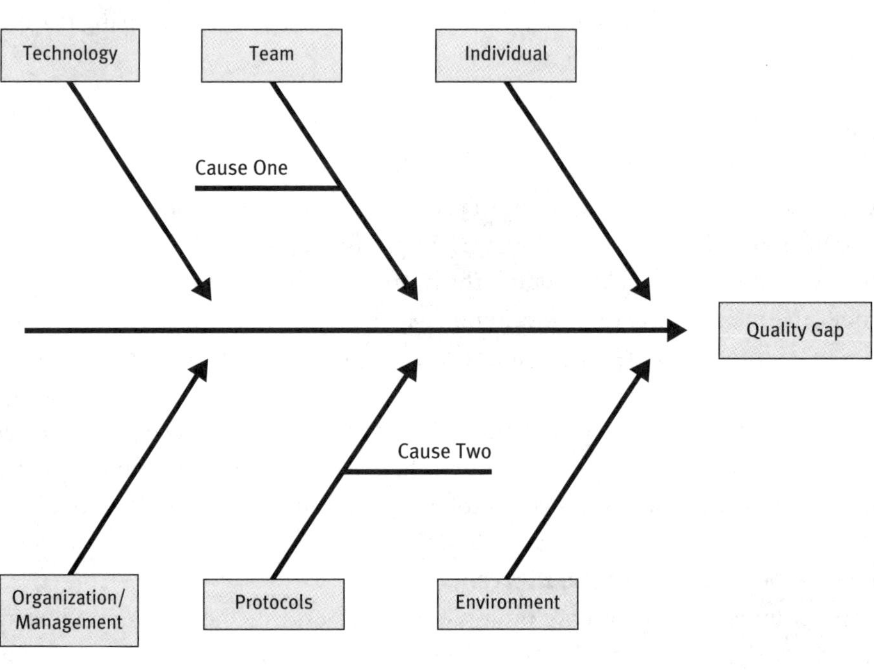

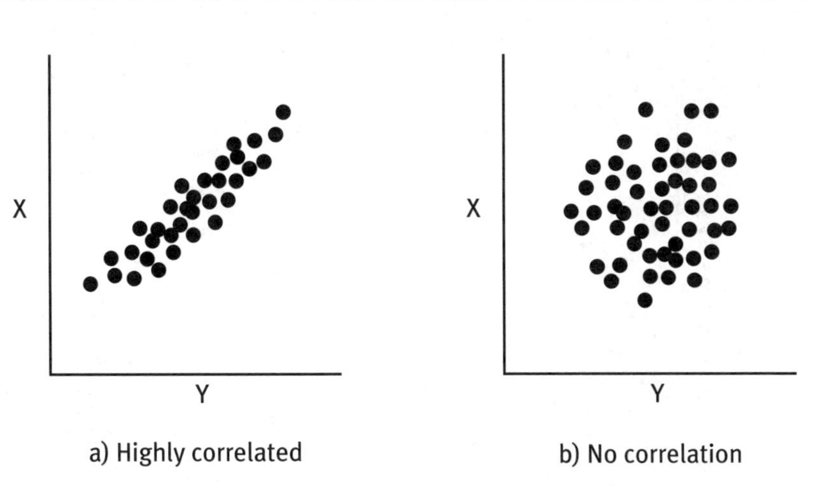

EXHIBIT 1.5 Scatter Diagrams Demonstrating Two Data Sets

Pareto Chart

The Pareto chart developed from the work of the Italian economist Vilfredo Pareto (1848–1923), who observed that 80 percent of the wealth in Italy was held by 20 percent of the population. Joseph M. Juran (1904–2008), working as an internal consultant to Deming with Western Electric on the subject of industrial engineering, applied this principle more broadly and proclaimed that 80 percent of the variation of any characteristic is caused by only 20 percent of the possible causes.

A Pareto chart displays the occurrence frequency for a range of causes of variation, demonstrating the small number of significant contributors to a problem. It enables a project team to identify the frequency with which specific errors are occurring and thus to concentrate resources appropriately (Tague 2004). Pareto charts overlay a histogram and a line graph, showing the contribution of each error or cause to the total variation in the system. The charts have two *x* axes, with frequency of occurrence on the left-hand axis and cumulative percentage on the right. Causes are arranged in descending order of frequency, and those on the right-hand side account for the majority of the variation in outcomes (see exhibit 1.6).

Process Analysis

Many improvement initiatives target changes in process to achieve better outcomes. Fully understanding an existing or proposed process is a vital step in improvement.

Flowchart

Flowcharts, also called *process maps,* are used to visually display the steps of a process in sequential order. As shown in exhibit 1.7, each step in a flowchart is

EXHIBIT 1.6
A Pareto Chart Showing the Frequency with Which Causes Contribute to Error

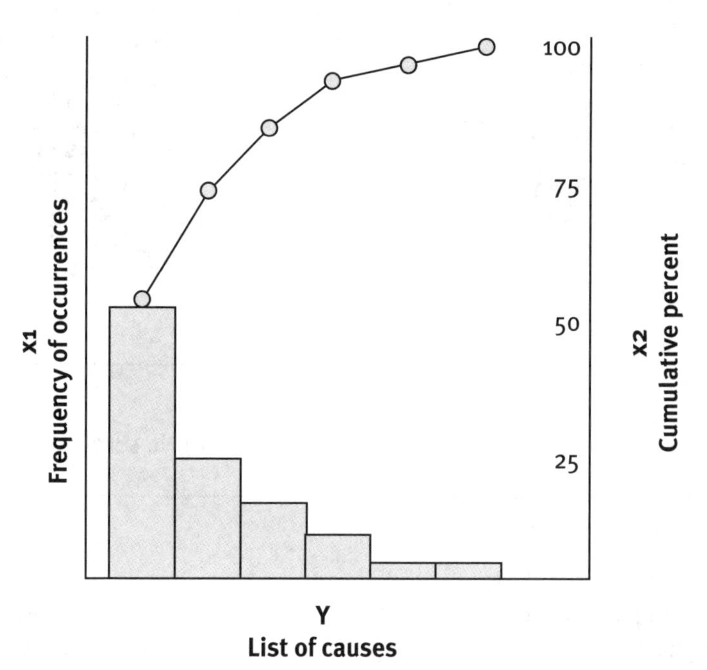

EXHIBIT 1.7
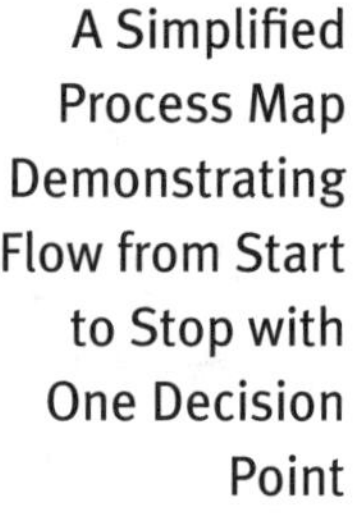
A Simplified Process Map Demonstrating Flow from Start to Stop with One Decision Point

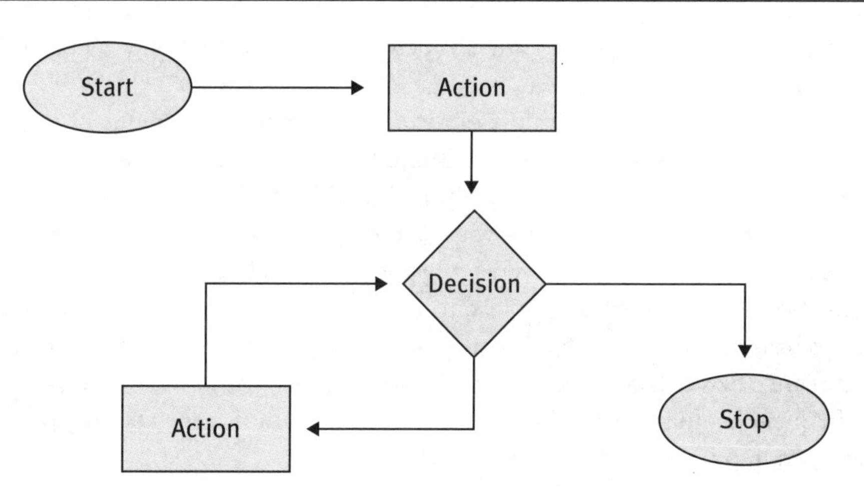

displayed as a symbol that represents a particular action (e.g., start/stop, process step, direction, decision, delay). Flowcharts are useful in quality improvement for identifying unnecessary or high-risk steps in a process, developing a standardized process, and facilitating communication between staff involved in the same process (Tague 2004). Specific improvement models include their own variations on flowcharts, such as value stream mapping in Lean.

Failure Mode and Effects Analysis / Mistake Proofing

Failure mode and effects analysis (FMEA) examines potential problems and their causes and predicts undesired results. Normally, FMEA is used to predict future product failure from past part failure, but it also can be used to analyze future system failures. By basing activities on FMEA, organizations can focus their efforts on steps in a process that have the greatest potential for failure before failure actually occurs. Prioritization of failure points, or modes, is based on the detectability of the potential failure, its severity, and its likelihood of occurrence.

Mistake proofing, or *poka yoke*, is a related concept developed in the 1960s by Japanese industrial engineer and TPS cofounder Shigeo Shingo (1909–1990). The goal of mistake proofing is to make a potential failure impossible, or at least to make failure easily detectable before significant consequences result. Mistake-proofing techniques can be used to address potential failures identified during FMEA.

Data Collection and Analysis

Identifying measures, setting benchmarks, and trending performance data lie at the heart of quality improvement. Various methods emphasize the ability to understand variation and recognize when trends represent true change.

SMART Aims

Improvement projects need to have SMART aims—aims that are specific (S), measurable (M), achievable (A), relevant (R), and time bound (T). A well-conceived aim allows a team to communicate with stakeholders, assess progress, galvanize efforts, and advertise its success.

Importantly, aims are not tied to a particular intervention. They do not specify how a team will achieve success, just what success will look like and by when. Usually, the initial aim for improvement is not to achieve a perfect performance. Instead, the aim represents a feasible incremental improvement—say, increasing the frequency of a positive outcome from 40 to 60 percent. When a team reaches its initial aim, a new one will be set. This technique emphasizes that improvement is a continuous process and that multiple improvement cycles are usually necessary to close quality gaps.

Run Charts and Control Charts

Run charts graph performance over time, as shown in exhibit 1.8. They can display process or outcome measures, and their ability to display change over time makes them more useful than simple "pre" and "post" data. Often, run charts display important events in a project (such as the interventions labeled in the exhibit), helping users to assess the impact of a process change and to identify or correct any problems that arise (Tague 2004). Statistical process

EXHIBIT 1.8 Run Chart Showing Performance on a Given Measure over Time

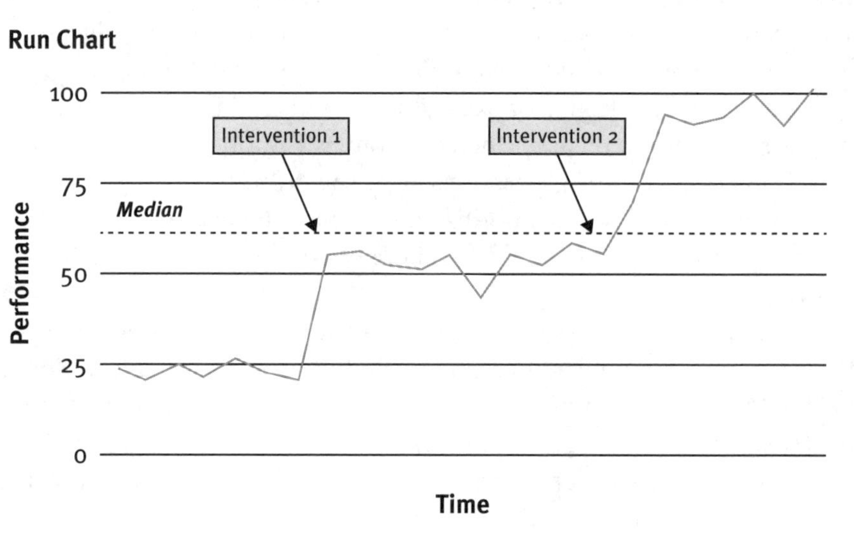

Note: Important events in a project can be added to the chart.

control charts, or simply control charts, are closely related to run charts. Control charts contain three lines: a central/control line (median), an upper control limit, and a lower control limit. These boundaries define statistically significant change and are used to monitor performance and variation.

Idea Creation

When a team is seeking solutions to a quality problem, stakeholders should be engaged and encouraged to think broadly. The best solution might not be the one the team thinks of first, and outside opinions might be necessary to better understand how a proposed solution will affect real people and processes. Not all ideas are created equal. Exhibit 1.9 presents a hierarchy for improvement, with strategies such as exhortation and education at the bottom and systems-based interventions such as checklists, automation, and forcing functions at the top. Proposed solutions to quality projects are sometimes referred to as *countermeasures.*

Project Planning and Implementation

Once a countermeasure is chosen, the team must begin implementing the new process or equipment. Depending on the nature of the countermeasure, this step may be extremely complex. Tools that help to organize, prioritize, and communicate are vital to keeping the team on track.

Stakeholder Analysis

In truth, stakeholder analysis should be listed as a quality improvement tool in each of the seven sections. From cause analysis to knowledge transfer and spread, the management of stakeholders is key to a successful improvement initiative.

EXHIBIT 1.9
Framework Showing Relative Strength of Interventions for Quality Improvement Initiatives

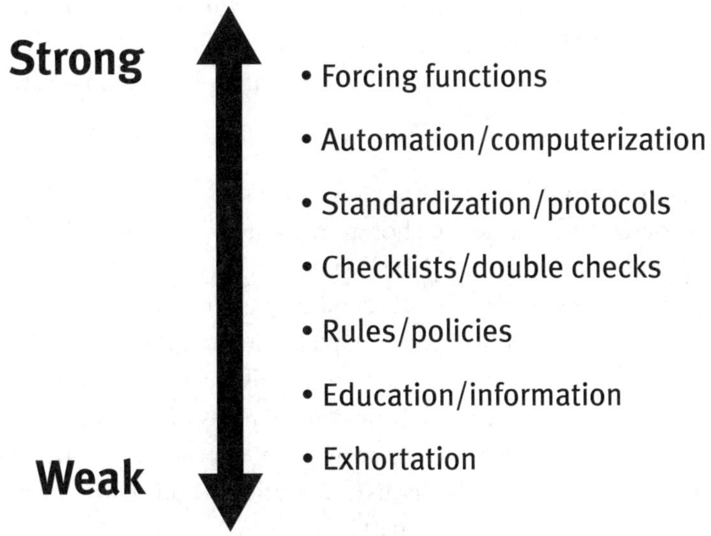

Source: Adapted from Gosbee and Gosbee (2005).

Engaging stakeholders early allows teams to better understand processes and problems from multifaceted perspectives. In healthcare, stakeholders usually consist of the "three *P*s": patients, providers, and payers.

Although stakeholder involvement is vital, it is important to recognize that not all stakeholders are of equal importance. Stakeholders can generally be broken down into three categories. The most important stakeholders *control* the success of the project. Others have *influence* on the project and should be kept informed. The third tier will simply be *interested* in the results. Teams can decide how to manage stakeholders by understanding which of the three categories each stakeholder group is in, as well as to what extent the stakeholders already support the work of the team. An individual with control who is strongly against the project will require intensive management. An interested party who is already moderately supportive is likely sufficiently engaged.

Checklists

Checklists are a generic tool with which to organize the steps of a project or process. They can also be used as countermeasures when improvement teams aim to standardize the workflow of frontline providers. For example, the surgical time-out before every surgery is a checklist step designed to prevent wrong-patient or wrong-site surgery and to establish a culture of safety in the operating room. Checklists can also be used to capture data measured repeatedly over time for purposes of identifying patterns, trends, defects, or causes of defects. Data collected through a checklist can be easily converted into performance tools such as histograms or Pareto charts (Tague 2004). The use of checklists reached near mythological status after the publication of Atul Gawande's (2010) *The Checklist Manifesto*, which revealed their ubiquity in highly reliable industries and demonstrated their potential in healthcare.

2×2 Matrix

The 2×2 matrix is a tool for comparing and organizing items according to two important criteria. Criteria can be chosen by the user, but they often compete or conflict in some way. Exhibit 1.10 shows a specific type of 2×2 matrix known as an *effort vs. impact matrix*, which compares the potential impact of a countermeasure versus the effort needed for implementation. Potential stakeholders can be sorted by how important they are to the success of the project versus how supportive they are of the team or countermeasure, and designs can be sorted by their potential utility versus their visual appeal. 2×2 matrixes enable team members to systematically discuss, identify, and prioritize ideas and to evaluate different strategies (ASQ 2014).

5S

A concept from Lean methodology, 5S is a systematic program that allows workers to take control of their workspace. The aim is for the workspace to help workers complete their jobs, rather than being a neutral or, as is commonly the case, a competing factor. The program is so named because each step, in Japanese, starts with the letter *S*:

EXHIBIT 1.10
2×2 Matrix Showing Effort Versus Impact

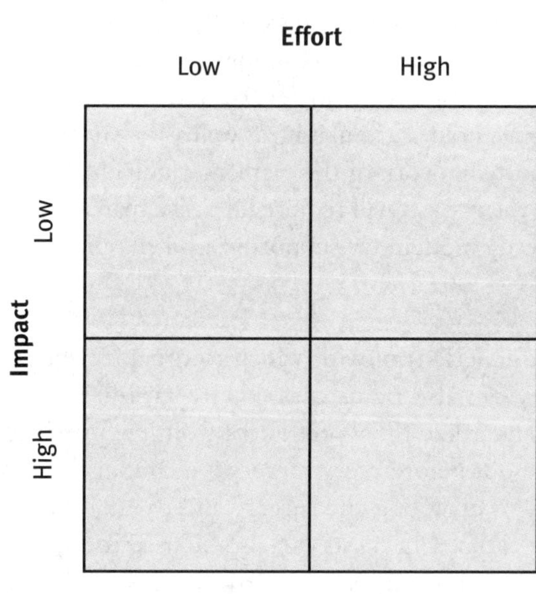

1. *Seiri* (sort) means to keep only items that are necessary for completing one's work.
2. *Seiton* (straighten) means to arrange and identify items so that they can be easily retrieved when needed.
3. *Seiso* (shine) means to keep items and workspaces clean and in working order.
4. *Seiketsu* (standardize) means to use best practices consistently.
5. *Shitsuke* (sustain) means to maintain gains and commit to continuing to apply the first four items.

Knowledge Transfer and Spread Techniques

A key aspect of any quality improvement effort is the ability to replicate successes in other areas of the organization. Failure to transfer knowledge effectively can cause an organization to produce waste, perform inconsistently, and miss opportunities to achieve benchmark levels of operational performance. Barriers to spread and adoption (e.g., organizational culture, communication, leadership support) can exist in any unit, organization, or system.

In 1999, the Institute for Healthcare Improvement (IHI) chartered a team to address this challenge, and IHI published a white paper titled "A Framework for Spread: From Local Improvements to System-Wide Change" in 2006. The report identified "the ability of healthcare providers and their organizations to rapidly spread innovations and new ideas" as a "key factor in closing the gap between *best* practice and *common* practice" (Massoud et al. 2006, 1). It identified the following important questions that organizations need to address when attempting to spread ideas to their target populations (Massoud et al. 2006, 6):

- Can the organization or community structure be used to facilitate spread?
- How are decisions about the adoption of improvements made?
- What infrastructure enhancements will assist in achieving the spread aim?
- What transition issues need to be addressed?
- How will the spread efforts be transitioned to operational responsibilities?

Kaizen Blitz/Event

Kaizen, which can be translated as "continuous improvement," was developed in Japan shortly after World War II, and it is a central concept in Lean thinking. Kaizen in any organization involves ongoing improvement that is supported and implemented at all levels of an organization. The key aspect of kaizen is the sustained focus on improving a system or process regardless of how well the system or process is currently functioning. A kaizen event, or "blitz," is a highly focused improvement effort aimed at addressing a specific problem. Kaizen events are short in duration—typically three to five days—and intended to produce rapid changes and immediate results. The approach taken during a kaizen blitz typically involves common improvement methodologies (e.g., DMAIC, PDSA, value stream mapping) and the participation of teams with decision-making authority from multiple departments and levels of leadership.

Rapid-Cycle Testing and Pilots

Two important characteristics of an effective spread model are (1) staff buy-in and (2) proof that the change will improve performance. Developed by IHI and shown in exhibit 1.11, rapid-cycle testing (or rapid-cycle improvement) uses various tests with small sample sizes and multiple PDSA cycles that build on lessons learned over a short period. The process is meant to concomitantly gain buy-in from staff involved in the change. Successful tests are applied to other units in the organization, whereas unsuccessful tests continue to be revised for potential spread and further implementation later.

Rapid-cycle testing is designed to reduce the cycle time of new process implementation from months to days. To prevent unnecessary delays in testing or implementation, teams or units using this approach must avoid overanalysis and remain focused on testing solutions. Rapid-cycle testing can be resource intensive, and it relies on flexibility and distributed autonomy. Therefore, it may require top-level leadership support.

Closely related to rapid-cycle testing is the act of conducting pilots. When piloting an intervention, the goal is to assess efficacy on a small scale and then modify and refine the approach before broad implementation. Pilots can

EXHIBIT 1.11 Example of Rapid-Cycle Testing

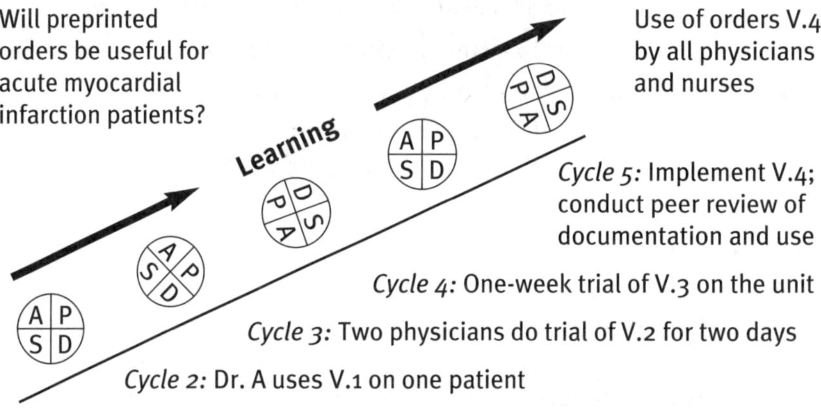
Using Rapid Cycle to Implement Preprinted Orders
Will preprinted orders be useful for acute myocardial infarction patients?
Use of orders V.4 by all physicians and nurses
Learning
A P S D
Cycle 5: Implement V.4; conduct peer review of documentation and use
Cycle 4: One-week trial of V.3 on the unit
Cycle 3: Two physicians do trial of V.2 for two days
Cycle 2: Dr. A uses V.1 on one patient
Cycle 1: Gather sample orders; have Dr. A provide feedback

help identify barriers to success and workarounds, presenting an opportunity to fix problems early. If successful, they can also provide quick wins that help build buy-in and goodwill among stakeholders.

Conclusion

An organization's success depends on the foundation on which it is built and the strength of the systems, processes, tools, and methods it uses to sustain benchmark levels of performance and to improve performance when expectations are not being met. Quality improvement theory and methodologies have been available since the early 1900s, but their widespread acceptance and application have been slower in healthcare than in other industries (e.g., manufacturing). Two landmark Institute of Medicine publications—*Crossing the Quality Chasm* (IOM 2001) and *To Err Is Human* (Kohn, Corrigan, and Donaldson 2000)—described significant concerns about the US healthcare system and prompted a movement that greatly increased healthcare institutions' focus on better care and patient safety (Leape and Berwick 2005). However, the combination of technical complexity, system fragmentation, a tradition of autonomy, and hierarchical authority structures presents, in the words of Leape and Berwick (2005, 2387), a "daunting barrier to creating the habits and beliefs of common purpose, teamwork, and individual accountability." Overcoming this barrier will require continued focus and commitment.

Sustainable improvement is further defined through will, ideas, and execution. Nolan (2007) writes: "You have to have the *will* to improve, you have to have *ideas* about alternatives to the status quo, and then you have to make it real—*execution*." The principles described in this chapter have demonstrated success in many healthcare organizations. As technology advances and access to care improves, healthcare must continue to build on these principles as it strives to reach and maintain benchmark levels of performance. Successful coordination of care across the healthcare continuum will consistently provide the right care for every patient at the right time.

Case Study: Mr. Roberts and the US Healthcare System

Note: This patient story was edited by Matthew Fitzgerald, director of the Center for Health Data Analysis at Social & Scientific Systems. It was originally composed by Heidi Louise Behforouz, MD, assistant professor of medicine at Harvard Medical School, associate physician in the Division of Global Health Equity at Brigham and Women's Hospital, and medical and executive director of the Prevention and Access to Care and Treatment Project.

(continued)

Mr. Roberts is a 77-year-old gentleman who is retired and living in Florida with his wife. A child of the Depression, he grew up to become an accomplished, affluent person. At age 13, he began working as a longshoreman and barracks builder. He started to experience back pain in his early 20s. At that time, he did not receive particularly good medical advice and did not pursue alternative therapies. World War II, 25 years in Asia, and life as a busy executive took priority, and the pain became a constant but secondary companion.

At age 50, the pain became unbearable. He returned to New York and spent the better part of a year "on his back." In 1980, he underwent the first of four major spine surgeries. Since then, he has had multiple intervertebral discs partially or completely removed. Despite these operations, his pain has been worsening over the past two to three years, and his functional status has been decreasing.

Living with pain is difficult, and Mr. Roberts is not sure he deals with it very well. He does not want to take narcotics, because they interfere with his ability to stay sharp and active, and he has stomach problems that prohibit the use of many nonnarcotic medications. Most of the time, he experiences only mild or temporary relief of his pain.

The pain is exhausting and limits his ability to do what he wants, but Mr. Roberts remains active and gets out as much as he can, even taking his wife dancing on Saturday nights. The worst thing about the pain is that it is changing—worsening—and he is uncertain of its future trajectory. As the pain increases, how will he survive? What are the possibilities that he will remain active and independent?

Mr. Roberts states that he has had "reasonably good" doctors. He is also well informed, assertive, and an active participant in his healthcare. He feels he is privileged because he has connections and advocates for himself, enabling him to expand his healthcare options and seek the best providers and institutions. Nonetheless, even though his overall experience in the healthcare system has been favorable, many instances of his care have been less than ideal.

Communication Deficits and Lack of a Team Approach

Mr. Roberts has observed that the lack of communication between providers is a huge problem. He has multiple specialists who care for different parts of his body; however, no one person is mindful of how these systems interact to create the whole person or illness. He is never sure whether one physician knows what the other is doing or how one physician's prescriptions might interfere or interact with another's. The physicians never seem inclined to "dig deeply" or communicate as team members treating one person. On many occasions, physicians have recommended therapies that have already been tried and failed. On other occasions, they disagree on an approach to a problem and leave Mr. Roberts to decide which advice to follow. No system is in place to encourage teamwork. "Unless the physician is extremely intelligent, on the ball, or energetic, it just doesn't happen," he says.

Seldom do physicians listen to his full story or elicit his thoughts before jumping to conclusions. Mr. Roberts suggests that physicians should carefully analyze their therapeutic personalities. They cannot assume that all patients are alike or that all patients will react similarly to a given intervention. Each patient needs to be treated as an individual, and service needs to be respectful of individual choice.

Record keeping and transfer of information are also faulty. Despite the fact that the physicians take copious notes, the information is often not put to use. Mr. Roberts has expended a great deal of time and energy ensuring that his medical records are sent to a new consultant's office, only to find within a few minutes of the encounter that the consultant has not reviewed the chart or absorbed the information. This realization has affected how he uses care. For instance, at one point, Mr. Roberts's stomach problems were worsening. His gastroenterologist was away on vacation for four weeks, and there was no covering physician. The thought of amassing his patient records for transfer to another physician (who likely would not review them and would suggest the same tests and therapies) was so unpleasant that he chose to go without care.

Removing the Question Mark from Patient–Provider Interactions

Mr. Roberts is particularly concerned with patients' inability to know the true qualifications of their physicians or evaluate their prescriptions. At one point, he was experiencing severe arm and finger pain. Assuming these symptoms were related to his spine, he sought the advice of a highly recommended chief of neurosurgery at a premier academic center. After eliciting a brief history and performing a short examination, the chief admitted him to the hospital.

The following day, an anesthesiologist came into the room to obtain his consent for surgery. Mr. Roberts had not been told that surgery was under consideration. He asked to speak to the neurosurgeon and insisted on additional consultations. Three days later, a hand surgeon reassured him that his problem was likely self-limiting tendonitis and prescribed conservative therapy. Within a few weeks, his pain had been resolved. Mr.

(continued)

Roberts was grateful that he had followed his instinct but was concerned for other patients who might not have asserted themselves in this manner.

Mismatch Between Supply and Demand

Mr. Roberts also noticed a profound disconnect between supply and demand in the healthcare system. In 1992, his pain had become particularly disabling, and his mobility was extremely restricted. His physicians suggested that he see a neurosurgeon, but there was only one neurosurgeon in the county. Despite his health emergency, he was not able to make an appointment to see this neurosurgeon for more than ten weeks. No other solutions were offered.

In pain and unable to walk because of progressively worsening foot drop and muscle weakness, he sought the help of a physician friend. This friend referred him to a "brash, iconoclastic" Harvard-trained neurologist, who in turn referred him to a virtuoso neurosurgeon at a county hospital 100 miles away. After only 20 minutes with this neurosurgeon, he was rushed to the operating room and underwent a nine-hour emergency procedure. Apparently, he had severe spinal cord impingement and swelling. The neurosurgeon later told him that he would have been a paraplegic or died had he not undergone surgery that day.

Mr. Roberts subsequently had a series of three more spinal operations. Postoperative care was suboptimal; he had to travel 100 miles to see the surgeon for follow-up. Eventually, this surgeon chose to travel to a more centralized location twice per month to accommodate patients in outlying areas.

Mr. Roberts states that we need to "overcome petty bureaucracies" that do not allow matching of supply with demand. The ready availability of quality care should be patient driven and closely monitored by a third party that does not have a vested interest in the market.

Knowledge-Based Care

Mr. Roberts is concerned about the status of continuing medical education. He guesses that physicians in large, urban teaching hospitals can easily to keep abreast of the latest diagnostic and therapeutic advances but that the majority of other physicians may not have similar opportunities. The system does not necessarily encourage physicians to keep up to date. This lack of current, in-depth knowledge is particularly important as issues of supply and demand force consumers to seek care in "instant med clinics." For example, Mr. Roberts believes "emergency care" to be an oxymoron.

On many occasions, he has gone to the emergency department and had to wait four to five hours before being treated. This experience is unpleasant and forces people to seek alternative facilities that may not provide the best care for complex, chronically ill patients.

Mr. Roberts also feels that we need to learn from our errors as well as from our successes and that groups of physicians should be required to regularly review cases and learn how to deliver care in a better way. This analysis needs to occur internally within institutions as well as externally across institutions. Ideally, the analysis would directly involve patients and families to gain their perspectives. In addition, the learning should be contextual; we should not only learn how to do better the next time but also know whether what we are doing makes sense within our overall economic, epidemiological, and societal context.

Mr. Roberts believes that high-quality healthcare is knowledge based. This knowledge comes not only from science but also from analysis of mistakes that occur in the process of delivering care. Patients should be involved in the collection and synthesis of these data. The transfer of knowledge among patients, scientists, and practitioners must be emphasized and simplified.

Nonphysician/Nonhospital Care

Mr. Roberts has been impressed with the quality of the care he has received from nonphysician clinicians, and he believes the growth of alternative healthcare provider models has been a definite advance in the system. As an example, Mr. Roberts cites the effectiveness of his physical therapists as healthcare providers; they have been alert, patient conscious, conscientious, and respectful. Mr. Roberts believes that their interventions "guide people to better life," and his functional status has improved as a result of their assistance. In addition, these providers are careful to maintain close communication with physicians. They function as members of a team.

Postoperative care also has improved. At the time of his first surgery more than two decades ago, Mr. Roberts spent two weeks in the hospital. Now, after three days he is discharged to a rehabilitation facility that is better equipped to help him recuperate and regain full function.

Mr. Roberts knows how crucial his family and friends are to his medical care. Without their support, recommendations, constant questioning, and advocacy, his condition would be more precarious. The system needs to acknowledge patients' other caregivers and involve them in shared decision making and knowledge transfer.

Case Study: Stopping Catheter-Related Bloodstream Line Infections at the Johns Hopkins University Medical Center and Hospitals Across the United States

Evidence indicates that medical errors result in part from the lack of a patient safety culture—a culture that encourages detection of quality problems—and from poor communication and teamwork in addressing quality problems. In response to these findings, in 2001 a team of researchers at the Johns Hopkins University Quality and Safety Research Group developed an innovative, comprehensive program to improve patient safety at the Johns Hopkins Hospital, a 1,015-bed tertiary care facility that treats more than 268,000 patients annually from across the United States and around the world. This case illustrates many of the improvement concepts and tools described in this chapter.

The efforts of the Johns Hopkins team led to the creation of the Comprehensive Unit-Based Safety Program (CUSP). CUSP is a program of continuous measurement, feedback, and improvement that was designed to

- be implemented sequentially in work units,
- improve the culture of safety,
- enable staff to focus safety efforts on unit-specific problems, and
- include rigorous data collection through which tangible improvements in patient safety are empirically derived to educate and improve awareness about eliminating central line–associated bloodstream infections (CLABSI).

It engages frontline staff and uses a combination of tools and compliance reports to achieve improvement goals.

Implementation of CUSP consists of five major steps:

1. Train staff in the science of safety (e.g., basic strategies for safe design, including standardized processes and independent checklists for key processes).
2. Engage staff in identifying defects (e.g., ask staff how the next patient could be harmed on their unit).
3. Perform senior executive partnership/safety rounds (i.e., have hospital executives interact and discuss safety issues with staff on hospital units).
4. Continue to learn from defects by answering four questions:
   a. What happened?
   b. Why did it happen?

c. What was done to reduce risk?
d. How do we know that risk was actually reduced?

5. Implement tools for improvement (e.g., morning briefs, daily goals checklists, operating room debriefings).

A detailed flowchart of CUSP is provided in exhibit 1.12.

EXHIBIT 1.12
Comprehensive Unit-Based Safety Program (CUSP) Flowchart

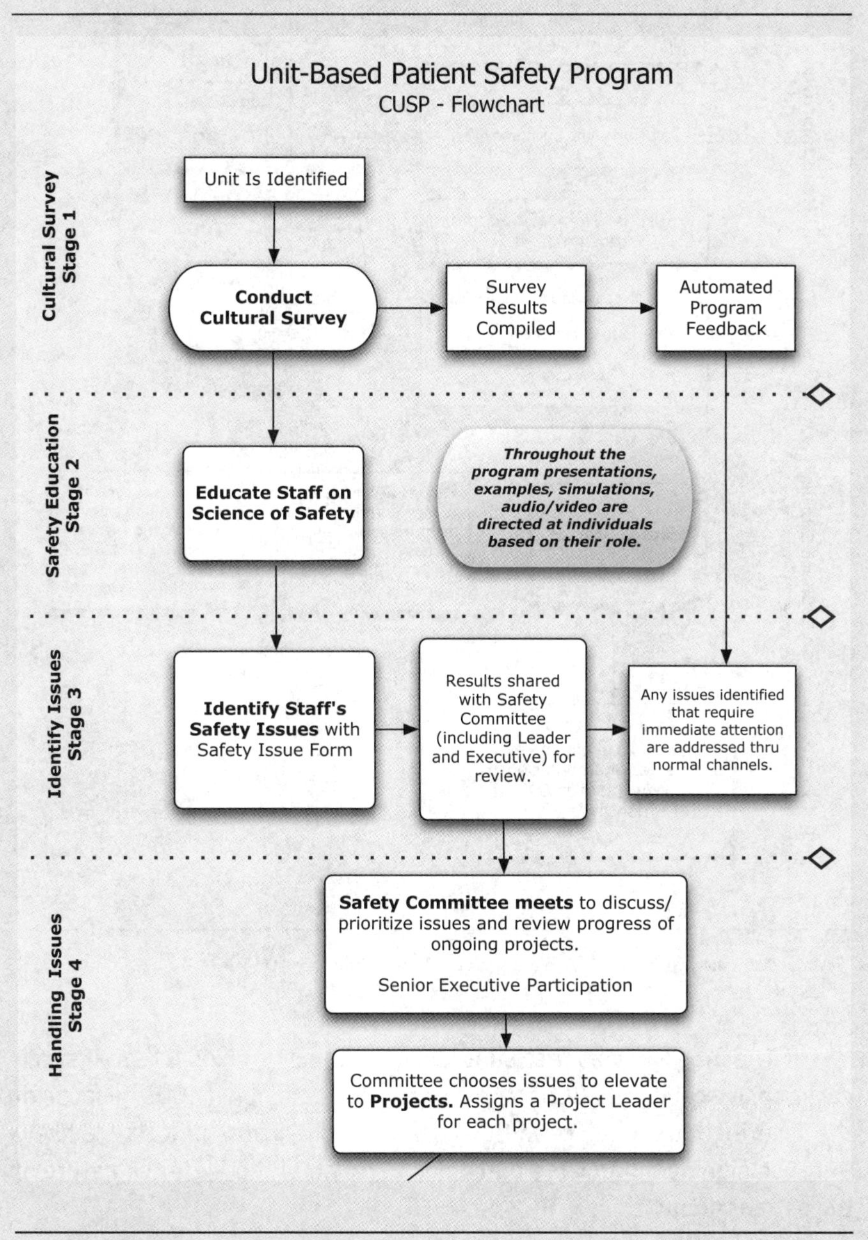

(continued)

EXHIBIT 1.12
Comprehensive Unit-Based Safety Program (CUSP) Flowchart *(continued)*

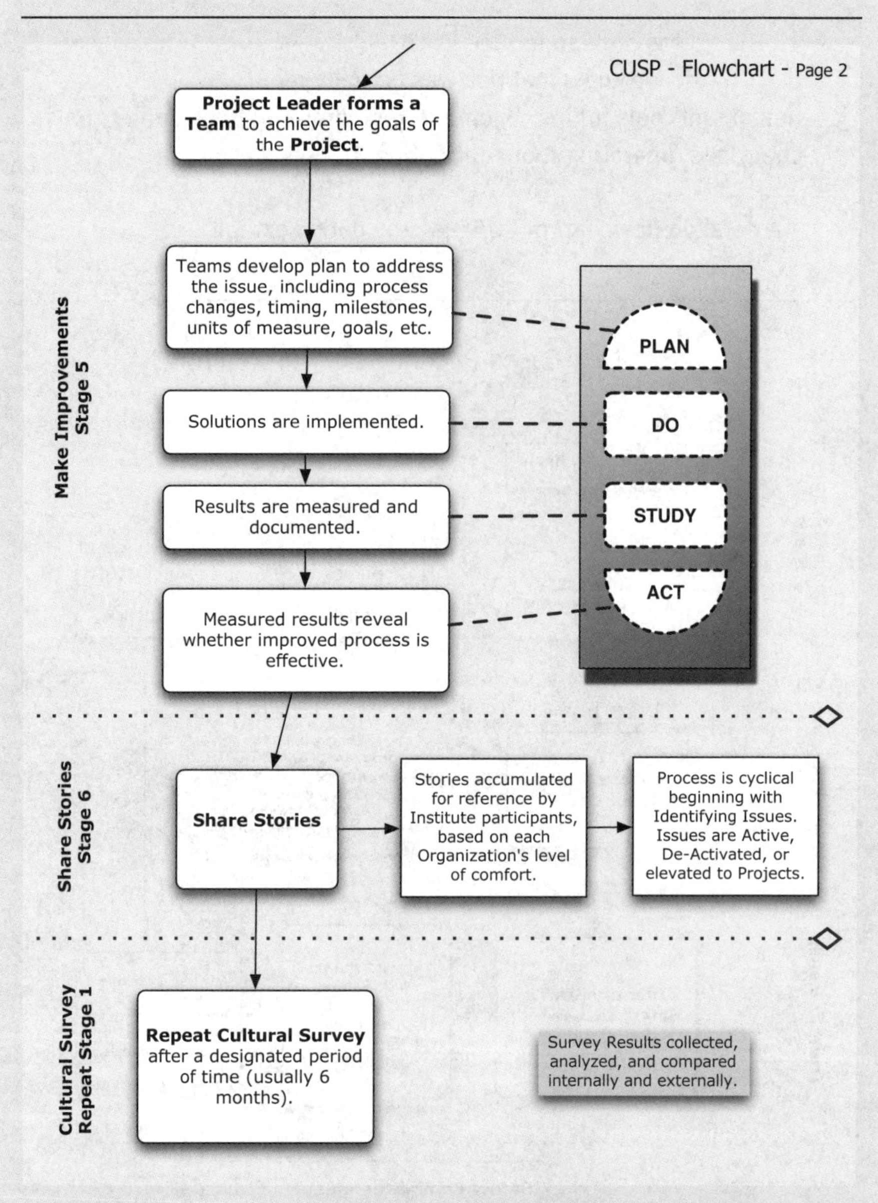
CUSP - Flowchart - Page 2
Project Leader forms a Team to achieve the goals of the Project.
Make Improvements Stage 5
Teams develop plan to address the issue, including process changes, timing, milestones, units of measure, goals, etc.
Solutions are implemented.
Results are measured and documented.
Measured results reveal whether improved process is effective.
PLAN
DO
STUDY
ACT
Share Stories Stage 6
Share Stories
Stories accumulated for reference by Institute participants, based on each Organization's level of comfort.
Process is cyclical beginning with Identifying Issues. Issues are Active, De-Activated, or elevated to Projects.
Cultural Survey Repeat Stage 1
Repeat Cultural Survey after a designated period of time (usually 6 months).
Survey Results collected, analyzed, and compared internally and externally.

Source: Published with permission of Johns Hopkins HealthCare LLC.

The program was first piloted in two Johns Hopkins Hospital surgical intensive care units (ICUs). Errors are more common in ICUs because of the severity of patients' conditions. Furthermore, errors in ICUs are likely to cause significant adverse outcomes because of the high-risk nature of the patient population.

In implementing the program, at least one physician and one nurse from each unit were required to participate. These individuals had to dedicate four to eight hours per week to CUSP implementation and serve on the improvement team. Program expenses were the costs associated with CUSP team members' time.

Upon initial investigation of the work, researchers uncovered encouraging findings:

- *Length of stay (LOS):* LOS decreased from 2 days to 1 day in one unit and from 3 days to 2.3 days in the other unit.
- *Medication errors:* The medication error rate dropped from 94 percent to 0 percent in one unit and from 40 percent to 0 percent in the other unit.
- *Nursing turnover:* The nurse turnover rate decreased from 9 percent to 2 percent in one unit and from 8 percent to 2 percent in the other unit.
- *Safety culture:* The percentage of staff who self-reported a positive safety climate increased from 35 percent to 52 percent in one unit and from 35 percent to 68 percent in the other unit.

Because of the considerable success of the pilot program, CUSP was implemented in approximately 170 clinical areas across the Johns Hopkins Hospital. Subsequently, CUSP was implemented at hospitals across the state of Michigan in collaboration with the Michigan Health and Hospital Association's Center for Patient Safety and Quality.

A total of 108 ICUs initially participated in the Michigan program. The program brought about dramatic decreases in CLABSI rates in Michigan hospitals, from a mean of 2.7 infections per 1,000 catheter days to 0 infections per 1,000 catheter days 18 months after implementation.

The success of the program did not go unnoticed. AHRQ awarded the Health Research and Educational Trust (HRET), a nonprofit research and educational affiliate of the American Hospital Association, an $18 million contract to spread CUSP to hospitals across the United States to reduce CLABSI. The new program—On the CUSP: Stop BSI—was implemented in 44 states as well as throughout Spain and England. More than 1,000 hospitals and 1,800 hospital units across the 44 states, the District of Columbia, and Puerto Rico have collectively reduced the national CLABSI rate from a baseline of 1.915 infections per 1,000 line days to 1.133 infections, a relative reduction of 41 percent (see exhibit 1.13).

(continued)

EXHIBIT 1.13 Average CLABSI Rates (infections per 1,000 catheter days) per Unit

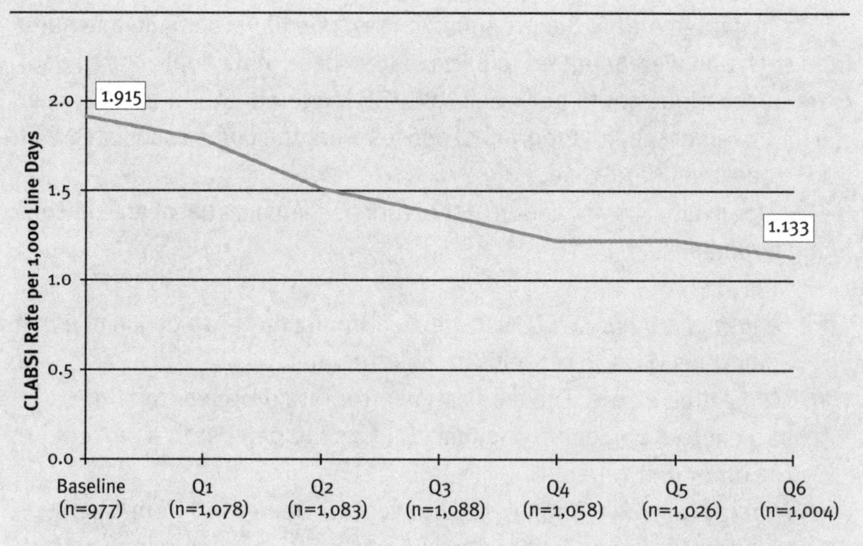

Source: AHRQ (2013). Used with permission.

EXHIBIT 1.14 Percentage of Reporting Units with CLABSI Rate of 0/1,000 or Less Than 1/1,000 Central Line Days

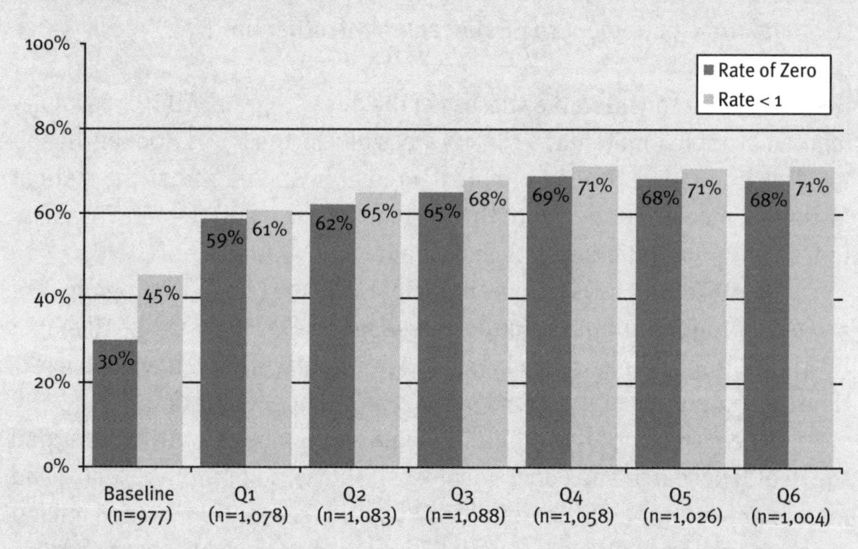

Source: AHRQ (2013). Used with permission.

The percentage of participating units with a 0 percent CLABSI rate also increased drastically, from 30 percent to 68 percent of all units (see exhibit 1.14). Additionally, the percentage of units reporting a CLABSI rate of less than one per 1,000 line days increased over time from 45 percent to 71 percent.

Building on the success of the On the CUSP: Stop BSI program, HRET also led the implementation of a neonatal CLABSI prevention program in partnership with the Perinatal Quality Collaborative of North Carolina. This effort resulted in a decrease in CLABSI rates from 2.043 at baseline in August 2011 to 0.855 in August 2012—a 58 percent relative reduction.

In addition to the expanded efforts to reduce CLABSI rates, the CUSP toolkit is now being applied to address other hospital-acquired infections, most notably catheter-associated urinary tract infections (CAUTI). HRET is working with numerous partners on the On the CUSP: Stop CAUTI project to reduce CAUTI rates by 25 percent over 18 months.

The path to improvement has not been simple; it has required collaboration between a variety of multidisciplinary stakeholders. Nonetheless, the perseverance of clinical leaders and organizations across the United States continues to make the On the CUSP: Stop BSI program and its many successive iterations a notable success.

Sources: AHRQ (2017); Health Research and Educational Trust, Johns Hopkins University Quality and Safety Research Group, and Michigan Health and Hospital Association Keystone Center for Patient Safety and Quality (2013, 2011); Johns Hopkins Medicine (2018); Patient Safety Group (2013); Pronovost et al. (2006).

Study Questions

1. Think of an experience you, a family member, or a friend has had with healthcare. Gauge the experience against IOM's six aims, and identify any opportunities for improvement.
2. Describe three instances in which outcomes would not be a good measure of healthcare quality, and explain why.
3. Do you agree that care can be both high quality and inefficient? Why or why not?
4. What are some of the challenges to spreading change? Identify two key questions/issues that need to be considered when applying change concepts in an organization or system.
5. How would a healthcare organization choose elements to measure and tools for measurement when seeking to improve the quality of care?
6. What are some of the key elements common to the various tools discussed in this chapter?
7. What is the difference between a quality improvement method and a quality improvement tool? Provide examples of each.

References

Agency for Healthcare Research and Quality (AHRQ). 2017. "AHRQ Safety Program for Improving Surgical Care and Recovery: A Collaborative Program to Enhance the Recovery of Surgical Patients." Published March. www.ahrq.gov/professionals/quality-patient-safety/hais/tools/enhanced-recovery/index.html.

———. 2016. *2016 National Healthcare Quality and Disparities Report*. Rockville, MD: AHRQ.

———. 2013. *Eliminating CLABSI, a National Patient Safety Imperative: Final Report*. Published January. www.ahrq.gov/professionals/quality-patient-safety/cusp/clabsi-final/index.html.

American Society for Quality (ASQ). 2014. "A. V. Feigenbaum: Laying the Foundations of Modern Quality Control." Accessed January 30. http://asq.org/about-asq/who-we-are/bio_feigen.html.

Berwick, D. M. 2002. "A User's Manual for the IOM's 'Quality Chasm' Report." *Health Affairs* (Millwood) 21 (3): 80–90.

Bodenheimer, T. S., and K. Grumbach. 2009. *Understanding Health Policy: A Clinical Approach*, 5th ed. New York: Lange Medical Books.

Brook, R. H., A. Davies-Avery, S. Greenfield, L. J. Harris, T. Lelah, N. E. Solomon, and J. E. Ware Jr. 1977. "Assessing the Quality of Medical Care Using Outcome Measures: An Overview of the Method." *Medical Care* 15 (9 suppl.): 1–165.

Chassin, M. R., and R. H. Galvin. 1998. "The Urgent Need to Improve Health Care Quality: Institute of Medicine National Roundtable on Health Care Quality." *Journal of the American Medical Association* 280 (11): 1000–5.

Cleary, P. D., and B. J. McNeil. 1988. "Patient Satisfaction as an Indicator of Quality Care." *Inquiry* 25 (1): 25–36.

Cochrane, A. L. 1973. *Effectiveness and Efficiency: Random Reflections on Health Services*. London: Nuffield Provincial Hospitals Trust.

Deming, W. E. 2000a. *The New Economics for Industry, Government, Education*, 2nd ed. Cambridge, MA: MIT Press.

———. 2000b. *Out of the Crisis*. Cambridge, MA: MIT Press.

Donabedian, A. 2003. *An Introduction to Quality Assurance in Health Care*. New York: Oxford University Press.

———. 1988a. "Quality and Cost: Choices and Responsibilities." *Inquiry* 25 (1): 90–99.

———. 1988b. "The Quality of Care: How Can It Be Assessed?" *Journal of the American Medical Association* 260 (12): 1743–48.

———. 1982. *Explorations in Quality Assessment and Monitoring. Volume II: The Criteria and Standards of Quality*. Chicago: Health Administration Press.

———. 1980. *Explorations in Quality Assessment and Monitoring. Volume I: The Definition of Quality and Approaches to Its Assessment*. Chicago: Health Administration Press.

———. 1966. "Evaluating the Quality of Medical Care." *Milbank Memorial Fund Quarterly* 44 (3): 166–206.

Donabedian, A., J. R. C. Wheeler, and L. Wyszewianski. 1982. "Quality, Cost, and Health: An Integrative Model." *Medical Care* 20 (10): 975–92.

Drummond, M. F., M. J. Sculpher, G. W. Torrance, B. J. O'Brien, and G. L. Stoddart. 2005. *Methods for the Economic Evaluation of Health Care Programs*, 3rd ed. New York: Oxford University Press.

Eddy, D. M. 2005. "Evidence-Based Medicine: A Unified Approach." *Health Affairs* 24 (1): 9–17.

———. 1996. *Clinical Decision Making: From Theory to Practice*. Sudbury, MA: Jones & Bartlett.

Evidence-Based Medicine Working Group. 1992. "Evidence-Based Medicine: A New Approach to Teaching the Practice of Medicine." *Journal of the American Medical Association* 268 (17): 2420–25.

Ferlie, E., and S. M. Shortell. 2001. "Improving the Quality of Healthcare in the United Kingdom and the United States: A Framework for Change." *Milbank Quarterly* 79 (2): 281–316.

Gawande, A. 2010. *The Checklist Manifesto*. New York: Metropolitan Books.

Gerteis, M., S. Edgman-Levitan, J. Daley, and T. L. Delbanco (eds.). 1993. *Through the Patient's Eyes: Understanding and Promoting Patient-Centered Care*. San Francisco: Jossey-Bass.

Gold, M. R., J. E. Siegel, L. B. Russell, and M. C. Weinstein (eds.). 1996. *Cost-Effectiveness in Health and Medicine*. New York: Oxford University Press.

Goode, A. P., C. Cook, J. B. Gill, S. Tackett, C. Brown, and W. Richardson. 2011. "The Risk of Risk-Adjustment Measures for Perioperative Spine Infection After Spinal Surgery." *Spine* 36 (9): 752–58.

Gosbee, J. W., and L. L. Gosbee (eds.). 2005. *Using Human Factors Engineering to Improve Patient Safety*. Oakbrook Terrace, IL: Joint Commission Resources.

Guinn, J. 2017. *Human-Centered Methods for Designing in Healthcare*. Philadelphia, PA: Digital Innovation and Consumer Experience, Thomas Jefferson University and Jefferson Health.

Harteloh, P. P. M. 2004. "Understanding the Quality Concept in Health Care." *Accreditation and Quality Assurance* 9: 92–95.

Health Research and Educational Trust, Johns Hopkins University Quality and Safety Research Group, and Michigan Health and Hospital Association Keystone Center for Patient Safety and Quality. 2013. *Eliminating CLABSI, A National Patient Safety Imperative: Final Report*. Published January. www.ahrq.gov/professionals/quality-patient-safety/cusp/clabsi-final/index.html.

———. 2011. *Eliminating CLABSI: A National Patient Safety Imperative. Second Progress Report on the National On the CUSP: Stop BSI Project*. Published September. www.ahrq.gov/professionals/quality-patient-safety/cusp/clabsi-update/clabsi-update.pdf.

Heim, K. 1999. "Creating Continuous Improvement Synergy with Lean and TOC." Paper presented at the American Society for Quality Annual Quality Congress, Anaheim, California, May.

Iezzoni, L. I. (ed.). 2013. *Risk Adjustment for Measuring Health Care Outcomes*, 4th ed. Chicago: Health Administration Press.

Institute of Medicine (IOM). 2002. *Unequal Treatment: Confronting Racial and Ethnic Disparities in Healthcare*. Washington, DC: National Academies Press.

———. 2001. *Crossing the Quality Chasm: A New Health System for the 21st Century*. Washington, DC: National Academies Press.

———. 1993. *Access to Health Care in America*. Washington, DC: National Academies Press.

———. 1990. *Medicare: A Strategy for Quality Assurance*. Washington, DC: National Academies Press.

Johns Hopkins Medicine. 2018. "The Comprehensive Unit-Based Safety Program (CUSP)." Accessed August 31. www.hopkinsmedicine.org/armstrong_institute/improvement_projects/infections_complications/stop_bsi/educational_sessions/immersion_calls/cusp.html.

Kohn, L. T., J. M. Corrigan, and M. S. Donaldson (eds.). 2000. *To Err Is Human: Building a Safer Health System*. Washington, DC: National Academies Press.

Langley, G., K. Nolan, T. Nolan, C. Norman, and L. Provost. 1996. *The Improvement Guide: A Practical Approach to Enhancing Organizational Performance*. San Francisco: Jossey-Bass.

Leape, L. L., and D. M. Berwick. 2005. "Five Years After *To Err Is Human*: What Have We Learned?" *Journal of the American Medical Association* 293 (19): 2384–90.

Lee, R. I., and L. W. Jones. 1933. *The Fundamentals of Good Medical Care: An Outline of the Fundamentals of Good Medical Care and an Estimate of the Service Required to Supply the Medical Needs of the United States*. Chicago: University of Chicago Press.

Makary, M., and M. Daniel. 2016. "Medical Error—The Third Leading Cause of Death in the US." *BMJ* 353: i2139.

Massoud, M. R., G. A. Nielson, K. Nolan, T. Nolan, M. W. Schall, and C. Sevin. 2006. "A Framework for Spread: From Local Improvements to System-Wide Change." IHI Innovation Series white paper. Cambridge, MA: Institute for Healthcare Improvement.

Muir Gray, J. A. 2009. *Evidence-Based Healthcare: How to Make Decisions About Health Services and Public Health*, 3rd ed. Edinburgh, UK: Churchill Livingstone.

National Academies of Sciences, Engineering, and Medicine. 2015. *Improving Diagnosis in Health Care*. Washington, DC: National Academies Press.

Nolan, T. W. 2007. "Execution of Strategic Improvement Initiatives to Produce System-Level Results." IHI Innovation Series white paper. Cambridge, MA: Institute for Healthcare Improvement.

Pande, P. S., R. P. Neuman, and R. R. Cavanagh. 2000. *The Six Sigma Way: How GE, Motorola, and Other Top Companies Are Honing Their Performance*. New York: McGraw-Hill.

Patient Safety Group. 2013. "Introduction—eCUSP." Accessed August 31, 2018. www.patientsafetygroup.org/program/index.cfm.

Pronovost, P., D. Needham, S. Berenholtz, D. Sinopoli, H. Chu, S. Cosgrove, B. Sexton, R. Hyzy, R. Welsh, G. Roth, J. Bander, J. Kepros, and C. Goeschel. 2006. "An Intervention to Decrease Catheter-Related Bloodstream Infections in the ICU." *New England Journal of Medicine* 355 (26): 2725–32.

Sofaer, S., and K. Firminger. 2005. "Patient Perceptions of the Quality of Health Services." *Annual Review of Public Health* 26: 513–59.

Straus, S. E., W. S. Richardson, P. Glasziou, and R. B. Haynes. 2005. *Evidence-Based Medicine: How to Practice and Teach EBM*, 3rd ed. Edinburgh, UK: Churchill Livingstone.

Strech, D., G. Persad, G. Marckmann, and M. Danis. 2009. "Are Physicians Willing to Ration Health Care? Conflicting Findings in a Systematic Review of Survey Research." *Health Policy* 90 (2–3): 113–24.

Tague, N. R. 2004. *The Quality Toolbox*, 2nd ed. Milwaukee, WI: ASQ Quality Press.

White, A., T. D. Thompson, M. C. White, S. A. Sabatino, J. de Moor, P. V. Doria-Rose, A. M. Geiger, and L. C. Richardson. 2015. "Cancer Screening Test Use —United States, 2015." *Morbidity and Mortality Weekly Report* 66 (8): 201–6.

Williamson, J. W. 1977. *Improving Medical Practice and Health Care: A Bibliographic Guide to Information Management in Quality Assurance and Continuing Education*. Cambridge, MA: Ballinger.

Womack, J. P., and D. T. Jones. 2003. *Lean Thinking: Banish Waste and Create Wealth in Your Corporation*. New York: Free Press.

Wyszewianski, L. 1988. "Quality of Care: Past Achievements and Future Challenges." *Inquiry* 25 (1): 13–22.

Wyszewianski, L., and A. Donabedian. 1981. "Equity in the Distribution of Quality of Care." *Medical Care* 19 (12 suppl.): 28–56.

CHAPTER

2

HISTORY AND THE QUALITY LANDSCAPE

Norbert Goldfield

Introduction

The extraordinary developments in the measurement and management of healthcare quality need to be placed into historical context. This chapter will first briefly highlight the many advances that have occurred in quality control in industry, as a whole, and in the healthcare system specifically between 1850 and 1960. As this discussion is purposely brief, readers wanting to learn more can refer to the numerous articles and books that have been written about this period. The remainder of this chapter focuses on the most fertile period of quality measurement and management in healthcare in the United States—the time since the enactment of Medicare and Medicaid in 1965.

Although many decry the profit motive that drives healthcare systems, the reality is that healthcare delivery is a critical part of the US economy, as it is in other countries. Many sectors—not just the insurance industry—enjoy substantial profits from the healthcare system. Healthcare spending represented 17.8 percent of the US gross domestic product (GDP) in 2015, and that figure is projected to rise to 19.9 percent by 2025—the highest of any country in the world (Advisory Board 2017). Financial incentives, such as those described in this chapter, are critical to the successful implementation of any quality measurement program. As numerous articles have documented, access to health insurance, the extent of its coverage, and socioeconomic disparities have a significant impact on quality of outcomes and important implications for the American healthcare economy. Typically, the people who suffer the most in terms of poor quality are the poor and nonwhite populations.

Perhaps the best way to counter the profit motive that exists in our present healthcare system is to tie transparent financial incentives of quality outcomes to organizational (as opposed to individual health professional) behavior. These financial incentives should be one leg of the "three-legged stool" of quality management. The other two legs are a focus on consumer empowerment, as discussed in detail later in this chapter, and payers' regular release of transparent, comparative outcomes data, which helps foster collaboration with payers.

If we were to implement this three-legged stool approach throughout the entire healthcare system, we could make tremendous progress in one absolutely critical intermediate outcome measure—namely, universal coverage. Universal coverage is a critical ingredient to the provision of quality care, as we have seen that, without insurance coverage, clinical outcomes are worse (Institute of Medicine 2001). Although we have made tremendous progress in improving access to healthcare coverage, those of us who believe that every American citizen deserves a "decent minimum" of healthcare coverage know that we still have a long way to go to achieve equity. The United States remains the only first-world industrialized country that lacks universal insurance coverage for its citizens, and prospects for achieving that important goal of quality management seem farther away than ever, at least at the national level.

Quality Measurement and Management Prior to 1965

The main themes of this chapter are an outgrowth of the period before 1965, the year that Congress passed Medicare and Medicaid into law. Over the past half century, our quality measurement tools have become much more refined, but the basic issues remain—we have reasonably good quality measures with inadequate implementation.

Historically, the principal approaches to quality measurement were developed outside the healthcare system, in the manufacturing sector. The giants in the field of industrial quality measurement and management were W. Edwards Deming, Walter Shewhart (Deming's teacher), and Joseph M. Juran (Deming 1982; Juran 1995). Deming pioneered the use of control charts, which had been developed by Shewhart (Best and Neuhauser 2006). Control charts are arguably the most important tool in the quality measurement armamentarium (though they are still not used enough in healthcare). Deming famously said, "Look for the trouble and its explanation and try to remove the cause every time a point goes out of control" (Clarke 2005, 36). Well before the *Dartmouth Atlas*, which will be described later in this chapter, it was Deming who declared that "uncontrolled variation is the enemy of quality" (Kang and Kvam 2012, 19).

Despite Deming's pioneering work, it was not until the late 1990s that we finally began to reverse many of the perverse incentives of paying more for poor quality outcomes (e.g., hospital complications)—and we are still only at the beginning! As Deming (1982, 11) said, "Defects are not free. Somebody makes them, and gets paid for making them." Deming clearly stated that a complete shift of financial risk from a payer to a provider means that the payer has abdicated any interest in quality (Schiff and Goldfield 1994).

Readers should keep in mind that effective medical interventions were few and far between in the early twentieth century. General anesthesia with tracheal intubation, the first antibiotics, and the discovery of insulin all occurred less than 100 years ago. The beginning of healthcare measurement and management can be attributed to the British nurse Florence Nightingale, who used statistics to document an improvement in the mortality rate after her sanitary interventions during the Crimean War in the 1850s. According to many, she paved the way for the first truly modern hospitals (McDonald 2014) with her use of statistics to identify opportunities for improvement (Kopf 1916), her focus on the most important quality measure (mortality), and her changes to managerial practices based on results.

In the early twentieth century, decades before Deming, surgeon Ernest A. Codman (1914, 496) was an early supporter of outcomes research:

> We must formulate some method of hospital report showing as nearly as possible what are the results of the treatment obtained at different institutions. This report must be made out and published by each hospital in a uniform manner, so that comparison will be possible. With such a report as a starting point, those interested can begin to ask questions as to management and efficiency.

Codman's arguments led to a hospital standardization program by the American College of Surgeons (ACS); however, in a 1918 survey, only 89 of 692 hospitals met the basic minimum standards. The results were announced at an ACS committee meeting at the Waldorf Astoria Hotel in New York City in 1919 (Wright 2017), but the leaders of the ACS burned Codman's papers so that the public would not find out which hospitals had failed his test (ACS 2018b).

Although Codman died a pauper, his research articles and short books remain among the most quoted in the healthcare quality measurement and management literature. Around the same time that Codman's efforts failed, Abraham Flexner was more successful in reforming America's medical schools—and hospitals in general—by creating standards for education and licensure of physicians and medical staff (Flexner 1910).

In the 1930s through 1950s, researchers documented the validity of yet another of Deming's beliefs, the presence of practice pattern variation in such procedures as tonsillectomies (Glover 1938) and hysterectomies (Doyle 1953). Leaders such as Mindel Sheps (1955), Cecil Sheps (Solon, Sheps, and Lee 1960), Leonard Rosenfeld (1957), Sam Shapiro (Berkowitz 1998), and Paul Lembcke (1956) developed new, preliminary approaches to quality measurement. Lembcke, for example, described a quality measurement technique he called "medical auditing," which is now called explicit chart review. In a remarkable article on the impact of medication on health and the importance of medication safety, Henry Beecher (1955) summarized the then scant research literature on the placebo effect. In an era with an unprecedented number of new medications and an increased focus on medication safety, Beecher summarized in a seminal article the 15 studies then extant documenting the placebo effect.

Around the same time, I. S. Falk, Odin Anderson, Milton Roemer, and Kerr White (White, Williams, and Greenberg 1961) published their research on the organizational and political aspects of quality management, including the connection between quality and the organization and financing of medical care. The first major efforts to provide health insurance coverage in the United States emerged in the 1930s—the same decade that witnessed the publication of findings by Falk and his group of researchers about the best organizational approaches to delivering quality care (Falk, Rorem, and Ring 1932). Based on many years of research, Falk's team concluded that the group practice model was the best approach for delivering quality medical care; at this time, most physicians were in solo fee-for-service practices. One of the most successful group practice programs is still in existence today: The Kaiser Permanente Medical Group started in the 1930s, became a medical group in the 1940s, and eventually evolved to a prototypical health maintenance organization (HMO) in the 1970s (Cutting and Collen 1992).

By the early 1950s, some aspects of Codman's dream began to become a reality (Mallon 2014), after the American College of Physicians, the American Hospital Association, the American Medical Association, and the Canadian Medical Association joined the American College of Surgeons to form the Joint Commission on Accreditation of Hospitals (Roberts, Coale, and Redman 1987). However, these were voluntary associations of professional organizations. The government had minimal involvement in quality improvement at the time, as its financial stake was minimal—another example of the Deming dictum of the relationships (or lack thereof) between interest in quality improvement and financial incentives. The Joint Commission and other voluntary associations took a "minimal standards" approach to quality measurement and management, and thus they did not adopt the quality management approaches that Codman and Deming would have supported.

In the 1960s, Sol Levine and other sociologists connected the political and organizational aspects of healthcare systems to quality measurement and management with their contributions to the rapidly developing field of medical sociology (Freeman, Levine, and Reeder 1963). In 1966, Levine became the founding member of the Department of Behavioral Sciences at Johns Hopkins University, and he came to exemplify the rare researcher who bridged the quality management and measurement fields. With his pioneering work in medical sociology, he paved the way for our understanding of the connections between nonhealthcare factors—such as housing, education, social class, and race—and healthcare outcomes. Levine was one of the first people to focus on such outcomes as quality of life and happiness. In addition to making voluminous contributions to our research understanding of these critical issues, he was also a teacher to hundreds around the world. His followers, in turn, have continued his legacy of advancing the science of quality measurement while connecting the findings to improvement of our healthcare system, particularly for the most vulnerable members of society.

Medicare, Medicaid, and Subsequent Developments

In 1965, the US Congress established the Medicare and Medicaid programs as Title XVIII and Title XIX of the Social Security Act. It was one of the most consequential legislative acts in US history, as it would lead to improved healthcare quality for more than one hundred million low-income Americans—particularly the elderly.

The immediate antecedents had begun in 1960. Working with Senator Robert Kerr of Oklahoma, Wilbur Mills, the powerful chairman of the House Ways and Means Committee, had attempted to stifle the drive toward Medicare by passing a limited program that provided means-tested health insurance to poor elderly citizens. The program would be administered by state and local governments that had chosen to participate. However, the guidelines for participation were so stringent that only 1 percent of the elderly received benefits. In 1964, Lyndon Baines Johnson won a landslide electoral and legislative victory over Barry Goldwater, delivering a critical electoral message that the country was ripe for Medicare and Medicaid. The Johnson administration revised its Medicare bill to include hospital insurance funded through Social Security taxes, a voluntary program covering physicians' costs paid for by contributions from beneficiaries and general revenue from the federal government, and an expanded version of the Kerr-Mills Act, administered by the states in a 50-50 match with the federal government. This expanded version would later be called Medicaid.

Along with the legislation came regulatory quality management bodies, beginning with Professional Standard Review Organizations (PSROs) and then, when the PSROs failed, Peer Review Organizations (PROs) in the 1980s. The federal government implemented a number of "screens" such as unscheduled return for surgery and adequacy of discharge planning. This profiling of physicians (Goldfield and Boland 1996) and healthcare institutions remains in place through the present federal, state, and private payer value-based purchasing programs that have replaced many of the federal programs of the 1960s.

Quality Measure Development Following the Passage of Medicare and Medicaid

Around the time Medicare and Medicaid were enacted, a series of scientific articles had a dramatic impact on healthcare delivery in the United States. Avedis Donabedian (1966) magisterially summarized and expanded upon the quality measurement literature with his voluminous contributions. In a seminal article titled "Evaluating the Quality of Medical Care," he provided a critique of the existing definitions of *quality* and approaches to the measurement of quality. In particular, he clarified the distinctions between structure, process, and outcomes measures. Donabedian (1966, 197) set forth a research agenda that many have followed ever since: "In addition to conceptual exploration of the meaning of quality, in terms of dimensions of care and the values attached to them, empirical studies are needed of what are the prevailing dimensions and values in relevant population groups."

Around the same time, an article by Sidney Katz and colleagues reported on the development of the activities of daily living (ADL) measure, one of the first in a veritable avalanche of validated measures that examine functional and mental health status from the perspective of either the patient or the provider (Katz et al. 1963). The ADL and IADL (instrumental activities of daily living) measures are still in use today—a testament to their durability. In the conclusion of their article, Katz and colleagues foreshadowed the enormous importance of the measurement of health status: "The index is proposed as a useful tool in the study of prognosis and the effects of treatment, as a survey instrument, as an objective guide in clinical practice, as a teaching device, and as a means of gaining more knowledge about the aging process" (Katz et al. 1963, 919).

Just a few years after the passage of Medicare and Medicaid, John Wennberg and Alan Gittelsohn (1973) at Dartmouth expanded on a fundamental Deming dictum pertaining to variation in medical practice patterns, noting that these variation patterns exist not just between the East Coast and West Coast of the United States but even within metropolitan areas such as New Haven, Connecticut, and Boston (Wennberg et al. 1989). The researchers not only documented the variations but also suggested ways of dealing with variations from clinical, financial, and organizational points of view. Over decades of subsequent research work, the Dartmouth group of researchers, including Wennberg and Gittelsohn, as well as Paul Batalden (Hayes, Batalden, and Goldmann 2015), Elliott Fisher (Lewis, Fisher, and Colla 2017), Robert Keller (1994), Eugene Nelson (Nelson et al. 2003), Jonathan Skinner (Skinner and Volpp 2017), and John Wasson (2017), among others, pioneered the use of the *Dartmouth Atlas*, the perspective of the consumer, the Deming philosophy as applied to healthcare, and many other quality measurement and management approaches. Specifically, Fisher developed the accountable care organization (ACO), and Wasson has worked to develop a truly consumer-focused vision of the patient-centered medical home.

Case Mix, Diagnosis-Related Groups, and Risk Adjustment

Case mix is defined as the scientific methodology of assigning like patients to the same category. The key is defining the dependent variable, which could be dollars expended, mortality, or complications. The case mix measurement and management tool with the most dramatic impact on the American healthcare system (and the systems of many other countries throughout the world) emerged in the late 1960s from a group at the Yale School of Management. At Yale, the industrial management professor Bob Fetter and the public healthcare expert John Thompson (a nurse by training) worked with two operations research graduate students—Rich Averill and Ron Mills—to develop diagnosis-related groups (DRGs). Averill focused on operationalizing the DRG concept, and Mills focused on building the analytic infrastructure (Mills et al. 1976; Thompson, Averill, and Fetter 1979; Fetter et al. 1980).

In 1977, after completing the first version of the DRGs, Fetter, Thompson, and Averill had a meeting with the senior staff of a major teaching hospital to present their findings on the significant variation (both within and between DRGs) in that hospital's lengths of stay and costs. They expected that the senior staff would be amazed by the findings and want to take immediate action to decrease the variation and improve the efficiency of care being delivered. However, the findings were simply ignored. Without a financial incentive, the institution had little interest in addressing variation in hospital lengths of stay and cost (Averill, pers. comm.).

After this experience, Fetter, Thompson, and Averill internalized and acted upon the Deming dictum that, without a financial stake in quality improvement, no organization would be interested. This understanding led the three researchers to take advantage of the uncontrolled Medicare costs that had emerged quickly after the passage of the program (Thompson, Averill, and Fetter 1979), and they worked to influence state and federal governments to take action. A successful interim trial of the DRGs in New Jersey in the 1970s led to national implementation of DRGs, also known as the Inpatient Prospective Payment System (IPPS), in 1982, as federal government officials sought to confront Medicare's dramatic cost overruns (Russell 1989). Ironically, the federal government under the conservative administration of President Ronald Reagan implemented the most regulatory government intervention ever undertaken in healthcare.

The IPPS had three objectives, as articulated in Public Law No. 98-21, the Social Security Amendments of 1983: "Restructure the economic incentives to establish marketlike forces, to Establish the Federal government as a prudent buyer of services, to Identify the product being purchased on behalf of Medicare beneficiaries." How were these objectives accomplished? The DRGs restructured hospital payment to be based on a clinically credible unit of payment (the DRG) that linked the clinical and financial aspects of care. Essentially, DRGs represent "a clinically meaningful product with a price that was payment in full, thereby providing the strong financial incentive for efficiency" (Schweiker 1982, 34). The program was so successful that no cost increases in the DRG payment were made for several years (Russell and Manning 1989). However, although the IPPS established a fair payment amount for hospital care (the DRG price), it did not attempt to adjust the payment amount for the quality of the care provided—a significant omission that is being addressed today. The IPPS was used to pay hospitals, but it has never to date, with the exception of a few demonstration projects, been used for physician payment. Amazingly but possibly not surprisingly, healthcare professional behavior has changed despite this lack of direct financial incentive.

In addition to its financial impact, DRG implementation had four important effects, all of which have impacted quality measurement and management across all aspects of the healthcare system. First, and most important, researchers and lobbyists alike expressed strong concerns about the potential negative effect of IPPS implementation on hospital quality of care (Coulam and Gaumer 1992). These concerns led to funding for the largest health services research project in US history, the RAND Health Insurance Study (HIS) (Brook et al. 1983). The study's team of researchers—which included Bob Brook, Shelly Greenfield, Joe Newhouse, and John Ware, to name a few—determined, among many other findings, that quality of hospital care under DRGs had not suffered; in fact, mortality rates went down after DRG implementation (Kahn et al. 1992).

The findings of the RAND HIS led to, as a second impact of DRGs, the development of a whole new generation of quality measures, particularly those focused on outcomes. Such measures included the Short-Form Health Survey (SF-36) and various ways of comparing mortality rates (Ware and Sherbourne 1992; Fink, Yano, and Brook 1989), among many others.

Third, because implementation needed validation of the DRG assignment, the federal quality assurance bureaucracy stepped into action (Dans, Weiner, and Otter 1985), and researchers developed additional quality measurement tools in response (Gertman and Restuccia 1981).

Finally, the financial success of the IPPS approach led to the development and implementation of prospective payment systems for virtually all aspects of the healthcare system, including ambulatory care (Averill et al. 1993), nursing home services (Fries and Cooney 1985), and rehabilitation care (Granger et al. 2007), along with the application of prospective payment or risk adjustment to managed care organizations (Ellis et al. 1996). The research and development needed to implement these new prospective payment systems, in turn, led to a large number of additional quality measures specific to such areas as rehabilitation, home health, and hospital outpatient ambulatory visits (Goldfield, Pine, and Pine 1996). Policymakers and researchers alike used these tools to adjust prospective payment and/or risk adjustment on an ongoing basis.

Adjusting Prospective Payment Case Mix Systems for Severity: A Key to Fair Comparisons of Quality Outcomes

Even though the DRGs had been developed, in the Deming tradition, as a management tool to increase hospital efficiency, federal officials implemented them largely as a financial cost-control intervention. Concurrent with the federal bureaucracy's increased efforts to retrospectively monitor hospital quality, many people demanded that policymakers adjust DRG payment to take hospital quality into account. First, however, researchers needed to develop much more detailed severity adjustment of the DRGs and decide whether claims-based data—the type of data readily available and used for payment for all healthcare encounters—were sufficient for making valid assessments of, for example, hospital quality. In the late 1980s and throughout the 1990s, researchers at several organizations—including the Centers for Medicare & Medicaid Services (CMS), which at that time was called the Health Care Financing Administration—developed severity adjustment algorithms for the DRGs (Iezzoni et al. 1993; McGuire 1991). Eventually, the Medicare severity DRGs (MS-DRGs) were implemented in 2007.

Claims-Based Versus Medical Records–Based Quality Metrics and Their Integration into DRG Payment: The Beginning of Value-Based Purchasing

Throughout the 1990s, a variety of researchers—such as Lisa Iezzoni (Iezzoni et al. 1993), Shukri Khuri (Best et al. 2002), Ed Hannan (Hannan et al. 2003), Patrick Romano (Romano et al. 2002), and others (Goldfield, Pine, and Pine 1996)—debated the advantages and disadvantages of claims-based metrics versus medical records–based outcomes metrics, such as complication and mortality rates. CMS retreated from the public disclosure of comparative hospital mortality rates in 1989 (Iezzoni 2012), but from a policy point of view, it made an implicit early decision to continue using claims-based measures in its assessment of Medicare quality. However, little could be done in terms of measure development to incentivize hospitals to improve quality, until policymakers mandated a "flag" on a claims form indicating whether a secondary diagnosis was present on admission. This seemingly innocuous piece of information was a critical first step in identifying whether a condition flagged as present or not present on admission could, for example, be considered a preventable complication.

Many researchers, including Pine and Romano, advocated for the "present-on-admission" flag. They pursued a state-based approach, and California became the first state to effectively implement the flag in the mid-1990s. The National Center for Vital Statistics followed suit, and the notation was implemented on the insurance claims forms in 2006 (Agency for Healthcare Research and Quality 2006). With the flag implemented, researchers in both the public and private sectors rushed to develop the first hospital complication measures (Zhan et al. 2009; Hughes et al. 2006), followed by measures to delineate preventable hospital readmissions (Krumholz et al. 2009; Goldfield et al. 2008).

Although some researchers still question the validity of claims-based metrics, the measures are well established in the policy world. In addition, new items are routinely collected from electronic medical records and then linked to claims data, thus increasing the claims-based metrics' scientific validity (Medicare.gov 2018). At the same time, however, a "parallel universe" has led to separate quality management efforts that rely largely on data abstracted from electronic medical records. Beginning with Hannan and Khuri, researchers have developed a significant number of quality measures using data typically abstracted from the medical record using a predefined form and trained abstractors. Although some states, notably New York, link the results of some of these medical records–based measures to payment, most use them for internal quality management (New York State Department of Health 2018). Khuri and his team encouraged the American College of Surgeons to embrace this internal quality improvement effort, and it has had a significant impact on surgical complications in thousands of hospitals (ACS 2018a).

Case Example: The Difficulty of Measuring Quality of Mental Health and Substance Abuse Services

Although significant advances have been made in quality measurement for surgery and other aspects of medical care, the development of meaningful quality metrics, especially outcomes measures, for mental health and substance abuse (MHSA) services has faced major challenges. Little progress was made in developing MHSA quality metrics until the aforementioned RAND HIS. During the early 1990s, researchers, including John Ware and Emmett Keeler, developed detailed process measures and initial outcomes measures that would be useful for severe mental health disorders such as schizophrenia and less severe ones such as mild anxiety or depression (RAND Corporation 2018). Ware and other researchers—including G. Richard Smith, Al Tarlov, Sol Levine, Gene Nelson, and Shelly Greenfield—built on this work in the Medical Outcomes Study, the successor study to the RAND HIS (Smith et al. 2002; Tarlov et al. 1989).

Don Steinwachs of Johns Hopkins University and Tony Lehman of the University of Maryland—along with Mady Chalk and Tom McLellan, both of the Treatment Research Institute—were among the many who advanced this research in MHSA services. As part of a new round of federally funded initiatives, the Patient Outcomes Research Teams, Steinwachs and Lehman focused on the outcomes of people with severe mental disabilities—especially those with socioeconomic disparities (Lehman et al. 2004; Kwan, Stratton, and Steinwachs 2017). The researchers addressed the challenges faced by this difficult-to-treat population head-on, pushing the boundaries of quality measurement and determining, for example, that nonhealthcare approaches such as subsidized housing and support for employment could lead to significantly improved outcomes (Lehman et al. 2002). Similarly, Chalk and McLellan, among others, emphasized the importance of housing and the positive impact of various types of counseling, including web-based and telephonic counseling, on outcomes (Dugosh et al. 2016).

Researchers have since tied these innovative MHSA quality measures to traditional measures, such as preventable hospital admissions and readmissions, based on the theory that interventions such as employment and web-based counseling can help with the management of expensive medical conditions (Dixon 2000). Despite these advances, much remains to be learned about both quality measurement and management (Goldfield et al. 2016).

New Quality Management and Measurement Research Institutions Since the Passage of Medicare and Medicaid

From a quality management perspective, the US healthcare system has moved, in fits and starts, toward a group practice model of care ever since the 1930s report from the Committee on the Costs of Medical Care. The movement accelerated with the passage of Medicare and Medicaid under President Lyndon B. Johnson and the subsequent push by President Richard Nixon to increase the number of HMOs. From a positive feedback loop perspective, this move toward HMOs led to the development of a number of organizations, such as preferred provider organizations (PPOs) in the 1990s, that policymakers thought could accomplish the same healthcare efficiencies as staff-model HMOs but without the brick-and-mortar expense. More recently, these efforts have culminated in the development of organizations such as ACOs that, in theory, would have an interest in improving population health for the communities they serve (Lewis, Fisher, and Colla 2017). New categories of healthcare professionals, such as case managers and community health workers, have emerged in response to these developments.

Recognizing these organizational and professional trends, foundations such as the Robert Wood Johnson Foundation, the Kaiser Family Foundation, and the John A. Hartford Foundation, together with the federal government, have supported the establishment of institutions that engage in quality measurement and management research aligned with an HMO model or a population health perspective. The Kaiser Permanente Center for Health Research is the oldest of these institutions. During the late 1980s, Don Berwick founded the Institute for Healthcare Improvement (IHI), which became the most important institution driving quality measurement research and the effective dissemination of quality management best practices. The Health Research and Educational Trust (HRET) and, over the past two decades, newer institutions such as the Jefferson College of Population Health have provided further support for innovative approaches to quality measurement and management. In addition, the internet has facilitated interinstitutional collaboration on quality measurement. For instance, the Cochrane Database of Systematic Reviews, easily accessible online, appraises and synthesizes research from diverse sources and has contributed significantly to the evaluation of quality measurement and management interventions.[1]

Medical Malpractice

The results of the Harvard Malpractice Study were reported more than a quarter century ago, but the study remains the gold standard for research on medical malpractice (Brennan et al. 1991). The study found that adverse events occurred in 3.7 percent of hospitalizations and that 27.6 percent of adverse events were caused by negligence. Although 70.5 percent of the adverse events gave rise to disabilities lasting less than six months, 2.6 percent caused permanently disabling injuries, and 13.6 percent led to death. After the Harvard study, the Institute of Medicine's 2000 report *To Err Is Human* was the next landmark event in our understanding of medical malpractice and what we can do about it (Kohn, Corrigan, and Donaldson 2000).

Quality measures that focus on medical malpractice, such as incident reporting, are now routine.[2] Researchers and managers have developed strategies for disclosing medical errors to the affected parties and providing up-front payment for the cost of the medical error (Kalra and Kopargaonkar 2018). They have also explored adverse events beyond surgical encounters (Mills et al. 2018). Many of the advances in electronic medical records, together with virtually all of the quality measurement tools highlighted in this chapter, can help lessen the occurrence of malpractice and reduce the impact of adverse events that do occur—but only if the quality tools are implemented correctly (Lepelley et al. 2018; McKenzie et al. 2017). Legal strategies relating to malpractice include alternative dispute resolution, evidence of compliance with guidelines, and administrative compensation (Sohn and Bal 2012). Limiting the right to sue and the amount of plaintiff damages that can be awarded has, not surprisingly, had a significant impact on total malpractice awards (Sage, Harding, and Thomas 2016).

The Era of the Consumer Has (Almost) Arrived

Twenty-five years ago, we paid scant attention to what is arguably the most important outcome—the perspective of the consumer (i.e., the patient or family unit). Since that time, we have made dramatic strides in the measurement of that perspective, and concomitantly, the management role of the consumer has increased dramatically. Nonetheless, we have a long way to go.

John Ware and Cathy Sherbourne (1992) specified two types of information we can obtain from consumers: patient reports (e.g., "Am I able to climb a flight of stairs?") and ratings (e.g., satisfaction with service provided in a hospital). Paul Cleary and others during the 1980s and 1990s established the science of consumer ratings in healthcare, particularly with regard to patient satisfaction with hospital services (Zaslavsky et al. 2001). Policymakers and payers have since implemented patient satisfaction as a cornerstone of value-based purchasing and other incentive programs for all parts of our healthcare system.[3]

Although patient satisfaction has remained an important metric, other patient-reported outcomes—particularly patient confidence, activation, and empowerment—have been developed and advanced. In preparation for these new measures, a number of researchers explored the relationship between patient satisfaction and the individual's perception of the extent of control over a chronic disease. For example, research by Larry Linn, from the late 1960s through the late 1980s, documented that "patient satisfaction measures are sensitive to and confounded by patients' perceived health, view of life and social circumstance" (Linn and Greenfield 1982, 425). During the 1990s, building on the research of Linn and others and together with the burgeoning consumer movement, Judith Hibbard and John Wasson developed patient reports of self-confidence in the management of patients' healthcare conditions (Greene et al. 2015; Wasson and Coleman 2014). A number of health systems and payers have implemented either the Wasson or Hibbard patient confidence or activation measures.[4] These patient-derived outcomes measures, particularly in the management of a chronic illness, represent a critical leg of the three-legged stool mentioned earlier in the chapter: patient activation; financial incentives; and payers' regular release of transparent, comparative outcomes data, which helps foster collaboration with payers.

Researchers studying factors related to patient confidence have documented the positive impact of shared decision making on, for instance, whether a patient decides to undergo a prostatectomy for prostate cancer (Arterburn et al. 2012). Kate Lorig developed the Stanford Chronic Disease Self-Management Program (Lorig and Holman 2003), which has been used to teach thousands of leaders and has contributed to significant improvement in chronic disease control, with attendant economic impact.[5] Nonetheless, even though the value of shared decision making is well known, payers still have not adopted a strong, consistent focus on improving consumer self-confidence.

Importantly, Medicare has begun reimbursing YMCAs throughout the country for implementation of a diabetes program that aims to increase self-confidence in the management of this extremely common disease.[6] However, payers and policymakers have barely scratched the surface of how these types of programs can improve patient self-confidence in the management of chronic illness. Instead, most health policymakers, especially at the federal level, continue to focus almost exclusively on the idea that placing a greater financial responsibility on the consumer will result in better quality—a questionable proposition that is not supported by the research literature (Hwang, Garrett, and Miller 2017). This tendency is largely the result of the increasingly politicized nature of the quality measurement and management debate.

Quality Management, Evidence-Based Medicine, and the Impact of Politics

It is commonly known among healthcare professionals that too many back surgeries are performed in cases of lumbar disc problems and that too many magnetic resonance imaging (MRI) scans are done in the early stages of diseases that often should simply be left alone (Furlan et al. 2015). In the late 1980s, the then Agency for Health Care Policy and Research (AHCPR) addressed these concerns with the release of evidence-based guidelines about the appropriate use of MRIs and the outcomes of back surgeries. However, the North American Spine Society—possibly motivated by financial incentives—disagreed with the findings (Chassin and Loeb 2011) and engaged in lobbying efforts against quality measurement and management. The society was nearly successful in eliminating funding for AHCPR. The agency survived, but it was told to change its focus and get out of the guideline business. Hence, it became the Agency for Healthcare Research and Quality (AHRQ) (Gray, Gusmano, and Collins 2003).

There is no point in having quality measures and an outstanding Deming-inspired quality management system if the evidence supporting medical interventions is not robust. Healthcare professionals and consumers alike must have a commitment to evidence-based medicine, which can be defined as the "conscientious, explicit, and judicious use of current best evidence in making decisions about the care of individual patients" (Sackett et al. 1996, 71). As stated by the National Academy of Medicine, "Evidence is the cornerstone of a high-performing health care system" (Patashnik, Gerber, and Dowling 2017, 6). The impact of technology on our healthcare system is everywhere; it is both facilitating the expansion of medical knowledge (Singer 2017) and becoming inextricably embedded into regular medical practice (Goldfield 2017).

Unsurprisingly, given our society's political polarization and the ever-increasing role of technology in medical practice, the politics of quality measurement and management have become more toxic, well beyond the aforementioned example of back surgery. Thus, we need to conclude this historical overview of quality measures and quality management with an explicit acknowledgment of the importance of politics in this area.

As highlighted in Patashnik, Gerber, and Dowling's (2017) book *Unhealthy Politics*, politicians of both major political parties, as recently as 2008, tried to argue in favor of the pursuit of evidence for both quality measurement and management. Some degree of bipartisan commitment to evidence can be seen, for instance, in the fact that both political parties acknowledge that any nuclear power plant must adhere to scientifically accepted safety standards mandated by the federal government. Along the same lines, the baseball executive Billy Beane and politicians Newt Gingrich and John Kerry (2008) wrote an article in the *New York Times* focusing on the common-sense need for greater attention to the evidence base for medicine. Reflecting what now seems like a bygone era of bipartisanship, Gingrich, a Republican, and Kerry, a Democrat, together wrote:

> Remarkably, a doctor today can get more data on the starting third baseman on his fantasy baseball team than on the effectiveness of life-and-death medical procedures . . . . Nearly 100,000 Americans are killed every year by preventable medical errors. We can do better if doctors have better access to concise, evidence-based medical information . . . . To deliver better health care, we should learn from the successful teams that have adopted baseball's new evidence-based methods.

However, as the authors of *Unhealthy Politics* point out, politicians tend to lose political clout when they fight with medical societies, device manufacturers, and hospital associations that lobby against evidence-based methods and in favor of ineffective procedures (Patashnik, Gerber, and Dowling 2017). For example, the American Medical Association, the North American Spine Society, various device manufacturers (e.g., AvaMed), and the Pharmaceutical Manufacturers Association, among many other groups, have had a long tradition of resisting efforts to research and promote the scientific basis for medical practice. As a consequence of these efforts, agencies critical to the development of valid quality measures and the best methods of quality management have lost significant funding—and, in some cases, been defunded completely (Patashnik, Gerber, and Dowling 2017).

New Outcomes Metrics and the Future of Quality Measurement and Management

The healthcare landscape has been transformed by numerous landmark events since the start of the twentieth century, and groundbreaking advances continue to take shape. Insulin and antibiotics were not in use 100 years ago, and dialysis and coronary artery bypass grafts were just beginning 50 years ago. Similarly, the SF-36 measure for patient-derived health ratings, measures of consumer empowerment, ways to identify potentially preventable readmissions, and the entire field of case mix and risk adjustments did not exist 50 years ago; many of these things did not exist even 25 years ago. The leaders mentioned in this chapter, along with many others, have made significant contributions to advance the field of quality measurement and management (Averill, Hughes, and Goldfield 2011; Texas Health and Human Services 2018).

In their joint *New York Times* article, Beane, Gingrich, and Kerry (2008) wrote that "the best way to start improving quality and lowering costs is to study the stats." However, we must also be cautious not to fetishize quality measurement. The idea that "if you can't measure it, you can't manage it" is a costly myth. Indeed, running a company on visible figures alone was one of Deming's seven deadly diseases of management (Deming 1982; Deming Institute 2018). The best way to avoid the fetishizing of statistics is for health policy leaders to loudly proclaim that quality outcomes measurement must be inextricably linked to quality management or organizational continuous quality improvement.

Several decades ago, early pioneers such as Donabedian at the University of Michigan and Shapiro at Johns Hopkins University established the underpinnings and key definitions of the quality measurement field, and later researchers have carried their work forward. Today's quality outcomes measures are increasingly scientifically valid, and alongside case mix and risk adjustment, they will get even better. Significant improvement will occur in three ways:

1. In the coming years, information abstracted from claims data will be linked easily to information from electronic medical records across the entire continuum of healthcare (McCullough et al. 2011).
2. Further advances in technology will provide us with additional information about not only individual consumers and their families (taking into account genetic predisposition to certain diseases) but also the communities in which these individuals live. Much if not all of this information will be available to consumers on a real-time basis.
3. Information will be available to predict, with increasing reliability, the potential occurrence of adverse events and risks that can be mitigated with action. Prediction science is already here for both inpatient and outpatient services, but it will get even better (Chang et al. 2011).

In the coming years, consumers, both individually and in organized groups and associations, will be able to use this increasingly precise information to generate report cards and evaluations of quality that reflect their own, not the government's or trade associations', priorities.[7] Even so, we need to recognize that quality measurement is and always will be, at least in part, an art. We are dealing with human beings as opposed to industrial assembly lines, and new challenges and complications are certain to emerge. At the start of 2018, for instance, the *New York Times* reported that senior administrators at some Veterans Affairs hospitals had been avoiding complicated, high-risk patients in an effort to raise the hospitals' quality ratings (Philipps 2018).

The quality landscape will be further shaped by three evolving trends. First, increased organizational consolidation of providers (e.g., hospital mergers, hospital acquisition of physician practices) with greater assumption of financial risk will bring a heightened focus to population health. Second, the degree to which quality measurement is politicized will determine the impact that the increasingly precise measures can have. Third, the number of Americans without health insurance coverage will influence the degree to which quality management and measurement have overall relevance to society.

Conclusion

We have addressed some of the drawbacks associated with today's political climate, in which leaders are breaking many long-held norms of decorum and behavior. However, this climate also offers a meaningful benefit: Researchers and institutional leaders in healthcare are increasingly acknowledging the need to be engaged in politics, with a small *p*, as it relates to issues of quality management and measurement. This engagement may take the form of, for example, lobbying for federal research funding.

One wild card is the potential role of consumers, their families, and the communities in which they live. Can empowered consumers (especially those newly covered under the Affordable Care Act (ACA), whether individually or in organized groups, fully exercise their big-*P* political power to encourage elected officials to improve quality in the healthcare system and begin to stabilize costs? Such activity might include, for example, fighting for or against the repeal of the ACA with direct support for political candidates. A historical analogy from a different field involves Senator Ted Kennedy and a rising movement of consumers who had become discontented with airline prices in the 1970s. Seeking to burnish his credentials with this group, Kennedy fought government regulations and was victorious over the airline industry (Patashnik, Gerber, and Dowling 2017). The deregulated airline industry is now very competitive (albeit with some challenges in quality of service).

Newly empowered consumers—along with groups of healthcare professionals and possibly a few health systems committed to population health—hold the key to a reformed healthcare system that is truly based on relentless quality management, using measures described in this chapter. As Lorig (2017, 188) stated in a slightly different context, "Patients can be true partners in care. More than forty years ago, Dr. Tom Ferguson said, 'doctors (*health professionals*) would get off their pedestals when patients got off their knees.' All of us, patients and health professionals, need to do a bit more to adjust our posture. It is not we against them. We are all in this together." Valid and reliable quality measurement, intertwined with effective quality management, will be the glue that binds us together and points the way toward a continuously improving healthcare system in the United States.

Notes

1. For more information about the founding of the Institute for Healthcare Improvement, see www.ihi.org/about/pages/history.aspx. For more information of the Cochrane Database of Systematic Reviews, see www.cochranelibrary.com/about/about-cochrane-reviews.
2. For an example, see the New York State Department of Health resource at www.health.ny.gov/professionals/doctors/conduct/.
3. See www.cms.gov/Outreach-and-Education/Medicare-Learning-Network-MLN/MLNProducts/downloads/Hospital_VBPurchasing_Fact_Sheet_ICN907664.pdf for information about the CMS Hospital Value-Based Purchasing Program.
4. See https://suffolkcare.org/pubfiles/NYDOH_PAMGuidelines_09.16.2015.pdf for information on the Patient Activation Measure used by the New York State Department of Health.
5. For more information on the Stanford program, see www.selfmanagementresource.com.
6. See www.ymca.net/diabetes-prevention/ for more information on the YMCA diabetes-prevention program.
7. The Healthcare Bluebook website at www.healthcarebluebook.com serves as one example of an initiative to support transparency and consumer empowerment.

Study Questions

1. What is the difference between patient reports and ratings of health and healthcare?
2. What tools and techniques for addressing malpractice have been implemented in the years since the Harvard Malpractice Study? Which do you agree with? What more needs to be done?
3. What do you see as the future in quality measurement? What is the role of technology? What other factors will be important?
4. What are the roles of competition and antitrust laws in the future of quality measurement? What other factors will be important?
5. How does the consumer fit in with the manifold changes taking place in our healthcare system?
6. In what ways should healthcare professionals become involved in today's polarized political environment?

References

Advisory Board. 2017. "CMS: US Health Care Spending to Reach Nearly 20% of GDP by 2025." Published February 16. www.advisory.com/daily-briefing/2017/02/16/spending-growth.

Agency for Healthcare Research and Quality (AHRQ). 2006. *The Case for the Present-on-Admission (POA) Indicator*. Healthcare Cost and Utilization Project Methods Series. Published June. www.hcup-us.ahrq.gov/reports/methods/2006_1.pdf.

American College of Surgeons (ACS). 2018a. "ACS National Surgical Quality Improvement Program." Accessed September 10. www.facs.org/quality-programs/acs-nsqip.

———. 2018b. "1918: Most Hospitals Fail to Meet Minimum Standards of College Hospital Standardization Program." Accessed September 24. http://timeline.facs.org/1913.html.

Arterburn, D., R. Wellman, E. Westbrook, C. Rutter, T. Ross, D. McCulloch, M. Handley, and C. Jung. 2012. "Introducing Decision Aids at Group Health Was Linked to Sharply Lower Hip and Knee Surgery Rates and Costs." *Health Affairs* (Millwood) 31 (9): 2094–104.

Averill, R. F., N. I. Goldfield, M. E. Wynn, T. E. McGuire, R. L. Mullin, L. W. Gregg, and J. A. Bender. 1993. "Design of a Prospective Payment Patient Classification System for Ambulatory Care." *Health Care Financing Review* 15 (1): 71–100.

Averill, R. F., J. S. Hughes, and N. I. Goldfield. 2011. "Paying for Outcomes, Not Performance: Lessons from the Medicare Inpatient Prospective Payment System." *Joint Commission Journal on Quality and Patient Safety* 37 (4): 184–92.

Beane, B., N. Gingrich, and J. Kerry. 2008. "How to Take American Health Care from Worst to First." *New York Times*. Published October 24. www.nytimes.com/2008/10/24/opinion/24beane.html.

Beecher, H. K. 1955. "The Powerful Placebo." *Journal of the American Medical Association* 159 (17): 1602–6.

Berkowitz, E. 1998. "History of Health Services Research Project: Interview with Sam Shapiro." US National Library of Medicine. Published March 6. www.nlm.nih.gov/hmd/nichsr/shapiro.html.

Best, M., and D. Neuhauser. 2006. "Walter A. Shewhart, 1924, and the Hawthorne Factory." *Quality and Safety in Health Care* 15 (2): 142–43.

Best, W. R., S. F. Khuri, M. Phelan, K. Hur, W. G. Henderson, J. G. Demakis, and J. Daley. 2002. "Identifying Patient Preoperative Risk Factors and Postoperative Adverse Events in Administrative Databases: Results from the Department of Veterans Affairs National Surgical Quality Improvement Program." *Journal of the American College of Surgeons* 194 (3): 257–66.

Brennan, T. A., L. L. Leape, N. M. Laird, L. Hebert, A. R. Localio, A. G. Lawthers, J. P. Newhouse, P. C. Weiler, and H. H. Hiatt. 1991. "Incidence of Adverse

Events and Negligence in Hospitalized Patients—Results of the Harvard Medical Practice Study I." *New England Journal of Medicine* 324: 370–76.

Brook, R. H., J. E. Ware Jr., W. H. Rogers, E. B. Keeler, A. R. Davies, C. A. Donald, G. A. Goldberg, K. N. Lohr, P. C. Masthay, and J. P. Newhouse. 1983. "Does Free Care Improve Adults' Health? Results from a Randomized Controlled Trial." *New England Journal of Medicine* 309 (23): 1426–34.

Chang, Y.-J., M.-L. Yeh, Y.-C. Li, C.-Y. Hsu, C.-C. Lin, M.-S. Hsu, and W.-T. Chiu. 2011. "Predicting Hospital-Acquired Infections by Scoring System with Simple Parameters." *PLOS One* 6 (8): e23137.

Chassin, M., and J. Loeb. 2011. "The Ongoing Quality Improvement Journey: Next Stop, High Reliability." *Health Affairs* 30 (4): 559–68.

Clarke, C. 2005. *Automotive Production Systems and Standardization: From Ford to the Case of Mercedes-Benz.* New York: Springer.

Codman, E. A. 1914. "The Product of a Hospital." *Surgery, Gynecology and Obstetrics* 18: 491–96.

Coulam, R. F., and G. L. Gaumer. 1992. "Medicare's Prospective Payment System: A Critical Appraisal." *Health Care Financing Review* 1991 (Suppl.): 45–77.

Cutting, C. C., and M. F. Collen. 1992. "A Historical Review of the Kaiser Permanente Medical Care Program." *Journal of the Society for Health Systems* 3 (4): 25–30.

Dans, P. E., J. P. Weiner, and S. E. Otter. 1985. "Peer Review Organizations: Promises and Potential Pitfalls." *New England Journal of Medicine* 313: 1131–37.

Deming, W. E. 1982. *Out of the Crisis.* Boston: MIT Press.

Deming Institute. 2018. "Seven Deadly Diseases of Management." Accessed September 11. https://deming.org/explore/seven-deadly-diseases.

Dixon, L. 2000. "Assertive Community Treatment: Twenty-Five Years of Gold." *Psychiatric Services* 51 (6): 759–65.

Donabedian, A. 1966. "Evaluating the Quality of Medical Care." *Milbank Memorial Fund Quarterly* 44 (3): 166–206.

Doyle, J. C. 1953. "Unnecessary Hysterectomies: Study of 6,248 Operations in Thirty-Five Hospitals During 1948." *Journal of the American Medical Association* 151 (5): 360–65.

Dugosh, K., A. Abraham, B. Seymour, K. McLoyd, M. Chalk, and D. Festinger. 2016. "A Systematic Review on the Use of Psychosocial Interventions in Conjunction with Medications for the Treatment of Opioid Addiction." *Journal of Addiction Medicine* 10 (2): 91–101.

Ellis, R. P., G. C. Pope, L. Iezzoni, J. Z. Ayanian, D. W. Bates, H. Burstin, and A. S. Ash. 1996. "Diagnosis-Based Risk Adjustment for Medicare Capitation Payments." *Health Care Financing Review* 17 (3): 101–28.

Falk, I. S., C. R. Rorem, and M. D. Ring. 1932. *The Costs of Medical Care: A Summary of Investigations on the Economic Aspects of the Prevention and Care of Illness.* Chicago: University of Chicago Press.

Fetter, R. B., Y. Shin, J. L. Freeman, R. F. Averill, and J. D. Thompson. 1980. "Case Mix Definition by Diagnosis-Related Groups." *Medical Care* 18 (2 Suppl.): iii, 1–53.

Fink, A., E. M. Yano, and R. H. Brook. 1989. "The Condition of the Literature on Differences in Hospital Mortality." *Medical Care* 27 (4): 315–36.

Flexner, A. 1910. *Medical Education in the United States and Canada: A Report to the Carnegie Foundation for the Advancement of Teaching.* New York: Merrymount Press.

Freeman, H. E., S. Levine, and L. G. Reeder. 1963. *Handbook of Medical Sociology.* Princeton, NJ: Prentice Hall.

Fries, B. E., and L. M. Cooney Jr. 1985. "Resource Utilization Groups: A Patient Classification System for Long Term Care." *Medical Care* 23 (2): 110–22.

Furlan, A. D., A. Malmivaara, R. Chou, C. G. Maher, R. A. Deyo, M. Schoene, G. Bronfort, and M. W. van Tulder. 2015. "2015 Updated Method Guideline for Systematic Reviews in the Cochrane Back and Neck Group." *Spine* 40 (21): 1660–73.

Gertman, P. M., and J. D. Restuccia. 1981. "The Appropriateness Evaluation Protocol: A Technique for Assessing Unnecessary Days of Hospital Care." *Medical Care* 19 (8): 855–71.

Glover, J. A. 1938. "The Incidence of Tonsillectomy in School Children." *Proceedings of the Royal Society of Medicine* 31 (10): 1219–36.

Goldfield, N. 2017. "Dramatic Changes in Health Care Professions in the Past 40 Years." *Journal of Ambulatory Care Management* 40 (3): 169–75.

Goldfield, N., and P. Boland. 1996. *Physician Profiling and Risk Adjustment.* Gaithersburg, MD: Aspen.

Goldfield, N., R. Fuller, J. Vertrees, and E. McCullough. 2016. "How Encouraging Provider Collaboration and Financial Incentives Can Improve Outcomes for Persons with Severe Psychiatric Disorders." *Psychiatric Services* 67 (12): 1368–69.

Goldfield, N. I., E. C. McCullough, J. S. Hughes, A. M. Tang, B. Eastman, L. K. Rawlins, and R. F. Averill. 2008. "Identifying Potentially Preventable Readmissions." *Health Care Financing Review* 30 (1): 75–91.

Goldfield, N., M. Pine, and J. Pine. 1996. *Measuring and Managing Health Care Quality: Procedures, Techniques, and Protocols.* Gaithersburg, MD: Aspen.

Granger, C. V., A. Deutsch, C. Russell, T. Black, and K. J. Ottenbacher. 2007. "Modifications of the FIM Instrument Under the Inpatient Rehabilitation Facility Prospective Payment System." *American Journal of Physical Medicine & Rehabilitation* 86 (11): 883–92.

Gray, B. H., M. K. Gusmano, and S. R. Collins. 2003. "AHCPR and the Changing Politics of Health Services Research." *Health Affairs* (Millwood) Suppl. W3: 283–307.

Greene, J., J. H. Hibbard, R. Sacks, V. Overton, and C. D. Parrotta. 2015. "When Patient Activation Levels Change, Health Outcomes and Costs Change, Too." *Health Affairs* (Millwood) 34 (3): 431–37.

Hannan, E. L., C. Wu, T. J. Ryan, E. Bennett, A. T. Culliford, J. P. Gold, A. Hartman, O. W. Isom, R. H. Jones, B. McNeil, E. A. Rose, and V. A. Subramanian. 2003. "Do Hospitals and Surgeons with Higher Coronary Artery Bypass Graft Surgery Volumes Still Have Lower Risk-Adjusted Mortality Rates?" *Circulation* 108 (7): 795–801.

Hayes, C. W., P. B. Batalden, and D. Goldmann. 2015. "A 'Work Smarter, Not Harder' Approach to Improving Healthcare Quality." *BMJ Quality & Safety* 24 (2): 100–102.

Hughes, J. S., R. F. Averill, N. I. Goldfield, J. C. Gay, J. Muldoon, E. McCullough, and J. Xiang. 2006. "Identifying Potentially Preventable Complications Using a Present on Admission Indicator." *Health Care Financing Review* 27 (3): 63–82.

Hwang, A., D. Garrett, and M. Miller. 2017. "Competing Visions for Consumer Engagement in the Dawn of the Trump Administration." *Journal of Ambulatory Care Management* 40 (4): 259–64.

Iezzoni, L. I. (ed.). 2012. *Risk Adjustment for Measuring Healthcare Outcomes*, 4th ed. Chicago: Health Administration Press.

Iezzoni, L. I., E. K. Hotchkin, A. S. Ash, M. Shwartz, and Y. Mackiernan. 1993. "MedisGroups Data Bases. The Impact of Data Collection Guidelines on Predicting In-Hospital Mortality." *Medical Care* 31 (3): 277–83.

Institute of Medicine. 2001. *Coverage Matters: Insurance and Health Care.* Washington, DC: National Academies Press.

Juran, J. M. 1995. *A History of Managing for Quality: The Evolution, Trends, and Future Directions of Managing for Quality.* Milwaukee, WI: Quality Press.

Kahn, K. L., D. Draper, E. B. Keeler, W. H. Rogers, L. V. Rubenstein, J. Kosecoff, M. J. Sherwood, E. J. Reinisch, M. F. Carney, C. J. Kamberg, S. S. Bentow, K. B. Wells, H. Allen, D. Reboussin, C. P. Roth, C. Chew, and R. H. Brook. 1992. *The Effects of the DRG-Based Prospective Payment System on Quality of Care for Hospitalized Medicare Patients.* RAND Corporation. Accessed September 10, 2018. www.rand.org/pubs/reports/R3931.html.

Kalra, J. J., and A. Kopargaonkar. 2018. "Quality Care and Patient Safety: Strategies to Disclose Medical Errors." In *Advances in Human Factors and Ergonomics in Healthcare and Medical Devices*, edited by V. Duffy and N. Lightner, 159–67. Cham, Switzerland: Springer International.

Kang, C. W., and P. H. Kvam. 2012. *Basic Statistical Tools for Improving Quality.* Hoboken, NJ: Wiley & Sons.

Katz, S., A. B. Ford, R. W. Moskowitz, B. A. Jackson, and M. W. Jaffe. 1963. "Studies of Illness in the Aged. The Index of ADL: A Standardized Measure of Biological and Psychosocial Function." *Journal of the American Medical Association* 185 (12): 914–19.

Keller, R. B. 1994. "Outcomes Dissemination. The Maine Study Group Model." National Institutes of Health grant. Accessed September 10, 2018. http://grantome.com/grant/NIH/R18-HS006813-04.

Kohn, L. T., J. M. Corrigan, and M. S. Donaldson (eds.). 2000. *To Err Is Human: Building a Safer Health System*. Washington, DC: National Academies Press.

Kopf, E. W. 1916. "Florence Nightingale as Statistician." *Publications of the American Statistical Association* 15 (116): 388–404.

Krumholz, H. M., A. R. Merrill, E. M. Schone, G. C. Schreiner, J. Chen, E. H. Bradley, Y. Wang, Y. Wang, Z. Lin, B. M. Straube, M. T. Rapp, S. L. Normand, and E. E. Drye. 2009. "Patterns of Hospital Performance in Acute Myocardial Infarction and Heart Failure 30-Day Mortality and Readmission." *Circulation: Cardiovascular Quality and Outcomes* 2 (5): 407–13.

Kwan, L. Y., K. Stratton, and D. M. Steinwachs (eds.). 2017. *Accounting for Social Risk Factors in Medicare Payment*. Washington, DC: National Academies Press.

Lehman, A. F., R. Goldberg, L. B. Dixon, S. McNary, L. Postrado, A. Hackman, and K. McDonnell. 2002. "Improving Employment Outcomes for Persons with Severe Mental Illnesses." *Archives of General Psychiatry* 59 (2): 165–72.

Lehman, A. F., J. Kreyenbuhl, R. W. Buchanan, F. B. Dickerson, L. B. Dixon, R. Goldberg, L. D. Green-Paden, W. N. Tenhula, D. Boerescu, C. Tek, N. Sandson, and D. M. Steinwachs. 2004. "The Schizophrenia Patient Outcomes Research Team (PORT): Updated Treatment Recommendations 2003." *Schizophrenia Bulletin* 30 (2): 193–217.

Lembcke, P. A. 1956. "Medical Audit by Scientific Methods: Illustrated by Major Female Pelvic Surgery." *Journal of the American Medical Association* 162 (7): 646–55.

Lepelley, M., C. Genty, A. Lecoanet, B. Allenet, P. Bedouch, M. R. Mallaret, P. Gillois, and J. L. Bosson. 2018. "Electronic Medication Regimen Complexity Index at Admission and Complications During Hospitalization in Medical Wards: A Tool to Improve Quality of Care?" *International Journal for Quality in Health Care* 30 (1): 32–38.

Lewis, V. A., E. S. Fisher, and C. H. Colla. 2017. "Explaining Sluggish Savings Under Accountable Care." *New England Journal of Medicine* 377 (19): 1809–11.

Linn, L. S., and S. Greenfield. 1982. "Patient Suffering and Patient Satisfaction Among the Chronically Ill." *Medical Care* 20 (4): 425–31.

Lorig, K. 2017. "Commentary on 'Evidence-Based Self-Management Programs for Seniors and Other with Chronic Diseases': Patient Experience—Patient Health—Return on Investment." *Journal of Ambulatory Care Management* 40 (3): 185–88.

Lorig, K. R., and H. Holman. 2003. "Self-Management Education: History, Definition, Outcomes, and Mechanisms." *Annals of Behavioral Medicine* 26 (1): 1–7.

Mallon, B. 2014. "Amory Codman: The End Result of a Dream to Revolutionize Medicine." Boston Shoulder Institute. Accessed September 10, 2018. http://bostonshoulderinstitute.com/wp-content/uploads/2014/07/Codman-Society-Bio.pdf.

McCullough, E., C. Sullivan, P. Banning, N. Goldfield, and J. Hughes. 2011. "Challenges and Benefits of Adding Laboratory Data to a Mortality Risk Adjustment Method." *Quality Management in Health Care* 20 (4): 253–62.

McDonald, L. 2014. "Florence Nightingale and Her Crimean War Statistics: Lessons for Hospital Safety, Public Administration and Nursing." Lecture for the Gresham College / British Society of the History of Mathematics Conference, October 2014. www.gresham.ac.uk/lectures-and-events/florence-nightingale-and-her-crimean-war-statistics-lessons-for-hospital-safety-.

McGuire, T. E. 1991. "An Evaluation of Diagnosis-Related Group Severity and Complexity Refinement." *Health Care Financing Review* 12 (4): 49–60.

McKenzie, E., M. L. Potestio, J. M. Boyd, D. J. Niven, R. Brundin-Mather, S. M. Bagshaw, and H. T. Stelfox. 2017. "Reconciling Patient and Provider Priorities for Improving the Care of Critically Ill Patients: A Consensus Method and Qualitative Analysis of Decision Making." *Health Expectations* 20 (6): 1367–74.

Medicare.gov. 2018. "Depression Screenings." Accessed September 10. www.medicare.gov/coverage/depression-screenings.html.

Mills, P. D., B. V. Watts, B. Shiner, and R. R. Hemphill. 2018. "Adverse Events Occurring on Mental Health Units." *General Hospital Psychiatry* 50: 63–68.

Mills, R., R. B. Fetter, D. C. Riedel, and R. Averill. 1976. "AUTOGRP: An Interactive Computer System for the Analysis of Health Care Data." *Medical Care* 14 (7): 603–15.

Nelson, E. C., P. B. Batalden, K. Homa, M. M. Godfrey, C. Campbell, L. A. Headrick, T. P. Huber, J. J. Mohr, and J. H. Wasson. 2003. "Microsystems in Health Care: Part 2. Creating a Rich Information Environment." *Joint Commission Journal on Quality and Safety* 29 (1): 5–15.

New York State Department of Health. 2018. "Cardiovascular Disease Data and Statistics." Accessed September 10. www.health.ny.gov/statistics/diseases/cardiovascular/.

Patashnik, E. M., A. S. Gerber, and C. M. Dowling. 2017. *Unhealthy Politics: The Battle over Evidence-Based Medicine.* Princeton, NJ: Princeton University Press.

Philipps, D. 2018. "At Veterans Hospital in Oregon, a Push for Better Ratings Puts Patients at Risk, Doctors Say." *New York Times.* Published January 1. www.nytimes.com/2018/01/01/us/at-veterans-hospital-in-oregon-a-push-for-better-ratings-puts-patients-at-risk-doctors-say.html.

RAND Corporation. 2018. "Mental Health Inventory Survey." Accessed September 12. www.rand.org/health/surveys_tools/mos/mental-health.html.

Roberts, J. S., J. G. Coale, and R. R. Redman. 1987. "A History of the Joint Commission on Accreditation of Hospitals." *JAMA* 258 (7): 936–40.

Romano, P. S., B. K. Chan, M. E. Schembri, and J. A. Rainwater. 2002. "Can Administrative Data Be Used to Compare Postoperative Complication Rates Across Hospitals?" *Medical Care* 40 (10): 856–67.

Rosenfeld, L. 1957. "Quality of Medical Care in Hospitals." *American Journal of Public Health* 47: 405–14.

Russell, L. B. 1989. *Medicare's New Hospital Payment System: Is It Working?* Washington, DC: Brookings Institution Press.

Russell, L. B., and C. L. Manning. 1989. "The Effect of Prospective Payment on Medicare Expenditures." *New England Journal of Medicine* 320: 439–44.

Sackett, D. L., W. M. C. Rosenberg, J. A. M. Gray, R. B. Haynes, and W. S. Richardson. 1996. "Evidence-Based Medicine: What It Is and What It Isn't." *British Journal of Medicine* 312: 71–72.

Sage, W. M., M. C. Harding, and E. J. Thomas. 2016. "Resolving Malpractice Claims After Tort Reform: Experience in a Self-Insured Texas Public Academic Health System." *Health Services Research* 51 (Suppl. 3): 2615–33.

Schiff, G. D., and N. I. Goldfield. 1994. "Deming Meets Braverman: Toward a Progressive Analysis of the Continuous Quality Improvement Paradigm." *International Journal of Health Services* 24 (4): 655–73.

Schweiker, R. S. 1982. "Report to Congress: Hospital Prospective Payment for Medicare." US Department of Health and Human Services. Published December. https://archive.org/details/reporttocongress00schw.

Sheps, M. C. 1955. "Approaches to the Quality of Medical Care." *Public Health Reports* 70 (9): 877–86.

Singer, N. 2017. "How Big Tech Is Going After Your Health Care." *New York Times*. Published December 26. www.nytimes.com/2017/12/26/technology/big-tech-health-care.html.

Skinner, J. S., and K. G. Volpp. 2017. "Replacing the Affordable Care Act: Lessons from Behavioral Economics." *JAMA* 317 (19): 1951–52.

Smith, G. R., T. L. Kramer, J. A. Hollenberg, C. L. Mosley, R. L. Ross, and A. Burnam. 2002. "Validity of the Depression-Arkansas (D-ARK) Scale: A Tool for Measuring Major Depressive Disorder." *Mental Health Services Research* 4 (3): 167–73.

Sohn, D. H., and B. S. Bal. 2012. "Medical Malpractice Reform: The Role of Alternative Dispute Resolution." *Clinical Orthopaedics and Related Research* 470 (5): 1370–78.

Solon, J. A., C. G. Sheps, and S. S. Lee. 1960. "Delineating Patterns of Medical Care." *American Journal of Public Health* 50 (8): 1105–13.

Tarlov, A. R., J. E. Ware Jr., S. Greenfield, E. C. Nelson, E. Perrin, and M. Zubkoff. 1989. "The Medical Outcomes Study: An Application of Methods for Monitoring the Results of Medical Care." *JAMA* 262 (7): 925–30.

Texas Health and Human Services. 2018. "Pay-for-Quality (P4Q) Program." Accessed October 12. https://hhs.texas.gov/about-hhs/process-improvement/medicaid-chip-quality-efficiency-improvement/pay-quality-p4q-program.

Thompson, J. D., R. F. Averill, and R. B. Fetter. 1979. "Planning, Budgeting, and Controlling—One Look at the Future: Case-Mix Cost Accounting." *Health Services Research* 14 (2): 111–25.

Ware, J. E. Jr., and C. D. Sherbourne. 1992. "The MOS 36-Item Short-Form Health Survey (SF-36): I. Conceptual Framework and Item Selection." *Medical Care* 30 (6): 473–83.

Wasson, J. 2017. "A Troubled Asset Relief Program for the Patient-Centered Medical Home." *Journal of Ambulatory Care Management* 40 (2): 89–100.

Wasson, J., and E. A. Coleman. 2014. "Health Confidence: An Essential Measure for Patient Engagement and Better Practice." *Family Practice Management* 21 (5): 8–12.

Wennberg, J. E., J. L. Freeman, R. M. Shelton, and T. A. Bubolz. 1989. "Hospital Use and Mortality Among Medicare Beneficiaries in Boston and New Haven." *New England Journal of Medicine* 321 (17): 1168–73.

Wennberg, J., and A. Gittelsohn. 1973. "Small Area Variations in Health Care Delivery." *Science* 182 (4117): 1102–8.

White, K. L., T. F. Williams, and B. G. Greenberg. 1961. "The Ecology of Medical Care." *New England Journal of Medicine* 265: 885–92.

Wright, J. R. Jr. 2017. "The American College of Surgeons, Minimum Standards for Hospitals, and the Provision of High-Quality Laboratory Services." *Archives of Pathology & Laboratory Medicine* 141 (5): 704–17.

Zaslavsky, A. M., L. B. Zaborski, L. Ding, J. A. Shaul, M. J. Cioffi, and P. D. Cleary. 2001. "Adjusting Performance Measures to Ensure Equitable Plan Comparisons." *Health Care Financing Review* 22 (3): 109–126.

Zhan, C., A. Elixhauser, C. L. Richards Jr., Y. Wang, W. B. Baine, M. Pineau, N. Verzier, R. Kliman, and D. Hunt. 2009. "Identification of Hospital-Acquired Catheter-Associated Urinary Tract Infections from Medicare Claims: Sensitivity and Positive Predictive Value." *Medical Care* 47 (3): 364–69.

CHAPTER

3

VARIATION IN MEDICAL PRACTICE AND IMPLICATIONS FOR QUALITY

David J. Ballard, Briget da Graca, David Nicewander, and Brett D. Stauffer

Medical practice remains empirical and is subject to considerable differences in process and outcome (Reinertsen 2003). For example, with regard to childbirth, the most common cause of hospitalization in the United States, the process measure of cesarean rates varies tenfold across hospitals and fifteenfold among women with low-risk pregnancies, after controlling for differences in patient risk (Kozhimannil, Law, and Virnig 2013). Looking at outcomes, rates of major obstetrical complications vary by 12 percentage points for vaginal deliveries and by 17 percentage points for cesarean deliveries (Glance et al. 2014). Similar variation can be seen from the population health perspective—a viewpoint of increasing importance as healthcare moves toward value-based structures that hold providers accountable for the health of the populations they serve. A 2016 Dartmouth Atlas Project report showed, for example, that the average number of healthcare system contact days in a year ranged from 10.2 for Medicare beneficiaries in Lebanon, New Hampshire, to 24.9 for those in East Long Island, New York (Bynum et al. 2016).

It is tempting to conclude that such variation indicates inconsistencies in the quality of care provided to different populations of patients. However, such a conclusion presumes that variation is undesirable and results largely from some providers following "best practices" and others not. More in-depth examination of clinical variation, however, suggests that the situation is far more complex, with multiple contributing influences and outcomes.

This chapter discusses the application of studies of variation in medical processes and outcomes to healthcare quality research and improvement, as well as to the developing field of population health. Exhibit 3.1 describes the types of variation relevant to healthcare quality.

Variation in Medical Practice

Variation in medical practice has excited interest since 1938, when Dr. J. Allison Glover's classic study on the incidence of tonsillectomy in schoolchildren in

EXHIBIT 3.1 Terminology of Variation in Medical Practice

Type of Variation	Definition and Relevance to Healthcare Quality Research/Improvement
Random variation	• Also called "common-cause variation" • An attribute of the event or process that adheres to the laws of probability and cannot be traced to a root cause • Generally considered "background noise"; seldom provides useful insight regarding quality of care
Assignable variation	• Also called "special-cause variation" • Arises from a single or small set of causes that can be traced and identified and then addressed or eliminated
Process variation	• Different usage of a therapeutic or diagnostic procedure in an organization, a geographic area, or another grouping of healthcare providers • Includes both use vs. nonuse of a procedure (e.g., screening for colorectal cancer vs. no screening) and differences in rates among multiple approaches that achieve approximately the same end (e.g., guaiac-based fecal occult blood testing, fecal immunochemical test, sigmoidoscopy, or colonoscopy for colorectal cancer screening)
Outcome variation	• Occurs when different results follow from a single process • Frequently the focus of healthcare quality research/improvement projects that seek to identify the process that yields optimal results • Requires rigorous adjustment for patient characteristics that affect outcomes • Faces a practical barrier in that outcome studies often require years or decades of follow-up, making it difficult to determine in real time whether the process being applied is, in fact, yielding optimal results
Performance variation	• The difference between any given result and the optimal result • Highly relevant to healthcare quality research/improvement: "the variation that is the greatest cause for concern is that between actual practice and evidence-based 'best practice'" (Steinberg 2003, 2681) • Faces a practical barrier in that it is only applicable where a best practice has been identified; one of the recurring themes in the discussion of variation in medical practice is the role of uncertainty, including uncertainty about what the best practice is in a given situation

England and Wales uncovered geographic variation that defied any explanation other than differences in medical opinion on the indications for surgery (Glover 1938). Subsequent studies have revealed similar variation internationally and across a variety of medical conditions and procedures (Katz et al. 1996; Lu-Yao and Greenberg 1994; McPherson et al. 1982; Rayner 2011; Sejr et al. 1991; Wennberg et al. 1996).

The degree of variation in utilization of a particular procedure relates more to the characteristics of that procedure than to the healthcare system in which it is performed. Similar degrees of practice variation are found in countries with different absolute rates of use (Wennberg, Barnes, and Zubkoff 1982; Westert et al. 2004) and variability in supply of healthcare services (e.g., the United States, where supply varies widely, and the Netherlands, where until recently the healthcare system was centrally planned and controlled to ensure consistency) (Westert and Faber 2011), as well as across diverse systems of healthcare organization and financing (e.g., health maintenance organizations, fee-for-service, national universal healthcare systems) (Wennberg, Barnes, and Zubkoff 1982).

Important procedural characteristics include the degree of professional uncertainty about the diagnosis and treatment of the condition the procedure addresses, the availability of alternative treatments, and controversy versus consensus regarding the appropriate use of the procedure. Differences among physicians in diagnosis style and in belief in the efficacy of a treatment contribute substantially to variation (McPherson et al. 1982).

The objective for healthcare quality researchers is not simply to identify variation but to determine its value. If variation reflects a suboptimal process, the task is to identify how the variation can be reduced or eliminated. If the variation is desirable, researchers need to understand how it can be applied across a system to improve quality broadly.

An important distinction to make when considering variation in medical practice is thus the difference between *warranted variation*, which is based on differences in patient preferences, disease prevalence, or other patient-related factors, and *unwarranted variation*, which cannot be explained by patient preference or condition or evidence-based medicine (Gauld et al. 2011). Although the former is a necessary part of providing appropriate and personalized care, the latter is typically a quality concern (Gauld et al. 2011). The effects of unwarranted variation include inefficient care (underutilization of effective procedures or overutilization of procedures with limited or no benefit) and its cost implications, as well as disparities in care between geographic regions or healthcare providers (Gauld et al. 2011).

John Wennberg, a leading scholar in the area of unwarranted clinical practice variation and founding editor of the *Dartmouth Atlas of Health Care*, identified three categories of care and the implications of unwarranted variation within each:

1. *Effective care* is care for which evidence has established that benefits outweigh risks and the "right rate" of use is 100 percent of the patients determined by evidence-based guidelines to need such care. In this category, variation in the rate of use within that population indicates areas of underuse (Smith 2011; Wennberg 2011).
2. *Preference-sensitive care* covers areas in which more than one generally accepted treatment is available, so the "right rate" depends on patient preferences (Smith 2011; Wennberg 2011). A challenge posed by this type of care is the uncertainty of whether patient preferences can be accurately measured—and if they can, whether measurement methods are so resource intensive that inclusion of patient preference is impracticable in large population-based studies (Mercuri and Gafni 2011). Nonetheless, active engagement of patients in decision making can help align rates of use with patient preferences (Greer et al. 2002; O'Connor, Llewellyn-Thomas, and Flood 2004; Wennberg 2011; Arterburn et al. 2012).
3. *Supply-sensitive care* is care for which frequency of use relates to the capacity of the local healthcare system. Studies have repeatedly shown that regions with high use of supply-sensitive care do not perform better on mortality or quality-of-life indicators than regions with low use, so variation in supply-sensitive services can provide evidence of overuse (Smith 2011; Wennberg 2011). Healthcare quality research in this context seeks (1) to acquire the evidence (through comparative effectiveness research) necessary to move procedures in the supply-sensitive care category to either the effective or preference-sensitive care category and (2) to adopt a pattern of use that achieves the best value (Ham 2011; O'Connor et al. 2009).

Effective care and preference-sensitive care are estimated to account for 15 percent and 25 percent, respectively, of healthcare services; the remaining 60 percent are supply sensitive (Smith 2011). The predominance of supply-sensitive care means that achieving meaningful improvements in the overall quality and value of healthcare will require more than just effective implementation of clinical decision-support tools and shared-decision-making tools, which target services in the effective and preference-sensitive categories. Instead, broader structural and policy-based changes are needed to create organized systems of care in which healthcare resources are matched to community need and in which undisciplined growth in capacity and spending is restrained (Smith 2011).

Sources of Unwarranted Variation in Medical Practice

Unwarranted variation in medical practice has been studied from the perspective of multiple frameworks, which have identified diverse underlying factors. These include

- inadequate patient involvement in decision making (Wennberg 2011);
- inequitable access to resources (Sepucha, Ozanne, and Mulley 2006);
- poor communication, role confusion, and misinterpretation or misapplication of relevant clinical evidence (Sepucha, Ozanne, and Mulley 2006);
- clinician uncertainty in defining disease, making a diagnosis, selecting a procedure, observing outcomes, assessing probabilities, and assigning preferences (Eddy 1984); and
- physicians' economic incentives (Davis et al. 2000).

Frameworks focusing on economic incentives—in which physicians are viewed as potentially taking advantage of their dual role as seller of a service and agent for the buyer (patient) to influence demand for a service (Davis et al. 2000; Wennberg, Barnes, and Zubkoff 1982)—emphasize marginal/deviant physician behavior as the key regulatory focus in addressing quality-of-care deficits, and they have strongly influenced public policy in the past. Such frameworks have, however, been criticized for underestimating the market implications of uncertainty in diagnosing and treating disease (Wennberg, Barnes, and Zubkoff 1982).

An alternative point of view is that the variation in demand among communities for specific procedures is better characterized as the result of different belief sets held by individual physicians (Wennberg, Barnes, and Zubkoff 1982). Factors influencing these belief sets—and thus potential sources of variation—are both endogenous (e.g., education, ability) and exogenous (e.g., reimbursement structures, organizational policies, patients' economic constraints) (Long 2002). The exogenous forces have the ability to overcome the endogenous to produce conformity with local practice (Long 2002). From this viewpoint, physicians demand resources consistent with their assessment of patients' clinical needs but modified by local exogenous influences, including patient–agency constraints (e.g., patients' financial resources and access to care), organizational constraints (e.g., policies, protocols), and environmental constraints (e.g., surgeons, hospital beds, or other resources per capita) (Long 2002). Physicians might choose to practice in a particular area or organization because it "suits" their practice style, or they might adapt to the style of the community where they settle. Physicians might also adapt their practices to local patient expectations and demands or to local market forces to maintain their income (e.g., shortening patient follow-up intervals when practicing in an area with a large number of physicians per capita, to keep a full schedule) (Sirovich et al. 2008).

Exogenous forces likewise exert influence at the organizational level, which then has an impact on individual physicians. For example, hospitals or medical group practices in high-spending, high-healthcare-density areas might be subject to greater competitive stresses and thus encourage the ordering of profitable services, whereas lesser availability of such services in low-density, low-spending areas could lead hospitals or group practices to dissuade physicians from ordering them (Sirovich et al. 2008). Certainly, although physicians are equally likely to recommend guideline-supported interventions across spending areas, those in high-spending areas see patients more frequently, recommend more tests of uncertain benefit, and opt for more resource-intensive interventions without achieving improved patient outcomes (Fisher et al. 2003; Sirovich et al. 2008).

Applying Evidence of Unwarranted Variation to Quality Improvement

Practice variation studies typically compare utilization rates in a given setting or by a given provider to an average utilization rate (Parente, Phelps, and O'Connor 2008). Policymakers and managers can use these data-driven studies to pinpoint areas of care in which best practices may need to be identified or implemented (Parente, Phelps, and O'Connor 2008). For example, exhibit 3.2 shows variation in 30-day risk-standardized mortality rates among heart failure admissions for hospitals within Dallas County, Texas. The rates range from less than 10.0 percent to almost 15.0 percent, and hospitals 2 and 3 show

EXHIBIT 3.2A Forest Plot Showing Variation in 30-Day Risk-Standardized Heart Failure Mortality in Medicare Patients for Hospitals in Dallas County (July 2013–June 2016)

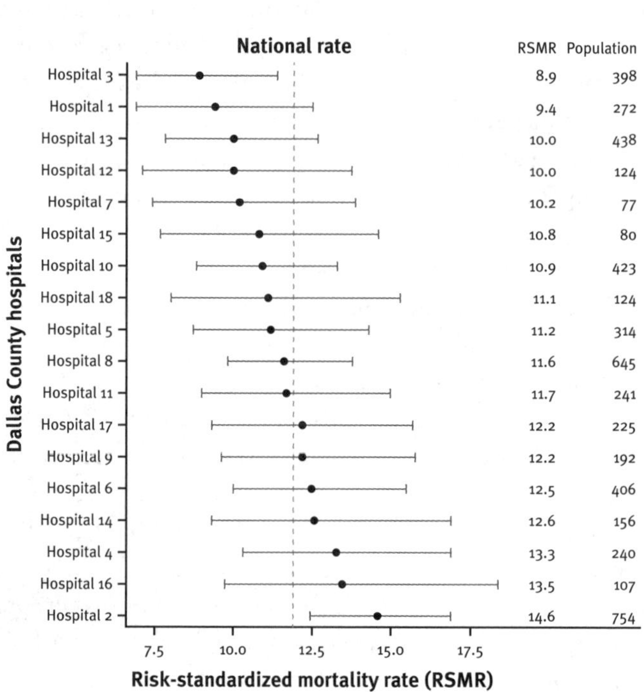

Note: Hospitals were assigned random number identifiers, in place of using names.

Source: Data from the Centers for Medicare & Medicaid Services "Hospital Compare" database.

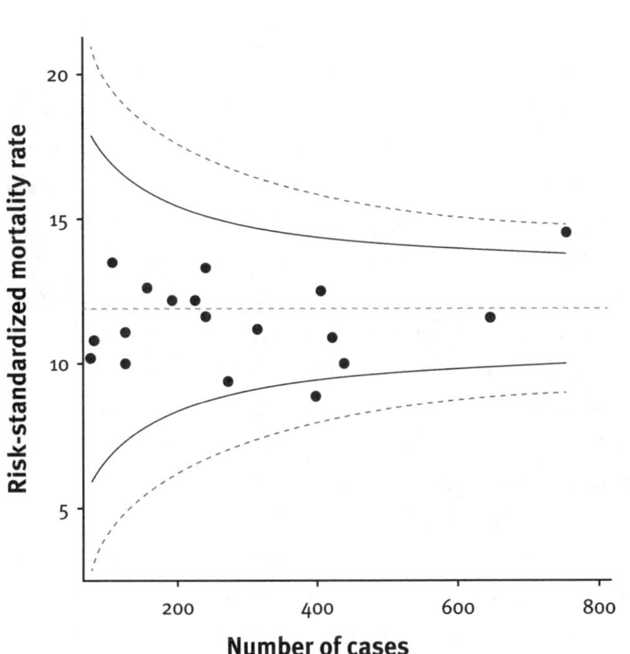

EXHIBIT 3.2B Funnel Plot Showing Variation in 30-Day Risk-Standardized Heart Failure Mortality in Medicare Patients for Hospitals in Dallas County (July 2013–June 2016)

Note: A normal approximation was applied to estimate the confidence intervals.
Source: Data from the Centers for Medicare & Medicaid Services "Hospital Compare" database.

mortality rates significantly different from the national average. The study of this variation can help poorer-performing hospitals—even those whose rates did not fall significantly below the national average—to improve, perhaps by cooperating with better-performing hospitals to investigate differences in practices and resources and developing improvement initiatives.

Where best practices have been identified (i.e., effective care), a common approach for decreasing unwarranted variation is the development of clinical guidelines (Timmermans and Mauck 2005). However, the availability of clinical guidelines is often insufficient to align practice with evidence-based standards (Kennedy, Leathley, and Hughes 2010; Timmermans and Mauck 2005). Moreover, the "evidence-based bandwagon" has become so popular, and so many competing guidelines have been produced, that the benefits of consistency can disappear under the confusion of overlapping, poorly constructed practice standards (Timmermans and Mauck 2005).

Other strategies to reduce unwarranted variation in effective care include benchmarking and report cards (Gauld et al. 2011). Such tools seek to create incentives for high performance—either through competition or by tying providers' compensation to performance.

Where unwarranted variation is identified in preference-sensitive care, improvement calls for comparative effectiveness research to elucidate differences between available treatment options, thereby enabling selection of the option that best addresses the patient's concerns and priorities. This research needs to be complemented by increased involvement of patients in treatment choices (Ham 2011). Much past research related to unwarranted variation has focused on provider behavior, treating patients as inert. However, quality improvement strategies aiming to address unwarranted variation in hospitals increasingly include initiatives to enhance patient engagement and education (Gauld et al. 2011; Greer et al. 2002), and research continues to pursue the development and implementation of effective shared decision-making aids (Savelberg et al. 2017; Hsu et al. 2017; Johnson et al. 2016). Ironically, although informed patient involvement can decrease unwarranted variation in preference-sensitive care (bringing utilization into line with patient preferences), it might increase total variation, because the preferences of patients, with their varied backgrounds and contexts, might be more diverse than those of their more educationally homogenous physicians (Greer et al. 2002).

With respect to unwarranted variation in supply-sensitive care, quality improvement strategies need to target the elimination of overuse. Such efforts must be supported by evidence from outcomes research that demonstrates equivalent patient outcomes (e.g., mortality, morbidity, quality of life) between areas of high and low use. Furthermore, to ensure that efforts to eliminate overuse do not drive practice into underuse, effectiveness or comparative effectiveness research is necessary to better understand the population that benefits from the care in question and the patient preferences that need to be considered in defining those benefits.

Analyzing Variation

The Challenge of Attribution

Historically, efforts to apply evidence of variation in healthcare to quality improvement, like healthcare quality measurement, have focused on the provider. However, the advent of accountable care organizations (ACOs) and the accompanying emphases on population health, coordination across the continuum of care, and availability of comprehensive and centralized data, have broadened the scope both for studying variation and for applying the findings to quality improvement efforts. These developments also, however, add their own complexities, particularly around the attribution to providers of patients whose need for, receipt of, or outcomes from care are being measured.

Ensuring that patients are attributed to the correct providers—and to the correct level/type of provider (e.g., individual physician vs. physician group or employing hospital)—is critical both for accurately assessing variation and for targeting any need for improvement that is identified. The complexity of this issue is highlighted by a 2010 study that used aggregated data from the four major commercial health plans in Massachusetts (covering more than one million enrollees) to assign physicians to categories of "low cost," "average cost," "high cost," or "low sample size." The study demonstrated that, compared to the retrospective attribution rule most commonly used by the health plans, 11 alternative rules—differing on (1) unit of analysis (patient vs. episode of care), (2) signal for responsibility (cost vs. number of visits), (3) number of physicians to whom a patient could be assigned (one vs. multiple), and (4) threshold for responsibility (majority vs. plurality of costs or visits)—assigned between 17 percent and 61 percent of physicians to a different performance category (Mehrotra et al. 2010). Similar effects of attribution rules have been demonstrated in the Medicare population (Pham et al. 2007).

These studies raise questions about the effectiveness of pay-for-performance and other incentive programs that assume a single provider to whom a patient is attributed can determine the quality of care received, when in fact most patients have patterns of care dispersed across multiple providers (Pham et al. 2007). Careful thought needs to go into the design of any retrospective attribution rule to ensure that the resulting performance measurement holds the relevant provider(s) accountable. It is conceivable that different attribution rules will need to be applied to different measures contributing to the overall evaluation of the quality of care provided to a single population.

Tools for Analyzing Variation Data

Multiple tools are available for analyzing variation, and care must be taken in selecting the appropriate one and in interpreting the results. For example, league tables (and their graphical equivalent, caterpillar charts) are often used to put providers in order from the lowest to highest performers on a chosen measure, using confidence intervals to identify providers with performance that is statistically significantly different from the overall average. League tables are frequently misinterpreted, however, because readers' instinct is to focus on the numeric ordering and assume, for example, that a provider ranked in the seventy-fifth percentile provides much higher-quality care than one in the twenty-fifth percentile. In reality, league tables fail to capture the uncertainty around each provider's point estimate, so much of the ordering reflects random variation. In some instances, providers who are widely separated in rank might have little or no significant difference (Woodall, Adams, and Benneyan 2012).

Forest plots, such as the one shown in exhibit 3.2A, provide a better, although still imperfect, performance comparison. Forests plots show both the point estimate for the measure of interest (e.g., risk-standardized heart failure 30-day mortality) and its confidence interval (represented by a horizontal line) for each provider, as well as a preselected standard (e.g., national average, represented by a vertical line) (van Dishoeck et al. 2011). By looking for providers for whom the *entire* confidence interval falls either to the left or to the right of the vertical line, readers can identify those with performance significantly better or worse than the selected standard.

Funnel plots are an even better approach for presenting comparative performance data, though they require greater statistical sophistication to produce (Spiegelhalter 2005). In a funnel plot, the measure of interest is plotted on the *y* axis, and the number of patients treated is on the *x* axis. The confidence interval bands on the plot are wide close to the origin (where numbers of patients are small) and narrow as the numbers of patients increase, creating the eponymous funnel shape. Providers with performance falling outside the confidence interval bands are outliers, with performance statistically significantly better or worse than the overall average. Because the funnel plot does not rank providers (beyond identifying the outliers), it is less open to misinterpretation by readers who fail to consider the influence of random variation. It also provides clear allowance for additional variability in institutions with small volume (Spiegelhalter 2005).

Exhibit 3.2B shows the funnel plot examining variation in 30-day risk-standardized heart failure mortality rates for the same Dallas County hospitals shown in the forest plot in exhibit 3.2A. As in the forest plot, one hospital has significantly higher mortality and one has significantly lower mortality than the national average when the 95 percent confidence interval limits are considered. At these limits, the hospital with the significantly higher mortality rate would need to be "on alert" to a quality problem; if any of the hospitals' data points fell above the upper 99.8 percent confidence interval limit, it would be considered an "alarm" pointing to a problem that requires urgent attention.

Statistical process control (SPC), an approach adopted from industrial manufacturing, appeals widely for healthcare improvement because it combines statistical significance tests with graphical analysis of summary data as the data are produced (Woodall, Adams, and Benneyan 2012). In this way, SPC can provide the time sensitivity so important to pragmatic improvement. Moreover, its methods and results—most often control charts, which plot measured points together with upper and lower reference thresholds (calculated using historical data) that define the range of the random variation—can usually be easily understood and applied by nonstatistician decision makers, making it a powerful tool for communicating with patients, other clinicians, administrative leaders, and policymakers. SPC does, however, have some important limitations (Thor et al. 2007):

- Statistical control does not necessarily equate to clinical control or desired performance.
- Patient risk factors must be adjusted for rigorously when healthcare outcomes are being examined.

- It is not well suited to analyzing rare events.
- It cannot typically identify the *cause* of any significant change it detects.

One complication in SPC is that different types of data require the use of different types of control charts; another is that different contexts require application of different rules to separate assignable variation from random variation. Exhibit 3.3 maps the most common data types and the assumed underlying statistical distributions to the appropriate control charts. The primary test for assignable variation is a data point that falls outside the upper or lower control limit.

The distance between the control limits on an SPC chart is set to balance the risk of falsely identifying assignable variation where it does not exist against the risk of missing it where it does. Typically, this distance is set at three standard deviations above and below the estimated mean of the measure of interest—a range expected to capture 99.73 percent of all plotted data. This wide net for the plotted points is necessary because the risk of a false positive applies to *each* plotted point, accumulating across the chart. Thus, in a control chart with 25 plotted points, the cumulative risk of a false positive is $1 - (0.9973)^{25} = 6.5$ percent when control limits of three standard deviations are used, compared to $1 - (0.95)^{25} = 72.3$ percent, for two standard deviations (Benneyan, Lloyd, and Plsek 2003).

Other patterns regarded as indications that a process is "out of control" or subject to assignable variation include the following (Benneyan, Lloyd, and Plsek 2003):

- Two out of three successive points more than two standard deviations from the mean on the same side of the center line
- Four out of five successive points more than one standard deviation from the mean on the same side of the center line
- Six successive points increasing or decreasing
- Obviously cyclical behavior

Ultimately, the quality of the information that can be obtained from any of the tools for analyzing variation depends on the quality of the data collection (including sampling and risk adjustment) and correct application of the methods. The data used for any quality assessment must be representative. Clinicians and administrators will be reluctant to accept results as valid or as indications to take action if they consider them to be based on data suffering from selection bias, collection errors, or other inaccuracies.

Unfortunately, both data collection and data analysis are frequently challenging in healthcare. For example, despite the impartiality of external record abstractors in gathering data from patient medical charts, critics may claim

EXHIBIT 3.3 Appropriate Control Charts According to Data Type and Distribution

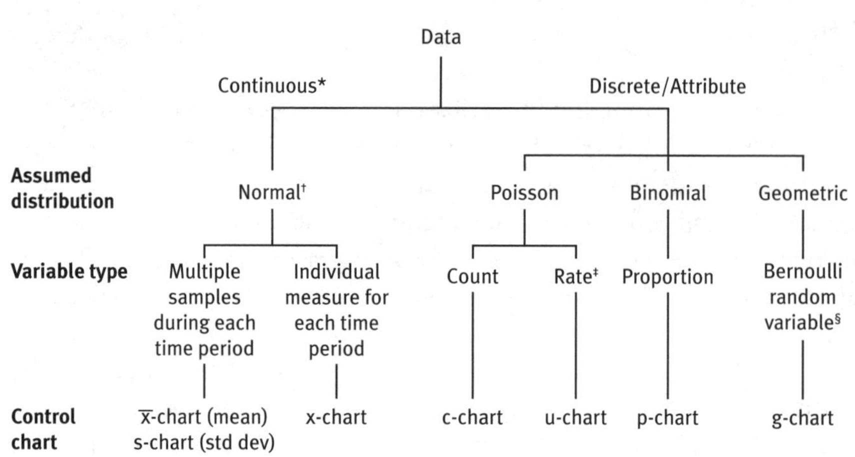

* Continuous data should not be collected as, or converted into, discrete/attribute data (e.g., categories, or a count of how frequently a particular standard was met); this causes unnecessary loss of information, which in turn causes loss of ability to detect important changes.

† For skewed continuous data (e.g., lognormal or exponential distribution) $\bar{x}$- and x-charts may not perform well, particularly if the sample taken at each time point is small. Calculate the limits from the appropriate distribution or, if appropriate, apply a normalizing transformation that will allow use of an $\bar{x}$- or x-chart.

‡ Rates are generally more informative than counts, particularly when the opportunity for the event varies over time (e.g., number of central line infections per 1,000 device-use days is more informative than just the number of central line infections).

§ The outcome of interest is known for each individual patient (e.g., whether each surgery patient developed a surgical site infection), so that each case can be considered a binomial variable with a sample size of 1. The g-chart assumes an underlying geometric distribution and would plot the total number of surgery patients until an infection occurs.

Source: Data from Woodall, Adams, and Benneyan (2012).

that these independent abstractors lack an insider's understanding or that they select data to fit an agenda, affecting the results unpredictably. Furthermore, healthcare outcomes are influenced by a wide range of demographic, clinical, societal, and environmental factors, which must be adjusted for to enable assignable variation to be identified—or, alternatively, must be investigated as potential causes of assignable variation. Similarly, when process measures are considered, the population in which delivery of that healthcare process is being measured must be accurately defined to ensure that it captures patients who will benefit while excluding patients who will not.

Additionally, many important healthcare measures violate assumptions on which analytic tools depend and therefore require special treatment. For example, autocorrelation—which violates the control chart's assumption that all data collected over time are independent—is a characteristic of many healthcare quality measures, which are frequently taken for the same patient or the same provider over time. Positive autocorrelation (in which large values tend to follow large values, and small values follow small values) causes some types of control charts (e.g., x-charts with limits based on moving ranges) to have high false positive rates for assignable variation. In these cases, more advanced statistical methods need to be applied, such as developing a time series model to predict values one step ahead of each measurement, allowing one-step-ahead forecast errors (or residuals) to be calculated from observed values and plotted on a control chart.

Using Variation Data to Drive Healthcare Quality Initiatives

A variety of indicators—including fiscal, service, and clinical indicators—are needed to capture the six domains of healthcare quality as defined by the Institute of Medicine (2001): safety, timeliness, effectiveness, efficiency, equity, and patient centeredness (Ballard et al. 2013). Variation in performance on these measures may be tracked internally over time by provider organizations to support local quality monitoring and improvement efforts, or it may be examined regionally or nationally as part of public reporting or value-based reimbursement programs intended to incentivize quality improvement.

Variability plays an obvious role in identifying, measuring, and reporting these quality indicators (Goldberg et al. 1994). For example, even within a single hospital system, differences in patient mix between facilities can create the appearance of variation in performance between hospitals if the adjustment for patient mix is inadequate. The same may be true for a single facility over time. Consequently, some healthcare administrators are reluctant to use quality indicators, perceiving them to be biased toward large academic medical centers or large healthcare organizations, which are less subject to changes in underlying factors such as patient mix (Miller et al. 2001). However, analytical techniques and appropriate indicators that are sensitive only to unwarranted variation can be successfully applied to small organizations, even single-physician practices, facilitating their efforts to improve quality of care (Geyman 1998; Miller et al. 2001).

Hospitals and healthcare systems, as well as health services researchers, are using variation data in a variety of ways and across many clinical fields to identify, implement, and evaluate quality improvement efforts. Variation data may be of interest for a variety of purposes (Neuhauser, Provost, and Bergman 2011), and the differing perspectives of various stakeholders may cause them to look at the same set of results and reach very different conclusions about the results' significance and the actions needed in response. For example, if research showed that age and sex predict patient outcomes following hip surgery and, in particular, explain 10 percent of the variation seen in early ambulation, a health services researcher might conclude that more variables need to be measured so that more variation can be explained and a better understanding of what influences this postsurgical outcome can be gained. Meanwhile, a healthcare manager focused on real-time quality improvement might note that 90 percent of the variation is unexplained by the variables investigated and thus could be the expected random variation, leading the manager to conclude that the process is sound and under control (Neuhauser, Provost, and Bergman 2011).

Examples of National Quality Improvement Efforts Applying Variation

Prominent examples of the application of variation data to the aim of widespread quality improvement include Medicare's Hospital Value-Based Purchasing (HVBP) program and Hospital Readmissions Reduction Program (HRRP), administered by the Centers for Medicare & Medicaid Services (CMS).

The HVBP Program, established as part of the Affordable Care Act (ACA) of 2010, reduces hospitals' base operating Medicare severity diagnosis-related group (MS-DRG) payments under the Inpatient Prospective Payment System by 2 percent and, at the end of the fiscal year, redistributes that 2 percent to hospitals based on their Total Performance Score (TPS). The TPS incorporates selected quality measures covering the following areas: (1) clinical care, (2) patient- and caregiver-centered experience of care / care coordination, (3) safety, and (4) efficiency and cost reduction (CMS 2017).

Medicare calculates two important thresholds for each measure in the TPS based on the performance of all participating hospitals: (1) the "achievement" threshold, set at the fiftieth percentile (median) performance during the baseline period and (2) the "benchmark" threshold, set at the mean performance of the top 10 percent of hospitals during the baseline period (Wheeler-Bunch and Gugliuzza 2018). Individual hospitals are awarded "achievement points" for each measure in the TPS based on the comparison of their performance to those two thresholds: Performance at or above the benchmark earns the hospital 10 points, performance from the achievement to the benchmark threshold earns the hospital 1 to 9 points, and performance below the achievement threshold earns 0 points (Wheeler-Bunch and Gugliuzza 2018). The hospital is also, however, rated against its own historical performance during the baseline period and can receive 0 to 9 "improvement points" for measures on which its performance falls between the benchmark threshold and the hospital's own performance during the baseline period (whether above or below the achievement threshold) (Wheeler-Bunch and Gugliuzza 2018). Medicare then counts the higher of the achievement or improvement points for the measure toward the hospital's TPS (CMS 2012).

A hospital's TPS is used to calculate its value-based incentive percentage, using a linear exchange function for which the slope is set so that the estimated total value-based incentive payments to all participating hospitals for that fiscal year will equal the 2 percent of the base operating payments withheld from all participating hospitals (CMS 2012). What hospitals earn, therefore, depends on the range and distribution of all eligible hospitals' TPS scores for the fiscal year. The value-based incentive payment for each discharge is then calculated by multiplying the base operating DRG payment amount for the discharge for the hospital by the value-based incentive payment percentage for the hospital (CMS 2012). A hospital's value-based incentive payment percentage may be less than, equal to, or more than its 2 percent reduction in base payments (CMS 2012).

In theory, as the financial incentives of the HVBP program encourage hospitals to identify and address quality issues related to the performance measures included in the TPS, the range and distribution of participating hospitals' performance will narrow to the point that the achievement and benchmark thresholds could no longer discriminate between good- and poor-quality care. In other words, once hospitals have addressed the factors underlying the assignable variation contributing to the performance range, only random variation would be left, essentially leaving the incentive payments (or penalties) up to chance. In practice, this scenario is avoided by replacing measures that have "topped out" (i.e., measures where almost all providers routinely achieve near optimal performance) with measures reflecting new priorities. For example, in fiscal year 2017, Medicare removed six "topped out" process-of-care measures from the clinical care domain and added two new safety measures (CMS 2015). "Refreshing" the measures in this way helps the program stay current with priorities and advances in healthcare quality. It also helps ensure that hospitals are evaluated on aspects of performance over which they have control.

The HRRP, likewise established as part of the ACA, applies a similar variation-based strategy for evaluating hospitals' performance. It focuses on 30-day readmissions for a chosen set of procedures and conditions: heart attack, heart failure, pneumonia, chronic obstructive pulmonary disease, hip/knee replacement, and coronary artery bypass graft surgery (Medicare.gov 2018). A hospital's readmissions are measured using a ratio, in which the hospital's number of "predicted" unplanned 30-day readmissions is divided by the number that would be "expected" based on an average hospital with similar patients. Hospitals that are determined to have "excess" readmissions are assessed a penalty of up to 3 percent of the hospital's base operating DRG payments (Medicare.gov 2018). Unlike the HVBP Program, the HRRP does not allow hospitals to earn an incentive payment for high performance; they can merely avoid the penalty. And because the HRRP is structured around performance relative to the national average, roughly half the hospitals will *always* face a penalty, and the overall magnitude of the penalty will remain much the same, even if, as hoped, all hospitals improve overall over time (*Health Affairs* 2013).

An example of a more detailed examination of variation data for the purpose of directing (rather than incentivizing) quality improvement involved the use of coronary angiography data collected from 691 US hospitals from

2005 to 2008 in the CathPCI Registry (for diagnostic catheterization and percutaneous coronary intervention [PCI] procedures). The data revealed that the rate of finding obstructive coronary artery disease (CAD) varied from 23 percent to 100 percent between hospitals (Douglas et al. 2011). Further investigation showed that the variation was not random but rather associated with the hospitals' patient selection and preprocedural assessment strategies. The study revealed opportunities to reduce the number of unnecessary procedures, which place patients at needless risk and incur unnecessary costs (Douglas et al. 2011). Specifically, if the finding rates for hospitals in the two lowest quartiles were raised to the national median (45 percent), the number of coronary angiographies without a finding of obstructive CAD would drop by 23 percent. Thus, variation data revealed that at least one-quarter of cardiac angiographies performed may be unnecessary, and their elimination could improve the safety and efficiency of care (Douglas et al. 2011).

Examples of Healthcare Systems Applying Variation to Quality Improvement

An organization's capacity for quality monitoring and improvement depends on its size and infrastructure. As value-based purchasing comes increasingly into play, an organization's survival will depend on its ability to monitor and improve its quality of care. Even prior to mandated minimum standards of quality in reimbursement schemes, a number of providers chose to apply quality threshold levels because of the compelling business case to do so: Satisfied patients return for additional care or recommend that others use the same services (Ballard 2003; Holz and DeVol 2013; Stroud, Felton, and Spreadbury 2003).

Planning the collection and analysis of suitable data for quality measures requires significant forethought to minimize the indicators' sensitivity to warranted variation and to ensure that changes detected truly relate to the quality of care provided. This planning involves selecting appropriate measures, controlling for case mix and other variables, minimizing chance variability, and collecting high-quality data (Powell, Davies, and Thomson 2003).

Intermountain Healthcare (IHC), a large healthcare delivery system in Utah, has effectively used variation data to identify and address opportunities for quality improvement. The quality improvement team started by looking at practice variation in common care processes, revealed by chart review. Although the team found no evidence that one physician's patients demonstrated greater severity or complexity than other physicians' patients, it saw "massive" variation in physician practices (James and Savitz 2011). Specifically, when the team examined patients with similar admissions and good outcomes, the highest rates of use of common care processes examined were 1.6 to 5.6 times higher than the lowest rates of use, and hospital costs per case (other than physician payment) varied twofold (James and Savitz 2011).

To address this variation, IHC focused on the processes underlying the particular treatments, implementing tools such as guideline-based checklists, order sets, and clinical flow sheets to help standardize practices (James and Savitz 2011). Following initial implementation, the team once again examined variation, this time looking at the adaptations clinicians had made to guidelines in applying them. These data were fed back to the patient care team, which led in some cases to modification of guidelines to more accurately reflect the realities of care and in other cases to modification of clinician practice.

For treatment of respiratory distress, this method achieved a reduction in guideline variance from 59 percent to 6 percent in four months, with an accompanying increase in survival in the subcategory of patients seriously ill with acute respiratory distress from 9.5 percent to 44 percent and a 25 percent decrease in the total cost of care (James and Savitz 2011). Similar success was observed for elective induction of labor: The proportion of elective inductions that did not meet strong indications for clinical appropriateness decreased from 28 percent to less than 2 percent (James and Savitz 2011).

Case Example: Baylor Scott & White Health

Substantial evidence indicates that heart failure (HF) mortality and morbidity can be reduced through angiotensin-converting enzyme inhibitor or angiotensin receptor blocker therapy, beta-blocker therapy, and other treatment modalities (CIBIS-II Investigators and Committees 1999; Fonarow et al. 2004; Hjalmarson et al. 2002; CONSENSUS Trial Study Group 1987; SOLVD Investigators 1991), and clinical practice guidelines strongly recommend such therapies as part of the standard care for HF (Hunt et al. 2009). Nonetheless, these evidence-based therapies were used inconsistently at the turn of the twenty-first century. Specifically, they were underutilized in HF patients who did not have contraindications (Fonarow 2002; Masoudi et al. 2004).

Baylor Scott & White Health (BSWH) is an integrated healthcare delivery system in Texas. While conducting routine monitoring of quality-of-care indicators, BSWH observed inconsistent use of evidence-based HF therapies in its hospitals, despite relatively constant characteristics of its HF patient population. Having previously had success in increasing compliance with treatment recommendations, as well as improving patient outcomes, through implementation of a standardized order set for pneumonia care (Ballard et al. 2008; Fleming, Masica, and McCarthy 2013; Fleming, Ogola, and Ballard 2009), BSWH decided to take a similar approach as part of its

(continued)

systemwide HF improvement initiative (Ballard et al. 2010). It established a standardized HF order set—developed internally but based on the prevailing American College of Cardiology / American Heart Association clinical practice guidelines—across its eight acute care and two specialty heart hospitals, and it deployed the order set via the intranet physician portal in December 2007 (Ballard et al. 2010).

Exhibit 3.4 presents BSHW performance on the "all indicated services" bundle measure for HF (covering the HF process-of-care measures CMS reports on its Hospital Compare website) before and after its implementation of the standardized order set. During the early preimplementation phase (July 2006 to December 2007), the process of care was not "in control," as demonstrated by the September 2006 data point falling below the lower control limit. Although the later months of the preimplementation period show generally better performance, and no evidence of assignable variation, the process of care still had room for improvement—and for consistency in good performance. Following implementation of the HF order set (January 2008 to June 2010), BSWH shows not only statistical control but also evidence of successful quality improvement. The mean performance line has risen closer to 100 percent, and the control limit range has narrowed, indicating reduced variability around that higher performance.

EXHIBIT 3.4
Proportion of Heart Failure Patients Receiving All Indicated Services Before and After Baylor Scott & White Health Deployed Its Standardized Heart Failure Order Set

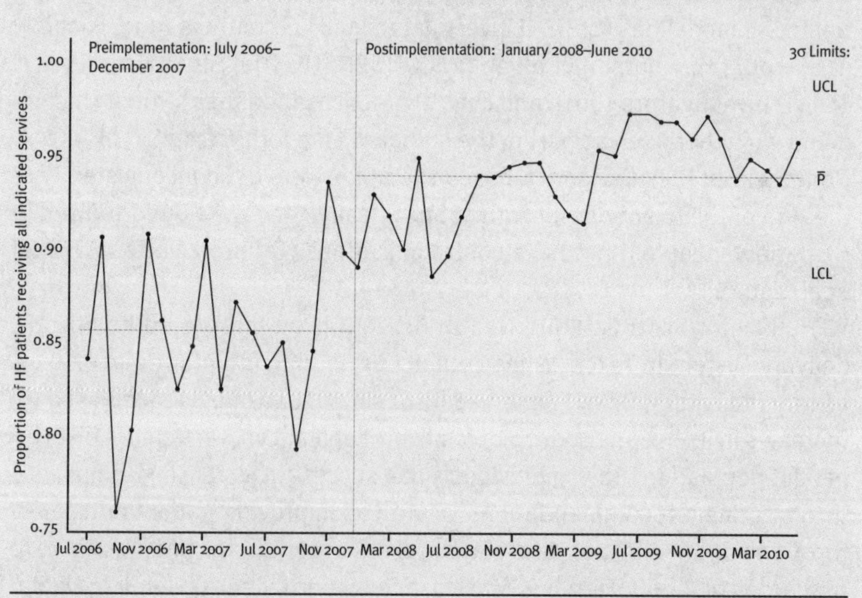

Source: Data from Baylor Scott & White Health.

Examples of Variation Data Being Applied for Population Health

As ACOs proliferated following passage of the ACA in 2010, new applications of variation data came into play to assist with the management of health at the population level, as well as the management of the financial risk that ACOs assume through risk-based contracts. One example of such an application is the patient-risk stratification process that Baylor Scott & White Quality Alliance (BSWQA)—the ACO affiliated with the Baylor Scott & White Health system—undertakes when it enters a contract to manage a new population (e.g., a Medicare Advantage plan, an employer-sponsored health plan). Using a combination of historical claims data from the payer and patient demographic and clinical data, BSWQA applies predictive algorithms to rank patients by likelihood of high healthcare resource utilization.

Using cutpoints, BSWQA assigns patients to appropriate levels of care coordination to support better disease management and preventive care, seeking to avert or mitigate the adverse health events that trigger high utilization. For example, as shown in exhibit 3.5, the 5 percent of the population with the highest risk for adverse health outcomes and/or high resource utilization would be assigned to a nurse care manager, who provides an assessment of the patient's current health status and compliance with evidence-based care guidelines to identify existing gaps in care (particularly around chronic disease management), performs medication reconciliation, and assists with health goal setting and care plan management (Couch 2016). The 15 percent with the next highest level of risk are assigned a medical assistant health coordinator, who provides a more limited set of care coordination services, focusing on closing

EXHIBIT 3.5
Example of Allocating Care Models in Accordance with Patient Risk

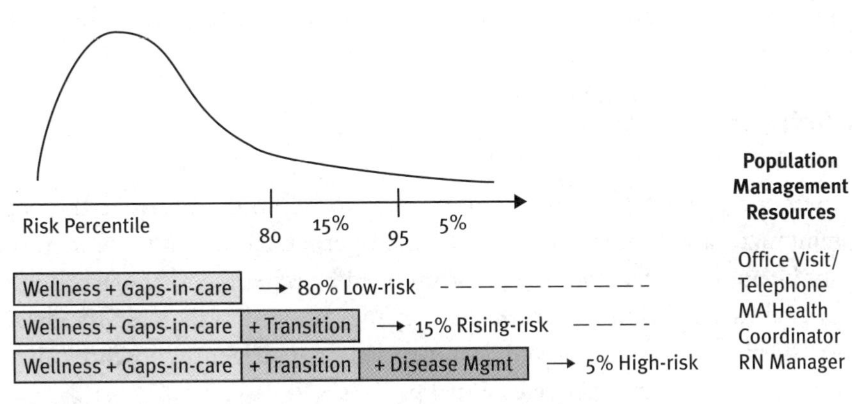

Note: MA = medical assistant; RN = registered nurse.

Source: Previously published in Couch, C. E. "Population Health." In *Accountable: The Baylor Scott & White Quality Alliance Accountable Care Journey*, edited by B. da Graca, K. M. Richter, and J. Sullivan. 131. Boca Raton, FL: CRC Press, 2016.

gaps in care related to preventive services and chronic disease management and ensuring the patient's regular connection with the primary care physician (Couch 2016). The remainder of the population is not assigned an individual care coordinator but receives reminders regarding recommended preventive or disease management services (Couch 2016).

The BSWQA strategy creates warranted variation, in which patients with different needs receive different services. Note that this risk stratification is conducted at the "contract population" level, rather than grouping all the BSWQA "covered lives" into a single population, which is important because the contract populations and the contracts themselves may differ widely. For example, if the ACO contracts with both a Medicare Advantage plan and an employer-sponsored health plan, combining the two populations would likely result in the 5 percent high-risk category and most of the next 15 percent category being swamped by members of the Medicare Advantage population, who, simply due to greater age, are much more likely to have multiple risk factors for adverse outcomes. Such an approach would leave essentially all of the employer-sponsored health plan population in the category that receives minimal care coordination—which may be insufficient to meet the health outcome targets set in the relevant contract. Depending on the degree of risk accepted by the ACO in the contract, failure to meet those outcome targets could be a critical issue for the ACO's viability.

Another important reason to perform risk stratification at the contract population level is that doing so allows the cutpoints for stratification to be adjusted as needed to account for both the population's characteristics and the degree of risk assumed by the ACO. For example, if the ACO has assumed a high level of financial risk, it may choose to place the cutpoints for care manager and health coordinator assignment at 8 percent and 20 percent, respectively.

Conclusion

Contemporary industrial quality improvement methods emphasize the need to minimize variation, if not eliminate it altogether. Although these methods might be appropriate in settings characterized by repetitive manufacturing of mass quantities of identical products, they may unnecessarily mask the details of variation in the healthcare environment and consequently obscure opportunities to change or improve essential processes of care.

The pursuit of high-quality healthcare focuses on the successful management—rather than elimination—of variation, and it requires the abilities to identify variation; to distinguish between random and assignable variation; to determine the meaning, importance, or value of an observed variation relative to some standard (i.e., to distinguish between warranted and unwarranted variation); and to implement methods that will take advantage of or rectify what the variation reveals. Ultimately, variation tells us what is working and what is not, and how far from optimal our healthcare processes are. Rather than avoid variation in pursuit of quality healthcare, we should embrace it as a useful guide on our pathway to success.

Study Questions

1. While exploring opportunities to improve processes of care for a group practice, you find no variability in compliance with the US Preventive Services Task Force's recommendations for colorectal cancer screening across the practice's physicians over time. Is this absence of variation optimal? Why or why not?
2. Distinguish between random and assignable variation. Discuss the relevance of each to measuring quality of care and to the design and evaluation of quality improvement initiatives.
3. Describe the three categories of care identified by Wennberg (2011), the possible opportunities for improvement that unwarranted variation might indicate for each of the categories, and the goals of health services research and quality improvement initiatives for each category.

References

Arterburn, D., R. Wellman, E. Westbrook, C. Rutter, T. Ross, D. McCulloch, M. Handley, and C. Jung. 2012. "Introducing Decision Aids at Group Health Was Linked to Sharply Lower Hip and Knee Surgery Rates and Costs." *Health Affairs* (Millwood) 31 (9): 2094–104.

Ballard, D. J. 2003. "Indicators to Improve Clinical Quality Across an Integrated Health Care System." *International Journal for Quality in Health Care* 15 (Suppl. 1): i13–i23.

Ballard, D. J., N. S. Fleming, J. T. Allison, P. B. Convery, and R. Luquire (eds.). 2013. *Achieving STEEEP Health Care: Baylor Health Care System's Quality Improvement Journey.* Boca Raton, FL: CRC Press.

Ballard, D. J., G. Ogola, N. S. Fleming, D. Heck, J. Gunderson, R. Mehta, R. Khetan, and J. D. Kerr. 2008. "The Impact of Standardized Order Sets on Quality and Financial Outcomes." In *Advances in Patient Safety: New Directions and Alternative Approaches*, vol. 2, edited by K. Henriksen, J. B. Battles, M. A. Keyes, and M. L. Grady, 255–69. Rockville, MD: Agency for Healthcare Research and Quality.

Ballard, D. J., G. Ogola, N. S. Fleming, B. D. Stauffer, B. M. Leonard, R. Khetan, and C. W. Yancy. 2010. "Impact of a Standardized Heart Failure Order Set on Mortality, Readmission, and Quality and Costs of Care." *International Journal for Quality in Health Care* 22 (6): 437–44.

Benneyan, J. C., R. C. Lloyd, and P. E. Plsek. 2003. "Statistical Process Control as a Tool for Research and Healthcare Improvement." *BMJ Quality & Safety* 12 (6): 458–64.

Bynum, J. P., E. Meara, C.-H. Chang, and J. M. Rhoads. 2016. *Our Parents, Ourselves: Health Care for an Aging Population.* Lebanon, NH: Dartmouth Institute for Health Policy & Clinical Practice.

Centers for Medicare & Medicaid Services (CMS). 2017. "Hospital Value-Based Purchasing." Updated October 31. www.cms.gov/Medicare/Quality-Initiatives-Patient-Assessment-Instruments/HospitalQualityInits/Hospital-Value-Based-Purchasing-.html.

———. 2015. "Fiscal Year (FY) 2016 Results for the CMS Hospital Value-Based Purchasing Program." Published October 26. www.cms.gov/newsroom/fact-sheets/fiscal-year-fy-2016-results-cms-hospital-value-based-purchasing-program.

———. 2012. "Frequently Asked Questions: Hospital Value-Based Purchasing Program." Updated February 28. www.cms.gov/Medicare/Quality-Initiatives-Patient-Assessment-Instruments/hospital-value-based-purchasing/downloads/HVBPFAQ022812.pdf.

CIBIS-II Investigators and Committees. 1999. "The Cardiac Insufficiency Bisoprolol Study II (CIBIS-II): A Randomised Trial." *Lancet* 353 (9146): 9–13.

CONSENSUS Trial Study Group. 1987. "Effects of Enalapril on Mortality in Severe Congestive Heart Failure. Results of the Cooperative North Scandinavian Enalapril Survival Study (CONSENSUS)." *New England Journal of Medicine* 316 (23): 1429–35.

Couch, C. E. 2016. "Population Health." In *Accountable: The Baylor Scott & White Quality Alliance Accountable Care Journey*, edited by B. da Graca, K. M. Richter, and J. Sullivan, 111–54. Boca Raton, FL: CRC Press.

Davis, P., B. Gribben, A. Scott, and R. Lay-Yee. 2000. "The 'Supply Hypothesis' and Medical Practice Variation in Primary Care: Testing Economic and Clinical Models of Inter-practitioner Variation." *Social Science & Medicine* 50 (3): 407–18.

Douglas, P. S., M. R. Patel, S. R. Bailey, D. Dai, L. Kaltenbach, R. G. Brindis, J. Messenger, and E. D. Peterson. 2011. "Hospital Variability in the Rate of Finding Obstructive Coronary Artery Disease at Elective, Diagnostic Coronary Angiography." *Journal of the American College of Cardiology* 58 (8): 801–9.

Eddy, D. M. 1984. "Variations in Physician Practice: The Role of Uncertainty." *Health Affairs* (Millwood) 3 (2): 74–89.

Fisher, E. S., D. E. Wennberg, T. A. Stukel, D. J. Gottlieb, F. L. Lucas, and E. L. Pinder. 2003. "The Implications of Regional Variations in Medicare Spending. Part

2: Health Outcomes and Satisfaction with Care." *Annals of Internal Medicine* 138 (4): 288–98.

Fleming, N. S., A. Masica, and I. McCarthy. 2013. "Evaluation of Clinical and Financial Outcomes." In *Achieving STEEEP Health Care: Baylor Health Care System's Quality Improvement Journey*, edited by D. J. Ballard, N. S. Fleming, J. T. Allison, P. B. Convery, and R. Luquire, 85–92. Boca Raton, FL: CRC Press.

Fleming, N. S., G. Ogola, and D. J. Ballard. 2009. "Implementing a Standardized Order Set for Community-Acquired Pneumonia: Impact on Mortality and Cost." *Joint Commission Journal on Quality and Patient Safety* 35 (8): 414–21.

Fonarow, G. C. 2002. "The Role of In-Hospital Initiation of Cardioprotective Therapies to Improve Treatment Rates and Clinical Outcomes." *Reviews in Cardiovascular Medicine* 3 (Suppl. 3): S2–S10.

Fonarow, G. C., W. T. Abraham, N. M. Albert, W. A. Gattis, M. Gheorghiade, B. Greenberg, C. M. O'Connor, C. W. Yancy, and J. Young. 2004. "Organized Program to Initiate Lifesaving Treatment in Hospitalized Patients with Heart Failure (OPTIMIZE-HF): Rationale and Design." *American Heart Journal* 148 (1): 43–51.

Gauld, R., J. Horwitt, S. Williams, and A. B. Cohen. 2011. "What Strategies Do US Hospitals Employ to Reduce Unwarranted Clinical Practice Variations?" *American Journal of Medical Quality* 26 (2): 120–26.

Geyman, J. P. 1998. "Evidence-Based Medicine in Primary Care: An Overview." *Journal of the American Board of Family Practice* 11 (1): 46–56.

Glance, L. G., A. W. Dick, J. C. Glantz, R. N. Wissler, F. Qian, B. M. Marroquin, D. B. Mukamel, and A. L. Kellermann. 2014. "Rates of Major Obstetrical Complications Vary Almost Fivefold Among US Hospitals." *Health Affairs* (Millwood) 33 (8): 1330–36.

Glover, J. A. 1938. "The Incidence of Tonsillectomy in School Children (Section of Epidemiology and State Medicine)." *Proceedings of the Royal Society of Medicine* 31 (10): 1219–36.

Goldberg, H. I., M. A. Cummings, E. P. Steinberg, E. M. Ricci, T. Shannon, S. B. Soumerai, B. S. Mittman, J. Eisenberg, D. A. Heck, and S. Kaplan. 1994. "Deliberations on the Dissemination of PORT Products: Translating Research Findings into Improved Patient Outcomes." *Medical Care* 32 (7 Suppl.): JS90–JS110.

Greer, A. L., J. S. Goodwin, J. L. Freeman, and Z. H. Wu. 2002. "Bringing the Patient Back In: Guidelines, Practice Variations, and the Social Context of Medical Practice." *International Journal of Technology Assessment in Health Care* 18 (4): 747–61.

Ham, C. 2011. "Review of the Week: A Roadmap for Health System Reform." *BMJ* 342: d1757.

Health Affairs. 2013. "Health Policy Brief: Medicare Hospital Readmissions Reduction Program." Published November 12. http://healthaffairs.org/healthpolicybriefs/brief_pdfs/healthpolicybrief_102.pdf.

Hjalmarson, A., S. Goldstein, B. Fagerberg, H. Wedel, F. Waagstein, J. Kjekshus, J. Wikstrand, D. El Allaf, J. Vitovec, J. Aldershvile, M. Halinen, R. Dietz, K. L. Neuhaus, A. Jánosi, G. Thorgeirsson, P. H. Dunselman, L. Gullestad, J. Kuch, J. Herlitz, P. Rickenbacher, S. Ball, S. Gottlieb, and P. Deedwania. 2002. "Effects of Controlled-Release Metoprolol on Total Mortality, Hospitalizations, and Well-Being in Patients with Heart Failure: The Metoprolol CR/XL Randomized Intervention Trial in Congestive Heart Failure (MERIT-HF). MERIT-HF Study Group." *JAMA* 283 (10): 1295–302.

Holz, K., and E. DeVol. 2013. "Alignment, Goal-Setting, and Incentives." In *Achieving STEEEP Health Care: Baylor Health Care System's Quality Improvement Journey*, edited by D. J. Ballard, N. S. Fleming, J. T. Allison, P. B. Convery, and R. Luquire, 23–28. Boca Raton, FL: CRC Press.

Hsu, C., D. T. Liss, D. L. Frosch, E. O. Westbrook, and D. Arterburn. 2017. "Exploring Provider Reactions to Decision Aid Distribution and Shared Decision Making: Lessons from Two Specialties." *Medical Decision Making* 37 (1): 113–26.

Hunt, S. A., W. T. Abraham, M. H. Chin, A. M. Feldman, G. S. Francis, T. G. Ganiats, M. Jessup, M. A. Konstam, D. M. Mancini, K. Michl, J. A. Oates, P. S. Rahko, M. A. Silver, L. Warner Stevenson, and C. W. Yancy. 2009. "2009 Focused Update Incorporated into the ACC/AHA 2005 Guidelines for the Diagnosis and Management of Heart Failure in Adults: A Report of the American College of Cardiology Foundation/American Heart Association Task Force on Practice Guidelines." *Journal of the American College of Cardiology* 53 (15): e1–e90.

Institute of Medicine (IOM). 2001. *Crossing the Quality Chasm: A New Health System for the 21st Century.* Washington, DC: National Academies Press.

James, B. C., and L. A. Savitz. 2011. "How Intermountain Trimmed Health Care Costs Through Robust Quality Improvement Efforts." *Health Affairs* (Millwood) 30 (6): 1185–91.

Johnson, D. C., D. E. Mueller, A. M. Deal, M. W. Dunn, A. B. Smith, M. E. Woods, E. M. Wallen, R. S. Pruthi, and M. E. Nielsen. 2016. "Integrating Patient Preference into Treatment Decisions for Men with Prostate Cancer at the Point of Care." *Journal of Urology* 196 (6): 1640–44.

Katz, B. P., D. A. Freund, D. A. Heck, R. S. Dittus, J. E. Paul, J. Wright, P. Coyte, E. Holleman, and G. Hawker. 1996. "Demographic Variation in the Rate of Knee Replacement: A Multi-Year Analysis." *Health Services Research* 31 (2): 125–40.

Kennedy, P. J., C. M. Leathley, and C. F. Hughes. 2010. "Clinical Practice Variation." *Medical Journal of Australia* 193 (8 Suppl.): S97–S99.

Kozhimannil, K. B., M. R. Law, and B. A. Virnig. 2013. "Cesarean Delivery Rates Vary Tenfold Among US Hospitals; Reducing Variation May Address Quality and Cost Issues." *Health Affairs* (Millwood) 32 (3): 527–35.

Long, M. J. 2002. "An Explanatory Model of Medical Practice Variation: A Physician Resource Demand Perspective." *Journal of Evaluation in Clinical Practice* 8 (2): 167–74.

Lu-Yao, G. L., and E. R. Greenberg. 1994. "Changes in Prostate Cancer Incidence and Treatment in USA." *Lancet* 343 (8892): 251–54.

Masoudi, F. A., S. S. Rathore, Y. Wang, E. P. Havranek, J. P. Curtis, J. M. Foody, and H. M. Krumholz. 2004. "National Patterns of Use and Effectiveness of Angiotensin-Converting Enzyme Inhibitors in Older Patients with Heart Failure and Left Ventricular Systolic Dysfunction." *Circulation* 110 (6): 724–31.

McPherson, K., J. E. Wennberg, O. B. Hovind, and P. Clifford. 1982. "Small-Area Variations in the Use of Common Surgical Procedures: An International Comparison of New England, England, and Norway." *New England Journal of Medicine* 307 (21): 1310–14.

Medicare.gov. 2018. "Hospital Readmissions Reduction Program." Accessed September 21. www.medicare.gov/hospitalcompare/readmission-reduction-program.html.

Mehrotra, A., J. L. Adams, J. W. Thomas, and E. A. McGlynn. 2010. "The Effect of Different Attribution Rules on Individual Physician Cost Profiles." *Annals of Internal Medicine* 152 (10): 649–54.

Mercuri, M., and A. Gafni. 2011. "Medical Practice Variations: What the Literature Tells Us (or Does Not) About What Are Warranted and Unwarranted Variations." *Journal of Evaluation in Clinical Practice* 17 (4): 671–77.

Miller, W. L., R. R. McDaniel Jr., B. F. Crabtree, and K. C. Stange. 2001. "Practice Jazz: Understanding Variation in Family Practices Using Complexity Science." *Journal of Family Practice* 50 (10): 872–78.

Neuhauser, D., L. Provost, and B. Bergman. 2011. "The Meaning of Variation to Healthcare Managers, Clinical and Health-Services Researchers, and Individual Patients." *BMJ Quality & Safety* 20 (Suppl 1.): i36–i40.

O'Connor, A. M., C. L. Bennett, D. Stacey, M. Barry, N. F. Col, K. B. Eden, V. A. Entwistle, V. Fiset, M. Holmes-Rovner, S. Khangura, H. Llewellyn-Thomas, and D. Rovner. 2009. "Decision Aids for People Facing Health Treatment or Screening Decisions." Cochrane Library. Published July 8. www.cochranelibrary.com/cdsr/doi/10.1002/14651858.CD001431.pub2/full.

O'Connor, A. M., H. A. Llewellyn-Thomas, and A. B. Flood. 2004. "Modifying Unwarranted Variations in Health Care: Shared Decision Making Using Patient Decision Aids." *Health Affairs* (Millwood) Suppl. Variation (2004): VAR63–VAR72.

Parente, S. T., C. E. Phelps, and P. J. O'Connor. 2008. "Economic Analysis of Medical Practice Variation Between 1991 and 2000: The Impact of Patient Outcomes Research Teams (PORTs)." *International Journal of Technology Assessment in Health Care* 24 (3): 282–93.

Pham, H. H., D. Schrag, A. S. O'Malley, B. Wu, and P. B. Bach. 2007. "Care Patterns in Medicare and Their Implications for Pay for Performance." *New England Journal of Medicine* 356 (11): 1130–39.

Powell, A. E., H. T. Davies, and R. G. Thomson. 2003. "Using Routine Comparative Data to Assess the Quality of Health Care: Understanding and Avoiding Common Pitfalls." *Quality and Safety in Health Care* 12 (2): 122–28.

Rayner, H. C. 2011. "Tackling Practice Variation: Lessons from Variation Can Help Change Health Policy." *BMJ* 342: d2271.

Reinertsen, J. L. 2003. "Zen and the Art of Physician Autonomy Maintenance." *Annals of Internal Medicine* 138 (12): 992–95.

Savelberg, W., T. van der Weijden, L. Boersma, M. Smidt, C. Willekens, and A. Moser. 2017. "Developing a Patient Decision Aid for the Treatment of Women with Early Stage Breast Cancer: The Struggle Between Simplicity and Complexity." *BMC Medical Informatics & Decision Making* 17 (1): 112.

Sejr, T., T. F. Andersen, M. Madsen, C. Roepstorff, T. Bilde, H. Bay-Nielsen, R. Blais, and E. Holst. 1991. "Prostatectomy in Denmark. Regional Variation and the Diffusion of Medical Technology 1977–1985." *Scandinavian Journal of Urology and Nephrology* 25 (2): 101–6.

Sepucha, K., E. Ozanne, and A. G. Mulley. 2006. "Doing the Right Thing: Systems Support for Decision Quality in Cancer Care." *Annals of Behavioral Medicine* 32 (3): 172–78.

Sirovich, B., P. M. Gallagher, D. E. Wennberg, and E. S. Fisher. 2008. "Discretionary Decision Making by Primary Care Physicians and the Cost of U.S. Health Care." *Health Affairs* (Millwood) 27 (3): 813–23.

Smith, R. 2011. "Medical Classics: Dartmouth Atlas of Health Care." *BMJ* 342: d1756.

SOLVD Investigators. 1991. "Effect of Enalapril on Survival in Patients with Reduced Left Ventricular Ejection Fractions and Congestive Heart Failure." *New England Journal of Medicine* 325 (5): 293–302.

Spiegelhalter, D. J. 2005. "Funnel Plots for Comparing Institutional Performance." *Statistics in Medicine* 24 (8): 1185–202.

Steinberg, E. P. 2003. "Improving the Quality of Care—Can We Practice What We Preach?" *New England Journal of Medicine* 348 (26): 2681–83.

Stroud, J., C. Felton, and B. Spreadbury. 2003. "Collaborative Colorectal Cancer Screening: A Successful Quality Improvement Initiative." *Baylor University Medical Center Proceedings* 16 (3): 341–44.

Thor, J., J. Lundberg, J. Ask, J. Olsson, C. Carli, K. P. Härenstam, and M. Brommels. 2007. "Application of Statistical Process Control in Healthcare Improvement: Systematic Review." *BMJ Quality & Safety* 16 (5): 387–99.

Timmermans, S., and A. Mauck. 2005. "The Promises and Pitfalls of Evidence-Based Medicine." *Health Affairs* (Millwood) 24 (1): 18–28.

van Dishoeck, A. M., C. W. Looman, E. C. van der Wilden-van Lier, J. P. Mackenbach, and E. W. Steyerberg. 2011. "Displaying Random Variation in Comparing Hospital Performance." *BMJ Quality & Safety* 20 (8): 651–57.

Wennberg, J. E. 2011. "Time to Tackle Unwarranted Variations in Practice." *BMJ* 342: d1513.

Wennberg, J. E., B. A. Barnes, and M. Zubkoff. 1982. "Professional Uncertainty and the Problem of Supplier-Induced Demand." *Social Science & Medicine* 16 (7): 811–24.

Wennberg, D. E., M. A. Kellett, J. D. Dickens, D. J. Malenka, L. M. Keilson, and R. B. Keller. 1996. "The Association Between Local Diagnostic Testing Intensity and Invasive Cardiac Procedures." *JAMA* 275 (15): 1161–64.

Westert, G. P., and M. Faber. 2011. "Commentary: The Dutch Approach to Unwarranted Medical Practice Variation." *BMJ* 342: d1429.

Westert, G. P., P. P. Groenewegen, H. C. Boshuizen, P. M. Spreeuwenberg, and M. P. Steultjens. 2004. "Medical Practice Variations in Hospital Care; Time Trends of a Spatial Phenomenon." *Health Place* 10 (3): 215–20.

Wheeler-Bunch, B., and M. Gugliuzza. 2018. "Hospital VBP Program: Overview of the FY 2019 Percentage Payment Summary Reports." Quality Reporting Center. Published August 7. www.qualityreportingcenter.com/wp-content/uploads/2018/07/04_VBP_PPSRWebinar_Slides_vFINAL508wointro-1.pdf.

Woodall, W. H., B. M. Adams, and J. C. Benneyan. 2012. "The Use of Control Charts in Healthcare." In *Statistical Methods in Healthcare*, edited by F. Faltin, R. Kenett, and F. Ruggeri, 253–65. Chichester, UK: Wiley.

PART

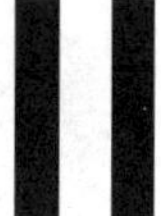

TOOLS, MEASURES, AND THEIR APPLICATIONS

Elizabeth R. Ransom

Quality improvement in healthcare has a long and illustrious history, dating back millennia to the work of Galen, Hippocrates, and others. Although physicians and other healthcare providers have always striven to improve care, only in the modern era have we become more diligent and consistent in our quest to analyze how we assess care, what outcomes we achieve, and how we use that information to drive change.

Improvement requires change, and without scientific analysis and recommendations, providers will rightly balk at making changes that may or may not have perceived benefits. In fact, one of the chief concerns in improving care is ensuring that the tools and measures we use to assess what we do are precise, understandable, and applicable.

The chapters in part II of this book hone in on precisely those issues. The aphorism that "what is measured is managed" holds true in the quality improvement landscape. As John Byrnes eloquently states in chapter 4, "Data provide the foundation of quality and patient safety." In today's healthcare climate, many organizations find themselves inundated with information. Electronic health records provide more information than clinicians have ever had about their patients, and payers keep fastidious claims records on every billable encounter for every patient. In the United States, the Centers for Medicare & Medicaid Services, the Department of Veterans Affairs, and public and private healthcare groups and organizations all track and measure different components of process, outcomes, and costs of care. Clinically integrated networks track numerous metrics in anticipation of using that information to drive improvement and achieve the resultant financial benefits from risk-based contracting. Employers use information in their decision making to achieve the highest value of care for their employees while balancing the cost of contracts with insurers.

The great challenge, however, is sifting through the deluge of information to find the truly valuable data that can be leveraged to improve the care provided to patients and communities. Byrnes addresses this task in chapter 4, on data collection. Among the first and most unavoidable considerations in the quantity and quality of data to analyze are the time and cost involved in gathering the information. Byrnes describes the value equation that weighs labor- and time-intensive chart review, along with broader administrative data review, while considering how the different methodologies can be complementary. He also highlights the importance of identifying what data will actually be informative and useful in driving change. He points out the universal tendency to gather as much information as possible *just in case* it might be valuable at a later time, noting how inefficient such an approach can be.

Byrnes also describes the diversity of data sources that currently exist. Organizations not only must decide from among the myriad sources but also must determine the chronological importance of the data. In other words, are the more prevalent sources of data that provide retrospective information (e.g., medical records, administrative databases) sufficient? Or is prospective information (i.e., information pulled from patients' records in real time) more critical? The collection of prospective information is usually accomplished by nursing staff, researchers, data analysts, and others, and it clearly is associated with higher costs.

Byrnes discusses the value and limitations of the increasingly prevalent and accessible administrative databases, including billing systems, health plan information, registration systems, and so forth. Administrative data can often be a starting point for identification of clinical issues that need to be investigated and addressed. Some worry that the data in these databases is unreliable, but such concerns can be mitigated by validation efforts, inter-rater reliability systems, and so on. Byrnes gives health plan databases, which are a subset of the larger category of administrative databases, a special focus. Information from health plans can be particularly valuable in population health efforts and disease management for groups of patients. Health plan databases also provide a unique insight into the total cost of care for specific procedures, and perhaps most importantly, they can be tapped to identify gaps in care for the plan's members.

Finally, Byrnes discusses the increasing abundance and sophistication of patient registries, which can be particularly rich sources of information because of their specific focus. Byrnes also highlights their versatility in terms of the types of information that can be captured.

Although data collection is key to ensuring quality of work, organizations must also be able to apply the appropriate statistical analysis to make the information meaningful. Davis Balestracci comprehensively evaluates statistical tools and methodologies in chapter 5, where he cogently argues that "the role of statistics in improvement is to expose variation and reduce inappropriate and unintended variation." To that end, he explains how variation can be categorized in two ways—as common cause, or systemic, variation or as special cause, or unique, variation. He goes on to describe the common pitfall of "tampering," which occurs when people react to common cause variation as if it were special cause. Tampering often results in added confusion and complexity.

Balestracci characterizes three types of statistics—descriptive, enumerative, and analytic—and explains the usefulness of run charts, along with the importance of using the median rather than the average. He then provides a thorough discussion of the importance of control charts in statistical analysis. Balestracci demonstrates the usefulness of the I-chart, which he considers the "Swiss Army knife" of control charts. Finally, he makes the critical point that, although statistics can be enormously helpful in driving process change and ultimately improving care, they must be applied to specific questions and problems. As he rightly states, "vague solutions to vague problems yield vague results."

The last 25 years have seen an explosion in the variety of tools, measures, and applications that can be used to drive performance in healthcare, along with a concomitant increase in the evaluation and analysis of physicians in multiple domains. In chapter 6, Bettina Berman and Richard Jacoby expertly tease out physician profiling and provider registries. They offer a comprehensive background on the genesis of profiling and registries, ultimately showing how their use spurs physicians to take a leading role in quality improvement. Berman and Jacoby explain the impact of value-based purchasing programs, the Medicare Access and CHIP Reauthorization Act (MACRA), and the Merit-Based Incentive Payment System (MIPS), as well as the efforts by private insurers to provide incentives for high quality and disincentives for poor performance.

Berman and Jacoby provide examples of various profiles and report cards, and they review the concept of benchmarking. Finally, they talk about the challenging but important aspects of profile development, including choosing the measures, collecting the data, interpreting the data, and disseminating the findings. The authors highlight many of the challenges to using profiles to drive change but point out that, ultimately, these tools are now a permanent part of the healthcare landscape.

The staggering pace of growth in information technology (IT) in healthcare represents a tremendous opportunity to improve the quality and safety of care provided across the country. The conundrum, however, is how to leverage emerging and existing technologies in ways that drive performance rather than clouding the landscape. In chapter 7, Sue S. Feldman, Scott E. Buchalter, and Leslie W. Hayes describe how healthcare organizations use healthcare IT in a three-part cycle of prevention, identification, and action. They report that these elements must form an ongoing cycle with no distinct beginning or end point—rather only an "insertion point."

The authors describe how IT can be used to prevent quality and safety problems through the use of checklists or clinical decision support tools such as alerts, guidelines, order sets, templates, and diagnostic support. They also convey the importance of IT's role in the initial identification of issues of quality, safety, or both. The opportunity for sophisticated algorithms and programs to recognize potential problems across systems is vastly improved with powerful applications. Finally, and importantly, the authors provide examples and case studies of how care can be improved with the appropriate use of specific IT solutions.

In chapter 8, Hyunjoo Lee and Dimitrios Papanagnou round out this part of the book with an overview of how simulation can be used to improve healthcare quality and safety. In particular, they highlight simulation's "intrinsic ability to expose, inform, and improve behaviors that are critical for effective communication and teamwork." The authors ground readers by providing an overview of the terminology specific to simulation and then describe the evolution of simulation, from the earliest cadaveric dissections reported by the Greeks to current-day technologies.

Lee and Papanagnou clarify the key point that simulation facilitates a paradigm shift away from the possibility of learners inflicting harm on patients. The authors also discuss how educational frameworks are applied to simulations, including the implications of adult-style learning, progression to higher levels of clinical assessment, and the importance of debriefing. Finally, they review the importance of team training and explain how crew resource management (CRM), a concept pulled from aviation and the military, has had a significant impact on improving safety in healthcare.

The chapters in part II provide a comprehensive examination of the measures, tools, and technologies that are needed to improve quality and safety in healthcare moving forward.

CHAPTER

4

DATA COLLECTION

John Byrnes

Data provide the foundation for quality and patient safety. Without data, improved performance is virtually impossible. Everywhere you turn, people want data. What do the data really mean? Where do you get data? Is chart review the gold standard, the best source? Are administrative databases reliable? Can they be the gold standard? What about health plan claims databases—are they accurate? What is the best source for inpatient data that reflect the quality of patient care from both a process and an outcome perspective? When working in the outpatient environment, where and how would you obtain data that reflect the level of quality delivered in physician office practices? These and other questions pose challenges for healthcare leaders as they try to develop quality measurement programs. This chapter will clarify these issues and common industry myths, and it will provide a practical framework for obtaining valid, accurate, and useful data for quality and patient safety improvement.

Considerations in Data Collection

Categories of Data: A Case Example

Data collected for quality measurements can be grouped into four categories or domains: (1) clinical quality (including both process and outcome measures); (2) financial performance; (3) patient, physician, and staff satisfaction; and (4) functional status. To report on each of these categories, one might need to collect data from several separate sources. The challenge is to collect as many data elements from as few data sources as possible, with the objectives of consistency and continuity in mind. For most large and mature quality improvement projects, teams will want to report their organization's performance in all four domains.

The clinical reporting (CR) system used by the author can serve as a case example to demonstrate the collection of data across the various categories. The CR system includes numerous disease- and procedure-specific dashboards—as shown in exhibit 4.1—that report performance at the system, hospital, and physician levels. Exhibit 4.2 shows one of the dashboards—for total knee replacement—which contains examples of clinical quality and financial performance measures.

To produce the CR system, our team used a variety of data sources, including extracts from finance and electronic health record (EHR) systems; applied a series of rigorous data-cleanup algorithms; adjusted for severity; and added industry benchmarks. The resulting report contains measures of clinical processes (e.g., antibiotic utilization, deep vein thrombosis prophylaxis, beta-blocker administration, autologous blood collection, blood product administration), financial performance (e.g., length of stay, total patient charges, pharmacy charges, lab charges, X-ray charges, intravenous therapy charges), and clinical outcomes (e.g., complications, readmissions, mortality, length of stay). From the more than 200 indicators available in the database, the team selected the measures deemed most important for assessing the quality and cost of care delivered. The team also included some Joint Commission core measures.[1]

To obtain patient experience information, we often use industry-standard patient experience surveys. An outbound call center administers the surveys by

EXHIBIT 4.1
Clinical Dashboards for High-Volume, High-Cost Medical Conditions and Surgical Procedures

Acute myocardial infarction (AMI)	Cervical fusion
Percutaneous coronary intervention (PCI)	Discectomy
Congestive heart failure (CHF)	Bariatrics—open and laparoscopic
Defibrillator	Colorectal surgeries—open and laparoscopic
Pacemaker placement	Diabetic emergencies
Pneumonia	Sepsis
Normal delivery	Respiratory failure
C-section	Chronic obstructive pulmonary disease (COPD)
Coronary artery bypass	Pulmonary embolism
Valve replacement	Deep vein thrombosis (DVT)
Transcatheter aortic valve replacement (TAVR)	Bowel obstruction
Cerebrovascular accident (CVA)—ischemic	Small intestinal resection
CVA—hemorrhagic	Esophageal and stomach surgery
Cranial neurosurgery	Gastrointestinal (GI) bleed
Total knee replacement	Pancreatitis
Total hip replacement	Prostate resection
Hip fracture repair	Transurethral resection of the prostate (TURP)
Total abdominal hysterectomy (TAH)—cancer	Abdominal aortic aneurysm (AAA)
TAH—noncancer	Carcinoembryonic antigen (CEA)
Vaginal hysterectomy	Peripheral vascular bypass
Cholecystectomy	Pediatric asthma
Lumbar fusion	Appendectomy
Lumbar laminectomy	Respiratory syncytial virus (RSV)/bronchiolitis

EXHIBIT 4.2
Clinical Dashboard for Total Knee Replacement

Administrative Data		Process											
Name	No. of Patients	Avg. Severity*	Average Age	1st Generation Cephalosporin	Vancomycin	Clindamycin	Coumadin	LMW Heparin	Coumadin or LMW Heparin	DVT/PE Rx (Minus Cellsaver)	DVT/PE SCD	DVT/PE RX & SCD	DVT Proph (Minus Cellsaver)
		1.65	65.8	90.4%	8.2%	5.1%	9.0%	82.7%	85.3%	85.6%	96.2%	82.3%	99.5%
		1.77	65.8	95.2%	13.1%	0.4%	6.8%	98.8%	99.2%	99.6%	98.0%	97.6%	100.0%
		1.67	65.8	91.1%	8.9%	4.4%	8.7%	85.1%	87.3%	87.6%	96.5%	84.5%	99.5%

* APR-DRG Average Severity of Illness (SOI) is calculated for inpatients only.

Administrative Data		Process				Outcome						
Name	No. of Patients	Beta Blocker	Autologous Blood Collected	Blood Product Given	Knee Revision	Hemorrhage	AMI as 2nd DX	Accidental Puncture or Laceration	AccPuncLac (Not Present on Admission)	UTI	UTI (Not Present on Admission)	Discharge to Home
		36.9%	0.0%	9.2%	10.8%	0.1%	0.1%	0.1%	0.1%	1.5%	0.7%	73.7%
		35.5%	0.0%	16.7%	6.0%	0.4%	0.8%	0.4%	0.4%	2.8%	1.6%	76.9%
		36.7%	0.0%	10.3%	10.1%	0.2%	0.2%	0.1%	0.1%	1.7%	0.9%	74.1%

Administrative Data		Outcome										
Name	No. of Patients	DVT	DVT (Not Present on Admission)	PE	PE (Not Present on Admission)	Sepsis as 2nd DX	Sepsis as 2nd DX (Not Present on Admission)	Unplanned Readmit 30 Days	Mortality	Mortality exc. Palliative Care	LOS	Health Grades Major Complicatons
		0.7%	0.6%	0.5%	0.5%	0.1%	0.0%	3.8%	0.0%	0.0%	3.73	3.4%
		1.2%	1.2%	1.2%	1.2%	1.2%	1.2%	2.4%	0.4%	0.0%	3.84	6.4%
		0.8%	0.7%	0.6%	0.6%	0.3%	0.2%	3.6%	0.1%	0.0%	3.74	3.9%

National Quality Measures* - Surgical Care Improvement Project							
Name	No. of Patients	Preop Dose (SCIP-INF-1e)		Antibiotic Selection (SCIP-INF-2e)		Post-op Duration (SCIP-INF-3e)	
	Varies	98.7%	n=226	99.6%	n=228	98.6%	n=220

*The number of patients included varies based on the measure.

Administrative Data		Joint Commission	
Name	No. of Patients	Acute Renal Failure	Ambulation 150 ft.
	1,482	0.6%	56.3%
	251	3.2%	70.5%
	1,733	1.0%	58.4%

Administrative Data		Direct Costs									
Name	No. of Patients	ICU Cost	Laboratory Cost	OR Cost	Pharmacy Cost	Radiology Cost	R&B Cost	Supplies Cost	Therapy Cost	Other Cost	Total Cost
		$25	$140	$2,676	$464	$90	$1,913	$5,157	$416	$67	$10,948
		$368	$172	$1,974	$355	$129	$1,700	$3,505	$468	$147	$8,818
		$75	$145	$2,574	$448	$96	$1,882	$4,918	$423	$78	$10,639

Administrative Data		Fully Allocated Costs									
Name	No. of Patients	ICU Cost	Laboratory Cost	OR Cost	Pharmacy Cost	Radiology Cost	R&B Cost	Supplies Cost	Therapy Cost	Other Cost	Total Cost
		$36	$207	$4,101	$693	$148	$2,991	$7,497	$612	$96	$16,382
		$569	$261	$2,964	$512	$203	$2,850	$5,241	$697	$214	$13,509
		$113	$215	$3,937	$667	$156	$2,971	$7,170	$624	$113	$15,966

Administrative Data		Potential Direct Cost Savings													
Name	No. of Patients	Hemorrhage		AMI as 2nd DX		DVT		DVT (Not Present on Admission)		PE		PE (Not Present on Admission)		Acute Renal Failure (Not Present on Admission)	
	Varies	($3,460)	n = 2	($93)	n = 1	$14,911	n = 10	$16,359	n = 9	$17,849	n=7	$17,849	n=7	$59,597	n=9
	Varies	$31,302	n = 1	$116,439	n = 2	$91,300	n = 3	$91,300	n = 3	$6,616	n=3	$6,616	n=3	$132,074	n=8
	Varies	$26,564	n = 3	$112,279	n = 3	$103,416	n = 13	$104,504	n = 12	$21,118	n=10	$21,118	n=10	$177,042	n=17

Administrative Data		Potential Direct Cost Savings												
Name	No. of Patients	Accidental Puncture or Laceration		Accidental Puncture or Laceration (NPOA)		UTI		UTI (Not Present on Admission)		Sepsis as 2nd Dx		Sepsis as 2nd Dx (Not Present on Admission)		Total Cost (Patients Above Average)
	Varies	$8,157	n = 1	$8,157	n = 1	$14,898	n = 22	$4,542	n = 11	$14,419	n = 2	$0	n = 0	$1,587,936
	Varies	$31,302	n = 1	$31,302	n = 1	$14,674	n = 7	$14,776	n = 4	$124,315	n = 3	$124,315	n = 3	$266,353
	Varies	$37,860	n = 2	$37,860	n = 2	$23,371	n = 29	$15,289	n = 15	$132,766	n = 5	$117,569	n = 3	$1,935,421

telephone within one week of a patient's discharge. The results can be reported by nursing unit or physician, are updated monthly, and can be charted over the past eight quarters.

To complete the measurement set, we include results concerning patients' functional status (following their treatments). This information can be obtained from patients' EHRs (if the desired information has been included) or through the use of survey tools during follow-up visits. Many hospital procedures are performed to improve patients' functional status. A patient who undergoes a total knee replacement, for example, should experience less knee pain when walking, have a good range of joint motion, and be able to perform activities of daily living that most of us take for granted.

In summary, quality improvement teams need to maintain a balanced perspective of the process of care through collection of data in all four categories: clinical quality, financial performance, patient experience, and functional status. Teams that fail to maintain this balance risk overlooking critical information. For instance, one health system in the Southwest initially reported that it had completed a series of successful quality improvement projects. Clinical care had improved, patient experience was at an all-time high, and patient outcomes were at national benchmark levels. However, subsequent review revealed that some of the interventions had negatively affected the system's financial outcomes. Several interventions had led to a significant decrease in revenue, and others had increased the cost of care. If financial measures had been included in the reporting process, the negative financial effect could have been minimized, and the same outstanding quality improvements could have resulted. In the end, the projects were considered only marginally successful because they lacked a balanced approach to process improvement and measurement.

Time and Cost Involved in Data Collection

All data collection efforts take time and money. The key is to balance the time and cost of data collection with the value of the data to your improvement efforts. In other words, is the collection of data worth the effort? Will the data have the power to drive change and improvement? Although this cost–benefit analysis might not be as tangible in healthcare as it is in the world of business and finance, the value equation still must be considered.

Generally, medical record review and prospective data collection are considered the most time-intensive and expensive ways to collect information. Many organizations reserve these methods for highly specialized improvement projects or use them to answer questions that have surfaced following review of administrative data sets. Administrative data[2] are often regarded as more cost-effective, especially because the credibility of administrative databases has improved and continues to improve as a result of coding and billing regulations and initiatives,[3] as well as rule-based software development. Additionally, third-party vendors can provide data cleanup and severity adjustment. Successful data collection strategies often combine both coded and chart-based sources into a data collection plan that capitalizes on the strengths and cost-effectiveness of each.

The following scenario illustrates how the cost-effective information from an administrative system can be combined with the detailed information available in a medical record review. A data analyst using a clinical decision support system (an administrative database) discovered a higher-than-expected incidence of renal failure (a serious complication) following coronary artery bypass surgery. The rate was well above 10 percent for the most recent 12 months (more than 800 patients were included in the data set) and had slowly increased over the past six quarters. However, the clinical decision support system did not contain enough detail to explain why such a large number of patients were experiencing this complication—whether the complication resulted from the coronary artery bypass graft procedure or was a chronic condition present on admission. To find the answer, the data analyst used chart review (1) to verify that the rate of renal failure as reported in the administrative data system was correct, (2) to isolate cases of postoperative incidence, (3) to identify the root cause(s) of the renal failure, and (4) to answer additional questions about the patient population that were of interest to the physicians involved in the patients' care. In this example, the analyst used the administrative system to identify unwanted complications in a large patient population (a screening or surveillance function) and reserved chart review for a much smaller, focused study (80 charts) to validate the incidence and determine why the patients were experiencing the complication.

Collecting the Critical Few Rather Than Collecting for a Rainy Day

Many quality improvement efforts collect every possible data element just in case such an element might be needed. This syndrome of stockpiling "just in case" as opposed to fulfilling requirements "just in time" has been studied in the field of supply chain management and has proved to be ineffective and inefficient, while also contributing to quality issues (Denison 2002). In short, it is one of the biggest mistakes a quality improvement team can make. Rather than provide a rich source of information, this approach unnecessarily drives up the cost of data collection, slows the data collection process, creates data management issues, and overwhelms the quality improvement team with too much information.

Quality improvement teams should collect only the data required to identify and correct quality issues. As a rule, in ongoing data collection efforts, the team should be able to link every data element collected to a report, thereby ensuring that teams do not collect data that will not be used (James 2003).

In the clinical reporting project from the case example earlier in the chapter, the hospital team was limited to selecting no more than 15 measures for each clinical condition. It also selected indicators that (1) had been shown by evidence-based literature to have the greatest effect on patient outcomes (e.g., for congestive heart failure, the use of angiotensin-converting enzyme

[ACE] inhibitors and beta blockers and evaluation of left ventricular ejection fraction); (2) reflected areas in which significant improvements were needed; (3) would be reported in the public domain (e.g., Joint Commission core measures, Leapfrog patient safety measures, and Healthgrades complication and mortality rates); and (4) together provided a balanced view of the clinical process of care, financial performance, and patient outcomes.

Inpatient Versus Outpatient Data

The distinction between inpatient and outpatient data is an important concern for planning the data collection process, because the data sources and approaches to data collection for the two types can be different.

Consider, for instance, the case of a team working on a diabetes disease-management project. First, disease-management projects tend to focus on the entire continuum of care, so the team needs data from both inpatient and outpatient settings. Second, the team needs to identify whether patients receive the majority of care in one setting or the other, and it needs to decide whether data collection priorities should be established with a particular setting in mind. For diabetes, the outpatient setting has the greatest influence on patient outcomes, so collection of outpatient data is a priority. Third, the team must select measures that reflect the aspects of care that have the greatest influence on patient outcomes. Aware of the need to collect only the "critical few" (as discussed in the previous section), the team would consult the American Diabetes Association guidelines for expert direction. Fourth, the team must recognize that the sources of outpatient data are much different from the sources of inpatient data and that outpatient data tend to be more fragmented and harder to obtain. However, with the advent of outpatient EHRs and patient registries, the ease of outpatient data collection is improving.

To identify outpatient data sources, the team should consider the following questions:

- Are the physicians in organized medical groups that have outpatient EHRs? Can their financial or billing systems identify all patients with diabetes in their practices? If not, can the health plans in the area supply the data by practice site or individual physician?
- Some of the most important diabetes measures are based on laboratory testing. Do the physicians have their own labs? If so, do they archive the lab data for a 12- to 24-month snapshot? If they do not do their own lab testing, do they use a common reference lab that would be able to supply the data?

Once the team answers these questions, it will be ready to proceed with data collection in the outpatient setting.

Sources of Data

The sources of data for quality improvement projects are extensive. Some sources are simple to access, whereas others require a complex undertaking; likewise, some data sources are relatively cheap to use, whereas others are expensive.

In the average hospital or health system, data sources include medical records, prospective data collection, surveys of various types, telephone interviews, focus groups, administrative databases, health plan claims databases, cost accounting systems, patient registries, stand-alone clinical databases, EHRs, and lab and pharmacy databases.

The following objectives are essential for any quality improvement project or data collection initiative:

- Identify the purpose of the data measurement activity (e.g., for monitoring at regular intervals, for investigation over a limited period, for a onetime study).
- Identify data sources that are most appropriate for the activity.
- Identify the most important measures to collect (i.e., the critical few).
- Design a common-sense strategy that will ensure collection of complete, accurate, and timely information.

By following these steps, project teams will gather actionable data and the information needed to drive quality improvements.

Medical Record Review (Retrospective)

Retrospective data collection involves identification and selection of a patient's medical record or group of records after the patient has been discharged from the hospital or clinic. Records generally cannot be reviewed until all medical and financial coding is complete, because codes are used as a starting point for identifying the study cohort.

Quality improvement projects may depend on medical record review for a variety of reasons. First, many proponents of medical record review believe it to be the most accurate method of data collection. They believe that, because administrative databases have been designed for financial and administrative purposes rather than for quality improvement, the databases contain inadequate detail, numerous errors, and "dirty data"—that is, data that make no sense or appear to have come from different sources.

Second, some improvement projects rely on data elements that are available from medical record review but not from administrative databases. For example, most administrative databases do not contain measures that require a time stamp, such as administration of antibiotics within one hour before surgical incision.

Third, several national quality improvement database projects—including the Healthcare Effectiveness Data and Information Set (HEDIS), Joint Commission core measures, Leapfrog Hospital Survey,[4] and National Quality Forum (NQF)[5] National Voluntary Consensus Standards for Hospital Care—depend on retrospective medical record review for a significant portion of the data elements required to be reported. The medical records not only contain measures that require a time stamp; they are also useful for measures that require the data collector to include or exclude patients on the basis of criteria that are not captured consistently in administrative databases. The percentage of patients with congestive heart failure (CHF) who are receiving an ACE inhibitor is one example of this type of measure. The use of an ACE inhibitor is indicated for all CHF patients with an ejection fraction of less than 40 percent, but the ejection fraction is not part of the typical administrative database. Sometimes this information is contained in a generally inaccessible, stand-alone database in the cardiology department; other times it is contained only in a transcribed report in the patient's medical record. Hence, accurate reporting of this measure, one of the most critical interventions that a patient with CHF will receive, depends completely on retrospective chart review. (NQF [2018] suggests that clinical importance should rate foremost among criteria for evaluating measures and that measures scoring poorly on feasibility[6] because of the burden of medical record review should not be excluded if their clinical importance is high.)

Fourth, focused medical record review is the primary tool for answering the "why" of given situations (e.g., why patients are experiencing a particular complication, why a certain intervention negatively affects patient outcomes).

Medical record review continues to be a key component of many data collection projects, but it needs to be used judiciously because of the time and cost involved. The best approach to medical record review involves a series of well-conceived steps, beginning with the development of a data collection tool and ending with the compilation of collected data elements into a registry or electronic database for review and analysis.

Prospective Data Collection

Prospective data collection also relies on medical record review, but it is completed during a patient's hospitalization or visit rather than retrospectively. The data are sometimes collected by nursing staff, although data collection can be time-consuming and may distract nurses from their direct patient care responsibilities. A better approach is to hire research assistants or full-time data analysts to collect and analyze the data. Because these individuals would have data collection and analysis as their primary responsibility, the accuracy would be greater. Also, if these individuals are responsible for presenting their analyses to various quality committees, they are likely to review the data more rigorously.

Obviously, this method of data collection is expensive, but if staff can minimize the time required for data entry, it can focus on accuracy and analysis/

reporting. One way to save time is by converting the data collection forms into a format that can be scanned. With this approach, data entry can be as simple as feeding the forms into a scanner and viewing the results on a computer screen. Successful execution hinges on careful design of the forms and careful completion, to ensure that the scanner captures all data elements. Alternatively, data collection forms can be developed for tablet technologies that automatically download the collected data to project databases. The most efficient data collection tools follow the actual flow of patient care and medical record documentation, whether the data are collected retrospectively or prospectively.

Prospective data collection has numerous advantages. First, it allows for the gathering of detailed information that is not routinely available from administrative databases. It can capture physiologic parameters, such as the range of blood pressures for a patient on vasoactive infusions or 24-hour intake and output for patients with heart failure. As noted earlier, it can also capture data requiring a time stamp. Timely administration of certain therapies (e.g., administration of antibiotics within one hour before surgical incision or within eight hours of hospital arrival for patients with pneumonia) has been shown to improve patient outcomes. The timing of "clot buster" administration to certain stroke patients can mean the difference between full recovery and no recovery, and the window of opportunity for these patients is small; they usually must receive thrombolytic therapy within three hours of symptom onset. For patients with acute myocardial infarction (AMI), the administration of aspirin and beta blockers within the first 24 hours is critical to survival.

Through prospective chart review, the data collection staff can spot patient trends as they develop rather than receive information after patients have been discharged. For instance, staff members may detect an increasing incidence of ventilator-associated pneumonia sooner, or they may spot an increase in the rate of aspiration in stroke patients as it occurs.

Unfortunately, the downside to prospective data collection is that it is costly and time consuming and often requires healthcare organizations to hire several full-time data analysts.

Administrative Databases

Administrative databases are a common source of data for quality improvement projects. Administrative data—including enrollment or eligibility information, claims information, and information about managed care encounters—are collected, processed, and stored in automated information systems. These data may relate to hospital and other facility services, professional services, prescription drug services, or laboratory services.

Examples of administrative data sources include hospital and physician office billing systems, health plan claims databases, health information management and medical record systems, and registration systems (for admission/discharge/transfer). Ideally, hospitals also maintain a cost accounting system that integrates the previously mentioned systems into a single database and provides the important elements of patient cost. Although each of these sources has unique characteristics, for the purposes of this discussion they will be considered collectively as administrative databases (with the exception of health plan claims databases, which are covered later in this chapter).

Administrative databases are an excellent source of data for reporting on clinical quality, financial performance, and certain patient outcomes. They are the backbone of many quality improvement programs, including the CR system described in the case example at the beginning of this chapter. The use of administrative databases is advantageous for the following reasons:

- They are less expensive to use, compared to alternative methods such as chart review or prospective data collection.
- They incorporate transaction systems already used in a healthcare organization's daily business operations (frequently referred to as *legacy systems*).
- Most code sets embedded in administrative databases are standardized,[7] simplifying internal comparison for multifacility organizations and external benchmarking with purchased or government data sets.
- Most administrative databases are maintained by individuals who are skilled at sophisticated database queries.
- Expert database administrators in information technology (IT) departments provide database architecture and support.
- The volume of available indicators is 100 times greater than that available through other data collection techniques.
- Data reporting tools are available as part of the purchased system or through third-party add-ons or services.
- Many administrative databases, especially well-managed financial and cost accounting systems, are subject to regular reconciliation, audit, and data cleanup procedures that enhance the integrity of their data.

Because of these advantages, many healthcare organizations use administrative data systems as the primary source for quality improvement projects.

This author typically uses two administrative data sources: the billing system and the medical record system. Information from these sources is extracted and subjected to extensive cleanup, and severity adjustment, statistical analysis, and benchmarks are applied. Using this approach, more than 50 of the most common clinical conditions (medical and surgical procedures) and at least 100 measures of clinical quality, financial performance, and patient outcomes are available for each condition. The decision support system contains a total of more than 5,000 standardized performance measures, with functionality to report performance at the system level, by individual hospital, by individual physician, by resident, and by nursing unit. The database can be updated daily, and historical data can be archived in its data warehouse for future quality improvement projects and clinical studies. The yearly cost to maintain this system is approximately $300,000—the equivalent of four to five data analysts' combined salaries—yet the system's reporting power surpasses anything that five analysts performing chart review would be able to accomplish. The system is a good value proposition because successful implementation of one or two quality improvement projects carefully selected from the many opportunities identified by the system can reimburse its full cost. For example, one of the first projects identified by the system addressed the need to improve blood product utilization. The savings realized as a result of this project were more than sufficient to cover the cost of the system for the first year.

A common criticism is that administrative data are less reliable than data gathered by chart review. However, when administrative data are properly cleaned and validated, when the indicator definitions are clear and concise, and when the limitations of the data are understood, they can be just as reliable as data from chart review. These conditions are central to the commercial outcome reporting systems available today. For example, the most common measures from the CR system described earlier in the chapter were validated using four approaches: (1) chart review with an appropriate sampling methodology, (2) chart review performed for the core measures, (3) comparison to similar measures in stand-alone databases that rely on chart abstraction or prospective data collection strategies (e.g., the National Registry of Myocardial Infarction), and (4) face validation performed by physicians with expertise in the clinical condition being studied. Results proved the administrative data sources to be just as reliable as chart review data. In fact, if systems (e.g., third-party audits) are not in place to ensure interrater reliability, chart review data can be highly inaccurate.

Patient Surveys: Satisfaction and Functional Status

Patient Experience Surveys

Patient experience surveys have long been a favorite tool of quality improvement professionals, especially those interested in the perceptions of patients, either in terms of the quality of care or the quality of service provided. However, the use of surveys to produce valid, reliable, relevant information is both an art and a science, and underestimation of the scientific complexity involved can lead to undesirable results. In addition, survey validation itself is a complicated and time-consuming undertaking. This section will provide a brief overview of the use of surveys; for more detailed information about survey development and validation—and discussion of the concepts of reliability, validity, sampling methodology, and bias—we recommend consulting one of the many excellent textbooks focused on the subject.

When an organization or a quality improvement team is considering the use of surveys, it has several choices for how to proceed. The team can design the survey tool itself, hire an outside expert to design the survey, or purchase an existing, well-validated survey or survey service. Usually, the fastest and least-expensive approach is to purchase an existing, well-validated survey instrument or to hire a survey organization to provide a solution.

The frequency with which surveys are conducted and reported to the organization is also important. When patient experience surveys are conducted on a continual basis, using a proper sampling methodology, the organization is best able to respond rapidly to changes in patients' wants and needs. It also can respond quickly to instances of poor service.

The ability to report survey results at an actionable level is critical; in most cases, *actionable level* means the specific nursing unit or location of service. Furthermore, full engagement at the management and support staff levels is important to ensuring that results are regularly reviewed and action plans are developed.

The point-of-service patient experience surveys at Lovelace Health System in the late 1990s provide an example of a successful survey project. During the project, any patient who received care within the system was able to comment on the quality of the care and service immediately following the encounter. The survey forms were concise (one page) and easy to read, and patients could complete them in a few minutes. The questions assessed the most important determinants of satisfaction (as selected by the survey research staff), and patients could provide comments at the end of the survey. Unit managers collected and reviewed the surveys on a daily or weekly basis to identify emerging trends and to quickly correct negative outcomes. Survey results were tabulated monthly and posted in the units for everyone—including patients in the clinics and inpatient areas—to see. Senior management reviewed the results on a unit-by-unit basis each month.

Patient experience surveys can be administered in a variety of ways. The Lovelace project used paper surveys, which enabled clinical leaders to easily review the results at the end of the day. In addition, the paper surveys could be scanned, allowing for the data to be uploaded to the database to facilitate additional analysis and reporting. Scanners are still in use at many organizations. They provide a turnkey solution that avoids the need for IT to "build an online solution," and they can help save the organization the hundreds of thousands of dollars that a vendor-based solution might cost. Scanners get surveys up and running quickly, for minimal expense, without the high IT price tag, and without the delays that often result when IT is heavily involved.

Surveys also may be administered using online tools, tablets, and smartphone applications. Millennials and other technologically savvy patients might enjoy completing surveys in this manner. However, the data might not be available in real time, limiting the ability of clinical leaders to make changes on a day-to-day basis—the true spirit of rapid cycle improvement. In addition, many Medicare beneficiaries and less technologically savvy users may be uncomfortable completing an online survey on an iPad. In many cases, "low tech" is preferable to "high tech."

Surveys also may be conducted via telephone. In fact, many vendors prefer this approach and feel it gets a much higher response rate than mailed paper surveys or online forms do. Once again, however, data collected via phone are not immediately available to physicians and clinical managers, and the turnaround time can significantly delay improvement efforts.

Functional Status Surveys

The measurement of functional status following medical treatment is another important category of data collection for clinical quality improvement projects. As a general rule, the purpose of medical treatments and hospital procedures is to improve patients' functional status or quality of life. For example, patients hospitalized for CHF should be able to walk farther, have more energy, and experience less shortness of breath following hospital treatment. Patients who undergo total knee replacements should have less knee pain when they walk, have a good range of joint motion, and be able to perform activities of daily living such as walking several miles, dancing, doing yard work, and performing normal household chores.

Functional status is usually measured before a treatment or procedure and at several points after. For some surgical procedures, such as total joint replacement, a baseline assessment is made before the procedure and then assessments are made at regular intervals afterward—often at 1, 3, 6, and 12 months postoperatively. The survey can be collected by several means, including mail, telephone, and internet.

The most widely recognized pioneer of functional status surveys is John Ware, the principal developer of the SF-36, SF-12, SF-8, and disease-specific health outcome surveys.[8]

Health Plan Databases—A Gold Mine for Population Health Management

Health plan databases can be an excellent source of data for quality improvement projects—particularly for projects that have a population health management focus. For many years, health plans have used a variety of means to collect data on their performance, to track the management of the care received by members, and to direct programs on disease management and care management. As a result, health plan data have become more and more reliable. Most health plans now have sophisticated data warehouses and a staff of expert data analysts.

Health plan databases are valuable because they contain detailed information on all care received by plan members. They track care through bills (claims), which are generated for all services provided to a patient. When bills are submitted to the health plan for payment, they are captured in a claims processing system. As a result of this process, all care received by the population of patients—including hospitalizations, outpatient procedures, physician office visits, lab testing, and prescriptions—is documented in the health plan claims database.

Why is this process so important? From a population management perspective, the health plan claims database is often the only source of information on the care received by a patient or, for that matter, an entire population of patients. It is therefore an excellent source for disease management teams whose goal is to improve the health of a specific population. It provides a comprehensive record of patient activity and can be used to identify and select patients for enrollment in disease management programs.

Claims databases are excellent tracking tools for examining the continuum of care, and until the advent of outpatient EHRs, they were the only available external source of information on physician office practice. In essence, a claims database is the single best source of information on the total care received by a patient.

EXHIBIT 4.3
Diabetes Provider Report

Rolling Calendar Year, July 1–June 30

PCP:
Provider Group:

I. Provider-Specific Data

Criteria	ADA Standards	Points	Tested	In Standard	Percentage
Education	1/2 year	48	42	42	88
Eye exams	Annual	48	30	30	63
Hemoglobin A1C ordered	Annual	48	45	45	94
Hemoglobin A1C level	≤7.0	48	45	37	82
Microalbumin ordered	Annual	48	31	31	65
Microalbumin >30	Rx filled	10	10	5	50
LDL ordered	Annual	48	42	42	88
LDL level	<100	48	42	31	73

*Patients in this report have had at least two diagnoses of diabetes.

EXHIBIT 4.3
Diabetes Provider Report *(continued)*

II. Percentage of Patients Within Standard

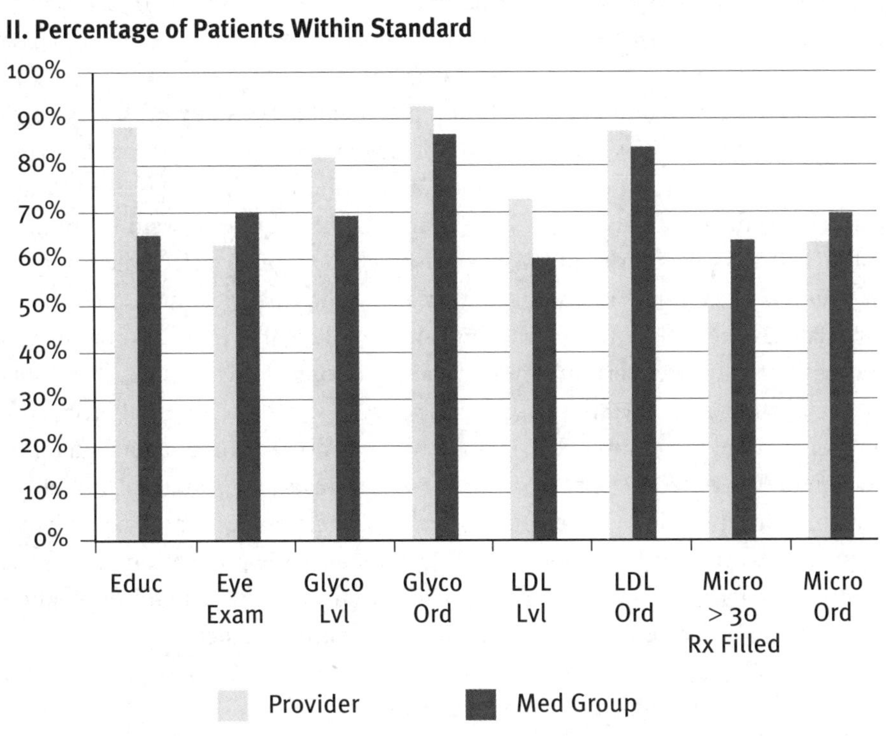

III. High-Risk Patient Detail—Patients Outside ADA Standards in Current Quarter

Criteria for inclusion - one or more of the following: 1) no education in past 24 months; 2) no eye exam in past 12 months; 3) Hemoglobin A1C > 7.0 or no Hgb A1C ordered in past 12 months; 4) no microalbumin in past 12 months; 5) microalbumin > 30 and no ACE/ARB filled; or 6) LDL > 100 or no LDL ordered in past 12 months.

Name	MR#	Phone #	email	Education	Eye Exam	Hgb A1C		Microalbumin		LDL	
						Ordered	Result	Ordered	> 30, Rx filled	Ordered	Result
Patient	#########	#########	#########	8/12/17	8/12/17	8/13/17	7	8/13/17	N	8/13/17	120
Patient	#########	#########	#########	7/12/17	1/12/17	7/12/17	7.3			8/13/17	132
Patient	#########	#########	#########	N	1/23/16		10.6	8/13/17	Y	8/14/17	166
Patient	#########	#########	#########	N	N		11.3			8/15/17	145
Patient	#########	#########	#########	N	N		12.4			8/16/17	150

Note: ADA = American Diabetes Association.
LDL = Low-density lipoprotein.
Source: J. Byrnes.

Health plan databases commonly are used to identify patients who have not received preventive services such as mammograms, colon cancer screening, and immunizations, or who are not receiving appropriate medications for chronic conditions such as heart failure and asthma. They also can be used to support physicians in their office practices.

Exhibit 4.3 provides an example of a report[9] for a diabetes disease management program. It provides participating physicians with a quarterly snapshot of (1) the percentage of their patients who are receiving all treatments and tests recommended by American Diabetes Association (ADA) guidelines, (2) the performance of individual physicians relative to that of their peers, and (3) all patients whose treatment has not met ADA standards in the previous quarter and who need recommended tests or treatments.

What are the limitations of health plan databases? Many of the concerns associated with hospitals' administrative databases apply to health plan databases as well, including questions of accuracy, detail, and timeliness. Users of health plan claims databases also must keep in mind that changes to reimbursement rules (and the provider's response to those changes) may affect the integrity of the data over time. Recoding may make some historical data inaccurate, especially as they relate to the tracking and trending of complication rates and the categorization of certain types of complications.

Furthermore, health plan databases track events, the types of procedure performed, and the completion of lab tests. They do not contain detailed information on the outcomes of care or the results of tests (e.g., lab tests, radiology examinations, biopsies). Nevertheless, health plan claims data are inexpensive to acquire, are available electronically, and encompass large populations across the continuum of care. Used properly, they are a rich source of data for population management, disease management, and quality improvement.

Patient (Specialty-Specific) Registries

Patient registries can be a powerful source of quality improvement data, especially for more sophisticated projects. Registries offer a straightforward design and the capacity for a high level of detail, and they may include data collected through all of the aforementioned approaches. Many organizations are driven to develop registries because they lack reliable sources of timely clinical information or wish to collect patient outcome information over several months following a hospitalization or procedure.

Patient registries are specialty or procedure specific. Common conditions and procedures for which specific registries are created include AMI, total joint replacement, coronary artery bypass graft, and CHF.

Patient registry use is advantageous for the following reasons:

- The registries are customized to serve as a rich source of information.
- They can collect all the data that the physician or health system considers most important.
- They can be used for quality improvement and research purposes.
- They are not subject to the shortcomings of administrative and health plan databases.
- They can combine a multitude of data sources and collection techniques to provide a complete picture of the patient experience, including the quality of care provided and long-term patient outcomes (often up to a year following the procedure).

Patient registries are versatile and flexible because they can be populated through just about any reliable data source or collection methodology, including administrative data, outbound call centers, prospective data collection, retrospective chart review, and various survey instruments (particularly those used to assess patient experience and functional status). However, with database projects, the volume of data collected, the insight they will provide, and the change they will drive must be weighed against the cost of collecting them. A team overseeing a registry must collect only the data necessary to the success of its project.

In-Home and Wearable Technology

With the continued evolution of digital technologies, data collection has become easier and more cost effective within a patient's home environment. For instance, patients with CHF can routinely monitor their daily weight using a scale at home that stores and reports the results. People are increasingly comfortable using glucometers at home. (I even use one for our dog, Tucker, who requires twice-daily insulin injections.) Wearable technology can do much more than just measure the number of steps we take in a day. Bracelets and finger sensors currently available can easily measure and report glucose levels. The continued development and improvement of in-home and wearable technologies are sure to have a major impact on data collection and quality improvement in the years ahead.

Conclusion: Returning to the Case Example

This chapter has described categories of data, key considerations for data collection, and the variety of data sources and data collection approaches from which healthcare organizations and quality improvement teams may choose. Rarely does one method serve all purposes, so teams need to understand the advantages and disadvantages of each option.

For an application of these concepts in a present-day hospital setting, recall the CR system introduced in the case example at the start of the chapter. It consists of a data mart assembled from a variety of sources and more than 50 disease-specific dashboards. The most commonly used reports include a clinical dashboard with health system–level and hospital-level data, as well as physician-level reports. Ideally, the executive leadership team and medical directors will review the executive dashboard monthly, and the relevant information will also be shared with the hospital quality committee and the board quality committee. The physician-level reports can contain any of the indicators in the database, including indicators generated for the hospital-level dashboard, and the information can be shared at medical staff or peer review committees. The data are adjusted for severity, to clearly identify patients considered "sicker" at hospital admission. The presentation format is similar to that of the hospital dashboard.

Such an approach, like all successful quality improvement initiatives, uses a combination of data and collection techniques, capitalizing on the strengths and minimizing the weaknesses of each. Understanding how to apply these concepts, with knowledge of the various data sources and techniques, will help you use data more effectively and efficiently in your own quality improvement efforts.

Notes

1. The Joint Commission core measures were developed as an initial attempt to integrate outcomes and performance measurement into the accreditation process by requiring hospitals to collect and submit 25 measures distributed across five core measurement areas.
2. Administrative data generally reflect the content of discharge abstracts (e.g., patient demographic information such as age, sex, and zip code; information about the episode of care, such as admission source, length of stay, charges, and discharge status; diagnostic and procedural codes). The Uniform Hospital Discharge Data Set and the Uniform Bill of the Centers for Medicare & Medicaid Services provide specifications for the abstraction of administrative/billing data.
3. Examples include the Health Insurance Portability and Accountability Act (HIPAA) of 1996 (Public Law 104-191); the International Classification of Diseases, developed by the World Health Organization; the Systematized Nomenclature of Medicine (SNOMED) project; and the Unified Medical Language System.
4. The Leapfrog Group is a coalition of more than 140 public and private organizations that provide healthcare benefits. It was created to help save lives and reduce preventable medical mistakes by mobilizing employer purchasing power to initiate breakthrough improvements in the safety of healthcare and by giving consumers information so that they can make better-informed hospital choices.
5. NQF is a private, not-for-profit membership organization created to develop and implement a national strategy for healthcare quality measurement and reporting. Its mission is to improve US healthcare through endorsement of consensus-based national standards for measurement and public reporting of healthcare performance data that provide meaningful information about whether care is safe, timely, effective, patient centered, equitable, and efficient.

6. Feasibility implies that the cost of data collection and reporting is justified by the potential improvements in care and outcomes that result from the act of measurement.
7. The Uniform Hospital Discharge Data Set standardizes the abstraction of administrative/billing data, including admission source, charges (national revenue codes), discharge status, and diagnostic and procedural codes.
8. For a description of available surveys, visit https://campaign.optum.com/optum-outcomes.html.
9. This report was developed as part of a diabetes collaborative. Lovelace Health System developed the original design in Albuquerque, New Mexico, as part of the Episode of Care Disease Management Program.

Study Questions

1. What are the notable advantages and disadvantages of using medical records as opposed to administrative sources for collecting quality data?
2. Give two examples of projects in which you have used a balanced set of measures from all four domains.
3. Have electronic health records (EHRs) improved data collection? Why or why not?

Acknowledgments

Special thanks go to Lori Anderson for her diligent review, suggestions, and contributions, as well as to Monica Carpenter for her editorial assistance.

Additional Resources

Byrnes, J. 2015. *The Quality Playbook: A Step-by-Step Guide for Healthcare Leaders.* Bozeman, MT: Second River Healthcare.

Byrnes, J., and S. Teman. 2018. *The Safety Playbook: A Healthcare Leader's Guide to Building a High-Reliability Organization.* Chicago: Health Administration Press.

Carey, R. G., and R. C. Lloyd. 2001. *Measuring Quality Improvement in Healthcare: A Guide to Statistical Process Control Applications.* Milwaukee, WI: ASQ Quality Press.

Eddy, D. M. 1998. "Performance Measurement: Problems and Solutions." *Health Affairs* (Millwood) 17 (4): 7–25.

Fuller, S. 1998. "Practice Brief: Designing a Data Collection Process." *Journal of the American Health Information Management Association* 70 (May): 12–16.

Gunter, M., J. Byrnes, M. Shainline, and J. Lucas. 1996. "Improving Outcomes Through Disease-Specific Clinical Practice Improvement Teams: The Lovelace Episodes of Care Disease Management Program." *Journal of Outcomes Management* 3 (3): 10–17.

Iz, P. H., J. Warren, and L. Sokol. 2001. "Data Mining for Healthcare Quality, Efficiency, and Practice Support." Presented at the 34th Annual Hawaii International Conference on System Sciences (HICSS-34), January 3–6.

Lucas, J., M. J. Gunter, J. Byrnes, M. Coyle, and N. Friedman. 1995. "Integrating Outcomes Measurement into Clinical Practice Improvement Across the Continuum of Care: A Disease-Specific Episode of Care Model." *Managed Care Quarterly* 3 (2): 14–22.

Micheletti, J. A., T. J. Shlala, and C. R. Goodall. 1998. "Evaluating Performance Outcomes Measurement Systems: Concerns and Considerations." *Journal of Healthcare Quality* 20 (2): 6–12.

Mulder, C., M. Mycyk, and A. Roberts. 2003. "Data Warehousing and More." *Healthcare Informatics*, March, 6–8.

References

Denison, D. C. 2002. "On the Supply Chain, Just-in-Time Enters New Era." *Boston Globe*, May 5.

James, B. 2003. "Designing Data Systems: Advanced Training Program in Health Care Delivery Research." Presented at Intermountain Healthcare, Salt Lake City, UT.

National Quality Forum (NQF). 2018. "Measure Evaluation Criteria." Accessed October 1. www.qualityforum.org/measuring_performance/submitting_standards/measure_evaluation_criteria.aspx.

CHAPTER

5

STATISTICAL TOOLS FOR QUALITY IMPROVEMENT

Davis Balestracci

Plotting measurements over time turns out, in my view, to be one of the most powerful devices we have for systemic learning. . . . [Y]ou have to ask . . . questions that integrate and clarify aims and systems all at once. . . . When important indicators are continuously monitored, it becomes easier and easier to study the effects of innovation in real time, without deadening delays for setting up measurement systems or obsessive collections during baseline periods of inaction. Tests of change get simpler to interpret when we use time as a teacher.

—Dr. Donald Berwick, from his plenary speech "Run to Space" at the 1995 Institute for Healthcare Improvement annual forum

Introduction

In 1989, Dr. Donald Berwick published his seminal editorial "Continuous Improvement as an Ideal in Health Care," in which he suggested that industrial quality improvement methods could be applied to healthcare. He followed that work in 1991 with "Controlling Variation in Health Care: A Consultation from Walter Shewhart," which cogently uses medical situations to zero in on the true enemy of quality: *variation.* (Note: These Berwick readings, along with many other works relevant to this discussion, are included in the list of additional resources at the end of the chapter.)

What has changed in the decades since Berwick's 1989 salvo? Everything . . . and nothing. Approaches such as Six Sigma and Lean have grown in importance in the healthcare field, but the original, elegant simplicity that had advanced critical thinking about basic tools and statistical theory has largely been usurped by more cumbersome tools and rigid formal structure. In reality, only 1 to 2 percent of improvement practitioners in any field actually need advanced statistical methods. The need for good data remains a constant, but the everyday world of confusion, conflict, complexity, and chaos—caused by human variation—creates issues that can invalidate statistics as traditionally taught. Whereas statistics is generally viewed as the science of analyzing data, when applied to improvement, it becomes the art and science of collecting and analyzing data, simply and efficiently.

Contrary to conventional wisdom, clinical trial statistics and statistics for improvement are very different. In the sanitized world of a clinical trial, one has the luxury of formally controlling variation. However, that luxury does not apply to the real world—your world—in terms of any trial result's applicability, or your attempts to experiment. Applying clinical trial findings to the real world is akin to studying lions in a zoo, making conclusions, and then trying to apply these conclusions to lions in the African wild.

Consider the result of a heavily controlled clinical trial from a state-of-the-art hospital with a carefully chosen group of patients (lions). Can a result from that setting be applied to a typical hospital—or a refugee camp in Tanzania—where such control is not possible? Isn't an everyday medical environment in some ways the equivalent of the African wild, containing not only lions but also tigers, leopards, panthers, and some nasty "predators" that were kept at bay during the research? What if a random person decides to apply the result to a "non-lion"? Do the results also apply to environments that aren't specifically African? What about mountain or desert areas that contain catlike animals such as mountain lions, jaguars, bobcats, lynx, and ocelots? Myriad opportunities exist for variation to manifest on a published result when control is inevitably relinquished.

Improvement statistics are designed to deal specifically with a seemingly chaotic environment by exposing its inherent variation and then taking actions to (1) reduce the variation that is *inappropriate* and *unintended* and (2) implement variation shown serendipitously to be beneficial.

Given that this book is an introduction to improvement in healthcare quality, the main objective of this chapter is to teach a robust mind-set rather than present an overly complicated tool set. Good critical thinking is the key to effective quality improvement. The content of this chapter runs counter to a traditional academic statistics course. Although the reasons are explained—and examples should help clarify them—some readers will still struggle as I did when I was first exposed to these ideas in the late 1980s. The ubiquitous "normal distribution" and any assumption of "normality" are unnecessary for the type of statistics used in quality improvement. The additional resources at the end of the chapter present a number of classic books and articles that were most helpful to me on my professional path to learning and assimilating the surprising power of this approach.

Process-Oriented Thinking: The Context for Improvement Statistics

The key framework for the type of statistics discussed in this chapter is process-oriented thinking—the idea that everything is a process and all work is a process.

All processes have potentially measurable outputs, many of which are captured routinely. Even when something seems to operate chaotically, a process is at work. Consider this brilliant observation by Henry Neave (1990, 125–26):

> [S]ystems are unlikely to be well-defined in practice unless they are both suitable and adequate for the jobs for which they are intended, *and are written down in a way comprehensible to all involved*. . . . [T]here can be big differences between what is written down—the way the system is intended, or thought, to operate—and what actually happens. . . . If a system cannot be written down, . . . it probably functions more on the basis of whim and "gut-feel" rather than on any definable procedure. This surely implies that the variation being generated is some scale of magnitude higher than really necessary, with the resulting (by now) well-known effect on quality.

Processes have six sources of inputs—people, methods, machines, materials, measurements (e.g., data reacted to), and the environment—each of which is a contributing source of variation. For example, in the zoo lions scenario from earlier, might you reach different conclusions depending on the specific zoo (environment) in which you observed the lions? What about the variation caused by the obviously different feeding methods or diets (materials) of zoo lions compared to those in the African wild? Do you see a parallel to data, analyses, and conclusions published in clinical literature, especially with regard to the additional dangers that arise when data from small studies are blindly combined to perform a common technique known as a statistical meta-analysis?

One idea that applies throughout this entire chapter should be incorporated into your daily work as you pursue organizational improvement: *Your current processes are perfectly designed to get the results they are already getting.* Ultimately, improvement tries to close what has been identified as an undesirable gap (variation manifesting as confusion, conflict, complexity, and chaos) between how a process actually works and how it should work. How does one expose the undesirable gap and reduce its inappropriate and unintended variation to make the process more predictable? (Learn more about the concept of processes and the 13 questions to ask about a process in Balestracci's "Can We Please Stop the Guru Wars?" from the list of additional resources.)

There are three types of statistics, and they can be applied to the zoo lions scenario as follows:

- Descriptive statistics: What can I say about this specific lion (or, in healthcare, the patient)?
- Enumerative statistics: What can I say about this specific zoo's lions (or, in healthcare, a specific group of patients within a health system, department, hospital, office, diagnostic category, clinical trial, or other group)? Enumerative statistics provide the inherent framework in most academic and basic statistics courses. However, applying enumerative

statistical methods to make causal inferences is usually asking for trouble. A computer will do anything it is programmed to do, but it won't necessarily result in a valid statistical analysis (see Mills's "Data Torturing" and Balestracci's "Can You Prove Anything With Statistics?" from the list of additional resources).

- Analytic statistics (new to most readers): What can I say about the process or processes that produced both this group (sample) of lions and its results? In healthcare, this type involves answering *how*—though not necessarily *why*—these particular patients were chosen, studying their resulting outcomes from a process of care, then making predictions for a future unknown group of patients. Analytic statistics represents the mindset of improvement statistics: *Improving quality = improving processes.*

Many improvement projects result from imposed external or desired internal goals. A failure to establish a good baseline estimate of the extent of the problem being addressed will almost always doom a project to failure. Data are vital for answering key questions in improvement: *What is our process "perfectly designed" to achieve compared to this goal? What is the most effective strategy to address the gap?*

Twentieth-century quality giant Joseph M. Juran advised that an initial step in any improvement project strategy should be to exhaust any in-house data. In addition to providing a look at historical performance and helping assess the possible need for improvement and clarification of data definitions and collection, these data can shed light on the extent of variation being experienced—something that can come as a shock when recognized for the first time. Once the baseline has been obtained, how should data be collected to test improvement theories and to answer the question, Did any of the changes we tried make a difference?

Variation: The Framework of This Chapter

W. Edwards Deming once stated, "If I had to reduce my message for management to just a few words, I'd say it all had to do with reducing variation" (*Economist* 2009).

In most healthcare settings, workers attend weekly, monthly, or quarterly meetings where performances are reported, analyzed, and compared to goals in an effort to identify trends. Reports often consist of month-to-month comparisons with "thumbs up" and "thumbs down" icons in the margins, as well as the alleged trend of the past three months and/or the current month, previous month, and 12 months ago.

The figures in exhibit 5.1 are typical of the type of performance data that leadership might discuss at a year-end review. Suppose the topic of interest is a key safety index indicator—for instance, some combination of patient falls, medication errors, pressure sores, and infections. The goal is to have fewer than 10 events monthly (less than 120 annually). In line with the craze of "traffic light" performance reporting, colors are assigned as follows:

- Less than 10 = green
- 10–14 = yellow
- 15 or higher = red

The 6.2 percent year-over-year drop in the performance measure (shown in exhibit 5.1) failed to meet the corporate goal of at least a 10 percent drop. Moreover, the upward trend over most of the last 12 months created additional concern (see exhibit 5.2).

Exhibit 5.2 presents two commonly used displays for these data: (1) the year-over-year line graph and (2) bar graphs for each of the past 12 months, with a fitted trend line. Typical reactions to these displays might include (1) "Month-to-month increases or drops in performance of five or greater need to be investigated—that's just too much"; (2) "Let's find out what happened to cause the most dramatic drop of 10 from March to April in year 2 and implement it"; or (3) "It looks like the root cause analyses we did on October and November's incidents broke the trend in December."

Although well intentioned, these kinds of statements derail improvement efforts and waste precious company resources. If leadership subsequently

EXHIBIT 5.1
Year-End Review Performance Data

	Jan	Feb	Mar	Apr	May	Jun	Jul	Aug	Sep	Oct	Nov	Dec	Total	
Year 1	10	14	9	12	8	11	14	11	9	8	9	15	130	
Year 2	11	10	16	6	7	8	8	12	7	14	15	8	122	↓6.2%

EXHIBIT 5.2
Two Common Displays of Year-End Review Performance Data

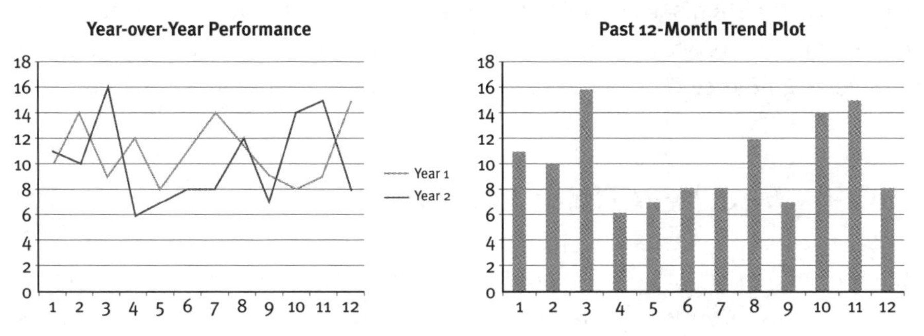

announces a "tough stretch goal" of reducing such incidents by 25 percent for the next year, the improvement efforts could go further off track, especially if fear is prevalent. The statements above reflect intuitive reactions to variation. When people see a number or perceive a pattern that exhibits an unacceptable gap (variation) from what they *feel* it should be, actions are suggested to close that gap. Whether or not they understand statistics, the people have just used statistics—decision making in the face of variation.

The fact is that no meaningful conclusions can be drawn from these commonly used data displays because of the human variation in how people perceive and react to variation, which clouds the quality of such data analysis. General agreement on each reaction and suggested solution will likely never be reached because decisions are based on personal opinions. (For further discussion of unwittingly destructive everyday data practices, see Balestracci's "Vital Deming Lessons STILL Not Learned" from the list of additional resources.)

The data in exhibit 5.1 were randomly generated from a single process—in other words, absolutely nothing changed during the 24 observations. This same conclusion, however, could be reached if the figures were actual recorded data. Moreover, goals such as "10 percent or greater reduction" in such situations cannot be met given how the work processes—and improvement efforts—are currently designed and being performed.

These data were generated through a process simulation equivalent to shaking up two coins in one's hands, letting them land on a flat service, observing whether two "heads" result, and repeating this process 39 more times. An individual result is the final tally of the total number of "double heads" in the 40 flips. One might calculate the odds of getting two heads as $\frac{1}{2} \times \frac{1}{2} = \frac{1}{4}$—that is, about 10 double heads in every 40 flips. This conclusion is true, but one also needs to consider the meaning of "about"—that is, what is the estimated expected range for any one set of flips? Human variation surfaces yet again: Each person will have a different opinion.

A group discussion might then try to decide what range would be "acceptable," which introduces another source of human variation—people making numerically arbitrary decisions rather than letting the processes and data speak for themselves. As will be shown using statistics, the actual range for this coin flip process is 1 to 20. Simple statistical theory addresses variation with clear guidance on how to react to it and deal with it appropriately.

Plotting Data over Time: The Run Chart

Exhibit 5.3 presents a time-ordered plot of the same two years' data, displayed as 24 months of output from a process. With the addition of the 24 months' data median as a reference line, the chart becomes more powerful. This type of chart, shown in exhibit 5.4, is known as a *run chart*.

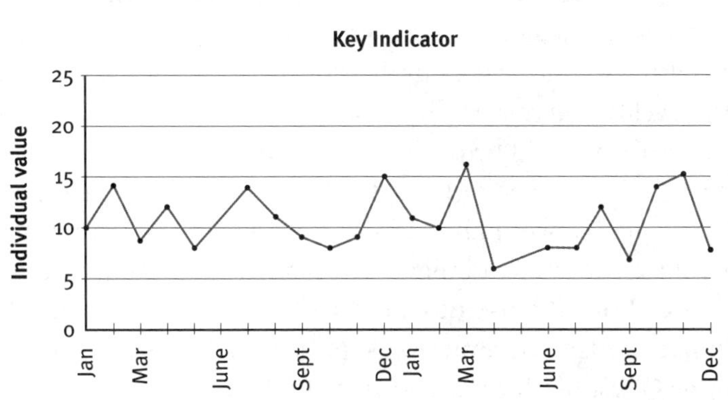

EXHIBIT 5.3
Time-Ordered Plot of Year-End Review Performance Data

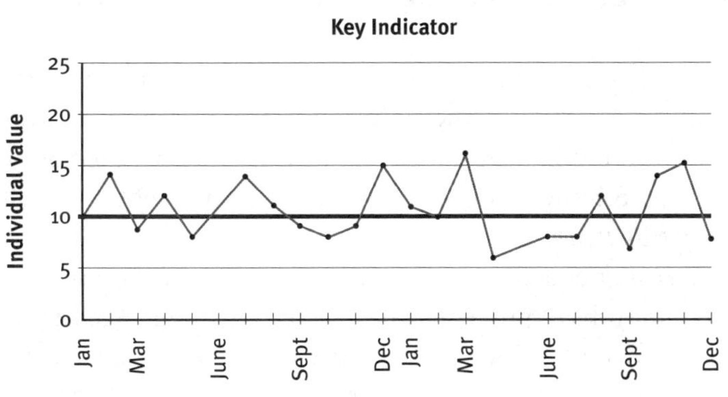

EXHIBIT 5.4
Run Chart of Year-End Review Performance Data

The median is the number that divides the data values in half when they are sorted from smallest to largest. Half of the numbers will be smaller than the median, and half will be larger. The median serves as the reference point for applying a statistical rule to determine whether any process shifts have taken place during the plotted time period. For n numbers, the median will be the value that occupies the position of $(n + 1) / 2$ in the sorted sequence.

The numbers from exhibit 5.1, in their original order, are as follows:

10, 14, 9, 12, 8, 11, 14, 11, 9, 8, 9, 15,
11, 10, 16, 6, 7, 8, 8, 12, 7, 14, 15, 8

Sorting from lowest to highest gives us this selection, from which we can identify the median:

6, 7, 7, 8, 8, 8, 8, 8, 9, 9, 9, **10, 10**, 11,
11, 11, 12, 12, 14, 14, 14, 15, 15, 16

In this case, n is an even number (24), so the median will be determined based on the formula of (24 + 1) / 2 = 12.5—meaning that we take the average of the twelfth and thirteenth numbers in the sorted sequence. For these data, both the twelfth and thirteenth numbers are 10, so the median is 10. If n were odd, the median would be one of the numbers. For example, if we were to add a value of 31 to the end of the data, the set of data would include 25 values, and the equation would be (25+1) / 2 = 13. In that case, the median would be the thirteenth value in the sorted sequence, or 10 once again.

For more about the use of run charts, see Balestracci's articles "An Elegantly Simple but Counterintuitive Approach to Analysis"—especially the "Three Routine Questions" section—and "Use the Charts for New Conversations," both included in the list of additional resources.

Common Causes Versus Special Causes of Variation

Using the same set of data, imagine that it represents a performance goal from the Centers for Medicare & Medicaid Services (CMS). Suppose CMS implemented an intervention in January of year 3 with an initial goal of increased reporting. Exhibit 5.5 shows the first month's postintervention result added to the previous run chart.

Clearly, the last data point differs from the previous one, as well as from the previous 23 months of process history. Most time sequences demonstrate normal up-and-down variation. Rather than simply reacting to one number being different from another, statistical improvement asks the question: *Is the process that produced the current number the same as the process that produced the previous number?*

EXHIBIT 5.5
Run Chart of Year-End Review Performance Data with First Postintervention Point Added

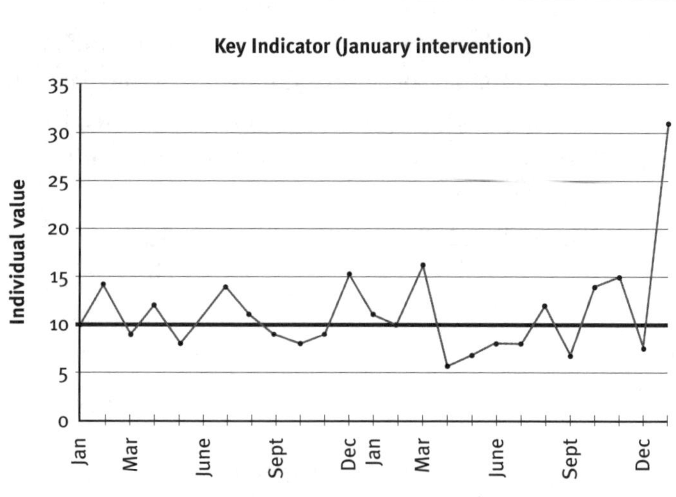

Given how the data were originally generated, the process that produced the year 2 March result of 16 was the same as the process that produced the 6 in April. However, the process that produced January's result of 31 was different from the one that produced December's 8, because a planned intervention had occurred to drive the number in that direction. This difference is known as a *special cause*, and it reflects a different process from the historical context preceding it.

The statistics of improvement can easily confirm these findings numerically. The 24 data points before the January special cause were all produced by the same process, and they exhibit variation from what is known as *common cause* (i.e., a "systemic" cause). Any process has an inherent common cause. It is what it is, and it can be calculated—it cannot be wished away or ignored because someone doesn't like it. The good news is that, regardless of its magnitude, strategies exist for the variation to be effectively addressed and improved. A baseline quantifying the common cause can be used as the means for determining whether a special cause above and beyond the inherently routine variation has occurred.

This simple run chart analysis illustrates the superiority of a process-oriented approach relative to quarterly, six-month, or annual data aggregations. A process-oriented approach leverages the elegantly simple power of plotting more frequent samples taken from shorter time intervals. Despite exhibiting variation that will be viewed by some as chaotic, subsequent effective actions will be clear.

Tampering

A common problem with current data use is that humans have a tendency to treat any and all variation as special causes that should somehow be explainable. Deming's term for reacting to common cause as if it were a special cause was *tampering*. Recall the initial reactions to the data in exhibits 5.1 and 5.2, where the perceived variations in the three data displays were treated as though they were all unique (special causes), required an explanation, and could actually be explained. Another complicating factor is that humans tend to be naively optimistic about the extent of common cause variation present in a situation or even deny its presence altogether.

Common cause variation can be addressed with relative ease—but only when it is properly identified as such. In the initial 24 months of data, any differences were *purely random*—even the drop from March to April in year 2, which some might consider significant because 10 seems like "too much." In this case, every data point results from a stable process: common cause. How does one reduce the human variation to come to this conclusion?

Two Rules for Determining Special Causes

Two simple rules can help you determine whether special cause variation is present in a run chart. These rules are based in statistical theory and are not arbitrary.

Run Chart Rule #1: Defining What a "Trend" Is and What It Is Not

First, the trend rule: A sequence of six successive increases or six successive decreases indicates special cause (when applying the rule with fewer than 20 data points, six can be lowered to five). An exact repeat of an immediate preceding value neither adds to nor breaks the sequence. Applied to the data in our example (shown in exhibit 5.3), the trend rule would indicate the following:

- Observations 7 to 10 (July through October of year 1) do *not* suggest a downward trend needing investigation, given that only three consecutive decreases occurred.
- Observations 16 to 20 (April through August of year 2) are *not* an upward trend, given that only three consecutive increases occurred (the July value, 8, is the same as the June value, so it neither adds to nor breaks the sequence).

Based on the trend rule, the 24 months of data do not include any series of six consecutive decreases that would indicate improvement.

Although the standard of six consecutive increases or decreases might seem excessive, this conservative approach is statistically necessary when reacting to a table of numbers with no common cause reference. In actual practice, this scenario will occur surprisingly rarely. The important benefit of this rule is curtailing the temptation to perceive trends in tabular data reporting. The common convention of using three points—whether all going up or all going down—does not necessarily indicate a trend. Other methods are more aggressive in finding special causes.

Run Chart Rule #2: Did a Process Shift Occur?

A run is a sequence of points either all above or all below the median, and a run is broken when a data point crosses the median. A special cause is indicated when one observes a run of eight consecutive data points either all above the median or all below the median. Points that are exactly on the median are simply not counted—they neither add to nor break the run.

Our run chart (shown in exhibit 5.4) shows runs of 1*, 1, 1, 1, 3, 3, 3*, 4, 1, 1, 2, 1 (an * indicates points on the median). Had there been a benefit from any efforts to improve the indicator's performance (i.e., achieve a decrease) over the two-year span, the data might show one or both of the following:

- A run of eight consecutive points all above the median early in the data
- A run of eight consecutive points all below the median late in the data

Neither is present. This finding, coupled with the lack of a downward trend, is an indication that process performance has not improved over the two years.

Example: Diabetes Guideline Compliance Data

A quality analyst was trying to implement a diabetes bundle guideline for providers in a five-state area. Compliance had been 50 percent, and the analyst's goal was to increase it to at least 75 percent. Exhibit 5.6 is a run chart of the last 20 months of performance, which included an intervention in December of year 1 (the seventh data point).

Applying the Run Chart Rules

When we apply the run chart rules to the diabetes bundle compliance data, rule #2 is triggered twice—first by the initial run of nine points below the median and then by the following run of eight points above the median. Only one of those signals was necessary to indicate a special cause. The data exhibit the desired increase—a process "needle bump" suggesting that the intervention was effective. Note that only three consecutive increases occur after the December intervention. This finding demonstrates the limitations of the trend rule and also suggests that, as a result of the intervention, the process changed *too fast* for six consecutive increases to occur. Nonetheless, the eight-in-a-row rule has demonstrated the special cause of an ongoing effective intervention.

Contrasting with the Use of Trend Lines

Contrast the use of statistically defined run chart rules with the common—but misguided—practice of applying a fitted trend line to the data. The trend line approach, as shown in exhibit 5.7, might elicit a reaction of, "Things are looking good for you to meet the goal in another three to four months!" Note how differently one's brain reacts to this inappropriate "trend analysis" as opposed to our earlier run chart analysis.

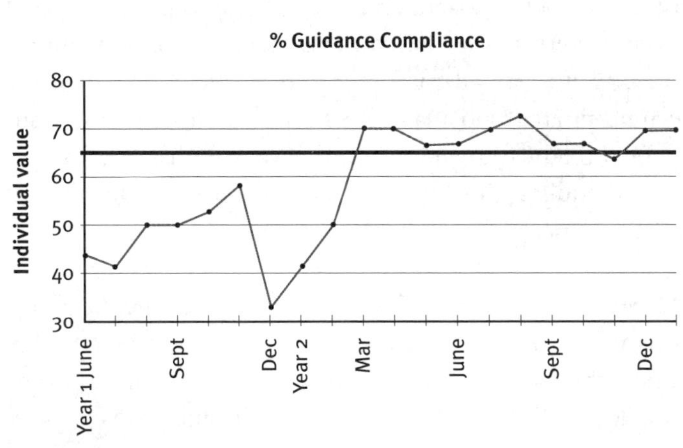

EXHIBIT 5.6
Run Chart of Diabetes Guideline Compliance Data

EXHIBIT 5.7 Diabetes Guideline Compliance Data with Fitted Trend Line

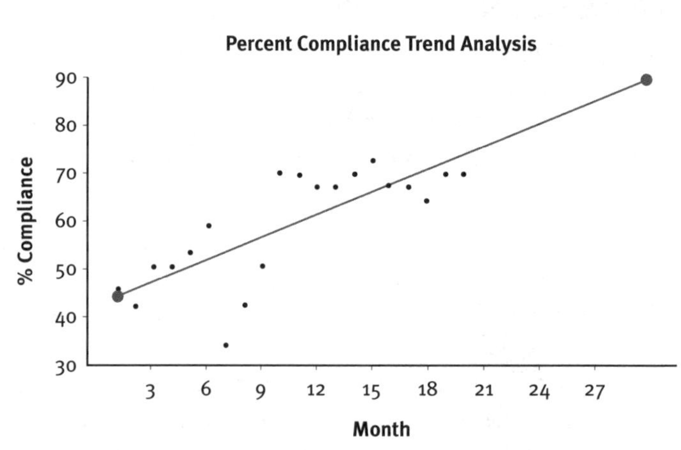

Analysis of the run chart in exhibit 5.6 clearly demonstrated both the benefits of process-oriented thinking and the limitations of trend thinking. Even when the trend rule is triggered, things can only *transition* to what the process is perfectly designed to achieve given its new inputs, which were changed for purposes of improvement. There is no guarantee that things will keep increasing (or even meet a future goal). The process will eventually stabilize and display only common cause variation around its new level.

The run chart presentation is helpful for developing the useful skill of looking at data *horizontally*. Imagine a horizontal "needle" in the first run (cluster) of nine points, and project it to the *y* axis: The initial process was perfectly designed to have a compliance rate of 50 percent. When an intervention changes the process inputs, the process transitions to what it is perfectly designed to achieve given the new inputs. Now, imagine another needle in the postintervention horizontal run (cluster) of eight points, and project it to the *y* axis. It seems to center around 68 to 69 percent—shy of the goal of 75 percent. Thus, achievement of the goal will require another intervention—best achieved using a common cause strategy!

If the quality analyst had based her improvement strategy on the misleading and inappropriate trend analysis (i.e., special cause strategy), she could easily have spent three to four more months working harder, implementing "good ideas," and adding unneeded complexity—while probably remaining at 68 percent compliance.

Why Use the Median for a Run Chart and Not the Average?

The run chart is an initial filter on a time sequence that can help to determine whether historical shifts (special causes) took place that either warrant investigation or correlate with known interventions. Its analysis is important for determining how best to calculate the average(s) of the data for further analysis and for constructing the correct expected common cause limits of performance. This analysis becomes especially useful in setting up a baseline of the most recent stable performance from which to measure an intervention's effectiveness.

Calculating an overall average can be misleading as an initial step. In the case of the diabetes guideline compliance data, calculating the average of the entire 20 months of performance data (58.6) makes no sense, because we actually have two averages: one for observations 1 through 9 (46.9) and another for observations 10 through 20 (68.2). The first average is based on what the initial process was perfectly designed to produce, whereas the second is a result of the postintervention process. The two processes' data cannot be averaged together. Only an initial run chart analysis could have discovered this issue and stopped the naïve use of the overall average as a process reference.

Multiple special causes in a time sequence and the presence of significant outliers can seriously affect the calculation of the data's average, skewing things to the point that the data are not divided "in half." The median, however, empirically divides the data in half, making each data point analogous to a fair coin flip. In other words, if you consider "heads" to be above the median and "tails" below the median, each point has a 50–50 chance of being one or the other. The eight-in-a-row rule is based on the fact that getting either eight heads in a row or eight tails in a row due solely to chance is very slim. Note: The median has no part in the trend analysis.

The Control Chart: A Very Powerful Tool

Determining how much process variation is present—and how much is "too much"—is the work of the powerful control chart. Revisiting the data from exhibit 5.1, its run chart (exhibit 5.3) had no special causes—one process had produced all the data points. Process-oriented thinking maintains that a process's overall performance can best be summarized by an appropriately calculated average (or two averages, as in the example of the diabetes guideline compliance data). Given exhibit 5.1's data and resulting run chart, the process performance is best summarized by the data's average of 10.5. When only common cause is present, the individually varying data points are indicative of this average only. Ignorance of the concept of an underlying process will miss this important point and try to improve a process by managing an individual month's results (i.e., treating each as the process "needle," or a special cause).

Once the run chart either determines that no special cause variation is present or reveals how to calculate the appropriate averages, the next step is to calculate the range of individual values that could be exhibited by the process's inherent common cause for any random time period. An additional calculation identifies how much difference between two consecutive periods is "too much"—another indication of a special cause. The difference between two consecutive data points—the absolute value of which is called the *moving range* (MR)—has statistical properties that allow calculation of the process common cause.

The 24 observations of exhibit 5.1 have been transferred to the column at the left of exhibit 5.8. The next two columns in exhibit 5.8 show the

EXHIBIT 5.8
Moving Range Calculations for Performance Data

Time-Ordered Data	Moving Range (MR) Calculation: ABSO ($x_i - x_{(i-1)}$)	MR	Sorted MR
10			
14	ABSO (14 – 10)	4	0
9	ABSO (9 – 14)	5	1
12	ABSO (12 – 9)	3	1
8	ABSO (8 – 12)	4	1
11	ABSO (11 – 8)	3	1
14	ABSO (14 – 11)	3	1
11	ABSO (11 – 14)	3	1
9	ABSO (9 – 11)	2	2
8	ABSO (8 – 9)	1	3
9	ABSO (9 – 8)	1	3
15	ABSO (15 – 9)	6	3
11	ABSO (11 – 15)	4	3 (median)
10	ABSO (10 – 11)	1	4
16	ABSO (16 – 10)	6	4
6	ABSO (6 – 16)	10	4
7	ABSO (7 – 6)	1	4
8	ABSO (8 – 7)	1	5
8	ABSO (8 – 8)	0	5
12	ABSO (12 – 8)	4	6
7	ABSO (7 – 12)	5	6
14	ABSO (14 – 7)	7	7
15	ABSO (15 – 14)	1	7
8	ABSO (8 – 15)	7	10

Note: ABSO = absolute value.

subtraction of each observation from its immediate predecessor in the naturally occurring time order, and all results are positive (i.e., absolute value). The 24 data points produce 23 MRs, given that the first point had no immediate predecessor. In the column at the right of the exhibit, the 23 MRs are sorted from smallest to largest to determine the median MR (MR_{med}). Based on the formula—(23 + 1) / 2—the twelfth value in the sorted sequence (3) is the MR_{med}. The MR_{med} contains all the information we need to understand the common cause variation of the process, regardless of the number of data points used to calculate it.

A process's common cause range for a typical result if the process continues to operate in a stable manner can be calculated as follows:

$$(\text{Process average}) \pm (3.14 \times MR_{med})$$

We know that the MR_{med} is 3, and because the previous run chart showed no special causes, we can use one process average: 10.5. Plugging those numbers into the formula, we can determine the common cause range for this process:

$$10.5 \pm (3.14 \times 3) = 1 \text{ to } 20$$

The maximum difference possible between two consecutive months solely due to common cause is the MR_{max}, and it can be calculated as follows:

$$MR_{max} = (3.865 \times MR_{med})$$

For our data, the MR_{max} is $3.865 \times 3 = 12$. (Note: The multipliers of 3.14 and 3.865 in these equations have been derived from statistical theory. They will never change, and they are used only with the MR_{med} calculations. In this instance, 3.14 has nothing to do with pi.)

We can now use the figures from these calculations to create a control chart, shown in exhibit 5.9. The chart shows the center-line average of 10.5 (control charts *always* use averages) along with a lower common cause limit of 1 and an upper common cause limit of 20.

A more specific name for this type of chart is a *control chart for individual values*, or *I-chart*. It can also be called a *process behavior chart*—a term favored by the applied statistician Dr. Donald Wheeler to avoid confusion associated with the word *control*. (The list of additional resources at the end of the chapter includes three articles by Wheeler; Balestracci's "Off to the Milky Way," which provides another example using falls data; and Brian Joiner's *Fourth Generation Management*, which has a clear explanation of control charts in chapter 9.)

EXHIBIT 5.9 Control Chart of Data from Exhibit 5.1

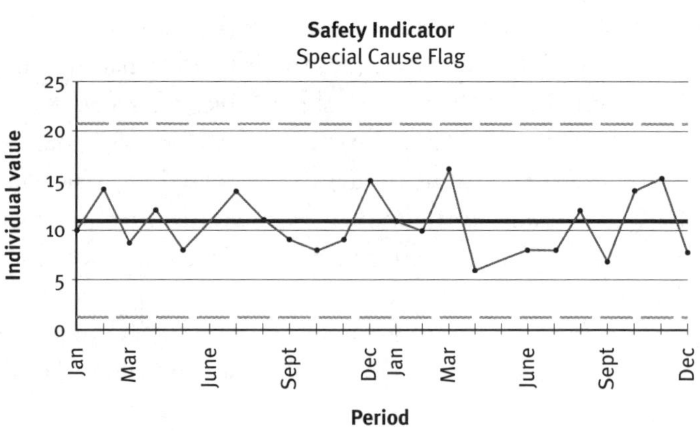

Process Summary Using Run and Control Chart Analyses

Based on our run and control chart analyses of the data introduced in exhibit 5.1, we can reach the following conclusions:

- As expected, all of the data points lie between the limits, indicating that the process is stable.
- The difference of 10 between March and April in year 2 is not a special cause because it is less than 12; the same applies for the decrease of 7 from November to December of year 2.
- The common cause range of 1 to 20 encompasses the entire original red (15 or higher), yellow (10–14), and green (less than 10) spectrum from exhibit 5.1; the color performance of any one month is essentially a lottery drawing.
- As presently designed, using the current criteria and the inherent special cause strategy, the process cannot consistently meet the monthly goal of keeping performance below 10; more than half of individual months' performances will be greater than 10.
- However, defined statistically (by the average), the process is meeting the goal. Each data point is, in essence, 10—the current estimate of the process average.
- If this special cause strategy is continued, the annual total number of events will most likely range from 98 to 142, but an occasional number as low as 87 or as high as 153 would not be unusual.

If the traditional special cause strategy (in reaction to individual incidents and monthly and annual results) continues, the process could not meet any proposed annual reduction goal—regardless of how "tough." However, in some circumstances, common cause variation could deceive one into thinking that it had!

Finally, recall the previous insertion of an additional data point (31) for January of year 3 (added for exhibit 5.5). That data point appeared to be a special cause, and we can now confirm that to be the case for two reasons: (1) Its value is greater than the upper limit of 20, and (2) its increase of 23 from December of year 2 is greater than the calculated MR_{max} of 12.

Some readers who have previous experience with this I-chart technique may have seen the limits derived from the average moving range (MR_{avg}) as opposed to the MR_{med}. Although the two multipliers used with MR_{avg} are different, the procedures are equivalent; the MR_{med} is taught here because it is easier to do by hand. Although the MR_{med} and MR_{avg} calculation results will not be identical, they will be close if only common causes are present. Most readers will eventually use a computer to obtain these charts, and most software packages default to using MR_{avg}. Good packages will have MR_{med} as an option, which would be advantageous in analyzing the data used to construct exhibit 5.5. The final special cause moving range of 23 would incorrectly inflate MR_{avg}, whereas MR_{med} would deal with it robustly and hardly affect the common cause calculation.

What Do These Common Cause Limits Represent in Terms of Standard Deviations?

The common cause limits are approximately three standard deviations on either side of the calculated average. Many people (especially researchers) struggle with this idea, because they are accustomed to using the criterion of two standard deviations, which is taught in most basic statistics courses. The limitation of using two standard deviations is that the criterion is always applied to a situation in which only one decision is being made. Such is not the case with a control chart, which has multiple points, each of which represents a decision and an opportunity for a false positive.

The criterion of three standard deviations was derived empirically by Walter Shewhart, the inventor of the control chart (and mentor to both Deming and Juran). He determined through experience that three standard deviations reasonably balanced the two risks inherent in any statistical decision: (1) the risk of declaring a difference when none is present and (2) the risk of not finding the difference when one indeed exists. The criterion has nothing to do with the normal distribution.

When seeking to obtain common cause limits, any statistical package that uses the standard deviation of observations as traditionally taught in basic statistics—commonly available as a spreadsheet column function—is seriously flawed. This calculation is virtually never used in statistical improvement work.

Common Mistakes Involving Calculation of Common Cause

The diabetes guidelines compliance data presented in exhibit 5.6—which contains a special cause—can be used to demonstrate several important concepts.

One common mistake that could be made in the analysis would involve constructing an alleged control chart using both the overall average and the standard deviation calculated from the 20 guideline performances (58.6 and 12, respectively). Exhibit 5.10 shows the chart that would result from such an approach, with limits set based on the calculation of 58.6 ± (3 × 12). Most readers will eventually encounter a chart like this one, and its only worth is in demonstrating the importance of doing a run chart first to identify special causes via the eight-in-a-row rule. Looking at the chart, some observers would determine that no special causes are present because all the data points are between the limits and none are even close to the extremes.

When using control charts, many healthcare stakeholders mistakenly cling solely to the "one point outside three standard deviations" rule to detect special causes. This tendency results in two common errors:

1. When looking at a control chart of historical data, the observers erroneously treat each point outside its limits as unique—in other words, every special cause signal is treated as a special cause. Suppose the data in exhibit 5.10 were put into typical statistical software to generate a chart by default. Most packages would generate the chart shown in exhibit 5.11 (note the narrower limits). Using that chart, some would consider points 2, 7, and 8 as individual special causes, each one needing its own investigation (or a root cause analysis) to find the causes for such "bad" performance. Astute analysts, however, would recognize immediately that the chart is not correct.
2. Some stakeholders will feel that the criterion of three standard deviations is too conservative for ongoing monitoring, which leads to

EXHIBIT 5.10 (Incorrect) Control Chart of Diabetes Guideline Compliance Data Using Overall Average and Standard Deviation

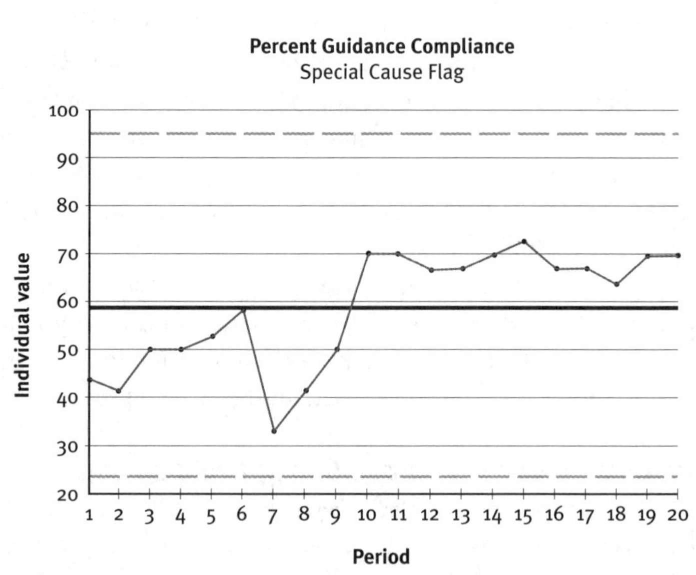

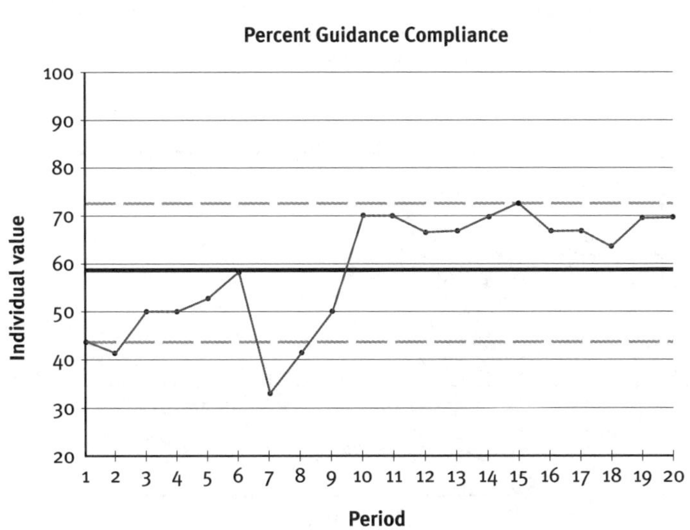

EXHIBIT 5.11 Control Chart of Diabetes Guideline Compliance Data Generated by Typical Statistical Software (average moving range used for limits)

ceaseless fretting governed by the mentality, "What if an outlier occurs? We should use fewer standard deviations to be extra careful!"

Another common practice is the addition of a line on the chart indicating two standard deviations as a "warning limit." However, this practice is not only misleading; it also encourages tampering and distracts from improvement efforts. It reflects a mind-set entrenched in healthcare, with a conventional statistical viewpoint at odds with the purpose of process analysis and, consequently, the use and interpretation of control charts. Through this lens, control charts are regarded narrowly as monitoring devices to provide an early warning of something going wrong, or as triggers for timely corrective action. At best, this approach maintains the status quo.

The traditional statistical viewpoint often uses the conventional calculation of standard deviation; if special causes are present, the calculation is seriously inflated. The frustration that results from this naïve use, in turn, contributes to a perceived need for relaxed standard deviation criteria to declare special causes. Rather than focusing on individual results or data points, improvement statistics is concerned with the process needle and the use of appropriate strategies to "bump" the process to a performance level where the feared outlier won't occur within its common cause range.

The Proper Summary of the Diabetes Guideline Compliance Data

The I-chart shown in exhibit 5.12 provides a good summary chart of the diabetes guideline compliance situation and its history. It adjusts for the successful intervention as identified in the run chart analysis. The three points that were outside the limits of the chart in exhibit 5.11 (which used the overall average)

EXHIBIT 5.12 Correct Control Chart of Diabetes Guideline Compliance Data

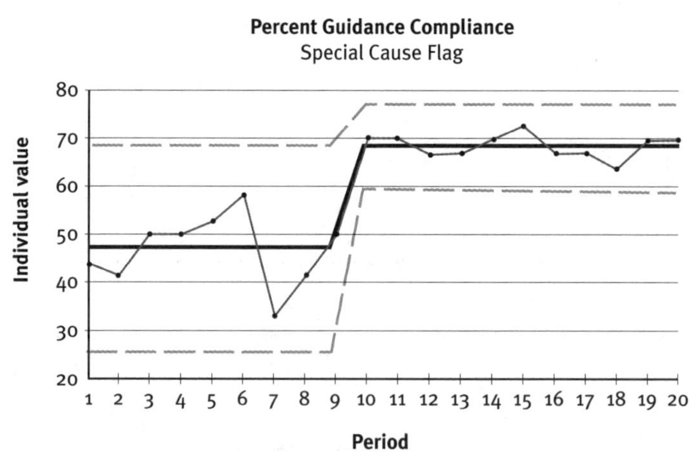

distracted from the fact that the only actual special cause was the one resulting from the intervention, which had been prompted by month 7's performance. The success of the intervention caused these three artificial signals of alleged special causes, which were actually common cause in the preintervention process.

The current analysis also yields two special cause moving range signals (greater than 11, though the calculation is not shown): (1) the drop of 25 from observation 6 to 7 (which was the significant drop in performance that provided motivation for the intervention) and (2) the upward bump of 19.4 from observation 9 to 10, which was an indication of the intervention's positive effect. Note how proper calculation of the standard deviation—reflected in limits using the moving range (± 9)—reduced the perceived variation of the limits calculated in the traditional manner (±36) by 75 percent.

The Goal Trap

Exhibit 5.12's chart warns of another trap, which may be exacerbated by the widespread use of "traffic light" interpretations. With the current performance as displayed in the chart, the 75 percent compliance goal will likely be achieved in occasional months—albeit randomly—and treated as special cause ("We met the goal!"). When subsequent months predictably fall below 75 (because the common cause range is 59 to 77 percent), disappointment will likely follow ("Why can't you do it every month?").

Goals are often expressed as a desired percentage performance. In the example of the diabetes guideline compliance data, the stated goal is 75 percent. However, the data show that the process has been perfectly designed (with its current inputs) to achieve 68.2 percent compliance over the past 11 months. It has also been perfectly designed for 32 percent noncompliance—common cause! An emphasis on goals contributes to two likely errors:

- All individual noncompliances tend to be treated as special causes, because the perception is that these instances "shouldn't happen."
- A "special cause" lens is used when analyzing the current month's overall performance and its deviation from the goal; the pervasive red/yellow/green traffic light scheme is commonly used to label and treat this variance as a special cause.

Thus, the tendency to focus on a goal does not help the improvement process. The process does not care what the goal is—its performance "is what it is."

For the diabetes guideline compliance data, the process has a common cause range of 59 to 77. Suppose a traffic light system assigns the color green for results of 75 or higher, yellow for 70 to 74, and red for results below 70. The individual noncompliances from a month in which performance is between the common cause limits and labeled red are no different (or "worse") than those from months in which performance is within the limits and labeled green. Isolating the red months' noncompliances because they occurred during "bad" months would be a limiting special cause strategy. Only one process is at work, and it is consistently producing 32 percent noncompliance.

Other Charts

Most statistical tool books include various other charts (e.g., c-charts, p-charts, and u-charts) and offer flow diagrams to help determine which of the charts should be used. However, this approach tends to be unnecessary and far too complex for the average user. Improvement statistics emphasizes taking the right action when faced with a given set of data. (For a more in-depth discussion of this issue, see Balestracci's "Right Chart or Right Action?" from the list of additional resources.)

Analysis: The I-Chart Is Your "Swiss Army Knife"

For any initial chart used to assess a process, the data should be presented in their naturally occurring time sequence, preferably as a run chart (i.e., a time-ordered plot with the median drawn in as a reference line). Usually, the most robust subsequent action is to create a follow-up I-chart. The I-chart—essentially the "Swiss Army knife" of control charts—tends to approximate the supposedly "correct" chart under most conditions, and it is much easier to understand and explain than the other chart options.

Two inevitable questions arise:

1. Under what conditions is the I-chart not correct?
2. How many samples do I need for an accurate chart?

However, in improvement statistics, it is more important to answer the following questions first:

1. What *actual* situation is making you ask this question?
2. Why is this situation important?
3. Do you have data available?
4. What ultimate actions would you like to take with these data?
5. *Exactly* how were these data collected?
6. Do you have a simple run chart of this indicator plotted over time?
7. Do you have enough information to convert it into an I-chart (i.e., as few as 7 to 10 data points)?

Answering these questions and following through with a data set that contributes to an appropriate action will demonstrate that the two "inevitable questions" are moot. You've also saved yourself a major side trip into the swamp of unnecessary calculation minutiae.

Many healthcare organizations participate in the Press Ganey patient satisfaction survey and feedback process. Questions are scored on a scale of 1 to 10, and individual question scores of 9 and 10 are considered superior, or "top box," performance. Tallies of how many respondents rated the organization a 9 or 10 divided by the total number of surveys received result in the important "percent top box" score. With the trend toward linking reimbursement to results, organizations have been under intense pressure to emphasize and increase top-box performance.

Results are supplied to participating organizations via tables with a red/yellow/green interpretation, along with a current percentile ranking. These results can easily be plotted over time. Many analysts would insist on using the percentage p-chart because it is regarded as "the technically correct chart for binomial data." Exhibit 5.13 shows one organization's data plotted on the allegedly correct p-chart and the I-chart.

In reviewing the charts, arguments about "which limits are more correct" are a waste of time (the limits are in very close agreement) and miss the point. The most important conclusion that can be drawn from these data is that no progress in performance has occurred over almost four years. Furthermore, there is little doubt that tampering has occurred in reaction to score summaries.

The purpose is not to have charts; the purpose is to use the charts. Wheeler (1996) wisely comments: "You get no credit for computing the right number—only for taking the right action. Without the follow-through of taking the right action, the computation of the right number is meaningless."

EXHIBIT 5.13
P-Chart and I-Chart of Press Ganey "Top Box" Data

P-chart of "9–10" / "Top Box" Performance

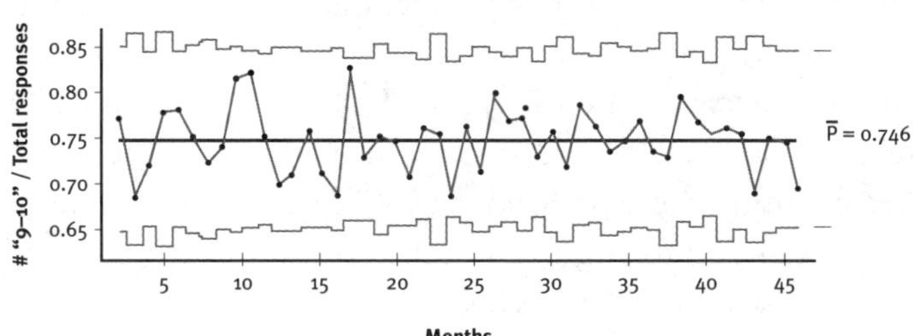

Months

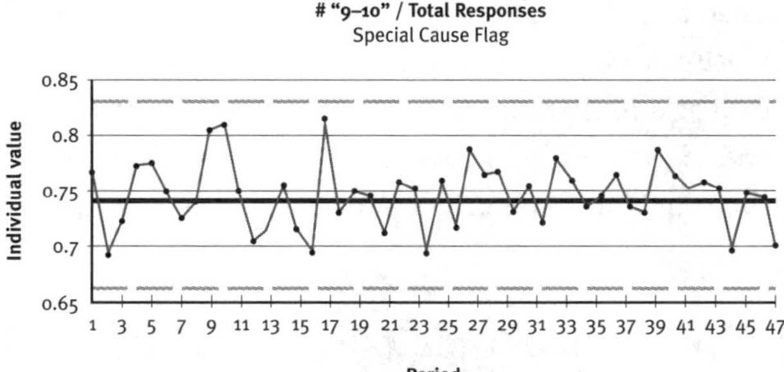

EXHIBIT 5.14
I-Chart of "Top Box" Scores' Percentile Rankings

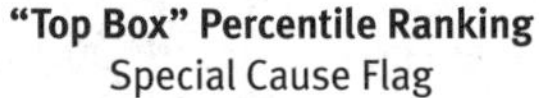

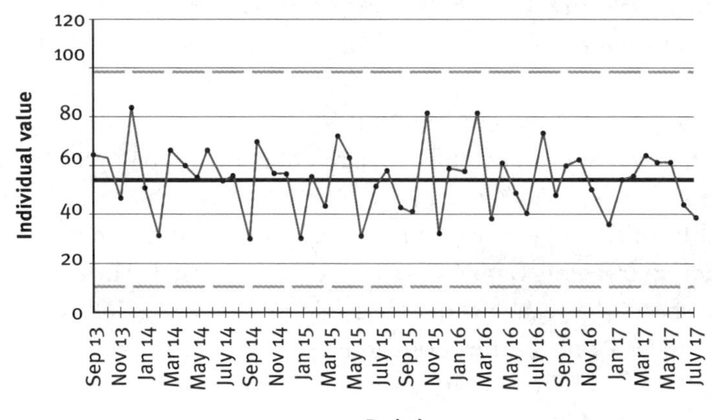

A common tendency is to concentrate on and react to the percentile ranking from the latest top-box percentage. Instead, consider the I-chart that results from plotting the corresponding percentiles of the data in exhibit 5.13, shown in exhibit 5.14.

As with the charts in exhibit 5.13, the I-chart in exhibit 5.14 shows no change in ranking in four years. The process (the ranking) has been stable, and it has exhibited common cause performance. Without a change in leadership's approach, the percentile ranking from month to month would continue to fluctuate randomly between 10 and 98.

Humans have a tendency to grossly underestimate the breadth of the common cause range. The desire for reduced variation and the temptation to justify tampering cause a great deal of distraction in meetings, waste time and resources, and increase staff cynicism. Because the process is stable, its four-year performance can be summarized as being perfectly designed to perform consistently at the 54th percentile, its average. Statistics on performance by themselves do not help to improve performance.

An Important Expansion of the Concepts of "Perfectly Designed," Common Cause, and Special Cause

People often associate working hard with making a difference, but a serious trap awaits a project team of smart people charged with fixing a persistent problem. Although they may have many ideas about how to improve the situation, many of the ideas are similar to those that have failed in the past. Vague solutions to vague problems yield vague results. Consider the following example involving an effort to reduce infections in a neonatal intensive care unit (NICU).

The NICU Conference Poster Session

A conference poster session proudly declared that a team had reduced infection rates in its NICU, and the team was eager to share the good ideas they had gleaned from the literature and their success with implementation. One of the poster requirements was to show how data were used. The first graph in exhibit 5.15 shows the team's choice of a side-by-side bar graph format with two separate scales—one for infections and one for patients—on the right and left axes. The second graph shows a similar display that is commonly used, with infections as a bar (left axis) and patients as a line graph (right axis). The team concluded that its improvement efforts had been successful because its members had performed 149 individual root cause analyses and worked very hard to implement everything they had learned.

However, with the left axis being a distinct integer "count" and the right axis its "area of opportunity" for occurrence, the correct representation

EXHIBIT 5.15
Typical Displays of Incident Data

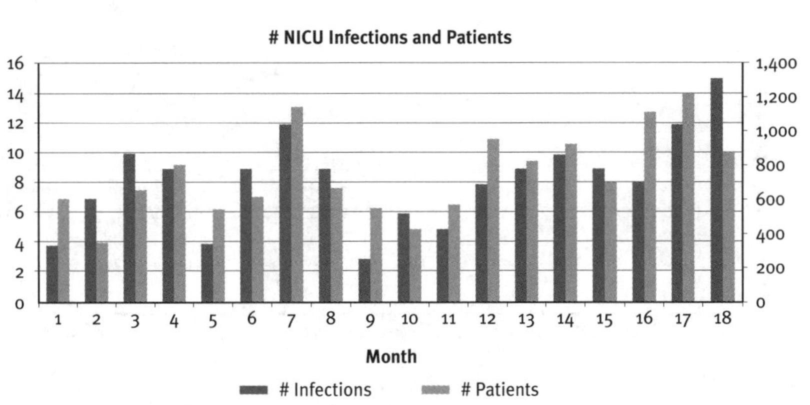

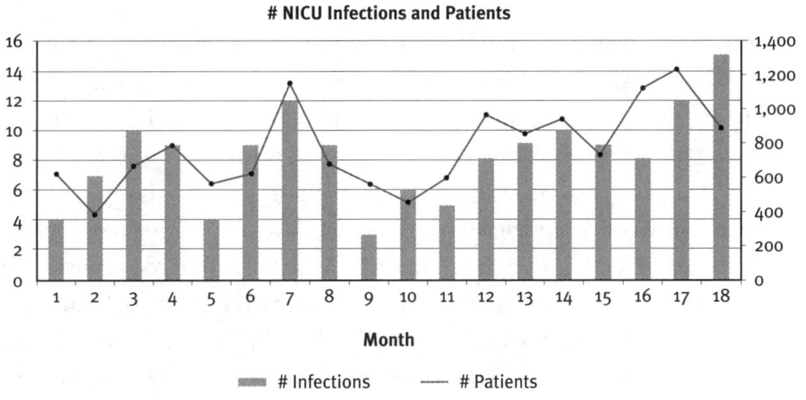

of the situation is to display the resulting *rate* obtained by dividing the former by the latter. The resulting run chart of the rate, shown in exhibit 5.16, demonstrates common cause. Despite the team's hard work, which included an extensive "best practice" literature review, the data provide no evidence of an overall effect. The team's root cause analysis approach treated every infection as a special cause, and the NICU unit appears "perfectly designed" to have these infections occur at the same rate. (For further discussion about dealing with count data, see Balestracci's "Count Data: Easy as 1-2-3? Hardly" from the list of additional resources.)

A Current Vague Healthcare Issue du Jour: Dealing with "Never Events"

Increasingly, public and private healthcare insurers are withholding payment of added costs for "never events"—that is, healthcare errors that, as determined by the National Quality Forum, should never occur. The theory is that, if people are held truly accountable, these events should not occur (special cause).

EXHIBIT 5.16 Run Chart of NICU Infection Rate (approximate common cause limits of 0 and 2.4)

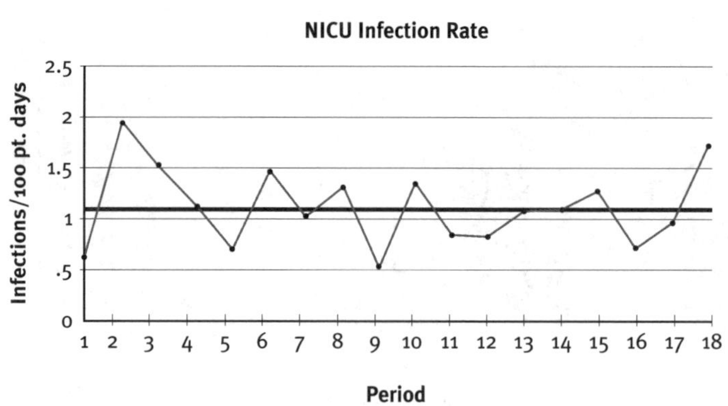

However, process-oriented thinking presents a broader, more robust perspective that raises the issue of whether organizations might be perfectly designed to have never events (common cause). One process-oriented definition of an incident is *a hazardous situation that was unsuccessfully avoided*.

The idea of organizations being perfectly designed for never events might create the *perception* of acceptance of neglectful actions and the inability to prevent them. The seemingly common-sense reaction is to redouble root cause analysis efforts and set "tough" goals; however, such a reaction uses special cause strategies and most likely amounts to tampering. (Although root cause analyses have a place in healthcare, they are overused and often poorly executed.) Furthermore, the cultural fear that results from these strategies may lead to decreased reporting.

Instead, why not exhaust in-house data and plot the number of occurrences of all events that could result in a root cause analysis (weekly, monthly, or quarterly)? If that plot is stable, as in the case of the 149 NICU infections from the previous example, a startling conclusion becomes apparent: If people continue to do what they have already done (i.e., reacting to common cause variation with special cause strategies), they are indeed being neglectful and accepting the inevitability of such events. They will experience occasional random numbers that are shockingly high as well as occasional instances of zero occurrences. Equally important, they will waste enormous resources of time and money by reacting inappropriately to common cause and by adding well-meaning, but unproductive, complexity. (For further discussion, see Leape's "Faulty Systems, Not Faulty People" from the list of additional resources.)

What Should "Root Cause" Really Mean?

Consider this useful analogy: Imagine that each patient is a spinning piece of Swiss cheese entering the invisible yet omnipresent "hazardous situations." Sometimes the holes line up just right to let the hazardous situation strike (e.g., an infection, a fall, a medical error)—like getting all the red lights on one's way to work. A root cause analysis dissects such occurrences to detect the specific "holes" and then deal with each one individually.

In the instance of encountering all red lights on the way to work, one might ask, "Why did I get all the red lights?" Isn't that an undesirable situation that was unsuccessfully avoided? Is it still present every day? Will it happen again? Can you say when? Won't there be days when you get all the green lights (zero incidents)?

Root cause analyses have the luxury of hindsight. With a known outcome, it is easy to oversimplify the inherent situational complexity and ignore the uncertainties of the circumstances faced by the potentially "blamable" person or people. It is easy to allow unrealistic perfection to become the standard and to react to human performance errors with disciplinary action or even public "shaming." It is easy to provide alternative scenarios after an undesired outcome has already occurred.

A better question might be, Could this have been common cause? In other words, are these the results the process was perfectly designed to have happen? The following questions are worth asking:

- Why did any decision make sense at the time?
- Could someone else just as easily have made this error if placed in this specific situation with its specific circumstances?
- Where else might something similar be waiting to happen?

Consider what a root cause analysis of *all* an organization's root cause analyses might uncover. The goal would be to categorize the discovered "Swiss cheese holes" more broadly—that is, without focusing on individual units, departments, facilities, or doctors. The likely culprits contributing to these events would most likely be systemic issues such as "fear," "lack of empowerment," "communication disconnect," "unreasonable delay," "doctor not available," "float on duty," or "lack of information."

The good news is that, even though one's current processes might be perfectly designed to get an undesirable result, one can aggregate *all* the performance of a stable period of common cause behavior to apply the common cause strategy of stratification—discussed in the next section—to further focus the problem.

There is no shame in discovering that a process is perfectly designed for undesirable things to occur. However, improvement might require a different strategy from what common sense would often dictate.

Common Cause Strategy: Stratification

Vague Projects Have Some Vague Issues

A wise saying, commonly attributed to Juran, goes something like, "There is no such thing as 'improvement in general.'" The NICU example described earlier illustrated the dangers of applying vague strategies (e.g., brainstorming possible causes, trying ideas obtained from people and published literature, engaging in well-intended root cause analyses) to a poorly defined problem or goal (e.g., "reduce NICU infections").

Juran was especially fond of what he named the Pareto Principle (also called the 80/20 rule): For a process needing improvement, 20 percent of the process causes 80 percent of the problem. An initial goal for any project, therefore, is to find this 20 percent so that improvement efforts can be focused to achieve the highest return. Consider the earlier example of the diabetes guideline compliance data and the final chart characterizing the current process (presented in exhibit 5.12). Exhibit 5.17 shows that chart again with the most recent stable history identified.

The use of "care bundles"—that is, the bundling of all aspects of treatment for an episode of, for instance, sepsis, pneumonia, or pressure sores—has increased in assessing provider performance and calculating reimbursement. Suppose the chart in exhibit 5.17 represents the overall percentage compliance to a bundle with seven necessary components for a six-hospital system. In line with the gap between the 75 percent goal and the current process average of 68 percent, this analysis shows the need for another intervention.

The system might be tempted to assemble a team and brainstorm the possible causes for noncompliance with the bundle. However, if not done carefully or if done prematurely, this step could easily result in an unwieldy cause-and-effect diagram in the vein of exhibit 5.18. (An American Society for Quality article about the design and construction of cause-and-effect diagrams—also called *fishbone diagrams* or *Ishikawa diagrams*—is included in the list of additional resources.)

The team will likely use this diagram to come up with and vote on improvement ideas and then "collect some data." Without careful planning,

EXHIBIT 5.17 Diabetes Guideline Compliance Data with Most Recent Stable History Identified

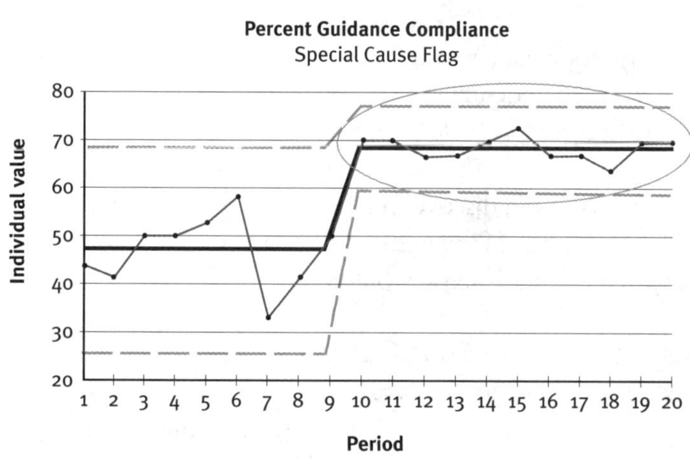

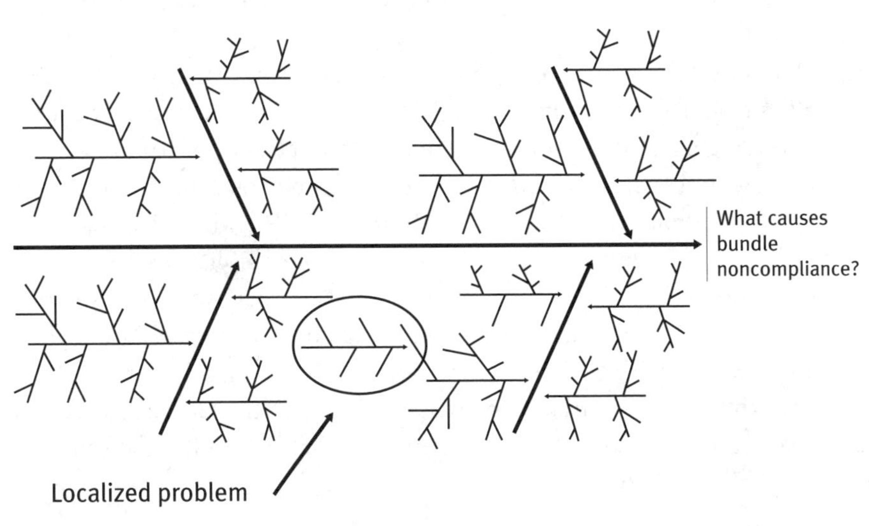

EXHIBIT 5.18
Typical Cause-and-Effect Diagram

these collections will have vague objectives and amass too much data; furthermore, the data collection will waste the time of frontline people.

Pareto Analysis

A better strategy is to exhaust all available in-house data sources before brainstorming. Often, this step will help establish an important baseline estimate of the problem. If detailed information beyond the overall performance baseline is not available, the next step should involve high-level, simple, efficient, formally planned data design and collection with the objective of localizing the problem—in other words, finding and subsequently focusing on "the 20 percent." Any such data should be both readily available and easy to collect. Data will be recorded for a brief time to make underlying issues evident, and the collection will not be permanent. (See Balestracci's "Four Data Processes, Eight Questions," parts 1 and 2, from the list of additional resources.)

Brainstorming may be useful at this point, while seeking possible categories for tallying data by process input to look for significant "clusters" of occurrence. This analysis will guarantee that the right people are subsequently involved in generating ideas for improvement. For example, from the most recent stable period of the bundle compliance data shown in exhibit 5.17, one could collect a reasonable number of noncompliances from each hospital—50 might be sufficient to reveal the problem—and analyze them to identify which element(s) of the bundle were not followed.

In improvement statistics (analytic), the issue of "sample size" does not apply. Instead, one collects just enough data to obtain an analysis that will yield a high degree of belief in the result, which can be tested further if necessary. Formal sample size issues are important only in academic (enumerative) statistics. In analytic statistics, the answer to "How much data?" is "Enough to characterize the underlying situation."

The next step would be to do a simple tally summary. A Pareto chart sorts tallies from largest to smallest and calculates the percentage contribution from each category. It then plots the sorted individual tallies as bar graphs (corresponding with the left axis) and the cumulative percentage line from category to category as a line graph (right axis). Exhibits 5.19 and 5.20 show Pareto charts of the total number of bundle element noncompliances both by the seven elements and by the six individual hospitals, respectively. (An American Society for Quality article about the design and construction of Pareto charts is included in the list of additional resources.)

In exhibit 5.19, bundle elements 3 and 5 seem to stand out as causing a large part (58.1 percent) of the problem. Hospitals B and E stand out (47.6 percent) in exhibit 5.20.

EXHIBIT 5.19 Pareto Chart of Guideline Noncompliances Compared by Bundle Element

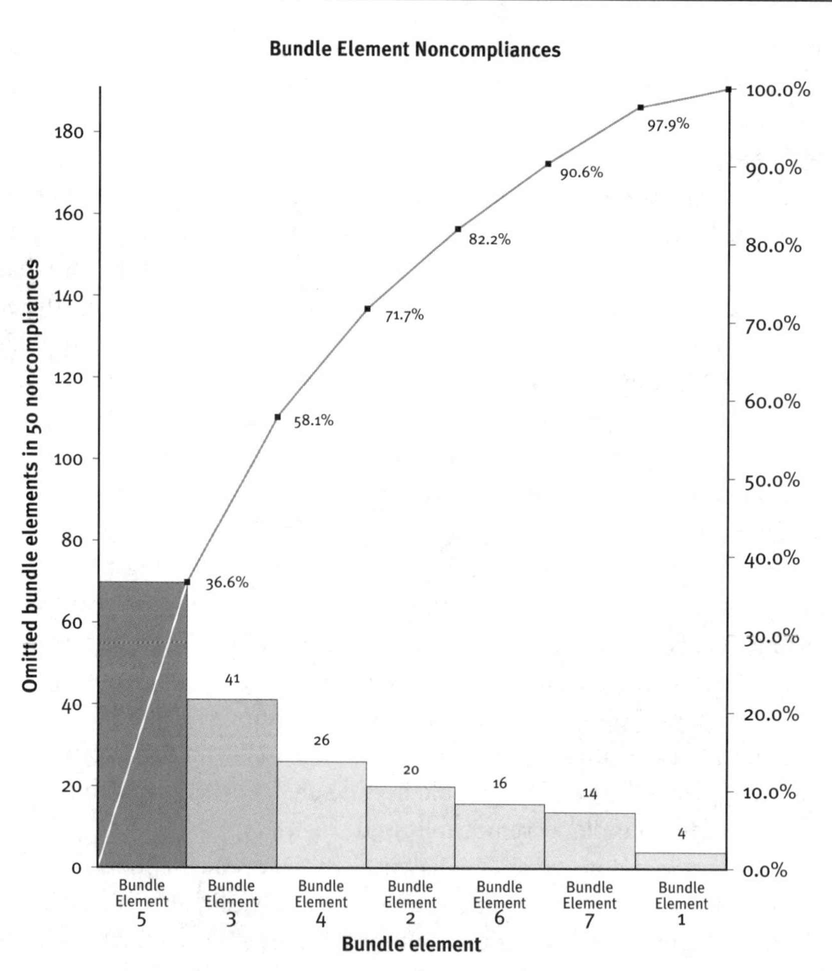

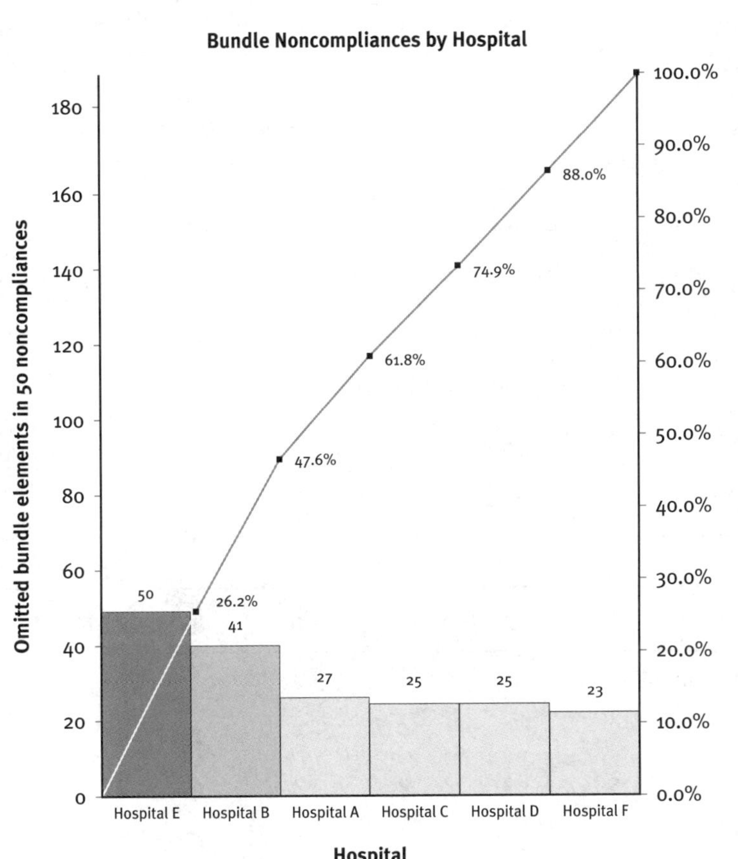

EXHIBIT 5.20 Pareto Chart of Guideline Noncompliances Tallied by Hospital

A clever Pareto analysis enhancement, called a Pareto matrix, comes from a 1980s video series titled "Juran on Quality Improvement," and it has proved to be a powerful tool. The goal with this type of analysis is to expose more deeply hidden special causes and allow for a laserlike focus on the 20 percent of the inputs causing 80 percent of the problems. The purpose of this tool is to expose *big* numbers.

Traditional Pareto analysis, as shown in exhibits 5.19 and 5.20, focuses solely on totals. In our example, a focus on bundle elements 3 and 5 and on hospitals B and E is a good start, but it misses a more important bigger picture. Exhibit 5.21 shows the same data in a two-dimensional matrix (bundle element × hospital) that stratifies the previous totals further.

The matrix quickly reveals that deeper special causes exist, highlighted in exhibit 5.22.

In the case of hospital B, the focused problem is bundle element 3. Notice that (1) the rest of hospital B's work is good and (2) no other hospital is having trouble with that bundle element. The possibility also exists that bundle

EXHIBIT 5.21
Pareto Analysis Data as a Two-Dimensional Matrix

Hospital	A	B	C	D	E	F	Total
Bundle element							
1	0	0	0	0	4	0	4
2	5	2	2	3	6	2	20
3	3	24	3	1	6	4	**41**
4	3	4	2	4	9	4	26
5	15	8	15	10	12	10	**70**
6	0	1	3	4	8	0	16
7	1	2	0	3	5	3	14
Total	27	**41**	25	25	**50**	23	191

EXHIBIT 5.22
Pareto Matrix Data with Special Causes Highlighted

Hospital	A	B	C	D	E	F	Total
Bundle element							
1	0	0	0	0	**4**	0	4
2	5	2	2	3	**6**	2	20
3	3	**24**	3	1	**6**	4	**41**
4	3	4	2	4	**9**	4	26
5	**15**	**8**	**15**	**10**	**12**	**10**	**70**
6	0	1	3	4	**8**	0	16
7	1	2	0	3	**5**	3	14
Total	27	**41**	25	25	**50**	23	191

element 3 simply does not apply to hospital B's particular patient population. Most likely, this issue can be resolved relatively quickly. The matrix presentation avoids the problem of treating special cause as common cause. Although the overall total for bundle element 3 is high (41), hospital B is the only hospital having problems with it (special cause). Had staff at all the hospitals been required to attend an in-service training (treating the bundle element 3 violations as common cause), the effort would have wasted a lot of time, angered many people, and expended unnecessary resources.

Hospital E's high total (50) tells a different story. The matrix shows no further obvious special cause, but the hospital seems to have problems with all the bundle elements. A likely culprit is the hospitals bundle implementation process (or lack of one). At this point, the data are too vague to suggest specific actions. Further data collection and analysis will be required—but only for hospital E. Similar data collection is not needed at this time for the other five hospitals. The other hospitals' performances indicate that knowledge exists within the system for relatively successful implementation.

In looking at the high total (70) for bundle element 5, no further special cause is evident. All hospitals are having trouble with it, which means that the overall system is perfectly designed for them to have trouble with it. The specific process redesign actions that the hospitals should take are unclear, but the analysis is becoming more focused. Issuing a general warning—such as, "There have been too many instances of bundle element 5 not being followed, so please be more alert and careful about it"—would be a mistake.

Had this Pareto analysis not taken place, and had the presentation of this data fallen into the current monthly trap of reacting to a deceptive, tampering-prone format, then

- hospital B would have unknowingly continued to have problems with bundle element 3;
- hospital E would have unknowingly continued its poor guideline process;
- all the hospitals would have unknowingly continued having problems with bundle element 5;
- all of these issues would predictably aggregate to the ongoing overall systemic level of 68.2 percent performance, manifesting in any one month as a number between 59 and 77 percent; and
- ultimately, nothing would change.

Focusing on the three targeted areas of exposed special causes would have the potential to reduce noncompliance by approximately 40 percent and attain a compliance level above 80 percent. The following points should be noted:

- At no point was the goal of 75 percent part of the improvement process. The underlying, hidden special causes that were exposed had nothing to do with the goal.
- 50 noncompliances were used for *each* facility. Each had the same "window of opportunity" for potential occurrences; therefore, comparisons between the individual counts were valid. 50 each was "enough" to show where to focus.

Did the Analysis and Action Make a Difference? Relaxing the Eight-in-a-Row Rule

Using the previous 11 bundle-compliance observations as a stable baseline, suppose the next five months of data looked like exhibit 5.23, a continued run chart showing performance following the analysis and intervention.

The eight-in-a-row rule—normally used when assessing the current state of a process (usually historically)—operates somewhat differently when following a planned intervention. In a specific case where we have (1) an established baseline and (2) a planned intervention intended to bump the needle in a specific direction, the eight-in-a-row rule can be relaxed to a *five-in-a-row* rule for points above or below the median in the intended direction. In this case, data points 12 to 16 satisfy the rule and therefore indicate a special cause—in other words, a successful intervention.

Exhibit 5.24 shows how using the control chart of the established baseline may indicate the desired result earlier—in this case, in the third month of the intervention, since the point is above the upper control limit.

Exhibit 5.25 demonstrates how continued subsequent plotting will show when the process has completed its transition to what it is now perfectly designed to achieve. Note that observations 15 to 18, analyzed statistically, are hardly indicative of a deteriorating trend.

A common misconception is that, if a process exhibits common cause only, a total process redesign will be necessary to improve it. This is usually not true. Often, an initial stratification, as can be achieved through a Pareto matrix, will yield surprising hidden opportunities.

Based on the chart in exhibit 5.25, further data collection and matrix analysis might not reveal more hidden opportunities—no individual cells or totals would stand out. The process is now at the level it is perfectly designed to attain.

EXHIBIT 5.23
Run Chart of Most Recent Baseline with Five Months of Intervention Data

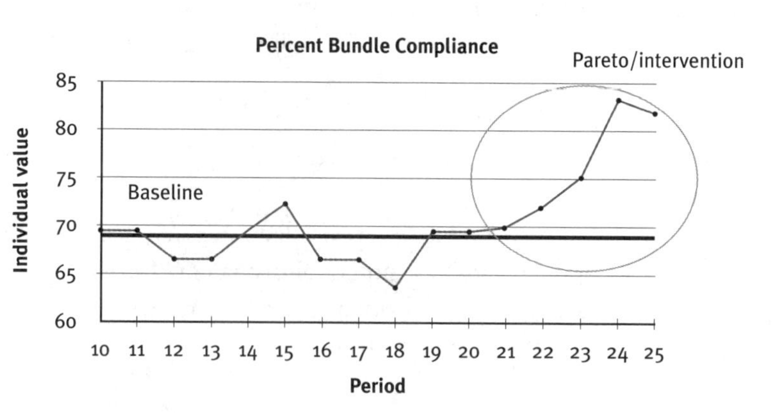

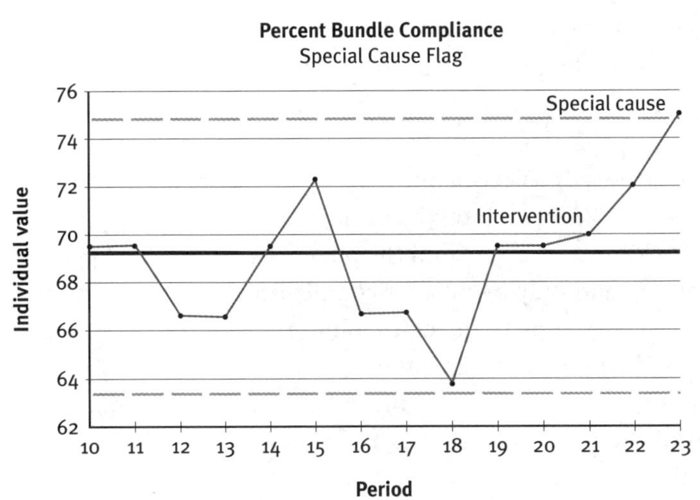

EXHIBIT 5.24 Control Chart of Baseline Data and the First Three Months of Intervention Data, Showing Beneficial Special Cause

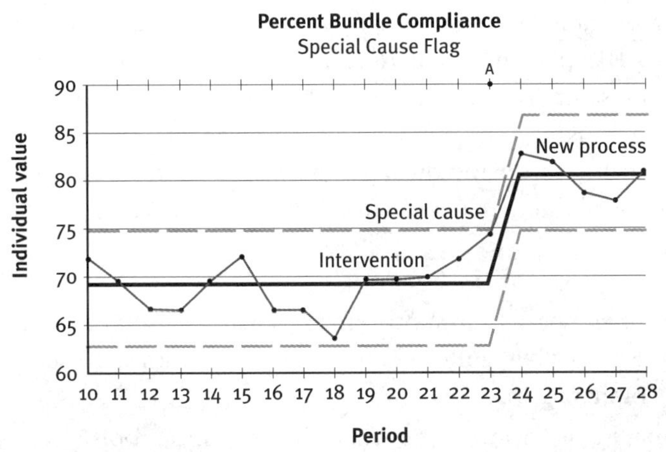

EXHIBIT 5.25 Control Chart of Baseline Data, Intervention, and Completed Transition

Before Jumping to Redesign . . .

Before jumping into a vague total redesign strategy, an effort should be made to understand and expose hidden special causes using this sequence:

1. Focus on stratification using in-house data or simple data collection.
2. Drill down deeper (process dissection) *only* on areas exposed by stratification (the vital "20 percent"). This step will usually involve more complicated data collection, dissecting processes into components and collecting work-in-progress data (especially the subprocess components of an overall time). The aim is to obtain enough data to focus and take action—simplicity and

efficiency in planning and collection are key. Even though this effort can be a major inconvenience, it *will* prove to be productive.

3. Only after points 1 and 2 have been completed, design and conduct some formal interventions with the intent of redesign.

This sequence achieves a much better use and focus of the right people's energy to initially generate categories for stratifying data, as opposed to simply asking them, for instance, to "find the reason why we had 72 percent compliance last month and only 64 percent compliance this month." It then focuses the right people's energy to generate solutions. (For further discussion of the need for good strategic use of initial common cause strategies, consult the list of additional resources—particularly the book by Joiner and Balestracci's articles on common cause strategies and resources.)

Summary

The role of statistics in quality improvement is to expose variation and to reduce inappropriate and unintended variation to make processes "go right," predictably, as close to 100 percent of the time as possible. The healthcare system is rife with data insanity. The key framework for dealing with this insanity is process-oriented thinking. The mind-set for improvement is that *everything* is a process. Essentially, improving quality = improving processes.

Regardless of whether people understand statistics, they are already using statistics.

- The statistical approach for improvement (analytic) is quite different from what is typically taught in basic academic courses and used in research (enumerative).
- Critical thinking is far more important than statistical tools.
- The presence of multiple uncontrolled sources of variation (and human variation) in an everyday work environment will invalidate most uses of traditional statistics.
- Plotting data over time is a crucial tool in analytic statistics.
- The normal distribution is not needed; its alleged importance is a myth.

Variation exists as one of two types: common cause (systemic) or special cause (unique).

- The human tendency is to treat *all* variation as special.

- Tampering involves reacting to common cause as if it were special cause. It generally makes things worse (certainly not better) and tends to add unneeded confusion, conflict, complexity, and chaos to a process.
- If something doesn't "go right," variation has occurred. Root cause analysis may inappropriately treat this variation as special cause.

All processes have an inherent common cause variation that can be determined only from the process itself. It has nothing to do with goals or what people *feel* it should be.

- Special causes due to process inputs (e.g., people, methods, machines, materials, measurements, environments) will aggregate to create a predictable process output exhibiting common cause only.
- Statistics on performance do not help to improve performance, but they can provide a useful baseline to test improvements.
- Even when variation seems chaotic or excessive, common cause strategies can expose the special causes to enable appropriate action to be taken.

Vague solutions to vague problems yield vague results.

- Many projects fail because they lack a good baseline estimate of the problem.
- People have a tendency early in projects to act on hunches ("good ideas") or to collect too much data.
- Existing data and/or simple and efficient data collection should be used in an effort to isolate the 20 percent of the process that causes 80 percent of the problem (the Pareto principle). The 20 percent could be different for each "environment."

Arbitrary numerical goals in and of themselves improve nothing and have no role in the actual improvement process.

- What is your process's "perfectly designed" performance compared to a goal? If it doesn't meet the goal, is that result due to common cause or special cause?
- Poor data displays—such as number tables, variance reports, traffic light reports, trend lines, bar graphs, and rolling averages—lead to time-wasting meetings rife with human variation, as well as unwittingly destructive actions resulting from tampering that treats deviations from goals as special causes.

Study Questions

1. Why is an expanded concept of "variation" necessary in statistical improvement? Is all variation necessarily numerical? How might this approach invalidate concepts and techniques taught in traditional basic statistics courses?
2. What are the advantages of initially plotting important data over time?
3. How might you improve the "everyday use of organizational data" process? Do you currently see it as a source of waste hampering your improvement efforts?
4. How should goals factor into improvement efforts?

Additional Resources

Classic Books and Articles

Berwick, D. M. 1991. "Controlling Variation in Health Care: A Consultation from Walter Shewhart." *Medical Care* 19 (12): 1212–25. Available at www.jstor.org/stable/3765991?seq=1#page_scan_tab_contents.

———. 1989. "Sounding Board: Continuous Improvement as an Ideal in Health Care." *New England Journal of Medicine* 320 (1): 53–56. Available at http://cds.web.unc.edu/files/2014/09/Berwick-1989.pdf.

Hacquebord, H. 1994. "Health Care from the Perspective of a Patient: Theories for Improvement." *Quality Management in Health Care* 2 (2): 68–75. Available at www.qualitydigest.com/IQedit/Images/Articles_and_Columns/December_2011/Special_Health/Heero_back_surgery.pdf.

Joiner, B. L. 1994. *Fourth Generation Management.* New York: McGraw-Hill.

Juran, J. M. 1964. *Managerial Breakthrough.* New York: McGraw-Hill.

Kerridge, D., and S. Kerridge. 1998. "Statistics and Reality" Unpublished draft, November 21. Available at http://docs.wixstatic.com/ugd/820c34_bd61780e55d9461881f4bdb8cbbb9272.pdf.

Leape, L. L. 1999. "Faulty Systems, Not Faulty People." *Boston Globe*, January 12. Available at www.ehcca.com/presentations/qualitycolloquium5/pc_article.pdf.

Mills, J. L. 1993. "Sounding Board: Data Torturing." *New England Journal of Medicine* 329: 1196–99. Available at www.google.com/url?sa=t&rct=j&q=&esrc=s&source=web&cd=2&ved=0ahUKEwj337Sa5LTXAhXEMyYKHQzpCzUQFggtMAE&url=http%3A%2F%2Flira.pro.br%2Fwordpress%2Fwp-content%2Fuploads%2F2009%2F03%2Fcomo-torturar-seus-dados.pdf&usg=AOvVaw363zTGUqIcXFRtkpzmoPia.

Nolan, T. W., and L. P. Provost. 1990. "Understanding Variation." *Quality Progress* 23 (5): 70–78. Available at http://apiweb.org/UnderstandingVariation.pdf.

Books

Balestracci, D. 2015. *Data Sanity: A Quantum Leap to Unprecedented Results*, 2nd ed. Englewood, CO: Medical Group Management Association.

Langley, G. J., R. D. Moen, K. M. Nolan, T. W. Nolan, C. L. Norman, and L. P. Provost. 2003. *The Improvement Guide: A Practical Approach to Enhancing Organizational Performance*, 2nd ed. San Francisco: Jossey-Bass.

Neave, H. R. 1990. *The Deming Dimension*. Knoxville, TN: SPC Press.

Scholtes, P. R., B. L. Joiner, and B. J. Streibel. 2003. *The Team Handbook*, 3rd ed. Madison, WI: Oriel.

Wheeler, D. J. 2012. *Making Sense of Data: SPC for the Service Sector*. Knoxville, TN: SPC Press.

———. 2000. *Understanding Variation*, 2nd ed. Knoxville, TN: SPC Press.

Articles by Davis Balestracci on Relevant Topics from This Chapter

On Analysis of Means

"What Do 'Above' and 'Below' Average Really Mean?" *Quality Digest*. Published June 14, 2017. www.qualitydigest.com/inside/statistics-column/what-do-above-and-below-average-really-mean-061417.html.

"New Results Equal New Conversations: A Data-Sane Alternative for Percentage Performance Comparisons." *Quality Digest*. Published July 17, 2017. www.qualitydigest.com/inside/statistics-column/new-results-equal-new-conversations-071717.html.

"Statistical Stratification with Count Data, Part 1." *Quality Digest*. Published September 11, 2014. www.qualitydigest.com/inside/quality-insider-column/statistical-stratification-count-data-part-1.html.

"Given a Set of Numbers, 25% Will Be the Bottom Quartile . . . or Top Quartile." *Quality Digest*. Published October 17, 2013. www.qualitydigest.com/inside/quality-insider-column/given-set-numbers-25-will-be-bottom-quartile-or-top-quartile.html.

"Understanding Variation: Can We Please Stop the Obsession with Rankings and Percentiles?" *Quality Digest*. Published May 15, 2017. www.qualitydigest.com/inside/statistics-column/understanding-variation-051517.html.

On Analytic Statistics

"Use the Charts for New Conversations." *Quality Digest*. Published March 20, 2012. www.qualitydigest.com/inside/health-care-column/use-charts-new-conversations.html.

"An Elegantly Simple but Counterintuitive Approach to Analysis." *Quality Digest*. Published March 5, 2012. www.qualitydigest.com/inside/quality-insider-article/elegantly-simple-counterintuitive-approach-analysis.html.

On Common Cause Strategies

"Wasting Time with Vague Solutions, Part 1." *Quality Digest.* Published September 14, 2012. www.qualitydigest.com/inside/quality-insider-article/wasting-time-vague-solutions-part-1.html.

"Wasting Time with Vague Solutions, Part 2." *Quality Digest.* Published September 18, 2012. www.qualitydigest.com/inside/quality-insider-column/wasting-time-vague-solutions-part-2.html.

"Wasting Time with Vague Solutions, Part 3." *Quality Digest.* Published September 19, 2012. www.qualitydigest.com/inside/quality-insider-article/wasting-time-vague-solutions-part-3.html.

"Another Strategy for Determining Common Cause." *Quality Digest.* Published November 5, 2012. www.qualitydigest.com/inside/quality-insider-column/another-strategy-determining-common-cause.html.

"The Final Common Cause Strategy." *Quality Digest.* Published December 14, 2012. www.qualitydigest.com/inside/quality-insider-column/final-common-cause-strategy.html.

"Dealing with Count Data and Variation." *Quality Digest.* Published August 19, 2014. www.qualitydigest.com/inside/quality-insider-column/dealing-count-data-and-variation.html.

"More Common Cause Subtlety." *Quality Digest.* Published July 28, 2014. www.qualitydigest.com/inside/quality-insider-column/more-common-cause-subtlety.html.

On Control Charts

"Right Chart or Right Action?" *Quality Digest.* Published June 11, 2014. www.qualitydigest.com/inside/quality-insider-column/right-chart-or-right-action.html.

"How Many Data Points Do I Need to Have a Good Chart?" *Quality Digest.* Published May 12, 2014. www.qualitydigest.com/inside/quality-insider-article/yet-another-predictable-question.html.

"Off to the Milky Way." *Quality Digest.* Published April 9, 2013. www.qualitydigest.com/inside/quality-insider-article/milky-way.html.

"Four Control Chart Myths from Foolish Experts." *Quality Digest.* Published March 30, 2011. www.qualitydigest.com/inside/quality-insider-article/four-control-chart-myths-foolish-experts.html.

On Data Collection

"Four Data Processes, Eight Questions, Part 1." *Quality Digest.* Published October 11, 2012. www.qualitydigest.com/inside/quality-insider-article/four-data-processes-eight-questions-part-1.html.

"Four Data Processes, Eight Questions, Part 2." *Quality Digest.* Published October 12, 2012. www.qualitydigest.com/inside/quality-insider-article/four-data-processes-eight-questions-part-2.html.

"Count Data: Easy as 1-2-3? Hardly." *Quality Digest.* Published August 14, 2017. www.qualitydigest.com/inside/statistics-column/count-data-easy-1-2-3-081417.html.

"Are You Unknowingly Reacting to the DATA Process?" *Quality Digest.* Published March 16, 2015. www.qualitydigest.com/inside/quality-insider-column/are-you-unknowingly-reacting-data-process.html.

On Data Sanity

"'Which of Deming's 14 Points Should I Start with?' Answer: None of Them." *Quality Digest.* Published November 14, 2016. www.qualitydigest.com/inside/management-column/111416-which-deming-s-14-points-should-i-start.html.

"'Unknown or Unknowable' . . . yet Shocking!" *Quality Digest.* Published December 19, 2016. www.qualitydigest.com/inside/health-care-column/112816-unknown-or-unknowable-yet-shocking.html.

"When the Indicators I Plot Are Common Cause, What Should I Do?" *Quality Digest.* Published February 13, 2017. www.qualitydigest.com/inside/statistics-column/when-indicators-i-plot-are-common-cause-what-should-i-do-021317.html.

"Vital Deming Lessons STILL Not Learned." *Quality Digest.* Published March 21, 2017. www.qualitydigest.com/inside/statistics-column/vital-deming-lessons-still-not-learned-032117.html.

"Can You Prove Anything with Statistics?" *Quality Digest.* Published December 14, 2015. www.qualitydigest.com/inside/statistics-column/121415-can-you-prove-anything-statistics.html.

"Are Your Processes 'Too Variable' to Apply Statistical Thinking?" *Quality Digest.* Published May 28, 2014. www.qualitydigest.com/inside/quality-insider-column/are-your-processes-too-variable-apply-statistical-thinking.html.

"The Universal Process Flowchart × 4." *Quality Digest.* Published April 7, 2014. www.qualitydigest.com/inside/quality-insider-column/universal-process-flowchart-4.html.

"Big Data Have Arrived." *Quality Digest.* Published October 13, 2014. www.qualitydigest.com/inside/quality-insider-column/big-data-have-arrived.html.

"'What's the Trend?' Wrong Question!" *Quality Digest.* Published August 11, 2014. www.qualitydigest.com/inside/quality-insider-column/what-s-trend.html.

"Control Charts: Simple Elegance or Legalized Torture?" *Quality Digest.* Published January 6, 2014. www.qualitydigest.com/inside/quality-insider-column/control-charts-simple-elegance-or-legalized-torture.html.

"Uh-oh . . . Time for the (Dreaded?) Third Quarter Review Meeting." *Quality Digest.* Published November 18, 2010. www.qualitydigest.com/inside/quality-insider-column/uh-oh-time-dreaded-third-quarter-review-meeting.html.

On Process

"A New Conversation for Quality Management." *Quality Digest.* Published August 2, 2011. www.qualitydigest.com/inside/health-care-column/new-conversation-quality-management.html. (Includes Joiner's "three levels of fix.")

"Finding the Unnecessary and Everyday Variation." *Quality Digest.* Published March 19, 2014. www.qualitydigest.com/inside/quality-insider-column/finding-unnecessary-and-everyday-variation.html.

"Can We Please Stop the Guru Wars?" *Quality Digest.* Published February 11, 2014. www.qualitydigest.com/inside/quality-insider-column/can-we-please-stop-guru-wars.html. (Includes 13 questions to ask about a process.)

"The 'Actual' vs. 'Should' Variation Gap." *Quality Digest.* Published March 10, 2014. www.qualitydigest.com/inside/quality-insider-column/actual-vs-should-variation-gap.html.

"There Is No Such Thing as 'Improvement in General.'" *Quality Digest.* Published October 4, 2013. www.qualitydigest.com/inside/quality-insider-column/customer-satisfaction-surveys-goal.html.

On Rapid Cycle PDSA

"Getting Real with Rapid Cycle PDSA." *Quality Digest.* Published February 16, 2016. www.qualitydigest.com/inside/management-column/021616-getting-real-rapid-cycle-pdsa.html.

"A More Robust 'P' for Any PDSA Cycle." *Quality Digest.* Published April 14, 2015. www.qualitydigest.com/inside/quality-insider-column/more-robust-p-any-pdsa-cycle.html.

"PDSA . . . or Rock of Sisyphus?" *Quality Digest.* Published April 16, 2014. www.qualitydigest.com/inside/quality-insider-column/pdsa-or-rock-sisyphus.html.

"'Just DO It!' Still Won't Do It." *Quality Digest.* Published January 29, 2014. www.qualitydigest.com/inside/quality-insider-column/just-do-it-still-won-t-do-it.html.

Helpful Articles by Donald J. Wheeler

"Working with Rare Events." *Quality Digest.* Published October 28, 2011. www.qualitydigest.com/inside/quality-insider-article/working-rare-events.html.

"What They Forgot to Tell You About the Normal Distribution." *Quality Digest.* Published September 4, 2012. www.qualitydigest.com/inside/quality-insider-article/what-they-forgot-tell-you-about-normal-distribution.html.

"What About *p*-Charts?" *Quality Digest.* Published September 30, 2011. www.qualitydigest.com/inside/quality-insider-article/what-about-p-charts.html.

Resources from the American Society for Quality

"Fishbone (Ishikawa) Diagram." Accessed October 18, 2018. http://asq.org/learn-about-quality/cause-analysis-tools/overview/fishbone.html.

"Pareto Chart." Accessed October 18, 2018. http://asq.org/learn-about-quality/cause-analysis-tools/overview/pareto.html.

References

Berwick, D. M. 1991. "Controlling Variation in Health Care: A Consultation from Walter Shewhart." *Medical Care* 19 (12): 1212–25.

———. 1989. "Sounding Board: Continuous Improvement as an Ideal in Health Care." *New England Journal of Medicine* 320 (1): 53–56.

Economist. 2009. "Guru: W. Edwards Deming." Published June 5. www.economist.com/news/2009/06/05/w-edwards-deming.

Neave, H. R. 1990. *The Deming Dimension.* Knoxville, TN: SPC Press.

Wheeler, D. J. 1996. "When Do I Recalculate My Limits?" *Quality Digest.* Published May. www.qualitydigest.com/may/spctool.html.

CHAPTER

6

PHYSICIAN PROFILING AND PROVIDER REGISTRIES

Bettina Berman and Richard Jacoby

Physician profiling and provider registries are a logical pairing for a book chapter. In its simplest conception, a physician profile, often displayed on a healthcare website, serves as a depiction of a particular physician as a professional in the field. Provider registries provide additional information about that physician or other provider (e.g., physician assistant, nurse practitioner), including data, displayed in various formats, that reveal performance on standard measures of quality. As such, registries are an integral part of the provider profile.

Physician profiles serve many functions. For patients seeking a physician, profiles provide a virtual introduction, where they learn something about the physician's background and practice, or get a sense for aspects of the physician's competence. For physicians and other providers, profiles can be used to measure and improve their own performance and to compare themselves to their peers. For payers and healthcare organizations that deliver clinical services, profiles provide a way to evaluate clinical performance, which may incorporate quality as well as costs. That evaluation may be used as a basis for rewarding or penalizing physicians by adjusting their reimbursement for billed services, or providing financial bonuses or penalties. The ultimate goal is to motivate physicians and other providers to meet the Institute for Healthcare Improvement (IHI) Triple Aim of improving the patient experience of care, improving the health of populations, and reducing the per capita cost of healthcare (IHI 2018). By their nature, physician profiles and provider registries can never be complete. As such, they are the subject of controversy.

Background and Terminology

Physician Profiling

Healthcare profiles may have varying emphases depending on the intended audience. As used by patients, a physician profile serves as an introduction to a physician. For patients seeking a physician online, a useful profile will contain a brief biographical sketch and other practical information. It may include basic contact information such as name, addresses, and phone numbers; gender; languages spoken; type of practice; whether the physician is part of a group practice; what schools the physician attended and degrees received; where and when the physician received clinical training; any specialty certifications, and whether the physician has maintained certification status. Hospital affiliation, state licenses, and participation in insurance plans are also frequently included. In addition to this basic information, a patient-oriented physician profile may also include information about the physician's participation in quality programs, along with some level of detail of how that physician performs on specialty-related quality measures. These measures of quality may be displayed in a variety of formats and for varying periods.

As used by physicians and payers, physician profiling involves the collection of provider-specific and practice-level data used to analyze physician practice patterns, utilization of services, and outcomes of care. Profile development enables a physician's treatment patterns to be assessed and evaluated. The near-term goal of physician profiling is to improve physician performance through accountability and feedback; a longer-term goal involves using this feedback to decrease practice variation through adherence to evidence-based standards of care.

Through profiling, physicians' performance can be measured against their colleagues' performance on local, state, or national levels. The idea is that physicians—who often tend to be highly driven, goal-oriented individuals—will be motivated to improve their performance in areas in which they do not currently rank the highest. Financial rewards and penalties also facilitate this motivation.

Since the 2001 publication of the Institute of Medicine's *Crossing the Quality Chasm*, which detailed problems with processes of care and unexplained clinical variation in the US healthcare system, stakeholders have increasingly been seeking information on which to base healthcare and provider choices. Information about provider performance assessments—made available through such resources as the Centers for Medicare & Medicaid Services (CMS) Physician Compare website—can help healthcare consumers make informed decisions based on quality.

Provider Registries

As used in this chapter, *registry* is a general term to describe a vehicle for presenting health-related clinical data. Sources of data include health records, billing records (for administrative claims data), and patient surveys. McIver (2017, 523) defines a registry as "an electronic system for uniform collection of information used to evaluate specified outcomes for a patient population defined by a particular disease, condition, or exposure." Of the various types of registries, CMS "recognizes qualified clinical data registries, which can be used to collect and submit physician quality reporting system measures data for a practice" (McIver 2017, 523).

Registries can take the form of a list (related items typically written one below the other), a table (data systematically displayed in rows and columns), a dashboard or scorecard, or another display. They can be used for tracking performance in a number of subject areas, including clinical quality, patient safety, patient satisfaction, and finances (e.g., charges billed for clinical services). People in the business world often state that "you can't manage what you don't measure," or that "you can't improve what you don't measure." True to those adages, the collection and display of accurate and meaningful healthcare data are critical functions for all decision makers.

Dashboards and scorecards are among the most common and useful tools for organizing and displaying healthcare data. For practical purposes, the terms *dashboard* and *scorecard* are often used interchangeably (with *report card* sometimes substituted for *scorecard*); strictly speaking, however, the tools are subtly different. A dashboard is best thought of, conceptually, as the term is applied to the elements displayed on the dashboard of a car. It provides real-time monitoring of processes occurring at a particular moment. For example, a speedometer tells you how fast a car is going, the engine light indicator tells the current temperature of the engine, and the fuel gauge gives the current amount of fuel in the car. In the healthcare setting, an example of a dashboard would be a patient monitor that displays a patient's current vital signs (e.g., pulse, blood pressure, temperature, respiration rate).

A scorecard, on the other hand, is more of a historical record of activities that have occurred in the past (Pugh 2014). For example, a baseball scorecard details aspects of what transpired during a baseball game. A golf scorecard is a summary of the scores recorded for each hole in a round of golf. Extending the dashboard example about the car, one could develop a scorecard of a car's performance on a trip by recording certain data points from the car's dashboard at set points in time. For simplicity's sake, we will use the term *scorecard* for the remainder of this chapter, as it more accurately reflects the temporal dimension of the data displayed for clinical quality measures—the most common form of scorecards in the healthcare setting.

CMS (2018) defines *quality measures* as follows:

> Quality measures are tools that help us measure or quantify healthcare processes, outcomes, patient perceptions, and organizational structure and/or systems that are associated with the ability to provide high-quality health care and/or that relate to one or more quality goals for health care. These goals include: effective, safe, efficient, patient-centered, equitable, and timely care.

"Effective" translates to measures of clinical quality. "Safe" translates to measures of adverse events, such as falls and medication errors. "Efficient" relates to utilization of resources and costs and is often reflected in financial measures. "Patient-centered" refers to measures of quality involving patient preferences and values, as measured and reported by healthcare institutions to CMS. "Equitable" refers to the delivery of care without discrimination. Finally, "timely" involves delivering care when it is needed. By measuring and tracking data in these domains, the full spectrum of healthcare services can be documented, analyzed, and improved.

In the context of a physician profile, quality measures relating to the actual clinical quality of the care delivered by a physician currently receive significant attention. Clinical quality measures have a long history, dating back at least to the early 1900s, when Ernest Codman (1914), a Boston surgeon, gained prominence as one of the initial champions of clinical outcomes measurement. Clinical quality measures, as classified originally by Avedis Donabedian (1966), can be divided into three types: structure, process, and outcome. Structure measures focus on the facilities, equipment, and other available services that affect the ability to deliver care. Process measures encompass all the steps in the actual delivery of care, including diagnosis, treatment, and preventive care. Outcome measures deal with the results or effects of the processes of care. Outcomes can be subclassified into clinical (e.g., morbidity, mortality), humanistic (e.g., quality of life), or economic (e.g., utilization, finance) categories.

The basic elements of a quality measure—also known as the *measure specifications*—typically include the population being measured (e.g., gender, age or age range), what is being measured (e.g., blood pressure), and time frame (e.g., in the previous calendar year). With these foundations in place, clinical quality measures may be developed for each clinical area in medicine, and for virtually any aspect of healthcare.

Organizations involved in the development and validation of clinical quality measures include CMS; the National Committee for Quality Assurance (NCQA), through its Healthcare Effectiveness Data and Information Set (HEDIS); and the National Quality Forum. All of these organizations have rigorous processes to ensure that measures that are developed and used meet the highest evidence-based clinical standards.

The Physician's Role in Improving Quality

Public reporting of quality data dates back to the 1980s, when the Health Care Financing Administration (the predecessor to CMS) began publishing mortality rates for the country's hospitals (James 2012). Nonetheless, despite advances in science and medical technology, healthcare in the United States is still characterized by uneven quality. A 2017 Commonwealth Fund study examined healthcare system performance in 11 high-income countries—focusing on domains of care process, access, administrative efficiency, equity, and healthcare outcomes—and the United States ranked last overall, despite having by far the highest costs (Schneider et al. 2017). Another comprehensive study of health system performance by the World Health Organization (2000) ranked the United States thirty-seventh out of 191 member countries.

Although clinical guidelines and best practices exist, a number of barriers prevent these practices from being implemented across the United States (Robert Wood Johnson Foundation [RWJF] 2009). The wide range of physicians' practice patterns has been shown to be a major contributor to unexplained clinical variation. The variation exists because evidence-based guidelines and standards exist for only a small portion of the care that is given in the United States (Kumar and Nash 2010). Even when such guidelines are available, physicians often fail to follow them.

Unexplained clinical variation exists among providers by specialty, geographic region, and practice setting, and it is associated with lower quality of care and worse health outcomes (Skinner and Fisher 2010). It exists for patients with a wide variety of conditions, from heart failure to orthopedic problems to cancer. Although variation may lead to similar outcomes, it can contribute to serious problems if, for instance, a patient develops an infection after a surgery that was not necessary.

Profiling compares providers' adherence to current evidence-based best practices in medicine and helps to reduce practice variation. Such feedback gives physicians the opportunity to make changes to their practice patterns and to improve patient outcomes. Performance measurement is a critical component of national and local efforts to improve care at the institutional as well as individual provider level. Provider profiles generated by these measurement efforts are currently used for public report cards, credentialing, and board certification, as well as in pay-for-performance programs that link quality rankings to financial incentives (Fung et al. 2010).

Although some of the elements that affect performance on quality measures are beyond physicians' control (e.g., patients' ability to pay for transportation to the doctor's office, patients' unwillingness to follow instructions), physicians are clearly "captains of the healthcare ship," playing a central and critical role in the decision making that drives the system. Their decisions with regard to diagnosis, treatment, prescriptions, diagnostic tests, laboratory tests, and referrals are the major influences on cost and quality. All providers face similar challenges with their patient populations. Therefore, as long as patient populations have been risk-stratified for socioeconomic, demographic, and severity-of-illness factors, it is entirely logical and appropriate for physicians' performances to be measured and compared, and for the results to be used as a basis for quality improvement.

Use of Physician Profiling and Provider Registries in Healthcare Organizations

Value-Based Purchasing

The provision of healthcare in the United States is becoming increasingly focused on value, or the relationship between quality and cost. With national healthcare expenditures projected to increase from 17.5 percent of the gross domestic product (GDP) in 2014 to 20.1 percent in 2025 (Keehan et al. 2016), the government, employers, and the public at large want to know whether healthcare providers offer high-quality, affordable care.

Quality metrics have been incorporated into financial incentives for providers under various programs of the Affordable Care Act (Doran, Maurer, and Ryan 2017). The repeal of Medicare's sustainable growth rate formula for physician payment and the passage of the Medicare Access and CHIP Reauthorization Act (MACRA) of 2015 changed many payment models from fee-for-service to value-based payment (Wilensky 2016). The MACRA legislation introduced the CMS Quality Payment Program with two tracks: the Merit-Based Incentive Payment System (MIPS) and Advanced Alternative Payment Models (CMS 2017b). Efforts to determine quality measures for hospitals and healthcare plans have been expanded to include measures relating to the performance of physicians. The MIPS program consolidated the Physician Quality Reporting System, a quality reporting program that encourages individual provider and group practice reporting to Medicare; the Electronic Health Records (EHR) Incentive Program, formerly called the Meaningful Use program; and the Value-Based Payment Modifier, an adjustment to claims payments based on value and cost of care provided to Medicare patients (Quality Payment Program 2018).

Private insurers are increasingly following the government's lead by providing financial incentives for high-quality care, thereby creating selective provider networks whose physicians score highly on measures of quality. Collaboration between health plans and providers include value-based purchasing models of various types, such as bundled payments for hip and knee surgery and episode-of-care payments for cancer care or heart surgery. These pay-for-performance models hold providers accountable for select patient outcomes, measured by quality metrics, in return for monetary incentives.

Because many employees receive health insurance through their employers, employers also have a stake in purchasing high-value healthcare. Evidence suggests that healthcare buyers are increasingly using value-based purchasing concepts in an attempt to control their healthcare spending. In addition to controlling costs, employers are also interested in incorporating outcomes and value into their decisions when selecting provider contracts.

Large employers can try to leverage their purchasing power by encouraging employees to select highly ranked care providers identified through profiling of hospitals and providers. Employers can also help educate their employees about partnering with providers to receive higher-quality care (RWJF 2013). These strategies can have a significant effect on physician practice patterns and decision making. Information about provider networks enables employers to make objective decisions about higher-quality care in the best interest of their employees. In addition, collection of reliable and accurate performance data gives purchasers an advantage in contract negotiations with physicians.

Examples of Profiles and Scorecards

As mentioned previously, the information included in a physician profile or scorecard depends on the intended audience. In 2010, CMS launched the Physician Compare website (to accompany its Hospital Compare site), providing a patient-oriented resource in which physician profiles are searchable using a combination of name, geographic location, and practice specialty (CMS 2017a, 2019). Physician Compare also provides a performance score derived from clinical quality measures (see exhibit 6.1).

Scorecards are commonly used by payers and institutions to look at elements of quality and cost. Exhibit 6.2 shows a scorecard appropriate for a primary care physician in a pay-for-performance program, and it consists predominantly of quality measures. The resource management portion of the scorecard looks at pharmacy management and relative cost of care index. Notice that two benchmarks are used as comparators: (1) the performance of regional peer groups and (2) the NCQA HEDIS 90th percentile performance benchmark (an indicator of high performance). Financial bonuses or penalties can be applied based on results.

EXHIBIT 6.1
Physician Compare Performance Scores

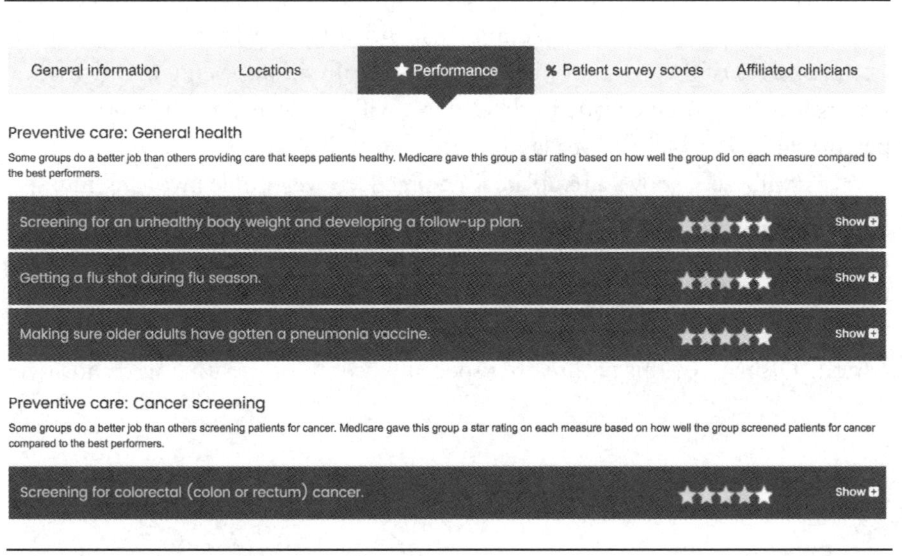

Source: Reprinted from CMS (2019).

EXHIBIT 6.2 Physician Profile, Pay for Performance (through third quarter)

Quality Measures	Target Local Peer Group Performance	Target HEDIS 90th Percentile Benchmark Performance	Physician C Results
Colorectal cancer screening	56.8%	63.5%	57.9%
Use of appropriate medications for people with asthma	91.8%	94.1%	89.5%
Breast cancer screening	70.6%	80.1%	73.0%
Comprehensive diabetes care: HbA1c control (<9.0%)	70.0%	86.1%	82.0%
Comprehensive diabetes care: Eye exam (retinal) performed	62.7%	69.3%	43.6%
Osteoporosis management in women who had a fracture	29.0%	30.4%	30.0%
Cholesterol management for patients with cardiovascular conditions	54.4%	56.5%	46.5%
Resource Management Measures			
Pharmacy management	53.18%	55.20%	52.8%
Relative cost of care index (episode treatment groups)			Calculated at year-end

Scorecards can also be used to compare the performance of various physicians on particular measures. The example in exhibit 6.3 appeals to providers' competitive nature by depicting their individual performance against the performances of their peers. The theory is that physicians, being highly trained professionals who take pride in their work, will be motivated to improve their performance if it is shown to lag behind.

Exhibit 6.4 shows a template for a practice-level profile involving multiple measures. Such a profile represents cumulative data from all physicians in a practice, and it can be used by experienced physician leaders and administrators to identify clinical practice patterns that may need to be improved.

Exhibit 6.5 shows selected cost and patient visit data over a defined period. Displays of this nature are especially useful for identifying trends over time.

EXHIBIT 6.3
Comparison of HbA1c Screening Rates by Provider

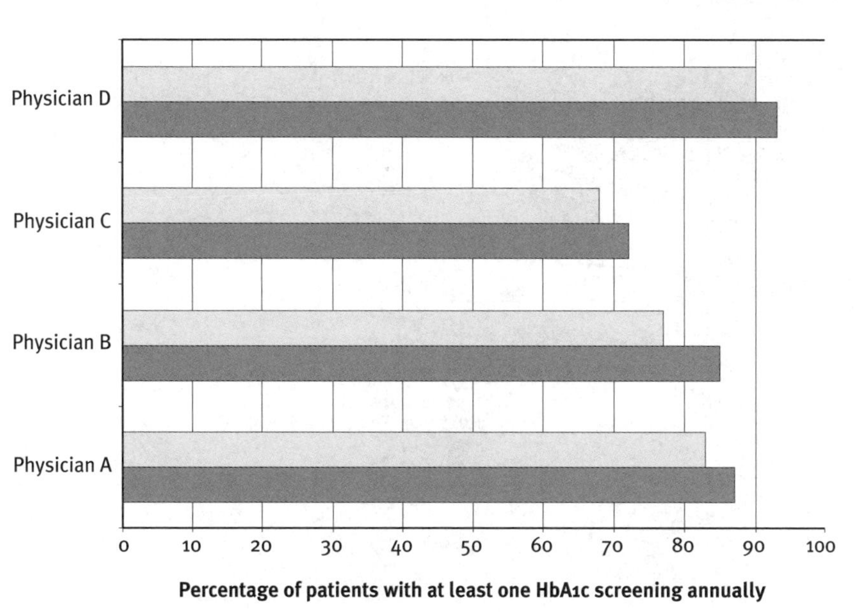

Note: HbA1c = glycohemoglobin.

EXHIBIT 6.4
Practice Profile Template

Demographic Summary

Site/Group	Unique Membership	% Female	% Male	Average Age	% 80 and over	Average PCP Visits per Patient
Practice X						
All Practices						

Risk & Rate Detail

Site/Group	HCC Risk Score	Inpatient Acuity (Case Mix)	7-Day Follow-Up Rate	All-Cause Readmission Rate	Generic Prescribing Rate	% AWV Completed	% Dual Eligible
Practice X							
All Practices							

Raw Utilization Detail

Site/Group	ED Visits	Observation Visits	Acute Admits
Practice X			
All Practices			

Risk-Adjusted Utilization Metrics

Site/Group	ED Visits/1,000	Observation Visits/1,000	Acute Admits/1,000	SNF Admits/1,000	PCP Visits/1,000	Specialist Visits/1,000	Urgent Care Visits/1,000
Practice X							
All Practices							

Source: Adapted from Jefferson Actuarial Informatics reports.

EXHIBIT 6.5
Practice Profile with Cost and Patient Visit Data

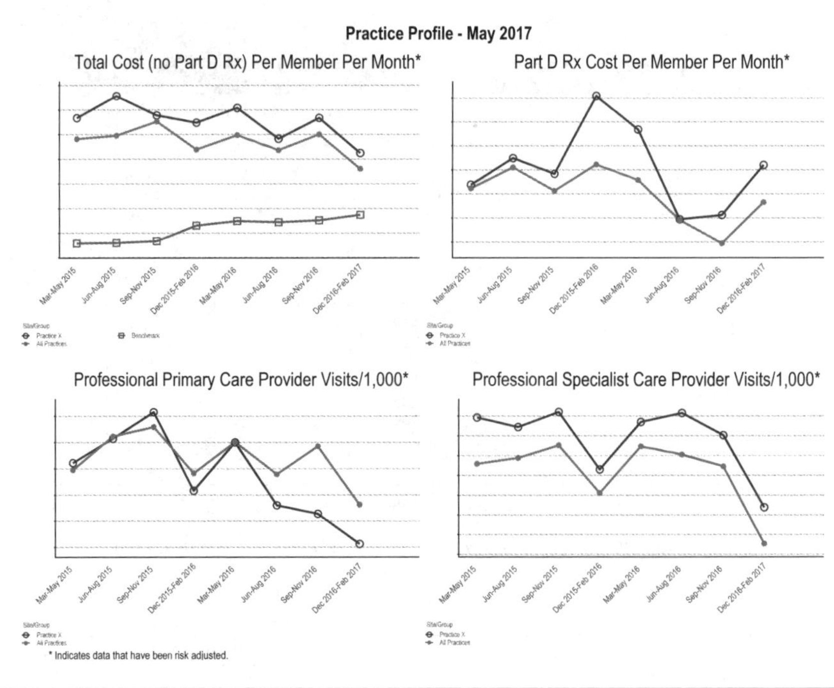

Source: Adapted from Jefferson Actuarial Informatics reports.

Benchmarking

Benchmarking involves comparing a physician's performance on a quality measure against a particular standard, or comparator. The comparator may be performance by peers in the same group or region, or it may be the level of performance defined as excellent by a recognized organization, such as NCQA. This latter type of benchmark is often represented as the "goal" on a scorecard issued by a payer or other healthcare organization. Ideally, a benchmark has been risk-adjusted to allow for an "apples-to-apples" comparison of the patient populations being measured.

Benchmarking uses quantitative measures of best practices (e.g., percentage of patients with hypertension under control) to evaluate physician performance. When physicians' performance is compared to the best practices of their peers, underperforming physicians are likely to be more willing to change their practice patterns. For example, in ambulatory care, achieving and maintaining an optimal blood level of glycohemoglobin (HbA1c) has been identified as an important measurement in controlling complications in patients with diabetes. If a physician's rate of achieving this level for diabetic patients lags behind that of the peer group, the physician can theoretically identify and rectify the causes so that subsequent measurements more closely resemble the best practices.

The Measurement and Implementation Process

Choosing the Measures

Many areas within a healthcare organization, including clinical processes of care and patient outcomes, lend themselves to quality improvement efforts. Examples may involve the appropriate prescribing of antibiotics (e.g., prescribing for the correct bacterial infection and not for viral infections), surgical outcomes (e.g., patients' functional ability after total knee and total hip surgery), blood pressure control, or patient satisfaction. The organization's quality improvement committee should identify the areas most appropriate for profiling and the areas in which performance needs to be improved. Committee members must understand that not all medical conditions are appropriate for profiling; they should profile only conditions for which evidence-based guidelines and endorsed measure specifications exist. The criteria for the profiles may come from nationally recognized practice guidelines or other practice parameters. Organizations are also inclined to choose metrics on which they are being tracked for payer contracts and governmental programs, such as the CMS Oncology Care Model and the Medicare Shared Savings Program.

Guidelines serve as a checklist of objectives against which the committee can compare its actions. Without guidelines, committee members cannot be sure that all components of the care process have been included. An emphasis on rational decision making will foster greater support from physicians and is more likely to bring about performance improvement.

Collecting the Data

The quality improvement committee should identify the techniques to be used in gathering and disseminating data. Traditional methods of data collection have relied on medical records and claims data; more recently, a significant amount of data are being collected via EHRs. Data collection by any method can be difficult. Organizations might find that information is unavailable or that discrete data are lacking for data pull from the EHR. In addition, as a result of healthcare mergers, committees often have to deal with multiple information systems that are not standardized and therefore not compatible (Agency for Healthcare Research and Quality [AHRQ] 2015).

The quality improvement committee must assess which data are most applicable for measuring performance. It also must determine how much data need to be gathered to produce valid results. Both hospitals and provider organizations have been investing large sums of money in the development of health information technology systems capable of generating large amounts of data. The challenge that remains is to translate these data into succinct and actionable information for leadership (Weiner, Balijepally, and Tanniru 2015). Leadership needs to be provided with the appropriate details to make informed decisions.

Data Interpretation

Once the data have been gathered, the quality improvement committee must develop an objective and appropriate way to interpret and validate the findings. Data validity depends on the sample size and the prevalence of the conditions measured in the physician's patient population (AHRQ 2015). Physician performance should be assessed in relation to the accepted national benchmarks for the condition or the target determined by the committee. Profiles should be developed only for physicians who have a large volume of patients with the condition. A physician who sees 200 patients with a certain condition is more likely to value data on her performance than will a physician who sees 20 patients with the same condition, because the data will provide a better representation of the entire population. To counteract issues with patient volume, most measures will be displayed at the physician practice level, rather than at the individual provider level (AHRQ 2015).

Physicians themselves can help the committee construct profiles by identifying areas with potential for improved treatment processes and outcomes, agreeing on benchmarks and gauges of quality, and encouraging other physicians to participate in the quality improvement process. The committee can then determine statistically and clinically significant outcomes. The data must be risk-adjusted to account for the diverse populations of patients that physicians encounter. Risk-adjusting will validate the physicians' results and improve the likelihood that physicians will accept the data. Finally, the measure selection process should be reevaluated periodically to ensure that areas of poor performance are monitored closely and that high-performance areas are deemphasized (Kondo et al. 2016).

Dissemination of Findings

After developing the profile, the quality improvement committee must decide what display format will be most valuable to the physician. Graphical presentations of data in scorecard format are easy to understand and allow physicians to view trends over a specific period. The information conveyed to the physician should be kept simple, and measure specifications and the methodology used to assess performance should be transparent to the providers (Damberg, Hymanm, and France 2014; Damberg and McNamara 2014). In addition, the committee must decide whether the information distributed in the profiles will be blinded or nonblinded. Some physicians may resent having their performance publicly available for other physicians to see, especially if they rank lower than their peers in certain areas. Ideally, physicians will use nonblinded information to identify physicians who have better outcomes and to learn ways to improve. Also, with a nonblinded format, physicians who rank lower will be motivated to improve because they will not want to be seen as performing at a lower level. For this part of the process, physician buy-in is crucial.

Committee meetings should be scheduled on a monthly or quarterly basis so that physicians have the opportunity to comment on how the profiling system is working. These meetings also will provide time for physicians to obtain feedback on their performance and to discuss ways to improve.

Keys to Success

Administrators and quality improvement committees seeking to develop profiles should work closely with physicians to determine an appropriate strategy. At the start of the project, teams should approach physician leaders who have expressed interest in quality improvement. The involvement of physicians who are open to change, respected by their peers, and knowledgeable about quality will increase the likelihood that other physicians in the organization will want to participate.

After developing a profile, the quality improvement committee should determine a time frame for all physicians to review the information before the profile becomes an official tool of the organization. If the committee allows physicians to participate in profile development, they may be more likely to approve of the profiling effort. Once the physicians have submitted their reviews, the committee should meet to finalize the profiles and set a date to begin using them.

Once the profiles have been in use for a defined period, the committee should present a series of educational sessions and organized follow-up activities to enhance provider understanding and acceptance. Modification of physician behavior is a process that will happen over time, and the organization needs to reassure physicians that the profiles are for educational and improvement purposes. Providing physicians with incentives to improve their performance, such as rewards and recognition, will also boost the improvement effort.

The profiling system should not be threatening to physicians. If profiles are to be successful in improving healthcare processes and outcomes, physicians must see them as nonpunitive, educational tools. Physicians have to believe that the profiling system is designed to help them improve their performance and target conditions that offer opportunity for improvement.

Challenges

As healthcare shifts from fee-for-service approaches to more value-based care, scorecards and physician profiles are proliferating. During this transition, the development of provider profiles and registries often presents a multitude of challenges.

Determining the metrics and the population can be a time-consuming process. Physicians generally want to measure their performance for all payers; however, organizations will receive comparative data by health plan, so collating the data may be difficult. Comparisons to regional as well as national benchmarks can be valuable but challenging, given that benchmarks are set by various payers and the organization might not have the same benchmarks for all insurance companies. Display of data, including graphical presentation, should be consistent across measures (Ward et al. 2014). Provider skepticism of data validity can to some extent be alleviated through risk adjustment, but the quality committee should be prepared for challenging questions about data accuracy and usefulness.

Stakeholders will have different preferences for what should be measured. Healthcare organizations will typically measure indicators deemed critical both to improved outcomes in care and to the financial bottom line. Insurers will measure provider performance for measures for which national accrediting bodies, such as NCQA, provide rankings (NCQA 2017). These measures often figure prominently in pay-for-performance contracts between the health plan and providers. The individual provider is likely to focus on measures of clinical or research interest, unless financial incentives are tied to the organizational measures.

Some providers still resist a strong focus on guideline-based measures, which they believe contributes to "cookbook medicine." As personalized medicine becomes more prevalent within specialties such as oncology, with treatment targeted to individual patients, providers might resist the population-based nature of scorecards for certain diseases, which do not allow the flexibility for individualized care. Some physicians also feel that performance measurement—particularly in instances where professional society guidelines and recommendations are translated into mandated quality metrics—can lead to unintended consequences of patient care, such as premature antibiotic treatment for suspected pneumonia (Esposito, Selker, and Salem 2015). Provider profiling could potentially lead to "cherry-picking" of patients with low risk for complications, and it may cause harm if patients are given inappropriate clinical care, if they are treated too aggressively, or if their preferences are not taken into account. Many providers are also concerned that quality improvement initiatives will be limited to improvement in documentation and not in actual patient outcomes (Hysong et al. 2017).

The increasing awareness of variation in quality of care has led to the proliferation of provider and organization scorecards. CMS has taken the lead with the creation of its Hospital Compare and Physician Compare websites, which use consumer-friendly star ratings (similar to those used in the hospitality industry) to encourage patients and consumers to make informed healthcare decisions. The ACA supported this trend by promoting the reporting of quality measures and accelerating Medicare's efforts to pay for healthcare based on *value* as opposed to *volume* of services (Findlay 2016). Information is also available through consumer sites such as Yelp and Healthgrades, where patients can rank providers and hospitals the way they rate restaurants, complete with reviews.

Overall, however, the public has not fully embraced these report cards. Some consumers may have difficulty accessing, understanding, or navigating the online information, and many people are accustomed to making healthcare choices based on personal recommendations from friends and family, rather than through an online search of databases. The design of publicly available report cards can also make them difficult to interpret. In addition, the quality indicators are often based on clinical practice and are not patient-centric. They might not seem relevant to the consumer, and concerns about data validity remain (Daskivich, Spiegel, and Kim 2017). Finally, with growing numbers of providers joining alternative payment models, such as accountable care organizations (ACOs), much of the data displayed might not reflect an individual provider's performance; rather, the data provide a summary at the ACO level.

Interest in online provider ratings based on patient satisfaction measures—such as likelihood to recommend a provider or hospital—has seen a faster growth, although these types of ratings can reduce the focus on standardized quality measures (Kanouse et al. 2016).

Physician Profiling and Provider Registries in a Changing Healthcare Landscape

Numerous attempts have been made to constrain the rapid growth in healthcare spending, and a heightened emphasis on value has led to a host of quality initiatives and value-based programs. CMS, with the goal of becoming an active purchaser of high-quality care, spearheaded the Physician Quality Reporting System in 2006. More recent programs include the EHR Incentive Program and the Value-Based Payment Modifier. The MACRA legislation of 2015 established the Quality Payment Program, which includes MIPS and the Advanced Alternative Payment Models (CMS 2017b). The vast majority of providers will be eligible for the MIPS program, which combines four performance categories—quality, advancing care information, improvement activities, and cost—into one composite score (Chen and Coffron 2017). Value-based purchasing is a key component of MACRA. As such, physician reimbursement will be directly tied to performance on quality metrics, and pay-for-performance programs will likely remain a focus of US healthcare for the foreseeable future (Mendelson et al. 2017; Jha 2017).

Measuring performance through the use of quality indicators has become a key part of efforts to reform healthcare delivery, and provider profiles generated by these efforts are increasingly being tied to financial incentives. To remain successful and competitive in a value-conscious era, providers and healthcare organizations must collaborate to create a culture of accountability that will lead to greater value. By measuring and improving the quality of care delivered to patients, we can take important steps along the road toward the overarching goal of achieving population health.

Study Questions

1. What are quality measures?
2. Describe the strengths and weaknesses of the profiles discussed in this chapter.
3. What challenges might a quality improvement committee encounter when attempting to measure physician performance?

References

Agency for Healthcare Research and Quality (AHRQ). 2015. "The Challenges of Measuring Physician Quality." Published February. www.ahrq.gov/professionals/quality-patient-safety/talkingquality/create/physician/challenges.html.

Centers for Medicare & Medicaid Services (CMS). 2019. "Physician Compare." Accessed November 3. www.medicare.gov/physiciancompare/.

———. 2018. "Quality Measures." Modified August 6. www.cms.gov/Medicare/Quality-Initiatives-Patient-Assessment-Instruments/QualityMeasures/index.html.

———. 2017a. "Hospital Compare." Accessed November 4. www.medicare.gov/hospitalcompare/.

———. 2017b. "Quality Payment Program." Accessed November 3. www.cms.gov/Medicare/Quality-Payment-Program/Quality-Payment-Program.html.

Chen, S. L., and M. R. Coffron. 2017. "MACRA and the Changing Medicare Payment Landscape." *Annals of Surgical Oncology* 24 (10): 2836–41.

Codman, E. A. 1914. "The Product of a Hospital." *Surgery, Gynecology and Obstetrics* 18: 491–96.

Damberg, C. L., D. Hyman, and J. France. 2014. "Do Public Reports of Providers Make Their Data and Methods Available and Accessible?" *Medical Care Research and Review* 71 (5): 81S–96S.

Damberg, C. L., and P. McNamara. 2014. "Postscript: Research Agenda to Guide the Next Generation of Public Reports for Consumers." *Medical Care Research and Review* 71 (5): 97S–107S.

Daskivich, T. J., B. Spiegel, and H. L. Kim. 2017. "Online Ratings Systems for Physicians and Institutions: Limitations of the Current State of the Art." *European Urology* 71 (3): 311–12.

Donabedian, A. 1966. "Evaluating the Quality of Medical Care." *Milbank Memorial Fund Quarterly* 44 (3 Suppl.): 166–203.

Doran, T., K. A. Maurer, and A. M. Ryan. 2017. "Impact of Provider Incentives on Quality and Value of Health Care." *Annual Review of Public Health* 38: 449–65.

Esposito, M. L., H. P. Selker, and D. N. Salem. 2015. "Quantity over Quality: How the Rise in Quality Measures Is Not Producing Quality Results." *Journal of General Internal Medicine* 30 (8): 1204–7.

Findlay, S. D. 2016. "Consumers' Interest in Provider Ratings Grows, and Improved Report Cards and Other Steps Could Accelerate Their Use." *Health Affairs* 35 (4): 688–96.

Fung, V., J. A. Schmittdiel, B. Fireman, A. Meer, S. Thomas, J. Hsu, and J. V. Selby. 2010. "Meaningful Variation in Performance: A Systematic Literature Review." *Medical Care* 48 (2): 140–48.

Hysong, S. J., R. SoRelle, K. B. Smitham, and L. A. Petersen. 2017. "Reports of Unintended Consequences of Financial Incentives to Improve Management of Hypertension." *PLOS ONE* 12 (9): e0184856.

Institute for Healthcare Improvement (IHI). 2018. "IHI Triple Aim Initiative." Accessed October 19. www.ihi.org/Engage/Initiatives/TripleAim/Pages/default.aspx.

Institute of Medicine (IOM). 2001. *Crossing the Quality Chasm: A New Health System for the 21st Century.* Washington, DC: National Academies Press.

James, J. 2012. "Public Reporting on Quality and Costs: Do Report Cards and Other Measures of Providers' Performance Lead to Improved Care and Better Choices by Consumers?" *Health Affairs.* Published March 8. www.healthaffairs.org/do/10.1377/hpb20120308.53696/full/.

Jha, A. K. 2017. "Value-Based Purchasing: Time to Reboot or Time to Move On?" *JAMA* 317 (11): 1107–8.

Kanouse, D. E., M. Schlesinger, D. Shaller, S. C. Martino, and L. Rybowski. 2016. "How Patient Comments Affect Consumers' Use of Physician Performance Measures." *Medical Care* 54 (1): 24–31.

Keehan, S. P., J. A. Poisal, G. A. Cuckler, A. M. Sisko, S. D. Smith, A. J. Madison, D. A. Stone, C. J. Wolfe, and J. M. Lizonitz. 2016. "National Expenditure Projections, 2015–25: Economy, Prices, and Aging Expected to Shape Spending and Enrollment." *Health Affairs* 35 (8): 1522–31.

Kondo, K. K., C. L. Damberg, A. Mendelson, M. Motu'apuaka, M. Freeman, M. O'Neil, R. Relevo, A. Low, and D. Kansagara. 2016. "Implementation Processes and Pay for Performance in Healthcare: A Systematic Review." *Journal of General Internal Medicine* 31 (Suppl. 1): 61–69.

Kumar, S., and D. B. Nash. 2010. *Demand Better! Revive Our Broken Healthcare System*. Bozeman, MT: Second River Healthcare Press.

McIver, J. S. 2017. "David B. Nash Advocates Better Outcomes and Lower Costs Through Population Health." *Pharmacy and Therapeutics* 42 (8): 522–26.

Mendelson, A., K. Kondo, C. Damberg, A. Low, M. Motu'apuaka, M. Freeman, M. O'Neil, R. Relevo, and D. Kansagara. 2017. "The Effects of Pay-for-Performance Programs on Health, Health Care Use, and Processes of Care." *Annals of Internal Medicine* 166 (5): 341–53.

National Committee for Quality Assurance (NCQA). 2017. "NCQA Health Insurance Plan Ratings 2017–2018." Accessed November 4. http://healthinsuranceratings.ncqa.org/2017/Default.aspx.

Pugh, M. D. 2014. "Dashboards and Scorecards: Tools for Creating Alignment." In *The Healthcare Quality Book: Vision, Strategy, and Tools*, 3rd ed., edited by M. S. Joshi, E. R. Ransom, D. B. Nash, and S. B. Ransom, 241–67. Chicago: Health Administration Press.

Quality Payment Program. 2018. "MIPS Overview." Centers for Medicare & Medicaid Services. Accessed October 22. https://qpp.cms.gov/mips/overview.

Robert Wood Johnson Foundation (RWJF). 2013. "How Employers Can Improve Value and Quality in Health Care." Published January. www.rwjf.org/content/dam/farm/reports/issue_briefs/2013/rwjf403361.

———. 2009. "Communicating with Physicians About Performance Measurement." Published December 1. www.rwjf.org/en/library/research/2009/12/communicating-with-physicians-about-performance-measurement.html.

Schneider, E. C., D. O. Sarnak, D. Squires, A. Shah, and M. M. Doty. 2017. "Mirror, Mirror 2017: International Comparison Reflects Flaws and Opportunities for Better U.S. Health Care." Commonwealth Fund. Published July. www.commonwealthfund.org/interactives/2017/july/mirror-mirror/.

Skinner, J., and E. S. Fisher. 2010. "Reflections on Geographic Variations in U.S. Health Care." Dartmouth Institute for Health Policy and Clinical Practice. Published March 31. www.dartmouthatlas.org/downloads/press/Skinner_Fisher_DA_05_10.pdf.

Ward, C. E., L. Morella, J. M. Ashburner, and S. J. Atlas. 2014. "An Interactive, All-Payer, Multidomain Primary Care Performance Dashboard." *Journal of Ambulatory Care Management* 37 (4): 339–48.

Weiner, J., V. Balijepally, and M. Tanniru. 2015. "Integrating Strategic and Operational Decision Making Using Data-Driven Dashboards: The Case of St. Joseph Mercy Oakland Hospital." *Journal of Healthcare Management* 60 (5): 319–30.

Wilensky, G. 2016. "Time to Hit the Pause Button on Medicare's Payment Demonstration Projects?" *JAMA* 316 (15):1535–36.

World Health Organization (WHO). 2000. "World Health Report: World Health Organization Assesses the World's Health Systems." Accessed January 23, 2018. www.who.int/whr/2000/media_centre/press_release/en/.

CHAPTER

7

HEALTH INFORMATION TECHNOLOGY IN HEALTHCARE QUALITY AND SAFETY: PREVENTION, IDENTIFICATION, AND ACTION

Sue S. Feldman, Scott E. Buchalter, and Leslie W. Hayes

Introduction

It has long been known and accepted that healthcare in the United States is too expensive and its outcomes are less than predictable (Marmor, Oberlander, and White 2009). The turn of the century brought with it a realization that healthcare, like other industries, could use data to increase our awareness of seemingly uncontrollable costs and unpredictable outcomes. After almost two decades of compiling, analyzing, and mashing up data and trying to make sense of how the data inform multiple layers of healthcare, the time has come to look beyond the awareness that the data provide and instead develop an understanding of how to use the data for predictable and actionable purposes, especially with regard to healthcare quality and safety.

The literature is mixed on the degree to which the tools, applications, and systems of health information technology (IT) contribute to actual savings and efficiencies (Buntin et al. 2011; Goldzweig et al. 2009; Marmor, Oberlander, and White 2009; Karsh et al. 2010). However, the area of healthcare quality and safety lends itself to many of the same business intelligence and predictability advantages that have been seen in the credit card industry (Jamal, McKenzie, and Clark 2009; McCullough et al. 2010; Parente and McCullough 2009).

Much as healthcare has its Triple Aim of per capita cost, population health, and experience of care (Institute for Healthcare Improvement 2018), the credit card industry strives for decreased costs (fraud), increased quality (better transactions), and increased satisfaction (happier merchants and happier cardholders). The credit card industry has used business intelligence to predict behavior that suggests fraud, developed process maps for transaction processing, and offered perks to merchants and cardholders. These parallels suggest an opportunity for healthcare to learn from the credit card industry to use healthcare intelligence for prevention, identification, and action related to quality and safety events.

Health IT in Healthcare Quality and Safety

The Institute for Healthcare Improvement (IHI) suggests that reliability around healthcare is a three-part cycle of failure prevention, failure identification, and process redesign, as shown in exhibit 7.1 (Nolan et al. 2004). However, a review of the literature suggests that healthcare organizations that are using health IT for quality and safety have replaced the word *redesign* with *action*, as shown in exhibit 7.2.

An understanding of this cycle helps create an awareness around where various applications of health IT find their "best fit" in improving the reliability of healthcare quality and safety. A distinct advantage of this being a cycle is that it really has no distinct and defined beginning or ending point—only an

EXHIBIT 7.1 Improving the Reliability of Healthcare

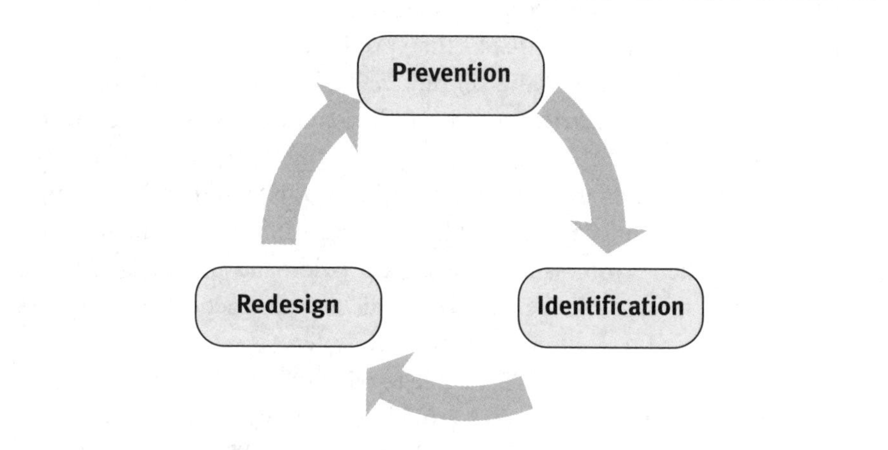

EXHIBIT 7.2 Improving the Reliability of Healthcare Quality and Safety

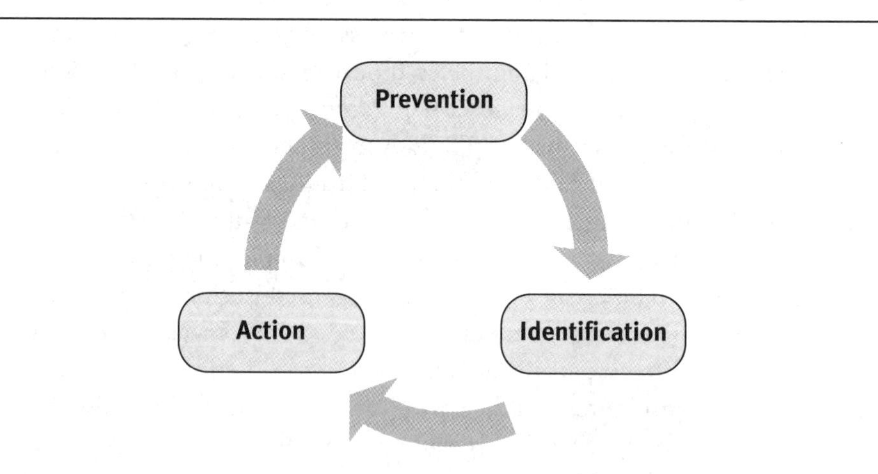

insertion point. The cycle should not be interpreted as starting with prevention and ending with action.

A scan of the literature suggests that organizations looking to devote health IT resources to quality and safety might get the most return on their investment by focusing on alerts and clinical decision support in terms of *what* to implement. In terms of *how* to implement, organizations need to recognize that culture and interface design have been identified as primary challenges. Detailed findings from that scan of the literature are the focus of the next section.

What Does the Literature Say About Health IT Use in Healthcare Quality and Safety?

The scan of the literature included 36 peer-reviewed studies dealing with how health IT was used in quality and safety efforts (see the table at the end of the chapter). Those articles included 92 mentions of health IT for prevention of healthcare quality and safety issues, 62 mentions of the use of health IT for identification of such issues, and 41 mentions of health IT for action. The challenges associated with health IT for healthcare quality and safety were mentioned 43 times.

Prevention

The first exploration focused on the literature that discussed health IT for prevention of quality and safety issues, to see exactly how organizations were reporting health IT use. The greatest areas of use were around alerts, clinical decision support, implementation, interface design, and customized health IT solutions. Customized health IT solutions included instances where the use of health IT was mentioned but without specificity, and they could be as simple as checklists or as complex as algorithmic diagnostic trees.

To clarify, alerts are a subset of clinical decision support. However, because so many of the mentions specified alerts and clinical decision support separately, they were coded separately. Clinical decision support, by definition, includes alerts, clinical care guidelines, condition-specific order sets, clinical reports and summaries, documentation templates, diagnostic support, and clinical reference support (Beeler, Bates, and Hug 2014).

Identification

The next exploration was across the literature that discussed health IT for identification of quality and safety issues—in other words, how health IT was being used to identify an issue once it had already happened. In this regard, alerts, clinical decision support, implementation, and customized health IT solutions were most prominent.

Action

The third exploration was across the literature that discussed health IT for action relative to quality and safety issues that had already happened—in instances where health IT had not detected the issue but was being used to act upon it. Relative to action, the major areas were documentation, implementation, and culture.

Co-occurrences

Using the three components of the "improving the reliability of healthcare quality and safety" model (introduced in exhibit 7. 2) and adding the challenges, six critical co-occurrences emerged (see exhibit 7.3). The first co-occurring code, implementation, appeared in the explorations of prevention, identification, and action, and the literature has also highlighted it as its own category as a challenge. Analysis of challenges suggests that the major areas are culture, implementation, and interface design.

The top co-occurring codes provide a macro-level view of how health IT was most commonly used for quality and safety relative to the model. However, we also must understand the full universe of ways in which organizations used health IT for quality and safety—in other words, the "art of the possible" when using health IT for these purposes. Network maps provide a mechanism by which to visualize all data coded across all the articles included in the analysis. These maps, along with some quantitative information, increase understanding at this universe level, which incorporates both macro and micro views.

In the network diagrams in exhibits 7.4 through 7.7, the letter *G* signifies the level of groundedness of the particular code. Groundedness indicates the frequency of the code relative to the code category. The letter *D* signifies the level of density, or connectedness, of the particular code—the number of other code categories with which a given code is connected.

EXHIBIT 7.3 Co-occurrence Codes in Descending Order

Code	Co-occurrences
Implementation	Prevention, identification, action, challenges
Alerts	Prevention, identification
Clinical decision support	Prevention, identification
Interface design	Prevention, challenges
Culture	Action, challenges (tattling)
Customized health IT solutions	Prevention, identification

EXHIBIT 7.4
Network Diagram—Action

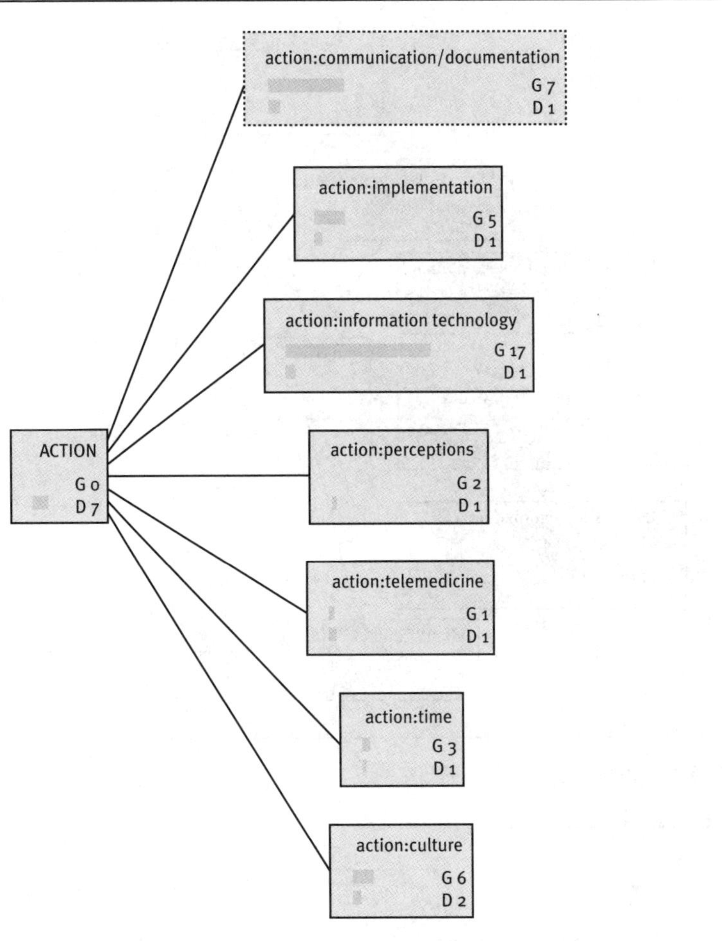

Note: G = groundedness, D = density.

EXHIBIT 7.5
Network Diagram—Outcomes

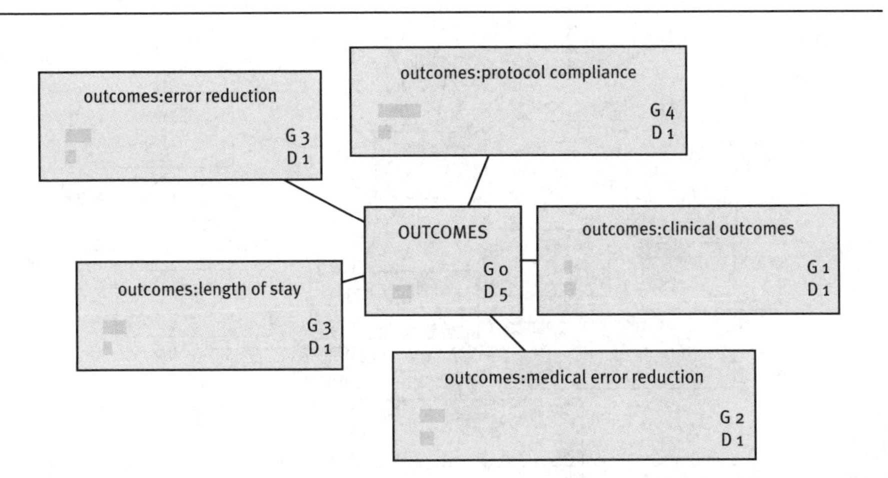

Note: G = groundedness, D = density.

EXHIBIT 7.6
Network Diagram—Identification

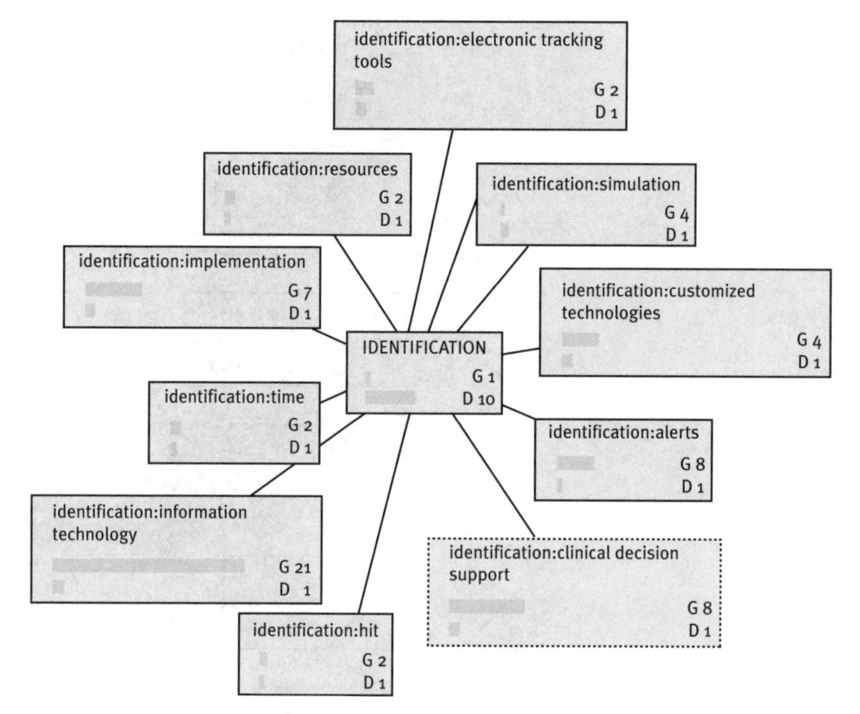

Note: G = groundedness, D = density.

EXHIBIT 7.7
Network Diagram—Prevention

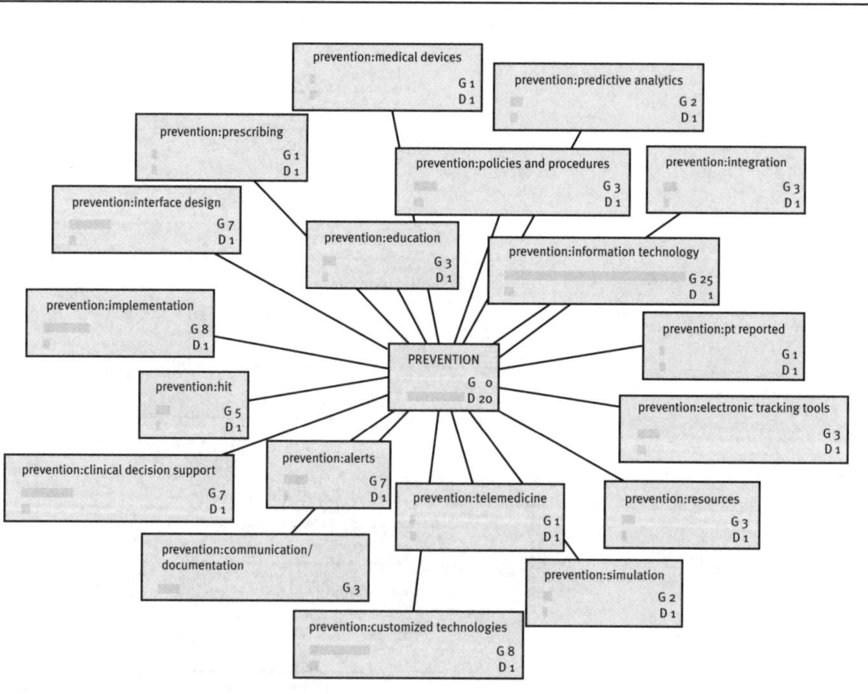

Note: G = groundedness, D = density.

For example, in the network diagram for action, "action" is the code category, and "action:culture" is the code for "culture" within that code category (this coding structure helps maintain alphabetical order). The "action:culture" code shows G6, D2, which can be read as follows: "Across all the articles, *culture* was mentioned six times relative to action and is connected to two code categories total." Specificity around the groundedness or the density is not shown in the exhibits, to avoid making the network diagrams unwieldy.

Improving Care Delivery Through Health IT: Case Studies

Health IT for Prevention

Automated reminders and alerts are useful for providing important information that supports safe and effective clinical decisions (Grissinger 2016). Such alerts within the EHR system are a common mechanism for the use of health IT for prevention of potential missed quality and safety events. For example, immunization alerts have led to a 12 percent increase in well-child and a 22 percent increase in sick-child immunization administration (Fiks et al. 2007). Similarly, drug alerts have been associated with a 22 percent decrease in medication prescription errors (Smith et al. 2006).

Case study 1 discusses the use of health IT in preventing safety events via soft- and hard-stop alerts. Soft-stop alerts can provide key information about a potential quality or safety issue and may offer alternative choices, but they usually require only that the user acknowledge the alert in order to proceed. A hard-stop alert, on the other hand, prevents the user from moving forward with a potentially dangerous order or intervention. Hard stops may allow continuation of the process only if a significant required action is taken by the user, such as a call or consultation with an expert (e.g., pharmacist, medical specialist). In some instances, soft stops may be ignored or overridden because of such issues as alert fatigue, poor implementation, or poor interface design (van der Sijs et al. 2006; Harrison, Koppel, and Bar-Lev 2007). Hard stops, when appropriately designed, have been shown to be more successful in changing an unsafe plan or preventing a potentially dangerous intervention (Strom et al. 2010; Eslami, de Keizer, and Abu-Hanna 2008).

Case Study 1: Prevention

Preventing High-Risk Safety Events Through Use of a Hard-Stop Alert

Effective implementation of an EHR requires that clinical and operational leaders understand effective clinical workflows and design care delivery processes that facilitate safe, effective, and efficient care (Walker, Bieber, and Richards 2005). This case study describes the use of an automated alert system for a contraindicated drug.

In one large academic health system, an active error-reporting process and surveillance system identified a patient safety event in which an elderly patient receiving levodopa to treat her Parkinson's disease was admitted for treatment of a urinary tract infection. When she developed some behavioral disturbances, she was given Haldol for three days. She subsequently became less responsive, requiring an admission to the intensive care unit (ICU). Haldol was discontinued, and the patient recovered to baseline function after an extended ICU stay. However, the risk to her health was substantial.

Haldol is an antipsychotic drug that blocks dopamine receptors in the brain, which can dramatically worsen the effects of Parkinson's disease and reduce the effectiveness of treatment with levodopa (Derry et al. 2010; Magdalinou, Martin, and Kessel 2007). When administered to patients with Parkinson's disease, it may result in serious mental status changes, a reduction in ability to respond, or even coma or death (Okun 2012, 2011). For these reasons, Haldol is contraindicated for elderly patients with Parkinson's disease.

In this case, a multidisciplinary team of clinicians, pharmacists, and health IT experts initially designed a soft-stop alert. However, the intervention did not significantly reduce the number of provider attempts to order Haldol for this patient population (suggesting alert fatigue). The team then designed a hard-stop alert that prevented providers from ordering Haldol for Parkinson's disease patients and allowed continuation of the process only after consultation with an expert pharmacist or medical specialist. The results of this health IT intervention are shown in exhibit 7.8.

The hard stop was initiated in the first quarter of 2014, during which 105 attempts were made to order Haldol for a patient with Parkinson's disease, resulting in 105 alert firings to abort the ordering. After this period, no patient safety events involving administration of Haldol to patients with Parkinson's disease were identified or reported. Thus, the hard stop proved extremely effective in preventing inadvertent unsafe care. In the months that followed, the health IT implementation substantially reduced the number of ordering attempts and subsequent alerts fired. We are not concerned that the alert firings have not dropped to zero; these results, combined with the lack of identified patient safety events, offer some reassurance that the alert is functional.

This case highlights the usefulness of health IT interventions such as hard stops in appropriate settings, given the complexity of medicine, the volume of knowledge that exists, and the human factors that can lead to

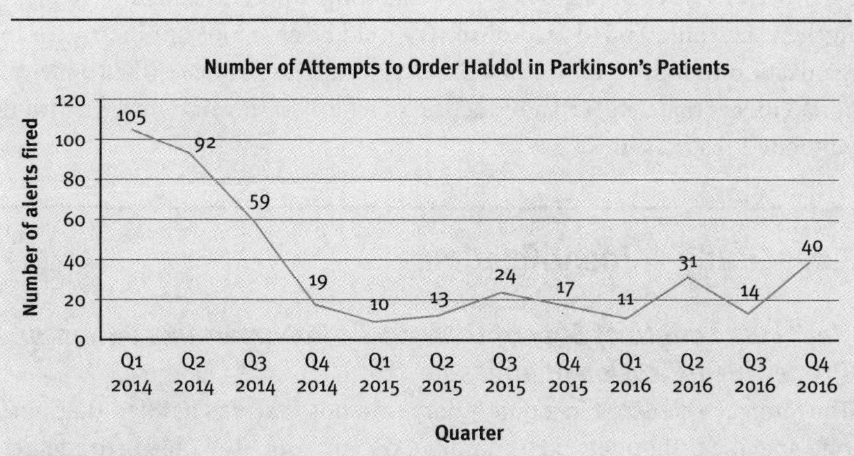

EXHIBIT 7.8 Stop-Order Results: Number of Attempts to Order Haldol for Parkinson's Patients

errors. It also stresses the importance of systemwide provider education, competency testing, and ongoing surveillance.

Case Study Discussion Questions

1. Describe the relationship between soft stops and hard stops as health IT interventions and ongoing surveillance.
2. In this situation, why was the hard stop more effective than the soft stop in preventing an error from reaching the patient?
3. What might be some pitfalls in using hard stops in a clinical setting? Might there be negative consequences that should be considered?

Health IT for Identification

Health insurance providers are placing increased pressure on healthcare systems to reduce the cost of care delivery and to improve patient outcomes. This pressure is often applied through tiered reimbursement structures that benefit those systems that meet or exceed certain performance benchmarks, as well as through nonreimbursement for care determined by the payer to be unnecessary or in excess of "standard care." Organizations can use health IT to identify problem areas and suggest changes that lead to better performance under these pressures. Health IT can help expose certain populations of patients, as segments of the overall inpatient population, that are strongly associated with a particular challenge or issue—for instance, length of stay.

During the implementation of any new process, organizations must give thoughtful consideration to balancing measures. In other words, they need to answer the question, What unintended negative outcomes could arise from the new process? For example, when implementing a process aimed at reducing length of stay, unintended readmissions would be an important metric for the organization to follow. Case study 2 describes the use of health IT to identify improvements that achieved a reduction in length of stay of four days with no unintended readmissions.

Case Study 2: Identification

Reducing Length of Stay of Orthopedic Postoperative Patients: Proper Identification of an Issue

The intensive care unit in a quaternary care hospital was notified that, for one specific orthopedic postoperative patient type (the only orthopedic patients in the ICU postoperatively), reimbursement would only be provided for three days after surgery. A review of the data for this patient population at the hospital revealed that the length of stay had historically been seven days—more than twice the number of days that would receive full reimbursement. Seeking to address the issue, the institution initiated a four-pronged approach:

- Form a team consisting of all key stakeholders in the care of these patients.
- Partner with both quality improvement and health IT to identify the specifics of the problem.
- Analyze the challenges with the current process (achieved through detailed process mapping and understanding of baseline data).
- Prioritize solutions for both an improved process and improved outcomes.

During the initiative, the team discovered that health IT actually played a larger role than anyone had anticipated; it actually underscored the entire project. Analysis of the data that were available in partnership with health IT enabled assessment of the extent of the current problem. Optimizing the skills of the health IT experts and quality improvement experts, the team determined that orthopedic postoperative patients represented a significant proportion of the admissions to one of the hospital's ICUs.

Exhibit 7.9 shows a Pareto chart—a histogram that prioritizes categories from most to least frequent in occurrence—demonstrating that a primary orthopedic diagnosis was the second most common ICU admission diagnosis in 2014. This group included 135 patients, or 12 percent of the total ICU patient population.

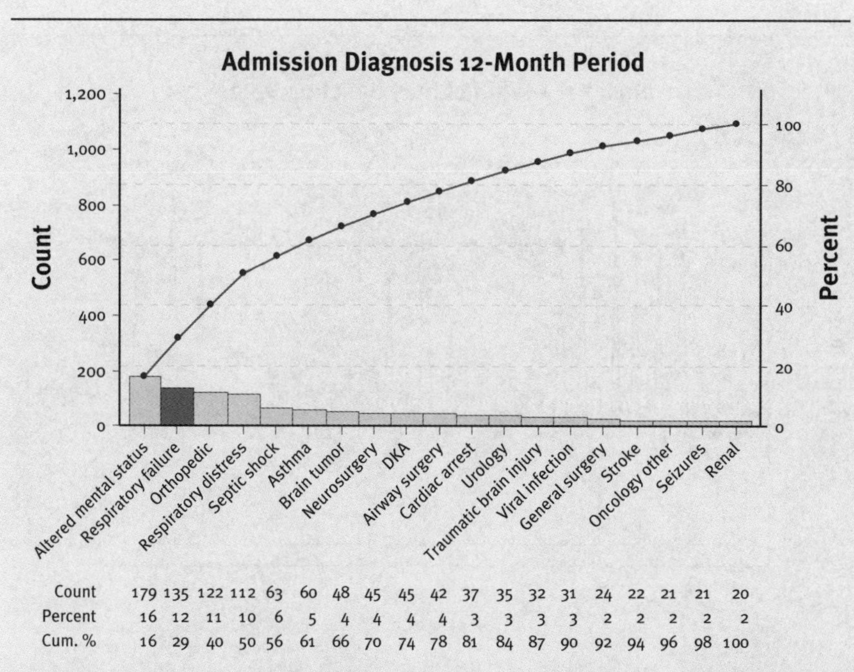

EXHIBIT 7.9
Pareto Chart Showing Intensive Care Unit Admission by Diagnosis (12-month period, 2014)

Detailed process mapping of the current process for admitting and caring for these patients revealed variation in practice, which contributed to delays in timely postoperative care. The strong partnership between health IT and quality improvement allowed for thorough analysis of all pertinent data; this analysis highlighted the current challenges of implementation and identified optimal solutions. Exhibit 7.10 shows a statistical process control (SPC) chart—a tool for analyzing data over time, focusing on how the data are distributed around the mean and the spread (standard deviation)—for overall hospital length of stay. The graph, representing all 135 patients, shows wide variation in length of stay, from 3 days to 18 days.

Health IT and quality improvement partnered with key stakeholders in the process to streamline care delivery, and they created a standard protocol for postoperative management that was initiated during surgery and continued throughout the hospital stay. The protocol was first piloted on paper, with immediate feedback sought from the healthcare delivery team and health IT to evaluate for additional improvements in terms of process and implementation. Within one month, the team reached the final version of the protocol, and health IT implemented the protocol in the EHR. The protocol has shown sustained improvement, as displayed in exhibit 7.11.

(continued)

EXHIBIT 7.10
Statistical Process Control Chart Showing Length of Stay for Patients with a Primary ICU Orthopedic Admission Diagnosis

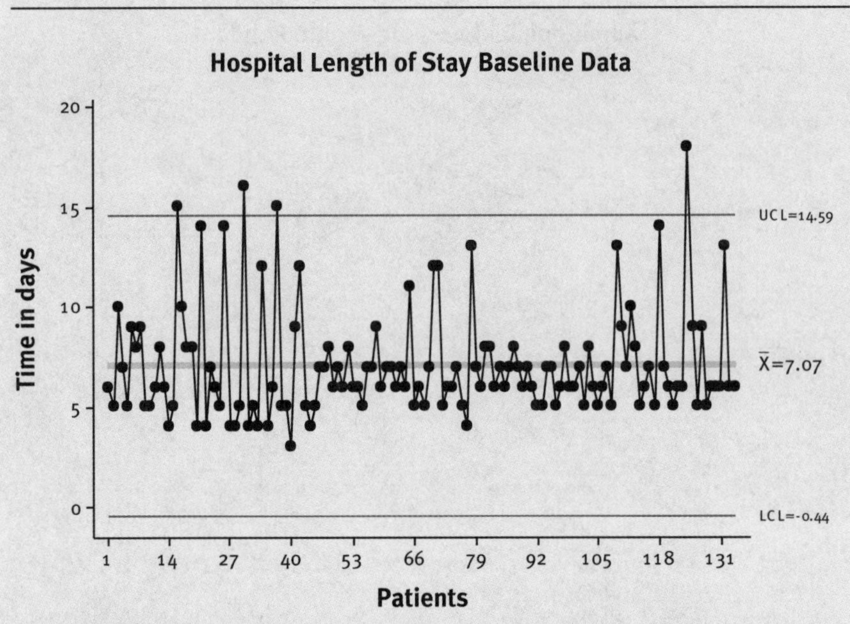

Note: Data here are for the same 12-month period as exhibit 7.9. UCL = upper control limit; LCL = lower control limit.

EXHIBIT 7.11
Length of Stay for Patients with a Primary ICU Orthopedic Admission Diagnosis, Before and After Implementation

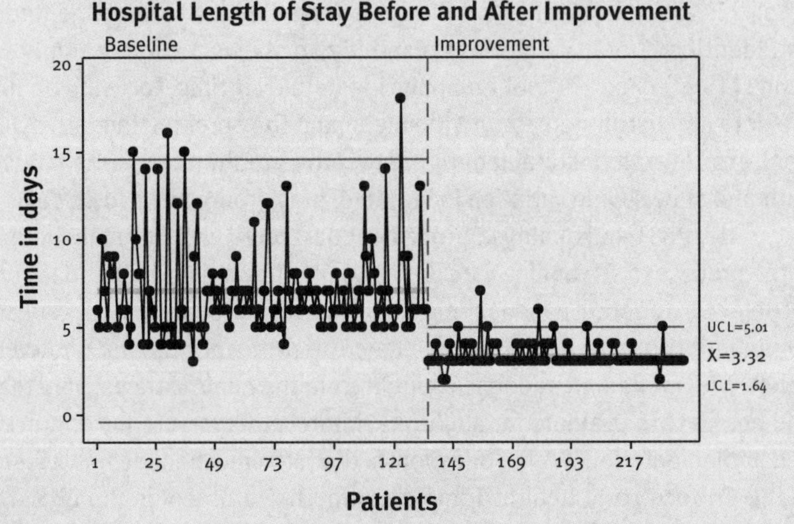

Note: Data here are for the same 12-month period shown in exhibits 7.9 and 7.10, followed by an additional 12-month postimplementation improvement period in 2015. UCL = upper control limit; LCL = lower control limit.

The initial improvement could not have been maintained without health IT involvement, which illustrates the importance of having health IT involved in quality and safety initiatives at the beginning of the process.

Case Study Discussion Questions

1. In this case, no barriers to improvement were identified, because all providers were motivated to improve care. How might you address resistance to improvement, if it existed?
2. Key to the success of this project was the immediate partnership among health IT, quality improvement, and the experts in patient care. How might the implementation of this protocol have been different without input from one of these groups?

Health IT for Action

Despite nearly two decades of advances in early sepsis care, sepsis outcomes remain poor, and sepsis continues to account for significant morbidity and mortality worldwide (Busund et al. 2002). The early identification and treatment of sepsis have therefore become the focus of a growing national push aiming to improve healthcare outcomes.

Patients with sepsis are some of the most critically ill patients admitted to hospitals, and their survival depends heavily upon timely administration of key interventions, followed quickly by assessment and action based on results of those interventions (Rivers et al. 2001). Examples of key interventions include administration of intravenous (IV) antibiotics and aggressive IV fluids within one hour (Rivers et al. 2001). Assessments of interventions often involve measurement of certain physical and laboratory values that provide key information about patient response. All too often, clinicians are faced with an overabundance of data, much of which may be necessary to collect but not relevant to the issue at hand. For example, lab results might be presented in their entirety even though, in practice, only three or four tests will drive decision making. Often, the quandary is how to separate the noise (i.e., data that are nonessential at that moment) from the signal (i.e., data that are essential at that moment). Health IT is often called upon to build dashboards and other solutions that put essential data in a primary viewing position and nonessential data in a secondary position (perhaps accessible via drill down, for example).

Case study 3 provides an example of health IT for action, and it illustrates the cooperation and collaboration of a healthcare delivery team, health IT, and quality improvement to address what might be the most important issue in sepsis care. This issue is not lack of knowledge about *what to do* in the treatment of a patient with sepsis but rather how health IT and quality improvement can make it efficient for healthcare teams to provide the care they intend to deliver.

Case Study 3: Action

Improving Mortality from Sepsis

One academic health system charged its health IT and quality improvement experts with analyzing the system's mortality outcomes from sepsis. The group chose percent mortality in sepsis (i.e., the percentage of patients with sepsis who died) as the key metric to evaluate. Exhibit 7.12 shows the baseline data for the institution's percent mortality in sepsis, showing that, on average, 39.25 percent of patients with sepsis died from it.

The partnership with health IT provided the baseline data needed to develop an action plan to improve outcomes. Along with the outcome metric shown in exhibit 7.12, multiple process measures were obtained, revealing clear gaps in performance and opportunities for improvement. Through detailed process mapping—incorporating both direct observations of the process and brainstorming sessions with the care delivery team to discuss barriers to timely interventions and assessments—the team developed a practical, visual algorithm that was ready to be "test-driven" on paper. The improvement was developed to blend into the workflow at the bedside and turn an often complex and chaotic process into a streamlined and predictable one. Still missing, though, was the anywhere/anytime access afforded by having this process embedded in the EHR.

EXHIBIT 7.12 Percent Sepsis Mortality over a 24-Month Period (2012–2013)

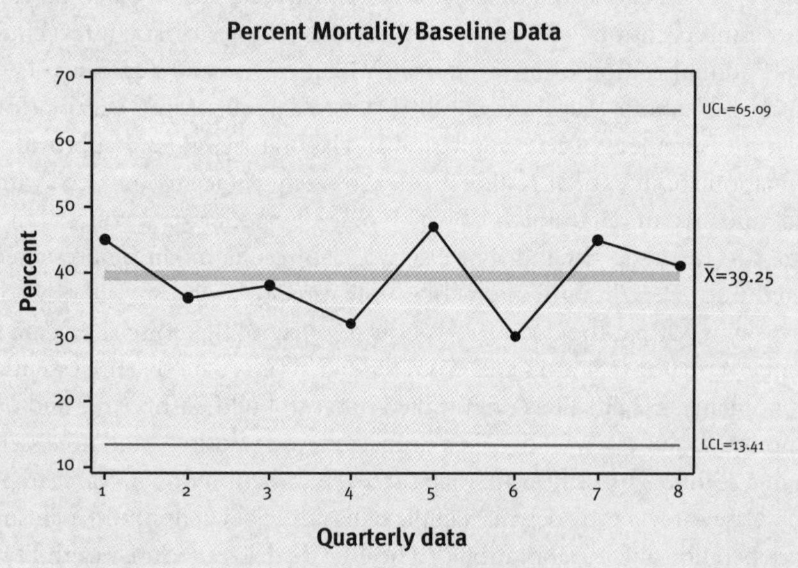

Note: UCL = upper control limit; LCL = lower control limit.

This collaboration led to the results shown in exhibit 7.13. With the improved process, an average of just 14.75 percent of the patients with sepsis died from it—a 62.4 percent reduction in mortality.

After proper testing of a paper solution, an algorithm-driven dashboard was embedded into the EHR. Doing so made the algorithm—which had previously been viewed in isolation without the benefit of other information—a sustainable, predictable, visible, and visual process. Exhibit 7.14 presents one key process measure—time to administration of antibiotics—that illustrates how algorithm-driven dashboards improve care delivery. The left side of the chart shows the baseline performance on time to administration of antibiotics, and the right side shows the improvement after health IT solutions were implemented. Whereas the baseline average time was 231.5 minutes, the average time after the improvement was 49.1 minutes—well within the standards of care for antibiotic administration in sepsis (Rivers et al. 2001).

The improvement described here is not typical for responses to healthcare problems. Commonly, action must be taken to educate providers and staff about what care needs to be delivered; in this case, however, the issue was not a knowledge deficit on the part of providers and staff. Instead, the action involved development of an improved process through

EXHIBIT 7.13
Percent Sepsis Mortality, Before and After Improvement Implementation (2012–2015)

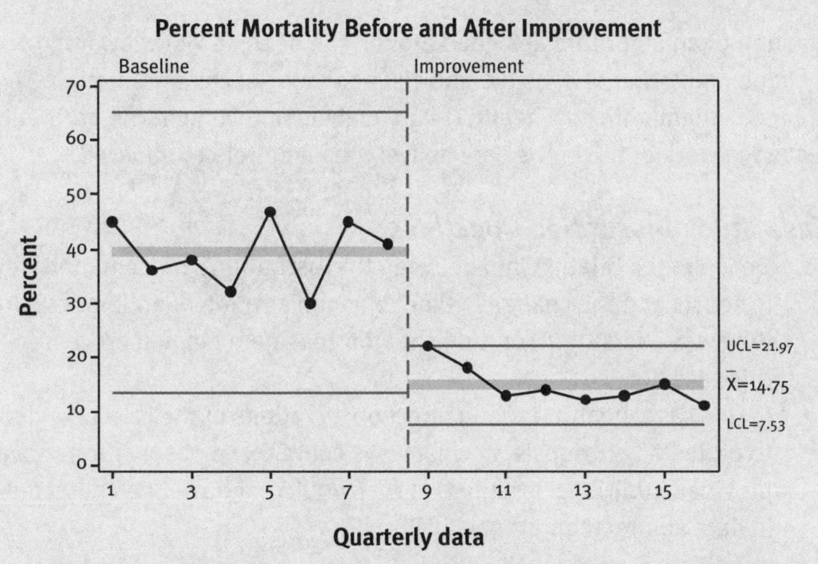

Note: Data here are for the same 24-month period shown in exhibit 7.12, followed by an additional 24-month postimplementation improvement period in 2014–2015. UCL = upper control limit; LCL = lower control limit.

(continued)

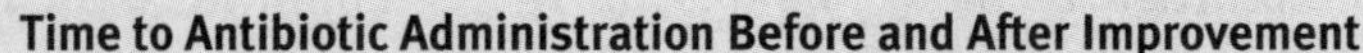

EXHIBIT 7.14
Time to Administration of Antibiotics (same 24-month period as exhibit 7.12, in 2012–2014; improvement is the 24-month period of 2014–2015)

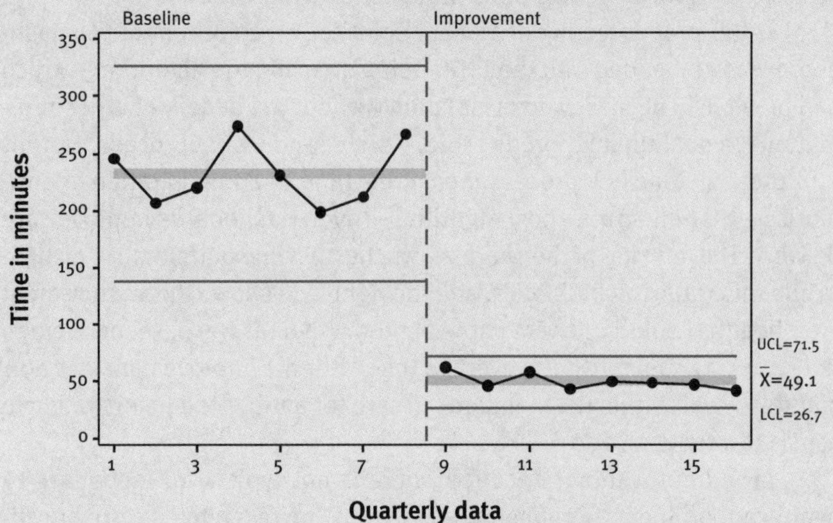

Note: Data here are for the same 24-month period shown in exhibit 7.12, followed by an additional 24-month postimplementation improvement period in 2014–2015. UCL = upper control limit; LCL = lower control limit.

creation of an algorithm designed around the bedside workflow, followed by implementation of a visible and visual display of the information. This approach highlights how health IT and quality improvement can partner to make the work of the entire care delivery team better coordinated.

Case Study Discussion Questions

1. Describe the relationship between the institution's percent mortality in sepsis and the change in time to administration of antibiotics. Why was a health IT solution superior to a more manual process in this case?
2. In this case, health IT made direct observations of the care provided to patients with sepsis. In what ways could these observations have provided additional information that would not have been detected in data abstracted from the EHR?

Conclusion

The information in this chapter can play an important role in helping organizations determine where they stand to get the most "bang for their buck" relative to health IT for quality and safety. Examples of common health IT interventions include reminders and alerts; decision support tools; checklists, including order sets and protocols; and soft and hard stops. Working from the three-part model introduced in exhibit 7.2 and incorporating the macro-level uses of health IT for quality and safety outlined in exhibit 7.3, organizations in the planning stages may want to begin with alerts and clinical decision support (with the understanding that alerts are a subset of clinical decision support).

The information presented in this chapter can also help with resource planning. Recall that implementation appeared as a concern for all three categories of the model (i.e., prevention, identification, and action), and culture was shown to be an additional challenge. Organizational leaders know that changing culture can be a long and intensive process. The findings both from the scan of the literature and from the case studies suggest that organizational champion leaders capable of shepherding implementation, influencing culture, and bridging knowledge with developers would be a valuable resource allocation to consider.

The case studies present real-world applications of health IT in prevention, identification, and action relative to healthcare quality and safety. To achieve optimal results, health IT must meet quality improvement at the intersection with care delivery. From a clinical perspective, efforts must span multiple levels, and solutions depend, in part, on the clinical problem being addressed. Although clinicians need to develop and pilot improvements on paper before embedding them in the EHR, the involvement of health IT partners early in the development process is vitally important for any quality improvement or patient safety effort, as it helps ensure a smooth transition to the IT system.

Overview of the Literature

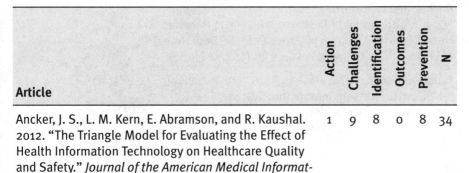

Article	Action	Challenges	Identification	Outcomes	Prevention	N
Ancker, J. S., L. M. Kern, E. Abramson, and R. Kaushal. 2012. "The Triangle Model for Evaluating the Effect of Health Information Technology on Healthcare Quality and Safety." *Journal of the American Medical Informatics Association* 19 (1): 61–65.	1	9	8	0	8	34

(continued)

Overview of the Literature *(continued)*

Arabi, Y. M., B. W. Pickering, H. M. Al-Dorzi, A. Alsaawi, S. M. Al-Qahtani, and A. W. Hay. 2016. "Information Technology to Improve Patient Safety: A Round Table Discussion from the 5th International Patient Safety Forum, Riyadh, Saudi Arabia, April 14–16, 2015." *Annals of Thoracic Medicine* 11 (3): 219–23.	0	0	3	2	1	6
Asch, E., S. H. Shah, S. Berkowitz, S. Mehta, R. L. Eisenberg, R. Jayadevan, C. Connolly, and P. J. Slanetz. 2017. "Resident Idea System: A Novel Tool to Engage Trainees in Quality Improvement at the Institutional Level." *Journal of the American College of Radiology* 14 (2): 256–61.	0	0	0	0	3	4
Badrick, T., S. Gay, E. J. McCaughey, and A. Georgiou. 2017. "External Quality Assessment Beyond the Analytical Phase: An Australian Perspective." *Biochemia Medica* 27 (1): 73–80.	0	0	0	0	0	0
Coiera, E., F. Magrabi, and J. Talmon. 2017. "Engineering Technology Resilience Through Informatics Safety Science." *Journal of the American Medical Informatics Association* 24 (2): 244–45.	0	1	0	0	1	3
Colicchio, T. K., J. C. Facelli, G. Del Fiol, D. L. Scammon, W. A. Bowes, and S. P. Narus. 2016. "Health Information Technology Adoption: Understanding Research Protocols and Outcome Measurements for IT Interventions in Health Care." *Journal of Biomedical Informatics* 63: 33–44.	4	0	0	0	0	0
El Morr, C., L. Ginsburg, N. V. Seungree, S. Woollard, and B. Hensen. 2016. "IT Integration and Patient Safety: The Case of a Software Tool." *Procedia Computer Science* 98: 534–39.	0	0	6	0	8	15
Every, N. R, S. D. Fihn, A. E. B. Sales, A. Keane, J. R. Ritchie, and QUERI IHD Executive Committee. 2000. "Quality Enhancement Research Initiative in Ischemic Heart Disease: A Quality Initiative from the Department of Veterans Affairs." *Medical Care* 38 (6): I49–I59.	0	0	7	0	1	10
Farzandipour, M., Z. Meidani, H. Riazi, and M. Sadeqi Jabali. 2016. "Nursing Information Systems Requirements: A Milestone for Patient Outcome and Patient Safety Improvement." *Computers, Informatics, Nursing* 34 (12): 601–12.	0	3	1	0	4	10
Gupta, M., and H. C. Kaplan. 2017. "Improving Quality Improvement in Neonatal-Perinatal Care." *Clinics in Perinatology* 44 (3): xvii–xix.	1	0	0	0	0	0

Overview of the Literature *(continued)*

Hoonakker, P. L., P. Carayon, and R. S. Cartmill. 2017. "The Impact of Secure Messaging on Workflow in Primary Care: Results of a Multiple-Case, Multiple-Method Study." *International Journal of Medical Informatics* 100: 63–76.	0	0	1	0	1	2
Jensen, S. 2015. "Patient Safety and Quality of Care: How May Clinical Simulation Contribute?" *Knowledge Management and E-Learning* 7 (3): 412–24.	1	4	2	0	5	12
Khullar, D., A. K. Jha, and A. B. Jena. 2015. "Reducing Diagnostic Errors—Why Now?" *New England Journal of Medicine* 373 (26): 2491–93.	1	0	0	0	0	0
Kim, M. O., E. Coiera, and F. Magrabi. 2017. "Problems with Health Information Technology and Their Effects on Care Delivery and Patient Outcomes: A Systematic Review." *Journal of the American Medical Informatics Association* 24 (2): 246–60.	0	1	0	0	6	7
Koppel, R. 2016. "The Health Information Technology Safety Framework: Building Great Structures on Vast Voids." *BMJ Quality and Safety* 25 (4): 218–20.	1	1	0	0	1	2
Lassere, M. N., S. Baker, A. Parle, A. Sara, and K. R. Johnson. 2015. "Improving Quality of Care and Long-Term Health Outcomes Through Continuity of Care with the Use of an Electronic or Paper Patient-Held Portable Health File (COMMUNICATE): Study Protocol for a Randomized Controlled Trial." *Trials* 16 (1): 253.	2	0	2	0	1	3
Levesque, E., E. Hoti, D. Azoulay, P. Ichai, D. Samuel, and F. Saliba. 2015. "The Implementation of an Intensive Care Information System Allows Shortening the ICU Length of Stay." *Journal of Clinical Monitoring and Computing* 29 (2): 263–69.	3	0	3	1	1	5
Magrabi, F., E. Ammenwerth, H. Hyppönen, N. de Keizer, P. Nykänen, M. Rigby, P. Scott, J. Talmon, and A. Georgiou. 2016. "Improving Evaluation to Address the Unintended Consequences of Health Information Technology: A Position Paper from the Working Group on Technology Assessment & Quality Development." *Yearbook of Medical Informatics* (1): 61–69.	1	0	0	0	0	0
Martin, B. S., and M. Arbore. 2016. "Measurement, Standards, and Peer Benchmarking: One Hospital's Journey." *Pediatric Clinics of North America* 63 (2): 239–49.	0	2	0	0	0	3

(continued)

Overview of the Literature *(continued)*

Mazur, L. M., P. R. Mosaly, C. Moore, E. Comitz, F. Yu, A. D. Falchook, M. J. Eblan, L. M. Hoyle, G. Tracton, B. S. Chera, and L. B. Marks. 2016. "Toward a Better Understanding of Task Demands, Workload, and Performance During Physician–Computer Interactions." *Journal of the American Medical Informatics Association* 23 (6): 1113–20.	1	0	0	0	1	1
Nakhleh, R. E. 2015. "Role of Informatics in Patient Safety and Quality Assurance." *Surgical Pathology Clinics* 8 (2): 301–7.	0	0	0	0	2	2
Peters, T. E. 2017. "Transformational Impact of Health Information Technology on the Clinical Practice of Child and Adolescent Psychiatry." *Child and Adolescent Psychiatric Clinics of North America* 26 (1): 55–66.	5	2	6	0	7	15
Popovici, I., P. P. Morita, D. Doran, S. Lapinsky, D. Morra, A. Shier, R. Wu, and J. A. Cafazzo. 2015. "Technological Aspects of Hospital Communication Challenges: An Observational Study." *International Journal for Quality in Health Care* 27 (3): 183–88.	0	4	0	0	3	11
Rizzato Lede, D. A., S. E. Benitez, J. C. Mayan III, M. I. Smith, A. J. Baum, D. R. Luna, and F. G. Bernaldo de Quirós. 2015. "Patient Safety at Transitions of Care: Use of a Compulsory Electronic Reconciliation Tool in an Academic Hospital." *Studies in Health Technology and Informatics* 216: 232–36.	2	1	1	0	2	4
Seblega, B. K., N. J. Zhang, T. T. H. Wan, L. Y. Unruh, and A. Miller. 2015. "Health Information Technology Adoption: Effects on Patient Safety and Quality of Care." *International Journal of Healthcare Technology and Management* 15 (1): 31–48.	2	0	6	2	7	17
Shy, B. D., E. Y. Kim, N. G. Genes, T. Lowry, G. T. Loo, U. Hwang, L. D. Richardson, and J. S. Shapiro. 2016. "Increased Identification of Emergency Department 72-Hour Returns Using Multihospital Health Information Exchange." *Academic Emergency Medicine* 23 (5): 645–49.	1	0	1	0	1	3
Skyttberg, N., J. Vicente, R. Chen, H. Blomqvist, and S. Koch. 2016. "How to Improve Vital Sign Data Quality for Use in Clinical Decision Support Systems? A Qualitative Study in Nine Swedish Emergency Departments." *BMC Medical Informatics and Decision Making* 16: 61.	0	2	3	1	4	14
Stanton, B. F. 2016. "Pediatric Safety, Quality, and Informatics." *Pediatric Clinics of North America* 63 (2): 15–16.	4	0	0	0	1	2

Overview of the Literature *(continued)*

Strickland, N. H. 2015. "Quality Assurance in Radiology: Peer Review and Peer Feedback." *Clinical Radiology* 70 (11): 1158–64.	0	0	0	0	0	0
Suresh, S. 2016. "The Intersection of Safety, Quality, and Informatics: Solving Problems in Pediatrics." *Pediatric Clinics of North America* 63 (2): 17–18.	0	1	1	0	2	6
Wang, H. F., J. F. Jin, X. Q. Feng, X. Huang, L. L. Zhu, X. Y. Zhao, and Q. Zhou. 2015. "Quality Improvements in Decreasing Medication Administration Errors Made by Nursing Staff in an Academic Medical Center Hospital: A Trend Analysis During the Journey to Joint Commission International Accreditation and in the Post-accreditation Era." *Therapeutics and Clinical Risk Management* 11: 393–406.	0	1	0	0	3	6
Weiner, S., and J. C. Fink. 2017. "Telemedicine to Promote Patient Safety: Use of Phone-Based Interactive Voice-Response System to Reduce Adverse Safety Events in Pre-dialysis CKD." *Advances in Chronic Kidney Disease* 24 (1): 31–38.	0	0	0	0	2	2
Whipple, E. C., B. E. Dixon, and J. J. McGowan. 2013. "Linking Health Information Technology to Patient Safety and Quality Outcomes: A Bibliometric Analysis and Review." *Informatics for Health and Social Care* 38 (1): 1–14.	2	0	0	0	0	0
Whitt, K. J., L. Eden, K. C. Merrill, and M. Hughes. 2017. "Nursing Student Experiences Regarding Safe Use of Electronic Health Records: A Pilot Study of the Safety and Assurance Factors for EHR Resilience Guides." *Computers, Informatics, Nursing* 35 (1): 45–53.	9	7	5	0	8	23
Yermak, D., P. Cram, and J. L. Kwan. 2017. "Five Things to Know About Diagnostic Error." *Diagnosis* 4 (1): 13–15.	0	0	0	0	0	0
Yu, X., J. Jiang, C. Liu, K. Shen, Z. Wang, W. Han, X. Liu, G. Lin, Y. Zhang, Y. Zhang, Y. Ma, H. Bo, and Y. Zhao. 2017. "Protocol for a Multicentre, Multistage, Prospective Study in China Using System-Based Approaches for Consistent Improvement in Surgical Safety." *BMJ Open*. Published June 15. https://bmjopen.bmj.com/content/7/6/e015147.info.	0	4	6	0	8	23
TOTAL	**41**	**43**	**62**	**6**	**92**	**245**

References

Beeler, P. E., D. W. Bates, and B. L. Hug. 2014. "Clinical Decision Support Systems." *Swiss Medical Weekly* 144: w14073.

Buntin, M. B., M. F. Burke, M. C. Hoaglin, and D. Blumenthal. 2011. "The Benefits of Health Information Technology: A Review of the Recent Literature Shows Predominantly Positive Results." *Health Affairs* 30 (3): 464–71.

Busund, R., V. Koukline, U. Utrobin, and E. Nedashkovsky. 2002. "Plasmapheresis in Severe Sepsis and Septic Shock: A Prospective, Randomised, Controlled Trial." *Intensive Care Medicine* 28 (10): 1434–39.

Derry, C. P., K. J. Shah, L. Caie, and C. E. Counsell. 2010. "Medication Management in People with Parkinson's Disease During Surgical Admissions." *Postgraduate Medical Journal* 86 (1016): 334–37.

Eslami, S., N. F. de Keizer, and A. Abu-Hanna. 2008. "The Impact of Computerized Physician Medication Order Entry in Hospitalized Patients—A Systematic Review." *International Journal of Medical Informatics* 77 (6): 365–76.

Fiks, A. G., R. W. Grundmeier, L. M. Biggs, A. R. Localio, and E. A. Alessandrini. 2007. "Impact of Clinical Alerts Within an Electronic Health Record on Routine Childhood Immunization in an Urban Pediatric Population." *Pediatrics* 120 (4): 707–14.

Goldzweig, C. L., A. Towfigh, M. Maglione, and P. G. Shekelle. 2009. "Costs and Benefits of Health Information Technology: New Trends from the Literature." *Health Affairs* 28 (2): w282–93.

Grissinger, M. 2016. "Small Effort, Big Payoff: Automated Maximum Dose Alerts with Hard Stops." *Pharmacy and Therapeutics* 41 (2): 82.

Harrison, M. I., R. Koppel, and S. Bar-Lev. 2007. "Unintended Consequences of Information Technologies in Health Care—An Interactive Sociotechnical Analysis." *Journal of the American Medical Informatics Association* 14 (5): 542–49.

Institute for Healthcare Improvement (IHI). 2018. "IHI Triple Aim Initiative." Accessed October 19. www.ihi.org/Engage/Initiatives/TripleAim/Pages/default.aspx.

Jamal, A., K. McKenzie, and M. Clark. 2009. "The Impact of Health Information Technology on the Quality of Medical and Health Care: A Systematic Review." *Health Information Management Journal* 38 (3): 26–37.

Karsh, B.-T., M. B. Weinger, P. A. Abbott, and R. L. Wears. 2010. "Health Information Technology: Fallacies and Sober Realities." *Journal of the American Medical Informatics Association* 17 (6): 617–23.

Magdalinou, K. N., A. Martin, and B. Kessel. 2007. "Prescribing Medications in Parkinson's Disease (PD) Patients During Acute Admissions to a District General Hospital." *Parkinsonism & Related Disorders* 13 (8): 539–40.

Marmor, T., J. Oberlander, and J. White. 2009. "The Obama Administration's Options for Health Care Cost Control: Hope Versus Reality." *Annals of Internal Medicine* 150 (7): 485–89.

McCullough, J. S., M. Casey, I. Moscovice, and S. Prasad. 2010. "The Effect of Health Information Technology on Quality in US Hospitals." *Health Affairs* 29 (4): 647–54.

Nolan, T., R. Resar, C. Haraden, and F. A. Griffin. 2004. "Improving the Reliability of Health Care." Innovation Series white paper, Institute for Healthcare Improvement. Accessed December 16, 2017. www.ihi.org/education/IHIOpenSchool/Courses/Documents/CourseraDocuments/08_ReliabilityWhitePaper2004revJune06.pdf.

Okun, M. 2012. "Hospitalization Tips: For Parkinson's Disease Patients." University of Florida Center for Movement Disorders and Neurorestoration. Published March 11. https://movementdisorders.ufhealth.org/2012/03/11/hospitalization-tips-for-parkinsons-disease-patients/.

———. 2011. "Parkinson's Treatment Tips on the Worst Drugs for Parkinson's Disease." University of Florida Center for Movement Disorders and Neurorestoration. Published September 22. https://movementdisorders.ufhealth.org/2011/09/22/parkinsons-treatment-tips-on-the-worst-drugs-for-parkinsons-disease/.

Parente, S. T., and J. S. McCullough. 2009. "Health Information Technology and Patient Safety: Evidence from Panel Data." *Health Affairs* 28 (2): 357–60.

Rivers, E., B. Nguyen, S. Havstad, J. Ressler, A. Muzzin, B. Knoblich, E. Peterson, and M. Tomlanovich. 2001. "Early Goal-Directed Therapy in the Treatment of Severe Sepsis and Septic Shock." *New England Journal of Medicine* 345 (19): 1368–77.

Smith, D. H., N. Perrin, A. Feldstein, X. Yang, D. Kuang, S. R. Simon, D. F. Sittig, R. Platt, and S. B. Soumerai. 2006. "The Impact of Prescribing Safety Alerts for Elderly Persons in an Electronic Medical Record: An Interrupted Time Series Evaluation." *Archives of Internal Medicine* 166 (10): 1098–104.

Strom, B. L., R. Schinnar, F. Aberra, W. Bilker, S. Hennessy, C. E. Leonard, and E. Pifer. 2010. "Unintended Effects of a Computerized Physician Order Entry Nearly Hard-Stop Alert to Prevent a Drug Interaction: A Randomized Controlled Trial." *Archives of Internal Medicine* 170 (17): 1578–83.

van der Sijs, H., J. Aarts, A. Vulto, and M. Berg. 2006. "Overriding of Drug Safety Alerts in Computerized Physician Order Entry." *Journal of the American Medical Informatics Association* 13 (2): 138–47.

Walker, J. M., E. J. Bieber, and F. M. Richards (eds.). 2005. *Implementing an Electronic Health Record System*. New York: Springer.

CHAPTER

8

SIMULATION IN HEALTHCARE QUALITY AND SAFETY

Hyunjoo Lee and Dimitrios Papanagnou

Introduction to Simulation

Medical simulation has been defined as "a technique—not a technology—to replace or amplify real experiences with guided experiences that evoke or replicate substantial aspects of the real world in a fully interactive manner" (Gaba 2004, i2). Oftentimes, simulation is equated with the use of advanced technologies such as high-fidelity patient manikins in healthcare, sophisticated flight simulators in aviation, and combat reenactment technologies for military training. At its core, however, simulation is a *pedagogy*, or an educational tool: It is the ability to recreate real experiences for the purpose of guiding learners toward predetermined goals. Simulation-mediated education offers learners a safe practice environment where they can engage in critical thinking without endangering themselves or others who might otherwise be subject to harm in a real-life event.

Simulation can also be used to assess how learners approach problem solving and to evaluate their critical thinking processes. Simulation affords its participants the opportunity to learn experientially from their errors and deliberately practice their skills to achieve mastery level within their respective practice domains. With this chapter, we hope to illustrate how simulation can be used to improve healthcare quality and safety, highlighting its intrinsic ability to expose, inform, and improve behaviors that are critical for effective communication and teamwork.

Simulation Terminology

Before we examine the applications of simulation for healthcare, patient safety, and quality, we first need to establish some of the terminology commonly used in the simulation landscape. Simulation creates an environment in which the learner can be immersed in a lifelike event with guided experience. Guidance may be provided during the simulation itself or in a debriefing that follows the simulation. The rationale for integrating simulation into a training program may be to learn something new, to develop a new skill, to practice or test a new concept or protocol, or to study an evaluation tool (Lopreiato et al. 2016).

The word *fidelity* is used to describe the degree of authenticity with which the simulation mimics the intended event and takes into account the physical, psychological, and environmental factors of the experience (Lopreiato et al. 2016). To this effect, a simulation may be termed *low fidelity* or *high fidelity* depending on its exactness in replicating reality. Low-fidelity simulation has a minimal level of realism, but it typically requires fewer resources and less external input and prompting than higher-fidelity simulation. Low-fidelity simulations often include role plays, reenactments, and procedural practice on replicas (e.g., human torso replicas for practicing chest compressions during cardiopulmonary resuscitation [CPR] training). High-fidelity simulation provides a much more realistic experience, and it often employs technology to replicate an event or an environment in which a real scenario may occur. In certain cases, the simulation can take place in an actual clinical or working environment where events occur (e.g., an operating room to practice procedural/technical skills; a patient's home for physical therapy training; an obstetrical suite to practice communication skills in delivery with shoulder dystocia).

The realism of a simulation is contingent on the effective integration and use of specific tools. A simulation can be as simple as reviewing a case study, facilitating a tabletop discussion, reenacting a case, or engaging in a role-play scenario. In such cases, educational simulation adjuncts might not be required. To heighten learning, however, a facilitator may choose to integrate a task trainer or partial task trainer into the program. Task trainers are devices that can be used by learners to practice a specific skill or procedure (Lopreiato et al. 2016). Typically, such devices are anatomic representations of a part of a larger system or body (e.g., a torso to practice safe chest thoracostomy or chest tube insertion).

If the facilitator wants to expose learners to heightened levels of realism, higher-fidelity simulators can be employed. These human patient simulators integrate technology and have the ability to replicate physical exam findings (e.g., breath sounds, heart sounds) and display vital signs on a digital monitor. The highest fidelity simulator is, naturally, a standardized patient (SP), or a human actor. Generally, an SP has been extensively trained to simulate an actual patient, from the words and body language used to communicate with the provider to the portrayal of certain symptoms and physical examination findings (Lopreiato et al. 2016). Depending on the scenario, the specific learning objectives of the instructor, and the learning level of the participants, the simulation may employ any or all of the aforementioned low- and high-fidelity modalities.

The mode of delivery is another simulation parameter that merits discussion. For example, with case studies, the learner often will *imagine* how she would experience the pertinent aspects of the case. With virtual reality, however, a computer software program can work in conjunction with technological adjuncts (e.g., headphones) to recreate an immersive three-dimensional world, and learners have the ability to directly *interact* with the simulation (Lopreiato et al. 2016). An often-cited example is the use of the flight simulator in the aviation industry. These simulators mimic the physical space and controls of an actual cockpit, and an instructor can remotely control the "scenes" and events of the simulated flight.

A unique type of virtual reality known as *augmented reality* creates a hybrid experience, where the learner's real world is modified with superimposed synthetic stimuli to challenge the learner (Lopreiato et al. 2016). The use of wearable eyeglass technology (e.g., Google Glass), for example, has the ability to superimpose pathologic visual displays (e.g., lacerations, physical deformities) onto a manikin or patient during a simulated encounter.

A particularly vital aspect of a simulation is the exercise of debriefing, or the reflective dialogue that follows the simulation; it is the stage where most, if not all, of the learning takes place. Following the simulation, the debriefing is led by one or two facilitators, typically the individuals responsible for designing the program. Debriefing allows learners to reflect on their participation and performance in the simulation, as well as to receive pertinent feedback (Lopreiato et al. 2016). As the observed events are being discussed, the facilitator can gain a better understanding of the learners' *frames* (i.e., their knowledge, assumptions, and feelings) and direct the conversation toward the overarching learning objectives (Fanning and Gaba 2007).

In addition to its uses in teaching and learning, simulation offers ample opportunities for practitioner assessment. A classic example is the objective structured clinical examination (OSCE) that has been integrated in the clinical training curricula across most health professions. In an OSCE, the competence of a learner is assessed in a structured and objective fashion through the use of checklists, direct observation, and/or follow-up presentations or exercises (Lopreiato et al. 2016).

Evolution and History

Simulation is not a new concept in healthcare. Early examples included anatomic models of the human body, including real pathologic specimens; cadaveric dissections; and practice of surgical skills on animals (Jones, Passos-Neto, and Braghiroli 2015; Ghosh 2015). Cadaveric dissections were first performed in Greece during the third century BCE. Centuries later, and after multiple iterations of change regarding procurement of bodies, cadaveric labs remain part of the educational curriculum in the health professions (Ghosh 2015).

Lessons learned from the aviation industry have guided both simulation device design and simulation program implementation in the health sciences.

The example of one of the original flight simulators is often retold. In the late 1920s, Edwin Albert Link created a prototype flight simulator composed of a cockpit and controls attached to a device that could mimic the motions produced during flight (Jones, Passos-Neto, and Braghiroli 2015). A few years later, in the 1930s, a series of fatal postal carrier crashes occurred as a result of poor weather conditions; even the US Army Air Corps could not safely navigate through these conditions (Jones, Passos-Neto, and Braghiroli 2015). The Army Air Corps invested in Link's flight simulators as a way to train their pilots to fly in rare, high-risk conditions without the fatal consequences. Today, flight simulation is ubiquitously incorporated into pilot training programs across the globe (Jones, Passos-Neto, and Braghiroli 2015).

Like flight simulation, medical simulation has evolved alongside advances in technology. In the 1960s, the toy manufacturer Laerdal created Resusci-Anne, a manikin used in the training of mouth-to-mouth ventilation using Dr. Peter Safar's head-tilt/chin-lift maneuver (Cooper and Taqueti 2008). Soon after, Laerdal added a compressible chest with a spring to allow for the simulation of chest compressions, giving birth to the CPR trainer that is still widely used today (Jones, Passos-Neto, and Braghiroli 2015). Resusci-Anne is a great example of a partial task-trainer, created to train individuals on the specific physical skills necessary for high-quality CPR.

Innovation in healthcare simulator devices did not stop with Resusci-Anne. In 1968, Dr. Michael Gordon unveiled Harvey, a manikin that functioned as a cardiology patient simulator (Cooper and Taqueti 2008). Harvey was able to generate a multitude of cardiac findings, including blood pressure, jugular venous distention, pulse, and respirations, as well as normal and abnormal cardiac sounds (Cooper and Taqueti 2008). With new innovations in technology, simulators continued to become more and more sophisticated.

Many of the advances seen in simulators related to physiology and pharmacology modeling came directly from the work of anesthesiologists. During the 1980s, Dr. David Gaba at Stanford University created the Comprehensive Anesthesia Simulation Environment, an advanced manikin simulator with the capability of reproducing and manipulating human vital signs and physiology (Cooper and Taqueti 2008). Similarly, Dr. Michael Good at the University of Florida created the Gainesville Anesthesia Simulator, a full manikin with the capability of interacting with an anesthesia machine and the ability to be preprogrammed to behave in a way that actually *responded* to a participant's interaction (Cooper and Taqueti 2008). Today, the simulation market is replete with various manikin-based simulators of varying fidelity and capability.

Integration into Educational Programming

The earliest form of education in the health professions revolved around an apprenticeship model. To some degree, this form of education has continued to the present day. After completing the first two preclinical years of medical school, for example, medical students transition into the clinical learning environment and interact with patients under the supervision and guidance of precepting physicians (i.e., faculty and/or senior residents). In post-graduate medical training (i.e., residency), resident physicians are given a significant amount of patient responsibility and autonomy, but they still remain under the supervision and guidance of an attending (or faculty) physician. The amount of supervision given by the attending physician typically varies depending on several factors: the resident's level of training, the availability of the supervising attending physician, the number of residents working with the attending physician, the comfort level and independence of the resident, and the level of patient acuity.

Often, in a busy clinical environment, the attending physician cannot possibly offer direct supervision and guidance to the student or resident in training 100 percent of the time. However, simulation can offer a multitude of opportunities to make up for this logistical limitation and to complement the clinical training of students and postgraduate trainees alike. Simulation provides a psychologically safe learning environment where trainees can learn from their errors without posing harm to patients. Its paradigm for training has significantly shifted from the traditional apprenticeship mind-set of "see one, do one, teach one."

Pedagogically, simulation enables educators in the health sciences to formally assess the student based on observed simulated patient encounters. Under the apprenticeship model, the apprentice would typically shadow the more experienced physician or have encounters with patients while the experienced physician observed the student's behaviors, with the physician later providing feedback. Not all patients, however, are comfortable, or even amenable, to repeated exams by multiple providers, particularly students.

Dr. Howard Barrows built on the concept of observed encounters with feedback but used standardized patients (Jones, Passos-Neto, and Braghiroli 2015). The involvement of trained SPs—capable of simulating specific signs and symptoms in a predictable and consistent manner for learner audiences—allowed for formalized/standardized simulation cases to be used for both teaching and assessment. Use of standardized cases was further enhanced by the advent of advanced manikin simulators with the capability of recreating physiological findings. The acuity level of these standardized cases can be easily adjusted for novice and advanced learners.

Given its educational adaptability, its technological enhancements, and its high safety profile, simulation has become widely used in crisis management training for health providers, particularly for the development of teamwork and communication skills. These efforts have been heavily influenced by lessons from crew resource management (CRM) in the aviation industry. One such program, the Anesthesia Crisis Resource Management program, has demonstrated simulation's potential for robust training in the areas of leadership, teamwork, and communication for anesthesiologists in the operating room and their interprofessional peers (Cooper and Taqueti 2008). Similar programs, with sophisticated simulation modalities, have been established to train learners across the entire spectrum (e.g., students, postgraduate trainees, practitioners) on critical event management.

Simulation Center Versus the Physical Workplace

The physical space in which simulations are conducted is yet another variable that contributes to the adaptability of simulation for education in the health professions. One of the major benefits of simulation is that it can be implemented virtually anywhere. It might take place in a staged room (e.g., an operating room), a set of staged rooms (e.g., a hospital suite), or even an entire building or training center dedicated to simulation activities and training. Although simulation at a dedicated training center can offer significant benefits to the educator or planner (e.g., control of the learning space and traffic, control over the scenario, protection from potential distractions), the level of realism or fidelity of the simulation might be limited.

One way to improve the fidelity of a simulation is to bring the simulation to the clinical environment—the actual environment where providers work on a daily basis. A simulation exercise that takes place in the real physical environment where the learner actually works is called an *in situ simulation*. In addition to improving scenario realism, in situ simulation offers natural methods for evaluating and troubleshooting the functioning of teams and systems in the workplace; identifying latent patient safety threats; and practicing high-stakes, low-frequency clinical events.

In situ simulations are an ideal vehicle with which to augment existing patient safety practices. For instance, the failure mode effects analysis (FMEA) is routinely used by patient safety and clinical quality champions, and it provides a step-by-step approach for identifying potential failures in a clinical space or process. In situ simulations allow patient safety champions the ability to identify failure risks and to adapt processes for continuous clinical improvement—thereby preventing failure and, more importantly, patient harm.

Applying Educational Frameworks to Patient Safety Simulations

Adult Learning and Its Implications on Simulation Training

Adult learning poses unique challenges and benefits. Adult learners are autonomous learners who come to work with accrued life experience and knowledge.

Studies have shown that they learn best in informal, nonthreatening environments. They are self-motivated and self-directed and, as such, learn best when they feel a need to know something. In general, adult learners are goal-oriented and practical.

Participatory learning experiences engage adults both cognitively and affectively. Adults are experiential learners at their core, and they learn from active participation and reflection on specific activities. David Kolb breaks down experiential learning into four discrete stages: (1) concrete experience, (2) observations and reflections, (3) formalization/generalizations of concepts, and (4) testing concepts in new situations. These stages of the learning cycle can be further simplified into the stages of feeling, watching, thinking, and doing, respectively (Taylor and Hamdy 2013).

Simulation naturally leverages this adult learning style, as shown in exhibit 8.1. By actively participating in a simulation, learners become engaged in the concrete experience. They then have the opportunity to reflect on that experience, in the form of a debriefing (following the simulation), which helps them to process what took place in the simulation as well as form generalizations based on that experience. These generalizations can then be applied to new situations as the learning cycle repeats.

Simulation is inherently structured to offer a student-centered approach to teaching and learning, making it the ideal modality for training and engaging adult learners. In addition to offering a safe, nonthreatening environment,

EXHIBIT 8.1
Kolb's Cycle of Learning

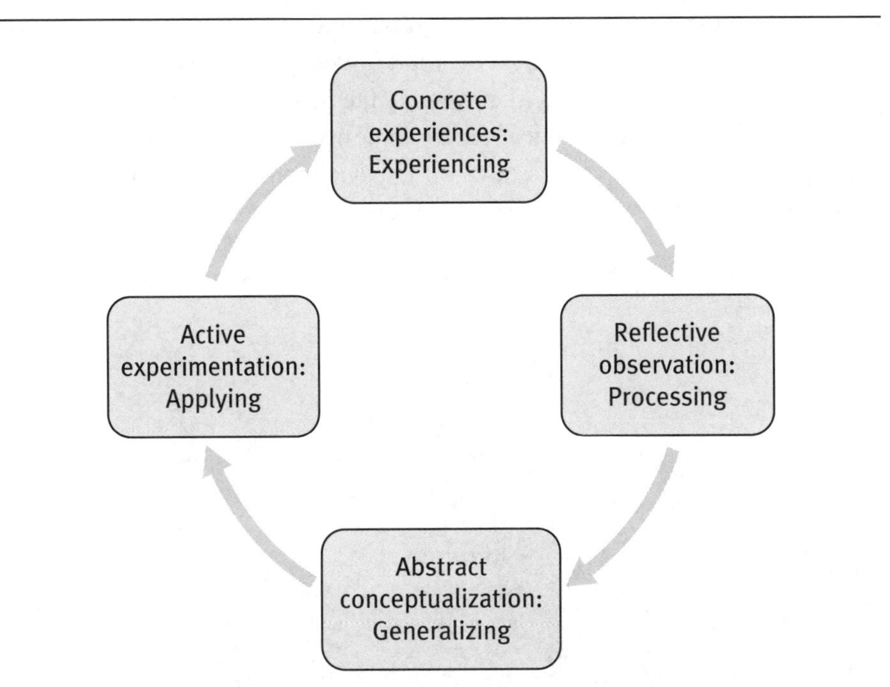

Source: Adapted from Taylor and Hamdy (2013).

simulation offers the opportunity for adult learners to troubleshoot their own errors and then immediately practice what they have learned. The debriefing that follows the simulation focuses on understanding the learners' critical thinking processes and internal motivations; offering opportunities for reflection through shared observations; and producing feedback for improved knowledge, skills, and practitioner performance. When facilitated well, the debriefing is student-centered; it encourages participants to actively contribute to the dialogue where decisions and actions are explored, assumptions are uncovered, and teaching opportunities are identified. The role of the facilitator is simply to guide learners through reflection, while linking the dialogue to the original objectives of the simulation.

Deliberate Practice for Procedural Training: Safety Through Mastery Training

"Knowing something" is simply not enough. The adult learner, particularly in the health professions, needs not just to have knowledge but also to display competence and perform at a level that appropriately reflects that competence.

George Miller (1990) proposed a conceptual framework, known as Miller's Pyramid, that describes the progression of higher levels of clinical assessment. The framework, shown in exhibit 8.2, consists of four levels: (1) *knows*, (2) *knows how*, (3) *shows how*, and (4) *does*. Miller's Pyramid assists clinical instructors by matching educational outcomes with expectations for what learners should be able to achieve at any stage. The *knows* level forms the base of the pyramid and represents the foundation for building clinical competence. The next level, *knows how*, builds on the knowledge that has been acquired and requires learners to apply that knowledge in various settings. The third level, *shows how*, requires the learner to demonstrate clinical skills. Finally, at the top of the pyramid, *does* focuses on behaviors and methods that provide an assessment of actual clinical performance (Miller 1990).

EXHIBIT 8.2
Miller's Pyramid of Assessment

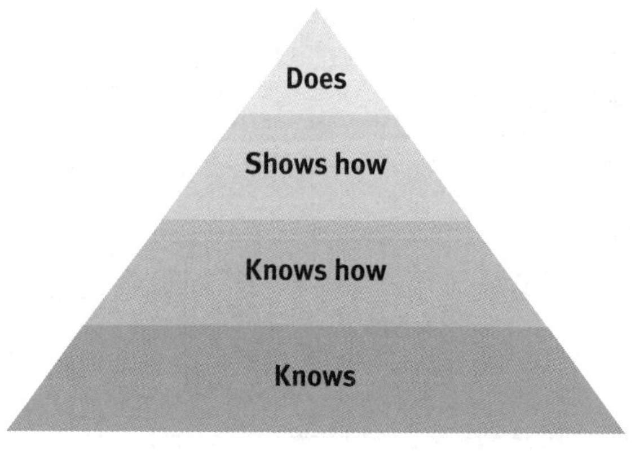

Source: Miller (1990).

Advancing from *knows* to *does* requires deliberate practice, which goes beyond simple repetition for improved performance. Deliberate practice allows learners to repeatedly practice a procedure under the guidance and supervision of someone with significant experience; to obtain specific feedback, in real time, every step along the way; and to immediately apply formative feedback into subsequent attempts. The overarching goal is to have the learner move toward technical proficiency. Simulation offers valuable opportunities for trainees to deliberately practice their skills. Whether through procedural practice on a low-fidelity task trainer or through team training, in situ, using a high-fidelity task trainer, simulation provides learning space with which trainees can practice procedures and apply feedback into their repertoire for improved performance and improved clinical outcomes.

Debriefing: Time for Reflection-in-Action and Reflection-on-Action

The ultimate success of experiential learning depends on the effectiveness of the reflective process. Debriefing is essentially a guided reflection—an activity that is student centered but executed in a way that allows the facilitator to bridge gaps in knowledge to optimize the learning experience and improve student behavior. To ensure a successful debriefing, the facilitator should first conduct a *prebrief* to establish the format for the conversation, to review the ground rules of the learning environment, and to delineate the objectives of the simulation (Fanning and Gaba 2007). Once the guided reflection begins, the facilitator assists learners as they recount a summary of the simulated experience; analyze pertinent aspects of the scenario; and, hopefully, contemplate the application of lessons to similar future experiences (Fanning and Gaba 2007).

Debriefing goes beyond adding to a learner's knowledge base. When faced with a new piece of data, learners have the opportunity to critically evaluate and compare the new information with what they already know; this step, in turn, helps them create a conceptual model to incorporate the new data into their existing schema. This process is commonly called *reflection-in-action*, and it can easily take place when the facilitator pauses a simulation to discuss what is actively taking place (Taylor and Hamdy 2013). Debriefing at the completion of a scenario, however, allows learners to delve into a more structured reflection and consider all the constituent pieces of the simulation as they occurred. This process is known as *reflection-on-action*, where learners process the events of the scenario and make generalizations for real clinical practice.

Simulation in the Patient Safety Landscape

Making the Case for Simulation

Simulation offers many benefits for patient safety. First and foremost, it opens an avenue for immersive, experiential education that fosters effective, active learning (Aggarwal et al. 2010). Simulation in healthcare can be used for clinical skills training, procedural training, and even team training. It allows participants to recreate low-frequency, high-stakes scenarios and assess clinicians' competence with the goal of working toward safer patient care (Aggarwal et al. 2010). In addition to enhancing performance at the individual provider level, simulation can be used to improve system performance and outcomes. The loftiest and most desired goal is improvement in patient safety and quality outcomes at the system level (Vincent et al. 2004).

Simulation is an adaptable educational tool, and it can be integrated anywhere. Although a dedicated simulation center has certain advantages (e.g., controlled environment and logistics), in situ simulations might offer more appropriate opportunities for patient safety efforts. Because they typically take place in real clinical/working environments, in situ simulations offer heightened fidelity and vital performance data on clinical workflow patterns. Additionally, participants do not need to leave their physical work environments to travel to the simulation center; the training is brought to them directly. Teamwork and communication can be practiced with other members of the interprofessional clinical team in the usual setting, and learners are more likely to perform as they normally would during a real situation. Another major advantage of in situ simulation is that participants and facilitators are able to better understand the nuances of their work environment and reveal latent system threats that had previously gone unidentified.

Procedural Training and Clinical Skills

Healthcare providers, particularly those in acute care settings, encounter clinical situations that require appropriate clinical skills and the ability to perform specific procedures. In the traditional apprenticeship model of "see one, do one, teach one," a healthcare professional might be called upon to perform a relatively high-risk procedure for the first time on a real patient. In addition to the obvious threat to patient safety, this paradigm imposes limitations on the operator's ability to learn the procedure. Effective procedural learning depends on the frequency with which the procedure is performed, yet the classic apprenticeship model offers minimal opportunity for deliberate practice and feedback on performance. Simulation enables practitioners to engage in the deliberate practice of procedures, which is especially valuable for those procedures that carry a significant patient risk.

Dankbaar and colleagues (2017) created and tested the abcdeSIM game as a way to train family medicine residents to appropriately handle emergency care. In the game, residents managed a simulated emergency department filled with virtual patients and were tasked with appropriately stabilizing those patients who were critically ill. Dankbaar and colleagues (2017) found that residents who played the game demonstrated higher clinical competencies than their counterparts who did not play it. Interestingly, the researchers also noticed that the group that played the game showed less variability in the level of competency. This initial difference in competency between "gamers" and "nongamers," however, was not observed two weeks later. This latter finding may suggest that a "ceiling" effect limits how much residents can learn through the simulation. Alternatively, it may highlight the need for continued reinforcement through the simulated game to prevent the decay of skills.

Simulation for the practice of procedural skills can offer varying levels of fidelity. Low-fidelity models can be used to train simple procedures—for instance, synthetic skin models can be used to practice suturing techniques. Health professionals can also learn specific tasks or procedures using partial task trainers, such as a modified thoracic model for practicing tube thoracostomy or a modified head-and-neck manikin for practicing endotracheal airway intubation. Cadaveric models offer yet another option for the practice of technical procedural skills. Procedural training can also be delivered through a fully immersive simulation of a real scenario with a high-fidelity manikin on which the learner can practice clinical procedures. Hybrid simulations are also possible. For instance, a patient manikin can be used for a simulated case scenario, with an emphasis on practicing teamwork and communication, and learners can then transition to a partial task trainer to perform a specific procedure. A key benefit of low-fidelity partial task trainers is their intrinsic ability to be used for deliberate practice with formative feedback by a supervising instructor; a high-fidelity simulator may be limited in its capacity for repetition of the task at hand.

Simulation offers an optimal environment for deliberate practice: Learners can learn and practice a procedure, receive timely feedback, and immediately apply the feedback they receive. Studies have repeatedly shown that practice that is spaced out over time to allow the brain to process the learned behavior results in significantly improved retention and performance (Moulton et al. 2006). Hence, simulation in isolation is not likely to improve patient care, but simulation that is incorporated into continuous educational programming has great potential to improve health providers' performance and skill.

Team Strategies and Tools to Enhance Performance and Patient Safety (TeamSTEPPS)

In fields where even a simple error carries dire consequences, such as in the aviation industry or the military, crew resource management has played a vital role in training individuals to be an effective part of a larger, more unified, higher-functioning team. Research has consistently shown that the quality of teamwork has a significant impact on safety outcomes (Lee et al. 2017). In an effort to enhance teamwork in healthcare, the US Department of Defense and the Agency for Healthcare Research and Quality have created a CRM program called Team Strategies and Tools to Enhance Performance and Patient Safety (TeamSTEPPS).

TeamSTEPPS is designed to address four key pillars of an effective team: leadership, mutual support, situation monitoring, and communication. Effective leadership requires the ability to assess the capabilities and progress of the team, coordinate the team, delegate tasks effectively, and create a positive atmosphere in which team members feel aptly involved and comfortable speaking up when appropriate (Lee et al. 2017). Mutual support requires that team members are readily familiar with the roles each person plays in the team and are cognizant of other team members' needs (Lee et al. 2017). Situation monitoring requires awareness that the clinical environment changes and a commitment to continuously monitoring team members' performance throughout specific activities (Lee et al. 2017). Arguably, communication is the most important pillar. Effective communication binds the other three pillars together.

Lee and colleagues (2017) studied the effects of TeamSTEPPS on teamwork behaviors in orthopedic surgery teams, which included orthopedic surgeons, operating room staff, nurses, and anesthesiologists. In the study, the researchers reinforced TeamSTEPPS through four types of interventions over a four-month period: (1) short 10- to 15-minute lectures on leadership during weekly meetings for nurses; (2) 5-minute discussions of leadership principles during monthly meetings for surgeons; (3) one-hour grand rounds on TeamSTEPPS principles for anesthesiologists; and (4) an online module on communication for nursing staff. After these interventions, the surgical team displayed significantly improved leadership and communication. In addition, the more reinforcement (specifically, active reinforcement) practitioners received, the more significant the improvement in leadership and communication was observed to be. For example, anesthesiologists whose only reinforcement consisted of the didactic one-hour grand rounds did not show a significant improvement in leadership or communication. On the other hand, nurses who had been provided with more reinforcement in the form of weekly short lectures on leadership and an online module on communication showed more significant improvements.

The study by Lee and colleagues (2017) demonstrates that a single educational intervention alone is not sufficient for instruction and maintenance of skills; continued reinforcement is essential for optimal improvement. The study also shows that active engagement is much more effective than passive instruction. Simulation has been shown to play a major role in reinforcing these necessary skills, with direct implications for patient care, quality, and patient outcomes (Reed et al. 2017).

Simulation has been used to engage and train health providers in the TeamSTEPPS principles and the collaborative practices that are vital for effective team functioning. Using immersive and multimodal learning opportunities, Reed and colleagues (2017) studied the effect of TeamSTEPPS training on nurses and fourth-year medical students. Students in the study engaged with the material in various ways. They first were introduced to TeamSTEPPS through a 45-minute interactive online module. Next, they were randomly assigned to a training arm that underwent a 10- to 15-minute high-fidelity patient simulation followed by a 30-minute debriefing on teamwork with TeamSTEPPS. The participants then had an hour-long discussion with the purpose of connecting their simulation experiences to concepts learned from the online modules and the principles of TeamSTEPPS. The process was then repeated with yet another simulation. The two simulations were evaluated, and student team performance was compared. The investigators found that simulation adequately and effectively reinforced TeamSTEPPS principles and, more importantly, positively affected team performance.

Systems Errors and Latent Threats

The delivery of high-quality, error-free healthcare depends on a variety of factors, including clinician knowledge, staff ability, equipment availability, and system infrastructure and resources. Excellent clinical skills, in isolation, do not predict excellent clinical care. "The environment in which health care is delivered also affects clinicians' ability to provide safe, effective, and timely care" (Kearney and Deutsch 2017, 1016).

Kearney and Deutsch (2017) suggest that a major focus of simulation should be on exposing latent safety threats (LSTs) to mitigate adverse effects on patient care. LSTs are system-based threats that affect patient safety but might not be obvious to clinicians or healthcare administrators. In situ simulations can be highly useful for evaluating teamwork and uncovering LSTs and other systems issues. According to Kearney and Deutsch (2017), the more realistic the in situ simulation is, the more useful the experience and debriefing will be. For optimal results, all clinical providers should participate in the simulation and learning experience, and they should use actual supplies and equipment that would normally be found in the real clinical environment where the case takes place.

A major limitation for conducting in situ simulations, however, is deciding when to actually conduct them. When first implementing an in situ simulation in a clinical unit, Kearney and Deutsch (2017) suggest running it at a scheduled time and checking in with unit leadership immediately before starting, to avoid potential interference with patient care duties (e.g., running the in situ simulation during times of high patient volume or acuity). When implemented correctly and mindfully, in situ simulation has the potential to identify LSTs before any patients are harmed.

Mock Codes

Simulation can be used for both educational and assessment purposes in healthcare training. Mock codes are one such way to leverage in situ simulation as a means to both educate and assess learners involved. A mock code is a unique form of in situ simulation, where a code scenario is conducted to help providers gain practical experience in the clinical workplace environment.

Delac and colleagues (2013) created the "Five Alive" program, an in situ simulation intended to improve nurses' responsiveness in the pivotal first five minutes of a resuscitation. Keeping in line with American Heart Society (AHA) standard recommendations of "one minute to CPR" and "three minutes to defibrillation," the researchers measured these times during monthly mock codes. Over the course of the mock code training, participants showed a 65 percent improvement in response time to CPR and a 67 percent improvement in time to defibrillation. In addition, the researchers found that nurses reported a higher confidence level with the emergency equipment and hand-off processes. Similarly, Herbers and Heaser (2016) ran quarterly unit-based mock codes over a two-year study period and found that CPR response time improved by 52 percent and time to defibrillation improved by 37 percent. The in situ mock codes in both of these studies were followed by debriefing sessions for reviewing AHA guidelines and deliberately practicing use of the equipment.

In situ simulations for mock codes offer several advantages. They give teams the experience of actually locating all the equipment and medications needed for a resuscitation; they make participants identify and practice protocols for escalating care and seeking assistance; and they provide participants with hands-on experience for relatively low-frequency, high-stakes events that require quick response times to ensure optimal patient outcomes.

Conclusion

Simulation is a learner-centered pedagogy rooted in the principles of experiential learning. It has consistently been associated with heightened learning outcomes, and it has long been used to address quality and safety issues in healthcare. Depending on the objectives of the educational program, instructors have a wide array of simulation options at their disposal, including low- and high-fidelity approaches, partial and full task trainers, and center-based and in situ modalities. Whether aiming to improve team performance, identify latent patient safety threats, or improve technical skills for specific procedures, simulation offers ample opportunities to augment training and development programs for patient safety and clinical quality.

Study Questions

1. How might you select and implement one or more of the simulation-based approaches described in this chapter at your institution?

2. What are some of the challenges you might encounter when using simulation to improve health outcomes and change the clinical landscape of your institution?
3. Identify three key questions or issues that would need to be considered when planning to implement healthcare-based simulation into your program or institution.
4. What are some simulation-based technologies that can be integrated into educational and training programs at your institution?
5. What are some quality improvement tools that can be linked with simulation-based education to augment training programs or interventions?

References

Aggarwal, R., O. T. Mytton, M. Derbrew, D. Hananel, M. Heydenburg, B. Issenberg, C. MacAulay, M. E. Mancini, T. Morimoto, N. Soper, A. Ziv, and R. Reznick. 2010. "Training and Simulation for Patient Safety." *Quality and Safety in Health Care* 19 (Suppl. 2): i34–i43.

Cooper, J. B., and V. R. Taqueti. 2008. "A Brief History of the Development of Mannequin Simulators for Clinical Education and Training." *Postgraduate Medical Journal* 84 (997): 563–70.

Dankbaar, M. E., M. B. Roozeboom, E. A. Oprins, F. Rutten, J. J. van Merrienboer, J. L. van Saase, and S. C. Schuit. 2017. "Preparing Residents Effectively in Emergency Skills Training with a Serious Game." *Simulation in Healthcare* 12 (1): 9–16.

Delac, K., D. Blazier, L. Daniel, and D. N-Wilfong. 2013. "Five Alive: Using Mock Code Simulation to Improve Responder Performance During the First 5 Minutes of a Code." *Critical Care Nursing Quarterly* 36 (2): 244–50.

Fanning, R. M., and D. M. Gaba. 2007. "The Role of Debriefing in Simulation-Based Learning." *Simulation in Healthcare* 2 (2): 115–25.

Gaba, D. M. 2004. "The Future Vision of Simulation in Health Care." *Quality and Safety in Health Care* 13 (Suppl. 1): i2–i10.

Ghosh, S. K. 2015. "Human Cadaveric Dissection: A Historical Account from Ancient Greece to the Modern Era." *Anatomy & Cell Biology* 48 (3): 153–69.

Herbers, M. D., and J. A. Heaser. 2016. "Implementing an in Situ Mock Code Quality Improvement Program." *American Journal of Critical Care* 25 (5): 393–99.

Jones, F., C. E. Passos-Neto, and O. F. M. Braghiroli. 2015. "Simulation in Medical Education: Brief History and Methodology." *Principles and Practice of Clinical Research* 1 (2): 56–63.

Kearney, J. A., and E. S. Deutsch. 2017. "Using Simulation to Improve Systems." *Otolaryngologic Clinics of North America* 50 (5): 1015–28.

Lee, S.-H., H. S. Khanuja, R. J. Blanding, J. Sedgwick, K. Pressimone, J. R. Ficke, and L. C. Jones. 2017. "Sustaining Teamwork Behaviors Through Reinforcement of TeamSTEPPS Principles." *Journal of Patient Safety.* Published October 30. https://journals.lww.com/journalpatientsafety/Abstract/publishahead/Sustaining_Teamwork_Behaviors_Through.99435.aspx.

Lopreiato, J. O., D. Downing, W. Gammon, L. Lioce, B. Sittner, V. Slot, A. E. Spain (eds.), and the Terminology & Concepts Working Group. 2016. *Healthcare Simulation Dictionary.* Accessed October 26, 2018. www.ssih.org/dictionary.

Miller, G. E. 1990. "The Assessment of Clinical Skills/Competence/Performance." *Academic Medicine* 65 (9): S63–S67.

Moulton, C. A., A. Dubrowski, H. Macrae, B. Graham, E. Grober, and R. Reznick. 2006. "Teaching Surgical Skills: What Kind of Practice Makes Perfect? A Randomized, Controlled Trial." *Annals of Surgery* 244 (3): 400–409.

Reed, T., T. L. Horsley, K. Muccino, D. Quinones, V. J. Siddall, J. McCarthy, and W. Adams. 2017. "Simulation Using TeamSTEPPS to Promote Interprofessional Education and Collaborative Practice." *Nurse Educator* 42 (3): E1–E5.

Taylor, D. C., and H. Hamdy. 2013. "Adult Learning Theories: Implications for Learning and Teaching in Medical Education: AMEE Guide No. 83." *Medical Teacher* 35 (11): e1561–72.

Vincent, C., K. Moorthy, S. K. Sarker, A. Chang, and A. W. Darzi. 2004. "Systems Approaches to Surgical Quality and Safety: From Concept to Measurement." *Annals of Surgery* 239 (4): 475–82.

PART

CULTURE AND LEADERSHIP

David B. Nash

As an observer of organizational culture in healthcare for more than 30 years, I consider myself a perennial student, particularly of the literature on leadership. One cannot have a meaningful discussion about how to improve healthcare quality and safety without a careful examination of the intersection of culture and leadership—the focus of part III of this book, which includes chapters 9 through 13.

In addition to studying the literature on leadership in healthcare, I have served on several hospital boards for almost two decades— including ten years for Catholic Healthcare Partners (now Mercy Health), a large multistate, multihospital nonprofit system headquartered in Cincinnati, Ohio, and nine years for Main Line Health, a multihospital community-based system in suburban Philadelphia. At both of these institutions, I chaired the hospital board's quality and safety committee. As a result, I have first-hand experience with the on-the-ground realities shared at board subcommittees, retreats, presentations, and the like.

I have also had the pleasure of serving, for more than 25 years, on the faculty of The Governance Institute (TGI), headquartered in San Diego, California, and now a part of NRC Health. TGI serves not-for-profit hospital and health system boards, executives, and physician leaders and supports their efforts to govern and lead their organizations. Under TGI's auspices, I have had the privilege of educating thousands of board members and healthcare professionals over the past three decades. This backdrop provides me with a real-world outlook that I hope will bring this section to life for our readers.

Chapters 9 through 13 form a wonderful story about the interplay of culture, communication, accountability, and transparency, and they highlight the urgent need for leadership in our field. For example, in chapter 9, Deirdre E. Mylod and Thomas H. Lee summarize the aspects of patient satisfaction and demonstrate that patients who have a better experience of care also tend to have better clinical outcomes (characterized by less harm and fewer errors).

This conclusion may seem obvious at first blush, but the reasons for it are actually somewhat complicated.

Based on a decade of research on Hospital Consumer Assessment of Healthcare Providers and Systems survey results, two things that patients care most about are care coordination and communication with and among providers. Patients assume (erroneously, in many cases) that providers will not harm them. The central take-home message of the patient experience is the expectation that providers will deliver patient-centric care each and every time. How close do we actually come to fulfilling this critically important expectation? Not nearly close enough.

Mylod and Lee also note an important difference between units of accountability and units of improvement. The individual delivering care, whoever that might be, is *accountable*, but the actual source for *improvement*, generally speaking, is at the system level. Upon discharge, for instance, a patient might give a negative review to a single clinician, but improving the individual patient experience requires collective concern and action. Health systems need greater alignment between the units of accountability and the units of improvement. Patient experience surveys in recent years have made clear that we have a long way to go in creating a truly patient-centric system.

In chapter 10, Craig Clapper, a national expert in and teacher of high reliability, reinforces some painful truths on safety and reliability. Our system needs to deliver care that is safe—that is, care that protects patients from harm. *Reliability* is defined as the probability that our complex socio-technical system will actually function correctly. Clapper illustrates the point with an equation, positing that reliability equals one minus system error.

Why should we care about the distinction between safety and reliability, and why should we devote an entire chapter to aspects of creating a high-reliability system? Reliability serves as a framework that, according to Clapper, optimizes results in all three spheres of safety, quality, and the patient experience. The distinction is important.

Zero preventable harm and 100 percent appropriate care—cornerstones of high reliability—are the basis, or the chassis, of a solid operating system. Unfortunately, most hospitals still cannot achieve these important goals. Patients have the right to assume we will give them such care, but they have little understanding of just how complex our systems are and of how critical the notion of high reliability must be as a watchword and goal for the future.

Chapter 10 also introduces us to the long-standing (though not always realized) concept of just culture. Organizations that practice high reliability also, in parallel, create a culture in which the person with the lowest stature can go against the authority gradient and play a central role in delivering care that achieves zero preventable harm. Clapper's work remains front and center today because of his clarity of presentation and the criticality of the goals he espouses.

Regrettably, by the time readers get to chapter 11, by David Mayer and Anne J. Gunderson, they may wonder if we will ever be able to produce a culture of high reliability when we continue to educate clinicians, including physicians, nurses, and pharmacists, in much the same paradigm that we used more than 35 years ago. In their chapter on education for healthcare quality and safety, Mayer and Gunderson trace the history of the education movement by outlining key milestone papers and symposia. We are left with the sense that not much has changed—that we are still putting the proverbial "lipstick on a pig" and thinking that the pig looks different.

This topic is of particular interest to me, as an active participant in the effort to reform and improve medical education at both the undergraduate and graduate level. I was honored to have participated in the 2009 white paper report from the Lucian Leape Institute in Boston (discussed in the chapter) and as a founding member of the Association of American Medical Colleges Integrating Quality Leadership Group (having served for nearly a decade on its related steering committee). Despite the efforts of many of my colleagues over the past 25 years, however, we cannot claim that medical education has pivoted and made a serious nationwide commitment to teaching the tenets of quality and safety.

Although Mayer and Gunderson provide a comprehensive review of the history and literature of reform, theirs is not a celebratory chapter lauding a job well done; alas, the conclusions reached in chapter 11 are a bit disheartening, to put it mildly. Perhaps a happier interpretation is that they have issued a rallying cry—a call to arms, if you will, that despite all of the key milestones noted therein, we have precious few pedagogic outcome measures to demonstrate improvement in education for quality and safety across all the key professional domains.

Chapter 12, by Michael D. Pugh, helpfully distinguishes between a dashboard and a scorecard. The former is the instrument panel, and the latter tracks progress against a goal or known benchmark. Pugh provides an important overview of the transition in our language from *quality assurance* to *quality control* and, ultimately, to *quality improvement*. He connects the dots by explicitly stating that the leadership system drives both organizational culture and alignment in daily work to achieve the desired level of performance. He also notes that, despite widespread implementation of electronic health records, we cannot say conclusively that they have led to significant improvements in quality and safety—although their use certainly improves the ability of organizations to track and collect certain quality and safety-related measures. Perhaps we can make this connection more clear in the next decade.

Pugh calls for hospital boards to peer through the haze and focus on what he labels the "vital few" initiatives. The test of a good strategy becomes, "Does successful deployment of the strategy actually lead to improved performance?"

Although it seems natural to expect all leaders, including board members, to look in the mirror and ask themselves this simple question, it is a very difficult exercise indeed! Pugh concludes his chapter with a discussion and accompanying visuals that link process and outcome measures to the strategic plan, from the level of the board of trustees all the way down to accountable entities within the organization. This chapter is an enduring contribution to the literature on culture and leadership.

Kathryn C. Peisert, a longtime leader within TGI, narrates part III's final chapter, which focuses on governance. She expertly traces the fiduciary responsibility of the board and delineates its central role in the quality and safety debate. The bottom line of chapter 13 is that it's all about the board! Boards bear the ultimate responsibility for *everything* in the healthcare organization, including quality and safety.

In reviewing the literature and the research evidence, Peisert notes that, when boards are effectively engaged in the quality and safety apparatus, all process and outcome measures move in the appropriate direction. She describes the progress that has been made over the last decade, after it was first discovered that nearly half of all community hospitals lacked a board committee devoted exclusively to the task of ensuring quality and safety. We have come a long way, at the governance level, to create a culture devoted to preventing harm and reducing waste. Chapter 13 also highlights the importance of the relationship between the CEO and the board chair—a relationship that serves as a lever to create alignment, improve visibility for quality, instill zero tolerance for harm, and provide a platform upon which to learn from the inevitable sentinel event.

The Institute of Medicine's 2001 *Crossing the Quality Chasm* report—a landmark work cited repeatedly throughout this book—outlined the so-called STEEEP goals of safe, timely, effective, efficient, equitable, and patient-centered care. Part III of our book will no doubt stimulate readers to ask how close we are to achieving these goals. Readers may ask, "What is the contribution of culture and leadership, from the governance level on down, for promoting these enduring 20-year-old goals?" Taken as a whole, these five chapters make me optimistic—despite the long road ahead—about our ability to make real progress toward these important aims.

CHAPTER

9

THE PATIENT EXPERIENCE

Deirdre E. Mylod and Thomas H. Lee

Over the past two decades, patient experience has moved beyond the purview of patient advocates to become a key strategic focus of major organizations. How and why did this change happen? What concerns do we have about the available data? How has the state of the science evolved? And how are the data being used to improve care and help organizations thrive? These questions will be central to this chapter's discussion.

The Patient Experience Emerges

The measurement of the patient experience is a relatively new business function. When providers first began measuring "patient satisfaction" in the 1980s, they had different goals. At that time, the prevailing attitude was that quality was difficult or impossible to measure, but it was assumed to be generally good. In this context, provider leaders—predominantly in hospitals—were interested in preventing patient complaints in hopes of avoiding malpractice suits. Hospitals also were interested in competing for market share by providing better service—often with the aim of providing "wow experiences." Such experiences might involve lovely settings, smiling and friendly personnel, good food, musicians in the lobbies, artwork on the walls, and easy parking. Clinical personnel were not opposed to such efforts, but they generally did not consider such matters relevant to what they considered quality.

Attitudes began to change in 2000, with the publication of *To Err Is Human,* a landmark Institute of Medicine (IOM) report on patient safety (Kohn, Corrigan, and Donaldson 2000), and its 2001 successor, *Crossing the Quality Chasm* (IOM 2001). In combination, these two reports revealed enormous problems in the quality of healthcare in the United States. What we had previously assumed to be consistently high-quality care was now revealed to be frequently unreliable and inadequate in meeting patient needs. Although much of the initial attention focused on patient safety, the reports—particularly the second one—also highlighted other issues. Recommendations included the following:

- Healthcare should be responsive to patients' needs at all times (i.e., 24 hours a day, every day).
- The care system should be designed to meet the most common types of needs, but also flexible enough to accommodate the needs and values of individuals.
- Patients should be the source of control, with all the necessary information and the opportunity to exercise as much control as they want over healthcare decisions that affect them.
- Clinicians and patients should communicate effectively and share information.
- The health system should anticipate patients' needs, not just respond to events.
- Clinicians and organizations should cooperate, communicate, and coordinate their efforts.

In the years that followed the publication of these reports, the federal government became increasingly interested in patient experience, and researchers worked with the Centers for Medicare & Medicaid Services (CMS) and the Agency for Healthcare Research and Quality to develop standardized, public-domain instruments to measure patient perceptions of care. The Hospital Consumer Assessment of Healthcare Providers and Systems (HCAHPS) survey, a standardized survey instrument that is administered to randomly selected patients after discharge from a hospital, was the first such instrument to be incorporated into required public reporting and, ultimately, value-based purchasing initiatives.

A game plan soon emerged for patient experience surveys to be used as an outcome measure to track and assess quality as changes were made to care models and payment structures. The HCAHPS survey was approved by the National Quality Forum in 2005 and adopted by CMS in 2006; voluntary public reporting of HCAHPS results began in 2008. HCAHPS then shifted from a voluntary program to a basic fact of life for hospitals. First, hospitals received a financial incentive for participating in HCAHPS ("pay for reporting"), and participation increased to nearly 95 percent. Then, with passage of the Affordable Care Act of 2010, a small portion of hospital Medicare reimbursement was tied to performance on HCAHPS, beginning with hospital discharges in 2012.

This same sequence is playing out—or has already been completed—for other sectors of healthcare delivery (e.g., home health, ambulatory care, emergency departments). Measures are developed, tested, and then implemented with the suffix *CAHPS*. For instance, the Home Health CAHPS (HHCAHPS) obtains patients' perspectives about home health care, whereas the Clinician and Groups CAHPS (CG-CAHPS) focuses on care provided in doctors' offices. Initially, use of the tools is voluntary, but adoption spreads as financial incentives for reporting are anticipated. Eventually, real use of the tools becomes mandatory, as financial incentives are tied to actual performance. Providers that "stand still"—that is, do nothing and have the same performance year after year—start to fall behind their competition.

A subtle yet important change that occurred in the years since the IOM reports was the replacement of the term "patient satisfaction" with "patient experience." The change reflects the realization that the challenges for healthcare go beyond meeting or exceeding the expectations of consumers (i.e., satisfying them); the real goal is to meet their needs with reliability, efficiency, and safety. Whereas "patient satisfaction" is based on whether the care conforms to patients' expectations, "patient experience" incorporates *everything* that directly or indirectly affects patients across the continuum of care, including the relief of their suffering, physical discomfort, and anxiety. Interestingly, some of the first validated measures of patient satisfaction within private industry, such as the Press Ganey instrument, evaluated a full complement of the patient experience (e.g., communication, respect, shared decision making, privacy, preparation for discharge). However, because early studies found that overall patient evaluation measures were associated with malpractice risk, much of the work was more narrowly focused on improving overall perceptions to avoid risk rather than enhancing quality for the various elements of patient care.

Since the advent of CAHPS measures, the range of questions considered most useful has expanded. CAHPS measures, designed for public reporting, are typically framed to represent the occurrence (expressed as *yes* or *no*) or frequency (expressed as *never*, *sometimes*, *usually*, or *always*) of behaviors. For each measure, the optimal response (e.g., *always*, *definitely yes*) is categorized as the "top box" response. For public reporting purposes, the measures are displayed in terms of the proportion of patients that responded with a top-box or optimal experience. Nationwide, the average top-box rating has continued to increase each year since the inception of public reporting (see exhibit 9.1).

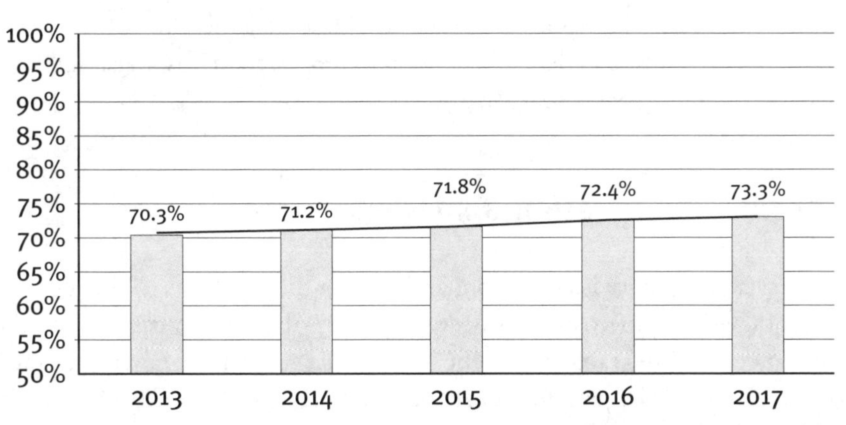

EXHIBIT 9.1
Trend in Median National Performance for Patients Evaluating Hospital Care as a 9 or a 10

Source: Press Ganey (2017). Used with permission. © 2017 Press Ganey Associates.

The patient experience, however, cannot be defined solely by the responses to a series of yes-or-no questions about whether certain processes have occurred (e.g., whether the patient received an explanation of test results). Patient experience as an outcome measure needs to incorporate patients' evaluation of the quality of the attributes of care. Thus, as opposed to a simple indication of whether a certain action has been performed, a more holistic measure might focus on patients' confidence that "everyone worked well together to care for me." This measure evaluates the quality of multiple interactions and represents a tougher challenge for clinicians.

The importance of evaluative measures—as opposed to measures that focus on the occurrence or frequency of a process—has been supported by analyses of the correlation between patients' overall ratings of their care and specific patient experience measures. For example, Press Ganey (2017) analyzed data from 1,882,559 patients at 1,733 facilities between January 1 and December 31, 2016, and found that the factors most strongly correlated with top ratings for hospitals included the following:

- How well the staff worked together
- Responsiveness to concerns and complaints
- Degree to which nurses kept patients informed
- Attention to special/personal needs

In multiple analyses of the independent drivers of patients' global ratings of care across various settings (e.g., inpatient, outpatient, emergency department), the measures that have consistently emerged as correlates are coordination of care, caring behaviors, and communication. Differences may exist from one setting to another—for instance, hospitalized patients tend to place great importance on perceptions of teamwork and nursing communication—but coordination, empathy, and communication are consistently important drivers. After these variables are taken into account, such factors as waiting time and amenities related to food or the environment are generally not statistically significant correlates of patients' likelihood to recommend hospitals, outpatient practices, or emergency departments.

Concerns About Patient Experience Data

For every action, there is a reaction, and among the reactions to the increased interest in patient experience has been skepticism about the measures and their importance. Providers worry that the measures reflect "hotel functions" rather than determinants of patients' health outcomes. They also express concerns that the data are not statistically valid because of inadequate samples and that the ability to adjust for variables that might skew the results is limited.

We divide these concerns into two categories. The first category, conceptual issues, encompasses, for instance, concerns that greater patient satisfaction might be linked to worse outcomes or that measurement of patient experience might actually worsen care. The second category, data issues, includes concerns about the validity of the information.

Conceptual Issues

Does measuring patient experience have potentially perverse effects? This question is often raised by physicians and others who are concerned that patients are unable to identify technically excellent care and that their opinions, therefore, are of uncertain value. Another concern is that patients sometimes have misguided ideas about what they need (e.g., magnetic resonance imaging for a headache) and might be critical of clinicians who do not order what they want.

One paper is brought up repeatedly to support the idea that higher patient satisfaction might actually worsen care. Fenton and colleagues (2012) analyzed data on 51,946 adult respondents to the national Medical Expenditure Panel Survey from 2000 to 2007. They looked at two years of data for each patient, including mortality data through the end of 2006. Patient satisfaction was assessed for the first year, with five items modeled after the CG-CAHPS survey but modified to ask about all care received in the prior 12 months rather than about a specific episode or care event. Correlations were sought with outcomes and healthcare utilization in the second year.

The analysis showed that patients in the highest quartile of patient satisfaction had lower rates of emergency department use, higher rates of hospitalization and medication use, greater total spending, and higher mortality compared to patients in the lowest quartile. Many people have cited these findings as an indication that higher patient satisfaction leads to higher death rates and higher costs.

In actuality, the authors drew no such conclusion. They noted the limitations in the data available to them, including the fact that they only had five questions regarding patients' assessments of their primary care physicians' performance on specific activities (e.g., listening carefully) for the entire prior year, along with a global assessment of all the care the patients received from all physicians and providers. These data were rolled together, with each item weighted equally, into a measure that was purported to represent year 1 satisfaction. As a result, they were unable to examine better-defined issues, such as whether patients' evaluation of their hospital care correlated with hospital mortality.

Even though the quartile of patients with the highest satisfaction also had the highest costs and worst mortality, there was no "dose–response" effect—that is, no trend suggesting the higher the patient satisfaction, the higher the mortality. The patients in the third quartile actually had slightly lower mortality than the patients in the second quartile. If higher satisfaction led to worse outcomes, one would expect the opposite. The same was true for hospital admissions. Seeking to explain these findings, Fenton and colleagues (2012, 408) wrote that "patient satisfaction may be a marker for illness, identifying patients who rely more on support from their physicians and thus report higher satisfaction." In short, sicker patients had more contact with their clinicians and, as a result, were more positive about their care.

The Fenton and colleagues paper is so often quoted—inaccurately, from our perspective—because it stands alone; it is the *only* paper with actual data raising the question of whether perverse effects might result from better patient satisfaction. The findings from other research studies overwhelmingly point in the opposite direction: Better patient experience correlates with better quality and better patient outcomes. For example, Jha and colleagues (2008) found that hospitals in the top quartile of HCAHPS ratings had better performance on quality metrics for all four clinical conditions examined—acute myocardial infarction, congestive heart failure, pneumonia, and prevention of surgical complications.

A study by Sacks and colleagues (2015), using data about more than 100,000 surgery patients from the American College of Surgeons National Surgical Quality Improvement Project, produced similar findings. The researchers evaluated the relationship between HCAHPS performance and well-documented clinical outcomes, including thirty-day postoperative mortality, major and minor complications, and hospital readmission. After adjustment for other clinical data, hospitals in the top quartile in HCAHPS performance were found to have a 15 percent lower risk of patient death compared to hospitals in the lowest quartile. The researchers' conclusion: "Using a national sample of hospitals, we demonstrated a significant association between patient satisfaction scores and several objective measures of surgical quality. Our findings suggest that payment policies that incentivize better patient experience do not require hospitals to sacrifice performance on other quality measures" (Sacks et al. 2015, 858).

The preponderance of evidence shows no tension between patient experience and other measures of quality; in fact, evidence suggests that the two concerns track in the same direction: Providers with better patient experience tend to have better outcomes and better patient safety records. But how and why?

When a group of researchers from Duke University considered this question, they noted that questions on the HCAHPS survey tend to focus on activities that are at the core of good medicine (Manary et al. 2013). Consider the following examples:

- Question 3, from the section on "Your Care from Nurses," asks: "During this hospital stay, how often did nurses explain things in a way you could understand?" The answer options are "never," "sometimes," "usually," and "always."

- Question 17, from the section on "Your Experiences in This Hospital," asks: "Before giving you any new medicine, how often did hospital staff describe possible side effects in a way you could understand?" Again, the answer options are "never," "sometimes," "usually," and "always."
- Question 20, from the section on "When You Left the Hospital," asks: "During this hospital stay, did you get information in writing about what symptoms or health problems to look out for after you left the hospital?" The answer options are "yes" and "no."

Such questions demonstrate that good, measured patient experience is inextricably intertwined with widely shared notions of excellent care delivery.

One specific conceptual concern involves the issue of whether measurement of pain management might lead to overuse of opioid analgesics, thereby fueling the current epidemic of opioid addiction and overdose deaths. However, a study of emergency department data by Schwartz and colleagues (2014) found no relationship between use of opioid analgesics and measures of patient experience. Furthermore, CMS removed existing pain control measures from value-based purchasing models beginning in fiscal year 2018 (Federal Register 2016) to address concerns about incentivizing pain control practices, and it developed new measures that instead ask about extent to which pain control options were discussed (Federal Register 2017). Although some patients with substance use disorder might express frustration or anger toward clinicians who follow judicious and appropriate prescribing practices, such patients have a low likelihood of completing a postdischarge survey. Thus, clinicians would be misguided to prescribe opioids based on the belief that doing so would help their pain management or other measures.

Data Issues

Creating an environment in which clinicians feel that patient experience data are being used to improve care—rather than to judge clinicians—is essential, because data collection will never be complete, and the ability to analyze data will never be perfect. Inevitably, clinicians will always feel somewhat judged by the measurement of patient experience, and every effort should be made to ensure fairness in the presentation of data. Concerns frequently articulated by clinicians include the following:

- The sample sizes are too small.
- The scores fluctuate.
- The data are old, and care has changed in the interim.
- The respondents are not representative of the overall population of patients who receive care from the clinician.
- The respondents really received care from many clinicians, so attributing the results to just one of them is inappropriate.

- The scores are too tightly packed. So many patients give high ratings that patient-reported data cannot be used to discriminate among providers.
- The interpretation of data and benchmarking do not have adequate adjustment for risk factors that may account for lower performance.
- Given the highly competitive environment, physicians or organizations with relatively high raw scores might rank as average or below average when compared to their peers.

Each of these concerns has some basis in reality, and each can and should be addressed and mitigated through various approaches. For example, concerns about small sample sizes can be addressed by collecting more data in a timely manner through a combination of modalities (e.g., email, telephone, mail). Such an effort could also address concerns about the recency and representativeness of data and the stability of measurement. With the rapid collection of larger amounts of data, the findings and patient comments become difficult to ignore.

For publicly reported measures and federal payment models, patient mix adjustment is applied to data to account for normative differences in patient responses related to patient-specific factors such as age, service line (e.g., medical, surgical, obstetrics [OB]), or language spoken at home. Patient mix adjustments are appropriate at the aggregate level to account for differences in the populations being served and to level the playing field across organizations. However, patient mix adjustment is less well suited for subgroups of data that are typically used for quality improvement purposes. For instance, a model that adjusts for more or fewer OB patients than average at a hospital cannot be appropriately applied to an individual OB unit. Additionally, we cannot possibly adjust for all the variables that might influence patient experience. Even if 100 percent of patients were to respond to surveys, comparisons among providers would always be susceptible to confounding.

Clinicians, therefore, should consider the goal of patient experience measurement to be *improvement*. They should view the data in the context of competition not with others so much as with themselves—trying to be better next year than they are now or, even more compelling, trying to be at their best with the next patient they see. Opportunities to learn and improve can be informed through the use of appropriate benchmarks, such as comparing performance against similar organizations, or against doctors of a similar specialty, or against patients with similar characteristics. Appropriate and specific benchmarking can account for differences in populations without requiring the statistical adjustment of the data used for quality improvement.

Survey response rates average about 20 to 25 percent, but they may vary from 10 to 60 across different patient populations. Clinicians worry that patients who are disgruntled or angry are more likely to respond than those who have had good experiences. On the contrary, however, patients tend to be generous graders and give providers high marks. Indeed, this tendency for responses to be at least moderately favorable supports an alternative criticism—that scores are distributed in a narrow portion of the upper range of performance. The prevalence of mostly positive responses reflects a state of care that has few absolute defects or failures; rather, it has care that is extremely reliable and care that is mostly reliable but lacks consistency across the episode or experience.

Although the preponderance of patient feedback is positive, a portion of patients do not give top-box responses for important outcomes, such as their likelihood to recommend care to others. According to the Press Ganey national database in 2017, only 21 percent of patients provided top-box ratings to every item on the HCAHPS survey. Nationally, patient responses to HCAHPS individual items or questions are optimal between 52 and 82 percent of the time (HCAHPS 2017).

In short, no providers are perfect, and plenty of opportunities exist to improve care. The key is to use the data to find them. So how can we resolve the tension between our need to improve and the imperfections in the data? The answer is by improving the measures, getting more data, and using the data appropriately.

Improving Patient Experience Measurement and Reporting

Many of the concerns described in the previous section have been mitigated—and sometimes even eliminated—through progress in patient experience measurement and reporting. The key areas of improvement are (1) measuring what matters to patients, (2) advances in data quantity and collection methods, and (3) advances in data analysis.

Measuring What Matters to Patients

As the healthcare system moves away from compensating providers purely on the basis of volume of services, the concept of patient-centered care is coming into focus. Patients' needs are not organized in patients' minds according to the traditional structure of medicine, based on areas of clinical expertise such as surgery or cardiology. Also, patients are not obsessed by whether individual clinicians are competent or reliable in their various roles. Rather, they assume this competence exists, and they are usually correct.

Instead of measurement of what providers do, patient-centered care requires measurement of providers' focus on meeting patients' needs. Clinicians' reliability is important, of course, but it is a means to an end. The end is defined by what actually happens from the perspective of patients—and patients are the only appropriate source of that information.

As expressed in multiple articles (Mylod and Lee 2013; Lee 2013; Kolata 2015; Press Ganey 2015), we believe that measurement of patient experience is part of the fundamental goal of healthcare, which is to recognize and reduce patients' suffering. Suffering, of course, can take a variety of forms, of which physical pain is just one; other forms include uncertainty, fear, and confusion. In approaching patient experience, we recommend "deconstructing" the notion of suffering into that which is *inherent* to the patient's medical condition, that which is *inherent* to the associated treatment, and that which is *avoidable* and results from dysfunction in the care delivery process.

The inherent suffering that patients experience as a result of either their specific medical problems or the necessary treatment is unavoidable; the role of providers is to anticipate, detect, and mitigate that suffering. Pain, discomfort, loss of function, and other physical symptoms are examples of the inherent suffering commonly associated with diseases or clinical conditions. Inherent suffering may also include fear, anxiety, and distress specifically related to patients' knowledge and concern over their condition. Furthermore, elements of treatment—even necessary and appropriate treatment—can also contribute to suffering. Surgery is frightening, can create pain, and often requires a difficult recovery. Medication often has side effects. Even the time spent receiving treatment—and the interruption it causes into patients' lives and responsibilities—can be considered a form of suffering. Anxiety often grows as patients wait for test results or for treatments to take effect, even when that wait has been appropriately minimized. Loss of autonomy and control is of great concern to patients, sometimes even more so than physical pain and discomfort.

If inherent suffering flows from patients' conditions and appropriate treatments, avoidable suffering stems from the dysfunction that exists within our systems today. Poor coordination, excessive waits, and lack of communication create uncertainty about what will happen next, erode patient trust, and contribute to anxiety, frustration, and fear. Each of these types of dysfunction is preventable, as evidenced by the relative lack of such dysfunction for patients regarded as "special" to healthcare providers. Preventing such dysfunction on a routine basis often seems beyond the control of individual personnel; hence, action at the organizational level is usually necessary. Reducing dysfunction and preventing avoidable suffering should be among the central goals of systems of care.

Current questionnaires used to measure patient experience do not directly ask patients about their level of suffering. However, they do ask patients to evaluate attributes of care, and the responses indicate the areas where patients view their care as optimal or less than optimal. This information helps providers understand where patients' needs are not being met and correct suboptimal experiences.

Exhibit 9.2 lists patient needs that may be primarily associated with either inherent suffering or avoidable suffering. For example, one of the basic needs

EXHIBIT 9.2
Examples of Patient Needs Within the Inpatient Setting

Inherent Patient Needs Arising from Disease and Treatment	Patient Needs That Stem from Dysfunction in Care Delivery
As part of having a health condition or receiving treatment, patients have a need for: • Skilled care providers • Pain control • Information • Responsiveness • Personalization • Empathy • Choice • Privacy • Preparation for discharge and self-care	When dysfunction exists, patients develop a need for: • Teamwork among caregivers • Courteous and respectful interactions • Reduced wait times • Comfortable environments • Service recovery • Adequate amenities

Source: Press Ganey (2015). Used with permission. © 2015 Press Ganey Associates.

of patients is information. Uncertainty is unnerving, and it causes suffering. Data on the extent to which physicians and nurses keep patients informed, the clarity of the communication, and the effectiveness of conveying to patients the side effects and purposes of tests and treatments all provide insight into how well this need is being met. Although the examples in the exhibit are from the inpatient setting, the implications are relevant to all patient care.

Advances in Data Quality and Collection

The traditional approach to the collection of patient experience data has been to use mailed surveys or to contact a modest sample of patients by telephone. This approach has enabled surveillance for major problems but does not provide enough data to drive improvement. CMS and other regulatory bodies still require data collection via these older methods, but data collection through email and other electronic approaches has become more prevalent.

Electronic methods allow for rapid and efficient data collection, and a growing number of hospitals and physician practices are trying to collect information from every patient after every encounter. Organizations now use "multimodality" systems in which a random sample of patients is invited to respond to surveys via an established mode, such as mail, and the balance of the population is then invited via an electronic survey. Statistical adjustments for differences in age and other factors enable the comparison of electronic survey results with data collected via traditional methods, so provider organizations can tell if they are improving or losing ground.

Response rates with e-surveys run about the same as with mailed questionnaires. However, because e-surveys are less costly, clinicians can get data from a much larger number of patients, which makes the findings difficult to dismiss. About half of the responses to e-surveys are made within 24 to 48 hours, so the data and comments provided to clinicians in this manner are considered "fresh."

Another interesting difference between the modes of feedback is that patients tend to have a lower threshold for writing comments and also write longer comments when responding via e-survey. Often, they provide multiple sentences that paint a clear picture of what they appreciated or disliked about their care. These comments are proving to be powerful drivers of improvement for clinicians. No one would argue that risk adjustment is needed for a vignette.

Many organizations are starting to use "point-of-care" data collection—for instance, using tablet computers to collect data from patients much more frequently, such as every day or even every shift during a hospitalization. Data collected in this manner can help overcome some of the challenges in attribution of information to individual clinicians.

Advances in Data Analysis: Benchmarking, Segmentation, and Attribution

Once data have been collected, they must be analyzed and reported in ways that have an impact. One of the changes associated with the arrival of patient-centered care is the increased recognition that not all patients are the same. Patients are infinitely heterogeneous, and improvement is more likely to occur when patients can be segmented into groups with similar needs. Patients are often segmented based on condition, but other categories are also useful. For instance, segmentation based on age group can help with addressing some of the coordination and information needs that differentiate older patients from younger ones (Press Ganey 2016).

The availability of more data on more patients has led to the revelation that no institution is "the best" at everything; when data are analyzed at the segment level, opportunities to improve and to learn from others inevitably arise. Thus, data need to be collected, analyzed, and reported for the levels at which accountability can be created and improvement can occur. However, just as individuals vary, so do groups. New Yorkers, for instance, have been found to be less likely to give high scores than Midwesterners (HCAHPS 2017). Given this complexity, large amounts of data from large numbers of providers are needed for benchmarking.

The need for large amounts of data is heightened when one considers that, ideally, data should be fed back at the level of "units of accountability" and "units of improvement." Units of accountability are those units that recognize responsibility for performance. Units of improvement are those that include the personnel and other components necessary to create permanent change for the better. To date, patient experience data have proved most effective when the units of accountability and improvement are the same, as is the case for an individual physician in the outpatient setting. Individual physicians usually understand that they are responsible for the experiences of their patients, and when they receive data and comments showing room for improvement, they are able to respond.

However, because modern medicine requires the input of multiple personnel with diverse skill sets, many issues arise for which the individual clinician cannot be the unit of accountability or improvement. For example, waiting time is generally not under the complete control of a physician, and coordination of care generally depends on the actions of many personnel, not one particular person. For such issues, the solutions lie with the organization, not with the measures and the data. If we approach medicine as a "team sport," we cannot possibly identify a unit of accountability if the teams do not actually exist, or if team members do not know that they are part of the team. Thus, organizations need to create units of accountability and motivate them to become units of improvement.

Consider, for example, the complaints that arise among virtually every hospitalist group from physicians who protest—with good reason—that the data attributed to them do not reflect the care that they actually deliver. Patients are surveyed after a hospitalization, and the data are analyzed based on the last physician who was overseeing the patient's care. This discharging physician might have been responsible for much of the patient's care—or very little. Frequently, the real "action" of the hospitalization occurred on someone else's watch. Such situations call for two potential solutions, which are increasingly being used.

The first solution is for the group of hospitalists to feel *collective* responsibility for their performance and to recognize that they are a team in which no individual's performance stands alone. The other solution is to collect more data throughout the hospitalization, so that patients can be asked to give feedback for personnel with whom they have interacted during the last day, or even the last shift. Some organizations have moved in this direction with the use of tablet computers that show photographs of the personnel to help patients identify them.

Using Patient Experience Data to Improve

Patient experience data are no longer tapped simply to assess whether care is adequate; rather, they have become a central focus at the core of strategy. Increasingly, healthcare organizations recognize that their "true north" is meeting the needs of patients and doing so with efficiency. Medicare provides a modest financial incentive for hospitals to improve patient experience, but the greater incentive for provider organizations is competition for market share. The overall trend in the market is steady improvement across the industry, which means that institutions that are not making progress are falling behind. For example, a hospital that was at the national median in 2013 would be at the 35th percentile in 2017 if it did not improve its performance.

Some of the key steps for driving improvement have been mentioned earlier in this chapter—for instance, collecting more data through electronic methods, doing so in a more timely manner, segmenting patients according to their needs, and organizing providers into teams that have accountability for the care of those segments. Another valuable approach is to focus organizations' efforts on the issues that are the most important drivers of patients' global ratings of care. A healthcare workforce will have difficulty responding to the message, "Get better at everything." Even though everything being measured in patient experience surveys does matter (otherwise the questions would not have been created), some issues matter more than others. These issues are the major drivers of patients' overall experience and, ultimately, the trust they have in the care they have received.

As noted earlier in the chapter, issues such as coordination, caring behaviors, and communication are consistently identified as independent correlates of patients' likelihood to recommend hospitals, physician practices, emergency departments, and other facilities. The importance of these issues has been apparent in analyses of drivers of performance in global ratings of hospitals. Exhibit 9.3 shows the variables that were most strongly associated with patients giving a top-box response (9 or 10) for a hospital's overall rating (Press Ganey 2017). This analysis was achieved using a driver index that incorporated two pieces of information: (1) correlation, or how strongly correlated the item is to the hospital's 0–10 overall rating; and (2) top-box ratio, the degree to which achieving a top-box score on that item was related to the likelihood of a patient giving the hospital an overall rating of 9 or 10. The array of survey items listed in the exhibit reflects the importance of coordination, communication, and empathetic behaviors, particularly from nurses in the inpatient setting.

Based on this knowledge, how do organizations spread these values and behaviors and make them cultural norms? Feedback that suggests opportunities for improvement is clearly necessary but often is not sufficient to motivate clinicians to be at their best reliably, either as individuals or as members of a team. The challenge of nudging clinicians to improve is, in some ways, "swimming upstream" against the multitude of forces contributing to burnout among doctors, nurses, and others in healthcare. In short, how do you foster an epidemic of empathy during an epidemic of burnout?

Much is being learned from healthcare organizations that are making the reduction of patients' suffering their core value. In the past, healthcare providers were so busy doing what they were sure was good work that they

EXHIBIT 9.3 Key Drivers of Patients' Overall Rating in the Inpatient Setting

Driver Rank	Survey Item	Correlation	Top-Box Ratio	Driver Index
1	Nurses treated you with courtesy/ respect (CMS)	0.57	3.08	87
2	Staff worked together to care for you (PG)	0.69	2.38	79
3	Friendliness/courtesy of the nurses (PG)	0.58	2.27	65
4	Skill of the nurses (PG)	0.59	2.2	63
5	Nurses listened carefully to you (CMS)	0.59	2.2	63
6	Attention to special/personal needs (PG)	0.62	1.97	61
7	Response to concerns/complaints (PG)	0.65	1.86	61
8	Nurses' attitudes toward requests (PG)	0.6	2.04	60
9	Staff did everything to help with pain (CMS)	0.55	2.2	55
10	Nurses kept you informed (PG)	0.62	1.93	58

Note: Sample size: 1.6 million surveys received Jan. 1, 2015 through Dec. 31, 2015.
(CMS) = measure from HCAHPS survey.
(PG) = measure from Press Ganey survey.
Source: Press Ganey (2017). Used with permission. ©2017 Press Ganey Associates.

might not have paid much attention to the mission and value statements of their organizations. In today's competitive marketplaces, however, providers can no longer ignore the constant refrain at the Mayo Clinic that "The needs of the patient come first," or the Cleveland Clinic's truncated version of the same statement, "Patients First." These institutions and many others often use the word *Way* to describe how they deliver care—for instance, the Mayo Way, the Cleveland Clinic Way, the Ascension Way, and so on. This trend reflects the organizations' realization that building culture is a critical part of improving patient experience and achieving business success.

Culture-building, of course, is an enormous topic appropriate for other chapters and other books. Here, we will simply describe one of the most powerful culture-changing tactics for improvement of patient experience—*transparency*. Led by the groundbreaking work at the University of Utah Health System, many US providers are now posting comments and ratings from patients online for all to see.

Although the posting of data and comments online may cause initial discomfort among physicians, evidence overwhelmingly indicates that consumers want such data. A 2013 Pew Research Center study found that 72 percent of adult internet users searched online for health information in the previous year (Thackeray, Crookston, and West 2013). Another study showed that 59 percent of American adults strongly consider online ratings when choosing a physician; furthermore, among individuals using online reviews, 35 percent reported choosing physicians based on positive reviews, and 37 percent reported avoiding physicians with negative reviews (Hanauer et al. 2014).

Unfortunately, many of the reviews that consumers encounter online may be deceptive. Researchers from the Massachusetts Institute of Technology and Northwestern University examined 325,869 consumer reviews online and found that 4.8 percent were submitted by customers with no confirmed transaction. These questionable reviews also included a higher proportion of negative comments than is normally found when patients are surveyed by vendors working for clients (Anderson and Simester 2014). In light of these concerns, many healthcare organizations are collecting and publishing quantitative and qualitative patient experience data via their own "find-a-doctor" sites.

The University of Utah Health System was the first system to post patient comments and ratings online. Although that system's experience is not reflective of a controlled experiment, key findings include the following:

- The percentage of the system's physicians who score highly in patient experience measures has improved dramatically. More than 25 percent of the providers ranked in the top 1 percentile in the Press Ganey national database (Mahoney 2014).
- The improvement was achieved without any financial incentives for physicians to improve patient experience. The nonfinancial incentives of peer pressure and the reward of seeing positive comments posted publicly were more effective for driving improvement than monetary rewards attached to specified patient experience results.
- The vast majority of patient comments (about 90 percent) at University of Utah Health are positive; other systems that have adopted this approach have seen similar results. Negative comments are taken quite seriously by most physicians, and the positive comments reinforce good behaviors.
- Every institution that has gone transparent in this way has an appeals process in which physicians are sent comments before they appear online. Physicians can also appeal after comments appear online, which can lead to the comments being taken down. However, the number of appeals has been low. For instance, University of Utah had 16 appeals in the first quarter and just 1 or 2 in most quarters since. About 99

percent of comments go online (excluding those with confidential or libelous information, or with feedback unrelated to the physician or the patient's experience).

- Search engines such as Google bring the officially hosted provider "find-a-doctor" sites to the top of the page when patients search on the names of physicians, because search engines prioritize sites that have more data and fresher data. Because provider organizations survey every patient, they tend to have many more results than the nonprovider alternative sites.
- Traffic to provider websites has increased, and the amount of time that viewers spend looking at the sites has increased. Providers believe that this approach has brought them more patients.
- Providers have more trust in organizationally hosted data sources, where patients are verified as having had a healthcare interaction, as opposed to public websites that collect consumer feedback in a voluntary ad hoc fashion.

Physicians often express concerns that transparency in patient experience will lead to dissemination of negative patient comments that paint a misleading, unflattering picture. The fact is, however, that patients want to think highly of their physicians, and the vast majority of the comments that come in are positive. The occasional negative comment (e.g., "He never looked at me—he was staring at the computer screen the entire visit") tend not to be repeated. Meanwhile, the positive comments remind physicians of what patients value in their interactions. Those behavior patterns are thus reinforced.

Because of these results, provider-driven transparency of patient experience is spreading rapidly. Some providers may still reject the idea of putting negative information about themselves online, but most understand that publishing only positive comments undermines the credibility of the information. Provider organizations are finding that transparency in patient experience not only meets patients' needs for information but also, even more important, is a powerful driver of improvement.

Study Questions

1. How has the patient experience evolved over time?
2. Describe three categories of patient suffering, and provide examples.
3. What are the benefits of using data collection technologies such as e-surveys to enhance traditional approaches?

References

Anderson, E. T., and D. I. Simester. 2014. "Reviews Without a Purchase: Low Ratings, Loyal Customers, and Deception." *Journal of Marketing Research* 51 (3): 249–69.

Federal Register. 2017. "Medicare Program; Hospital Inpatient Prospective Payment Systems for Acute Care Hospitals and the Long-Term Care Hospital Prospective Payment System and Policy Changes and Fiscal Year 2018 Rates." Accessed November 30. www.federalregister.gov/documents/2017/08/14/2017-16434/medicare-program-hospital-inpatient-prospective-payment-systems-for-acute-care-hospitals-and-the.

———. 2016. "Medicare Program: Hospital Outpatient Prospective Payment and Ambulatory Surgical Center Payment Systems and Quality Reporting Programs." Accessed November 30, 2017. www.federalregister.gov/documents/2016/11/14/2016-26515/medicare-program-hospital-outpatient-prospective-payment-and-ambulatory-surgical-center-payment.

Fenton, J. J., A. F. Jerant, K. D. Bertakis, and P. Franks. 2012. "The Cost of Satisfaction: A National Study of Patient Satisfaction, Health Care Utilization, Expenditures, and Mortality." *Archives of Internal Medicine* 172 (5): 405–11.

Hanauer, D. A., K. Zheng, D. C. Singer, A. Gebremariam, and M. M. Davis. 2014. "Public Awareness, Perception, and Use of Online Physician Rating Sites." *Journal of the American Medical Association* 311 (7): 734–35.

Hospital Consumer Assessment of Healthcare Providers and Systems (HCAHPS). 2017. "Summary of HCAHPS Survey Results: January 2016 to December 2016 Discharges." Published October 27. www.hcahpsonline.org/globalassets/hcahps/summary-analyses/results/2017-10_summary-analyses_states-results.pdf.

Institute of Medicine. 2001. *Crossing the Quality Chasm: A New Health System for the 21st Century.* Washington, DC: National Academies Press.

Jha, A. K., E. J. Orav, J. Zheng, and A. M. Epstein. 2008. "Patients' Perception of Hospital Care in the United States." *New England Journal of Medicine* 359 (18): 1921–31.

Kohn, L. T., J. M. Corrigan, and M. S. Donaldson (eds.). 2000. *To Err Is Human: Building a Safer Health System.* Washington, DC: National Academies Press.

Kolata, G. 2015. "Doctors Strive to Do Less Harm by Inattentive Care." *New York Times.* Published February 17. www.nytimes.com/2015/02/18/health/doctors-strive-to-do-less-harm-by-inattentive-care.html.

Lee, T. H. 2013. "The Word That Shall Not Be Spoken." *New England Journal of Medicine* 369 (19): 1777–79.

Mahoney, D. 2014. "Rising to the Transparency Challenge." *Partners*, September–October, 8–15.

Manary, M. S. E., W. Boulding, R. Staelin, and S. Glickman. 2013. "The Patient Experience and Health Outcomes." *New England Journal of Medicine* 368 (3): 201–3.

Mylod, D. E., and T. H. Lee. 2013. "A Framework for Reducing Suffering in Health Care." *Harvard Business Review*. Published November 14. https://hbr.org/2013/11/a-framework-for-reducing-suffering-in-health-care.

Press Ganey. 2017. "Performance Insights: Health Care Improvement Trends." Accessed December 1. http://healthcare.pressganey.com/2017-Health-Care-Improvement?s=White_Paper-Web.

———. 2016. "Patient Experience in the Very Elderly: An Emerging Strategic Focus." Accessed November 30, 2017. http://healthcare.pressganey.com/research-note-elderly.

———. 2015. "Measuring Patient Needs to Reduce Suffering." Published July 13. www.pressganey.com/resources/white-papers/measuring-patient-needs-to-reduce-suffering.

Sacks, G. D., E. H. Lawson, A. J. Dawes, M. M. Russell, M. Maggard-Gibbons, D. S. Zingmond, and C. Y. Ko. 2015. "Relationship Between Hospital Performance on a Patient Satisfaction Survey and Surgical Quality." *JAMA Surgery* 150 (9): 858–64.

Schwartz, T. M., M. Tai, K. M. Babu, and R. C. Merchant. 2014. "Lack of Association Between Press Ganey Emergency Department Patient Satisfaction Scores and Emergency Department Administration of Analgesic Medications." *Annals of Emergency Medicine* 64 (5): 469–81.

Thackeray, R., B. T. Crookston, and J. H. West. 2013. "Correlates of Health-Related Social Media Use Among Adults." *Journal of Medical Internet Research* 15 (1): e21.

CHAPTER

10

SAFETY SCIENCE AND HIGH RELIABILITY ORGANIZING

Craig Clapper

Since the start of the twenty-first century, patient safety, workforce safety, and the patient experience have taken on considerable strategic importance for most major healthcare organizations, and the concepts of *safety science* and *high reliability organizing* have emerged as a result. How and why did this change happen? What is safety science? What is high reliability organizing? How can both of these bodies of knowledge be used to drive improvement and ensure the safety, quality, and positive experience of care? These questions are the major foci of this chapter.

Safety and Reliability

The National Academy of Medicine (NAM)—formerly the Institute of Medicine—defines *safety* as "freedom from accidental injury" (Kohn, Corrigan, and Donaldson 2000, 4). The Joint Commission takes a broader view of patient safety through its efforts to monitor and prevent *sentinel events*—defined as unanticipated events in a healthcare setting that result in death or serious physical or psychological injury to a patient or patients, not related to the natural course of illness. Sentinel events specifically include the loss of a limb or gross motor function, as well as any event for which a recurrence would carry the risk of a serious adverse outcome. Safety thus involves protecting patients from sentinel events while they are receiving care and avoiding *iatrogenic injury*—that is, injury induced inadvertently by medical treatment or diagnostic procedures.

Regardless of how the term is defined by a particular healthcare organization, safety necessitates protecting patients from *harm*—which can be defined as any adverse outcome caused by and/or allowed to occur in the course of helping patients to achieve their best possible outcome. Some types of harm, such as medication errors, are closely associated with direct patient care. Other types of harm, such as falls and pressure ulcers, are more likely to be associated with being in a healthcare setting. Still other types are not closely associated with patient care at all but are classified as patient safety events only because the harm happened to a patient—one such example might be assault by a physician. Exhibit 10.1 shows the many types of possible patient harm.

EXHIBIT 10.1
Categories of Patient Harm

Direct Patient Care	Related to Patient Care	Patient Security
Procedure on wrong patient	Infections	Discharge to wrong person
Procedure on wrong site	Falls	Elopement
Wrong procedure on patient	Pressure ulcers	Suicide or attempt
Preventable procedural complications	Restraint entanglement	Discharge to wrong care setting
Medication errors	Burns	Abduction
Hemolytic reactions	Wrong or toxic gases	Sexual assault
Hypoglycemia	Contaminated drugs	Physical assault
Delay in diagnosis or treatment	Contaminated devices	

In its landmark report *To Err Is Human*, published in 2000, the Institute of Medicine (IOM) stated that the number of patient deaths caused by human error ranged between two earlier estimates of 44,000 and 98,000 per year (Kohn, Corrigan, and Donaldson 2000)—meaning that a patient death may be caused by errors in care as often as once every 5 minutes, 22 seconds. More recent estimates of patient harm have placed the number of deaths even higher. A team led by John James (2013), using triggers to systematically scan electronic health records, places the number of patient deaths in the range of 210,000 to 440,000 per year—potentially one patient death every 50 seconds. A more recent estimate places medical error as the third leading cause of death in the Unites States (after heart disease and cancer), with 251,000 deaths per year (Makary and Daniel 2016)—or one patient death every 2 minutes, 6 seconds. The risk of dying from an error in care is much higher than many other well-known risks. For example, the probability of dying in a scheduled airline flight is 10^{-6} per departure, and the probability of dying in a nuclear power plant accident is 10^{-8} per year. By contrast, the probability of dying as a patient in a hospital setting because of an error in care is one in 1,000 admissions, or 10^{-3} per year.

The safety of caregivers and providers is also a concern, given the substantial number of injuries that occur in the healthcare workplace. According to the Bureau of Labor Statistics (2017), the total case injury rate for hospitals in 2016 was 5.9 incidents per 200,000 hours worked—meaning that nearly 6 of every 100 people working in hospitals are injured in a given year. This injury rate is significantly higher than that of many other high-risk industries. Workforce safety has had a major negative impact on the quality of healthcare and has resulted in high costs for worker compensation claims. One tenet of safety culture in healthcare is that workforce safety and patient safety must be led and managed as one and the same.

Safety science is a modern name for all the aspects of safety management systems that work to ensure that care is provided without harm to patients or to the workforce, caregivers, and providers. Despite the alarming statistics about healthcare-related injuries and deaths, currently no comprehensive resource is available for implementing safety management systems in healthcare. Based on lessons learned in aviation (Stolzer, Halford, and Goglia 2011) and nuclear power (Institute of Nuclear Power Operations 2013), a complete safety management system for healthcare would include the following elements:

1. *Policy*—to communicate the importance of safety, to maintain a goal of zero harm and zero defects, and to establish a just culture that emphasizes transparency and learning without affixing blame
2. *Safety culture*—to teach safety skills to leaders, caregivers, and providers
3. *Safety promotion*—to identify critical safety practices, to disseminate lessons learned, and to inform healthcare providers about safety policy in the workplace
4. *Learning systems*—to measure patient harm and workforce injury, assess safety practices, and improve safety practices by learning from events that resulted in harm.

Safe systems must be reliable. *Reliability* can be defined as the probability that a sociotechnical system will perform correctly. A sociotechnical system is any complex organization that involves the interaction of people and technology in a workplace (Trist and Bamforth 1951); hence, all healthcare settings are sociotechnical systems. Reliability is not the same as repeatability: A repeatable system merely performs the same way every time, whereas a reliable system performs *correctly* every time. System reliability is typically expressed as a probability:

$$\text{System reliability} = 1 - \text{System error}$$

Reliability is sometimes expressed in terms of the frequency (per unit of time) with which infrequent bad outcomes occur—for instance, one patient fall with serious injury might occur every 30 days, or one patient fall resulting in death might occur every 90 days. Using the system reliability equation, error and reliability can be quickly determined. A perfectly reliable system has zero system error. If the rate of system error increases to 5 percent, then system reliability is reduced to 95 percent. Conversely, if system reliability increases from 95 percent to 99 percent, then system error is reduced from 5 percent to 1 percent.

Because a reliable system performs correctly every time, the question becomes, what is *correct*? For healthcare delivery systems, correct care is care that is safe, effective, and patient centered. Reliable care, therefore, is care that is consistently safe, meaning zero harm to patients; effective, meaning the care is 100 percent appropriate; and patient centered, meaning the care is always compassionate and consistent with patient preferences, needs, and values.

A focus on "safety first" is necessary but insufficient to achieve zero harm. Even with safety as the top priority, variation in the system can still result in system-caused human error that leads to patient harm. To achieve zero harm—to achieve safe, effective, and patient-centered care—requires both safety and system reliability, with the ability to execute consistently over time.

History of the Modern Safety Movement

Safety has always been a key component of patient care. The Hippocratic Oath, written between the fifth and third centuries BCE, requires physicians to provide treatment to the best of their ability and to strive to avoid causing injury or wrongdoing. A line commonly associated with the oath—"First, do no harm"—appeared in the seventeenth century and is derived from the Latin phrase *primum non nocere*. Historically, safety was regarded as a skill acquired by the individual caregiver or provider. Well-trained individuals were considered safe, and poorly trained individuals were deemed unsafe. Today, however, care delivery systems are so complex that safety is beyond the skill set of any one individual. Safety is an emergent property of the complex system that must be ensured using systems of safety.

The modern patient safety movement was reignited with the release of the IOM's aforementioned *To Err Is Human* report. That report included two earlier studies of patient harm—one estimating 44,000 patient deaths every year and the other providing the oft-cited statistic of 98,000 patient deaths (Kohn, Corrigan, and Donaldson 2000). These figures brought the issue of patient harm to the attention of healthcare thought leaders, the media, and the public, making clear that something needed to be done. The cases of several high-profile patients attracted significant scrutiny:

- Betsy Lehman, a 39-year-old *Boston Globe* health reporter who died of a chemotherapy overdose at the Dana-Farber Cancer Institute in 1994
- Willie King, a 52-year-old man who had the wrong foot amputated at University Community Hospital of Tampa in 1995
- Josie King, an 18-month-old girl who died of dehydration and a wrongly administered narcotic at Johns Hopkins in 2001

- Mary McClinton, a 69-year-old retired teacher who died when chlorhexidine, an antiseptic, was used to irrigate her catheterization site at Virginia Mason in 2004

Following the release of the report, institutions had both the will and the ability to drive changes and to provide solutions within healthcare, as well as in other high reliability industries (e.g., aviation, manufacturing, nuclear power). Changes affecting healthcare included the following:

- The Agency for Healthcare Research and Quality (AHRQ) became an important source of research, safety practices, and learning, including findings from the Hospital Survey of Patient Safety (HSOPS).
- The National Patient Safety Foundation (NPSF) became a leader in safety practices, learning, and innovation.
- The National Quality Forum (NQF) became a leader in measurement and learning.
- The Institute for Healthcare Improvement (IHI) became a leader in learning and innovation, as demonstrated by the 100,000 Lives Campaign and the 5 Million Lives Campaign.
- The Institute for Safe Medication Practices (ISMP) became a clearinghouse for safety practices and the measurement of harm resulting from medication errors.
- The Joint Commission developed practices and standards for safety (including the National Patient Safety Goals) and for high reliability through the creation of the Center for Transforming Healthcare.
- Healthcare innovations included the development of safety practices, an increased awareness of the role of human factors, automated processes such as bar-code scanning, smart infusion pumps and automated dispensing units, and electronic health records (EHRs).
- Aviation contributed to an improved safety culture by developing concepts related to cause analysis methods, human factors, and teaming (including crew resource management).
- Manufacturing contributed ideas relating to process management, process improvement, human factors, and automation.
- The nuclear power industry made contributions in safety culture, cause analysis methods, leadership skills for safety, and nontechnical skills for safety and high reliability.

Exhibit 10.2 presents a timeline of emerging concepts and thought leaders, as identified by Healthcare Performance Improvement, related to safety science and high reliability. Key concepts in the body of knowledge are shown in larger type, and the corresponding thought leaders (in some cases,

EXHIBIT 10.2 Timeline of Safety Science and High Reliability Organizing

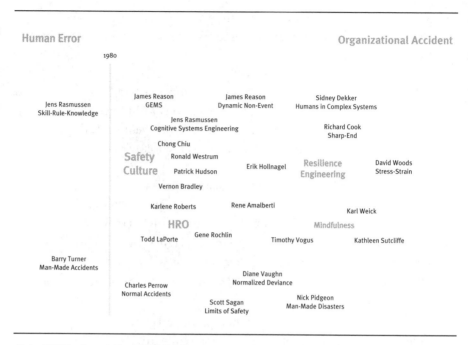

Note: GEMS = Generic Error Modeling System; HRO = high reliability organizing.

Source: Used with permission from Healthcare Performance Improvement.

with key ideas) are shown in regular type. The chronology is from left to right. Before 1980, safety experts were primarily focused on the human error that leads to harm and on ways to prevent such error. Later, however, virtually all safety experts placed the blame on what James Reason called the *organizational accident*. The focus then shifted to ways of preventing these more complex organizational (systemic) issues.

Vernon Bradley of Dupont and Ronald Westrum and Patrick Hudson, who collaborated for the Shell Oil Company, were strong champions of safety culture. Over time, high reliability organizing (HRO) emerged as a field related to safety culture, led by a "Berkeley group" consisting of Karlene Roberts and colleagues and a "Michigan" group headed by Karl Weick and Kathleen Sutcliffe. (The initials *HRO* may refer to the body of knowledge of high reliability organizing or to the high reliability organizations that grow out of that body of knowledge.) The concept of resilience engineering—which seeks to create systems that anticipate problems and adjust performance to meet new demands to prevent adverse events—emerged from both safety culture and HRO, led by Erik Hollnagel.

Today, three robust bodies of knowledge have converged to form state-of-the-art thinking in safety, quality, and reliability, as shown in exhibit 10.3. The top circle is the traditional quality movement, founded on the Donabedian (1988) model in which the definition of quality encompasses safety, effectiveness,

EXHIBIT 10.3
Three Bodies of Knowledge for Improvement

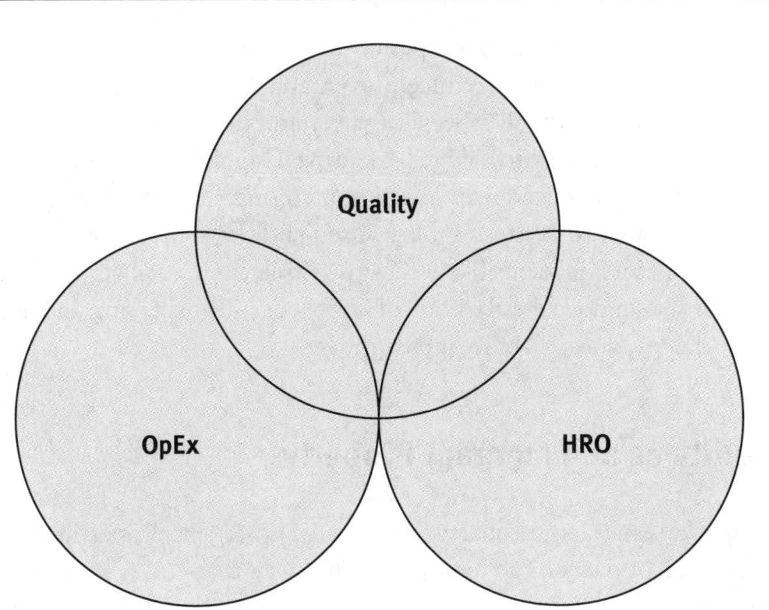

Note: OpEx = Operational Excellence; HRO = high reliability organizing.
Source: Used with permission from Healthcare Performance Improvement. Copyright 2017 Healthcare Performance Improvement.

and patient centeredness. Outcomes are the best measure of quality, and positive outcomes are produced by the best combination of structure and process. The traditional quality movement—shown at the 12 o'clock position—still dominates the structure of modern safety, quality, and reliability.

The second circle, at the 8 o'clock position, reflects the rise of the Lean methodology and Operational Excellence (OpEx). Lean, originally a manufacturing approach, is a collection of daily operating systems and improvement methods derived from the Toyota Production System (TPS). OpEx, closely related to Lean, has come to dominate contemporary thinking about how to improve efficiency and reduce the resources required to achieve desired levels of safety and quality. OpEx was first applied to support systems in healthcare that closely resemble linear processes, such as supply chain and sterile supply, but it has now been applied to all patient care systems, including perioperative and intensive care. Although OpEx efforts are not exclusively intended to improve safety and quality, the reliability improvements they create have made important contributions to all aspects of patient care.

The last of the three bodies of knowledge, shown in exhibit 10.3 at the 4 o'clock position, is high reliability organizing. The concept of HRO originated in high-risk industries, such as aviation and nuclear power, that demanded good safety records. HRO seeks to explain why some complex systems are able to manage their complexity and deliver high reliability, whereas other systems cannot and continue to experience adverse events. At first, HRO in healthcare aimed primarily to reduce preventable harm, though its uses have since expanded to address all aspects of safety and quality.

All three bodies of knowledge have proved highly effective in healthcare. To a large extent, the differences in opinion among the practitioners of each appear to be limited to the terminology used and the sources for attribution. In the coming years, it seems likely that the three circles will converge at the center to form a single, cohesive body of knowledge for managing and improving safety, quality, and reliability in healthcare.

Reliability as an Emergent Property

Reliability is an emergent property of a system. Emergent properties arise out of interactions of parts of a system in such a way that the system produces an effect that cannot be assigned to any single part. Safety is not a part of a complex system; rather, it arises out of the interactions of parts of the system. Reliability, too, is not a part of the system; it cannot be purchased or installed as a system improvement. It arises out of the numerous interactions of the parts. One healthcare leader said, "We do the big things well—we just have trouble with the little things." Safety and reliability depend on many "little things" being done consistently well.

Reliability emerges from the right mix of behavior-shaping factors. The Sharp-End Model, first described by James Reason (1997) and later illustrated by Richard Cook and David Woods (Cook 2002), provides further explanation. According to the model, the "blunt end" of the system includes behavior-shaping factors for caregivers and providers at the "sharp end." Blunt-end factors include

- organizing arrangements that define job functions and task-collaboration mechanisms;
- processes that define tasks and the sequencing of tasks;
- policies and protocols—including checklists—that define work rules;
- human factors in the environment of care and in equipment, devices, and technology; and
- culture that defines the actions and interactions of people—including knowledge, skills, and attitudes (KSA).

In human-based systems such as healthcare, culture is the strongest of these behavior-shaping factors. In such a system, people and culture occupy the largest space and hold all of the other factors together. Put another way, a safe surgery checklist in the operating room is not enough to keep patients safe; people in the operating room, thinking together as a team using a safe surgery checklist, keep patients safe. Bar code scanning in and of itself does not keep patients safe; caregivers scanning medications and thinking about the signals from the bar code scanners keep patients safe. Behind each system of behavior-shaping factors is a person who thinks and cares about safety and quality.

The role of the healthcare safety and quality leader is to know the right mix of behavior-shaping factors in the system for each caregiver or provider in each task. Safety and reliability—and quality for that matter—emerge from the adjustment of behavior-shaping factors over time. Process improvement essentially makes adjustments to behavior-shaping factors. Root cause analysis following a harm event and other learning methods also make adjustments to those factors, albeit after the fact for the patient who was harmed. But what is too late for that one patient might be just in time for future patients.

Overreliance on technology and on standardization of process, protocol, and practice can make a system brittle. A system that is robust yet brittle will rarely experience harm or defects, but when a single defect does occur, it causes severe and widespread harm. For comparison, imagine an oak tree that does not bend in the wind until it suddenly breaks in half. A resilient system, meanwhile, is like a palm tree that bends in the wind but does not break. Resilient systems can bounce back from individual defects to prevent harm. The system resilience equation shows an inverse relationship with brittleness:

$$\text{Resilience} = 1 \;/\; \text{Brittleness}$$

Healthcare systems are best when they combine the robust reliability from automation and standardization with the resilient reliability of people who can think independently and also as part of a team. The best reliability and resilience result from automation as the first line of defense, people and teams in the middle, and automation again as the last line of defense. The effects of people-only systems, automated systems, and combination systems can be summarized as follows:

1. People-only systems—low reliability and resilient
2. Automated systems—high reliability and brittle
3. Combination systems—high reliability and resilient

Resilience engineering—a body of knowledge within safety science and high reliability organizing—identifies sources of system resilience to be retained through thoughtful change management and detection and correction of drift in organizational performance. Resilience engineering also aims to systematically increase the resiliency of systems through thoughtful human factors integration and the use of information systems to predict system changes while there is still time to adjust and "bounce back" (Hollnagel 2013).

Descriptive Theories of High Reliability Organizations

The HRO concept gained prominence through research at the University of California, Berkeley, during the 1980s. Karlene Roberts, along with Todd LaPorte and Gene Rochlin, examined high-risk sociotechnical systems to understand why some complex systems performed with few failures. Examples of such systems included US Navy carrier aviation (the USS Carl Vinson, CVN 70); US nuclear power (the Diablo Canyon Power Plant operated by Pacific Gas and Electric); and commercial aviation (including an air traffic control center). Later research examined wildland firefighting command, healthcare (the Loma Linda Hospital pediatric intensive care unit), and electric power transmission (the California independent system operator). Karl Weick and Kathleen Sutcliffe, along with David Obstfeld, organized the body of knowledge using the principle of collective mindfulness (Weick, Sutcliffe, and Obstfeld 1999).

High reliability organizing was more of a discovery than an invention. The organizations practicing these principles had developed their practices over time, often in response to recurring failures. None of the organizations studied referred to itself as an HRO or used the phrase *high reliability*. All of the organizations based their thinking and messaging on safety, or on both safety and quality. High reliability was found to be a property underpinning systems that could perform in highly complex, fluid, and dangerous conditions, while being safe and successful in achieving the organizational purpose. Today, safety science and high reliability organizing provide several descriptive theories.

Karlene Roberts from Berkeley and Carolyn Libuser from the banking industry identified five characteristics of HROs (Roberts 1990; Roberts and Libuser 1993; Ciavarelli 2008):

1. *The use of process auditing*—to find defects and process problems that lead to defects
2. *Vigilant monitoring for quality degradation*—to detect declines in performance
3. *Reward systems*—to provide recognition aligned with organizational goals
4. *A heightened awareness of risk*—to ensure that latent (hidden) risks are identified and action is taken to reduce risk
5. *Command and control*—for effective leadership and system operation

Subsequent work by Roberts elaborated on the concept of command and control, describing situational awareness by leaders, decision making that includes operational experts, reduced authority gradients that enable leaders and teams to think collaboratively, the value of redundancy in people and safety systems, and standardized work and procedures.

Ronald Westrum and Patrick Hudson were the principal developers of the Shell Oil Company's Hearts and Minds campaign, which facilitated a successful and large-scale safety culture transformation. Westrum (1993) and Hudson (1999) identified five characteristics of successful workforce safety cultures:

1. *Communication* with high frequency and closed loops for vertical information flow and lateral integration
2. *Organizational attitudes* that are based on respect, allowing leaders and staff to work together to fix systemic problems
3. *Health safety environmental (HSE) programs* that are "owned" by staff, with a few safety professionals in advisory roles
4. *Organizational behavior* with safety considered to be as important as production; an emphasis on trust among leaders and staff; and frequent dialogue on the importance of working safely and improving work systems
5. *Working behavior* that allows staff to provide the safe environment in which leaders can share lessons learned

Rene Amalberti, a French professor of medicine, physiology, and human factors in aviation and later healthcare, identified another five characteristics of safety cultures and reliable organizations (Amalberti et al. 2005):

1. *Accepting limits* on discretionary action, such as deference to expertise, adherence to protocol, and complying with safety limits
2. *Abandoning autonomy* by being mindful of others and coordinating with various people, activities, processes, and systems
3. *Transitioning* from the role of "craftsman" to an equivalent actor through the use of standard work based on evidence-based best practices
4. *Sharing risk vertically* in the organization by communicating problems, both past and future, to leaders
5. *Managing the visibility of risk* by using visual management techniques and information systems to predict failure and adjust operations to prevent failure

Karl Weick and Kathleen Sutcliffe (2007) created the best-known descriptive theory of HROs, described in their best-selling book *Managing the Unexpected*. Their five elements of high reliability—the "Weick and Sutcliffe five"—are so well known that most practitioners think they represent the only characteristics of HROs. The list is divided into elements of anticipation and elements of containment—anticipation to keep systems running smoothly and containment to fix problems as soon as the system encounters trouble. Anticipation has three elements:

1. *Preoccupation with failure*. To avoid failure, look for early signs.
2. *Reluctance to simplify interpretations*. Use critical thinking, and look past easy explanations to provide situational awareness.
3. *Sensitivity to operations*. Systems are dynamic and nonlinear, so leaders provide direct oversight to adjust to unpredicted interactions.

Containment has the next two elements:

4. *Commitment to resilience*. The organization maintains function(s) during high demands. Resilience has three components:
   - Absorb demands and preserve functions.
   - Maintain the ability to return to service after untoward events.
   - Learn and grow from untoward events.
5. *Deference to expertise*. Decision making requires people with knowledge and experience, regardless of rank or status.

More recently, Christine Sammer, a nursing leader and researcher with Adventist Health System, organized a large body of literature into seven domains, or subcultures, of safety culture (Sammer et al. 2010):

1. *Leadership*. Safety culture leadership starts with the chief executive officer and permeates the organization.
2. *Teamwork*. A multidisciplinary and multigenerational approach crosses all ranks, layers, and individuals of the organization.
3. *Evidence-based practice*. Best-practice medicine is delivered using best-practice methods such as protocols, checklists, and guidelines.
4. *Communications*. Structured communications and transparency create shared situational awareness and organizational learning.
5. *Learning environment*. Learning is data driven and includes medical staff; lessons are deployed using performance improvement methods.
6. *Just culture*. Accountability is strong in a blame-free environment.
7. *Patient-centered culture*. Care is compassionate, is focused on the patient, and engages the patient and the family.

Across these descriptive theories, the significant overlap in the themes of leadership, thinking as a team, learning, and so forth is reassuring. The difficulty with a descriptive theory is that it merely tells what the organization should look like after the change has been made; it does not reveal how to make the change in practice. Healthcare today is in urgent need of a theory of change that can be used to build HROs for safety and quality.

Why Should We Care?

Healthcare leaders should care about safety and high reliability for three main reasons. First, zero preventable harm is not achievable without safety science and high reliability organizing. Healthcare systems are too complex for safety to be ensured solely by the competency of providers and caregivers; systems of safety are also required. Even then, the system-caused human error by caregivers and providers can still result in harm. Both safety science and high reliability are essential.

Second, high reliability can serve as a chassis, or common framework, for safety, quality, and a satisfactory experience of care. This effect is shown in exhibit 10.4. The top row shows that a safety focus coupled with high reliability increases the likelihood of zero preventable harm. After high reliability

EXHIBIT 10.4
The High Reliability Chassis

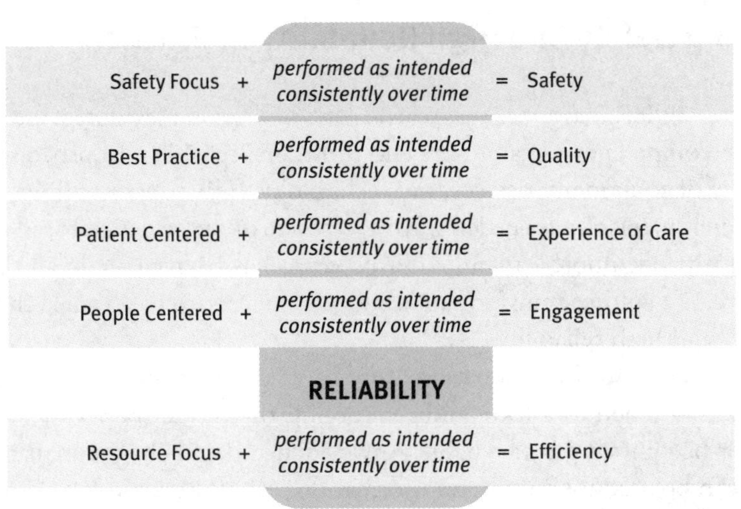
Safety Focus + performed as intended consistently over time = Safety
Best Practice + performed as intended consistently over time = Quality
Patient Centered + performed as intended consistently over time = Experience of Care
People Centered + performed as intended consistently over time = Engagement
RELIABILITY
Resource Focus + performed as intended consistently over time = Efficiency

Source: Used with permission from Healthcare Performance Improvement. Copyright 2009 Healthcare Performance Improvement.

in the sociotechnical system has been developed for safety, that reliability can be used for everything. Best-practice medicine, often in the form of clinical bundles, coupled with high reliability results in improved quality. Patient centeredness coupled with high reliability results in a more compassionate and connected experience of care. The effect is also seen in terms of engagement among staff and medical professionals—in other words, in the relationship between an organization and its members. An employee who is fully engaged takes positive action to advance the organization's mission. Safety is a good producer of engagement, and in return, engagement is a good producer of safety. People centeredness coupled with high reliability leads to engagement. This effect is also seen with efficiency. Resource focus—that is, stewardship of the community's healthcare resources—coupled with high reliability leads to greater efficiency.

The third reason that healthcare leaders should care about safety and high reliability is that a culture of "safety first" and high reliability ends the suboptimization effect that has plagued modern healthcare. When healthcare leaders embark on improvement efforts, they often make the newest goal their most important objective, targeting it with special messaging, attention, and auditing. This focus on the newest goal tends to improve a targeted area somewhat but at the detriment of other aspects of patient care. In other words, the system is compromised by the efforts to achieve the newest goal. However, when high reliability is used as a chassis for safety, quality, experience, engagement, and efficiency, the solution does not sacrifice one aspect of care in the service of another.

Creating Safety and High Reliability in Practice

The theory of HRO assumes that several parts of the complex system are already in place: competency of caregivers and providers; reliability of processes; and reliability of equipment, devices, and technology. If these assumptions are not true, then remediation is needed with at least one of the evidence-based models for performance improvement. After progress has been made in all three of those areas, a culture transformation model is necessary to advance the goals of safety and high reliability.

Culture transformation models are based on establishing a target behavior, usually framed as a tool, and reinforcing that target behavior until the behavior becomes a practice habit. Any evidence-based change management model can be used for culture transformation. All of these models share three fundamental principles:

1. Establish the target behavior as an expectation.
2. Enable people by providing the knowledge and skills necessary for them to perform the behavior.

3. Align reward systems and accountability systems so that the target behavior becomes a practice habit.

Target behaviors are often grouped together in bundles, with one set of tools particularly for healthcare leaders or another set for caregivers and providers. The general approach starts with a focus on characteristics of a safety culture or an HRO—such as preoccupation with failure and sensitivity to operations, as described in the Weick and Sutcliffe model. Next, a leader practice is identified that puts these characteristics into action—for instance, implementing a daily check-in for safety, a form of hospitalwide safety huddle (Stockmeier and Clapper 2011). Such a practice can then be deployed through the change management model.

In this general approach, several of the safety culture and HRO characteristics can be activated as manageable sets of leader tools. These bundles of leader tools are often selected through a systematic study of leader practices within an organization. The steps may occur as follows:

1. Study organizational performance (analysis of safety culture survey, assessment of system capability, and common cause analysis of harm events).
2. Inventory existing leadership tools and practices, and assess each for efficacy.
3. Form a culture design group comprising leaders and other stakeholders.
4. Choose leader tools that are evidence based in that particular healthcare setting, indicated by the study, and compatible with existing leader practices that are evidence based and effectively deployed.
5. Choose methods to educate and train leaders to use the tools.
6. Identify accountability systems to help leaders practice using the tools regularly so that they become habits.

These leader bundles are most effective when the tools are comprehensive and cover the full scope of leader functions described in safety science and HRO theory. Leader bundles for safety and high reliability often encompass messaging on safety, guiding operations through briefings and huddles, reinforcing safe practices through rounding, applying just culture principles through progressive discipline, and leading local learning efforts through huddles and learning boards. The following are three leader behaviors or tools for every leader safety or high reliability bundle:

1. *Start every meeting with a safety moment.* For every meeting that has a prepared agenda, open with a discussion that shapes the culture of

safety and high reliability. Often, these moments are stories about patient harm. Use a simple three-part structure that starts with the purpose of the message, delivers the message in a short and concise manner, and then finishes by restating the purpose of the message for emphasis.

2. *Use rounding to influence (RTI).* RTI is not a rounding program; rather, it is a leader skill that can be used in existing rounding programs. RTI opens a short dialogue with a caregiver or a provider; promotes a behavior that is important to safety or high reliability; reinforces that behavior; and provides a simple action, tailored for that caregiver or provider, to promote better practice of that behavior.
3. *Lead local learning systems.* Local learning systems improve performance at the unit or team level. Process improvement is often done for large, shared processes during monthly meetings, but local learning can be done by unit or team leaders every day. In theory, learning every day is 30 times faster than learning once a month, and small incremental improvement is often easier than large-scale change (as the old saying goes, "improvement by the inch is a cinch—improvement by the yard is hard"). Local learning systems most often use displays of unit or team performance metrics and a learning board that captures errors or defects. The learning boards also identify actions to correct the local system causes of those errors or defects.

Just culture, which necessitates more than a single leader behavior or tool, is discussed in greater detail later in the chapter.

The same general approach can be used for creating safety and high reliability in practice for caregivers and providers. Start with characteristics of safety culture or HRO, such as reluctance to simplify interpretations and deference to expertise from the Weick and Sutcliffe model. Next, identify a behavior, skill, or tool that, when practiced as a habit, promotes those characteristics—for instance, a questioning attitude coupled with speaking up for safety. That behavior, skill, or tool can then be implemented using the change management model. Much like the leader tools, these universal skills for caregivers and providers are often bundled as safety behaviors or error prevention techniques. These bundles of universal skills are often selected by a systematic study of practices within an organization. The steps may occur as follows:

1. Study harm in the sociotechnical system.
   - Study culture (by survey), system capability, and common causes of harm events (Clapper and Crea 2010).
   - Rule out specific or assignable system causes and knowledge/skill deficiencies as major causes before proceeding.

2. Form a culture design group comprising leaders, caregivers, and providers.
3. Choose universal skills that are evidence based in that specific healthcare setting and are indicated by the study.
4. Choose methods to educate and train all leaders, caregivers, and providers on the universal skills.
5. Strengthen accountability systems so that these skills become practice habits for all. Best practices include
   - deploying evidence-based leadership for safety culture and HROs;
   - deploying caregivers as peer coaches, sometimes called *safety coaches*, and providers as physician champions; and
   - recognizing peer checking and peer coaching as a universal skill.

As is the case with the leader bundles, the universal skill bundles are most effective when they are comprehensive—meaning that the behaviors, skills, and tools cover the full scope of human reliability. Most if not all of the bundles include the following:

1. *Attention.* Self-checking with the stop-think-act-review (STAR) technique is most commonly used. In using STAR, one stops for a moment to focus attention on performing the task. STAR was developed by the Jefferson Center for Character Education to promote thinking skills among schoolchildren, and it has become widely used in the nuclear power and transportation industries for self-checking.
2. *Communication.* Several techniques can be used, given that a variety of communication skills are needed to ensure quality and safety. A simple tool might be the three-way repeat-back to ensure authenticity of communication—in other words, making sure the receiver has correctly heard what the sender said. Other tools may involve phonetic or numeric verification or asking clarifying questions. More complex tools, such as situation-background-assessment-request (SBAR), have also been designed to provide both clarity and context. SBAR was developed by Kaiser Permanente to bridge the gap in communication styles between caregivers and providers.
3. *Critical thinking skills.* Critical thinking can and should be used by both individuals and teams. When used in teams, critical thinking is coupled closely with communication skills. Critical thinking skills, including those articulated in the emerging field of cognitive debiasing, are said to be too numerous to deploy in universal skills bundles. The tool of "a questioning attitude" is most commonly deployed—in many cases, it is the only critical thinking tool in the bundle.

4. *Checklist and protocol use*. The use of policies, protocols, checklists, and other guidance documents is a universal strategy in the fields of aviation and nuclear power, and many have argued that it should be adopted universally in healthcare. The use of checklists and protocols is an expectation more so than a tool, and it is often communicated in two scenarios: (1) as reference use for guidance that is well known, such as established policy, and (2) for continuous use with guidance that is complex or high risk, such as a flow sheet or checklist.
5. *Speaking up for safety*. Speaking up for safety requires both communication skills, for clarity and context, and an environment of psychological safety (i.e., comfort), for caregivers or providers who ask questions in the face of a higher authority. United Airlines developed the mechanism known as CUS—for *concerned*, *uncomfortable*, and *stop*—which has since been distributed by the Agency for Healthcare Research and Quality (AHRQ) through the Team Strategies and Tools to Enhance Performance and Patient Safety (TeamSTEPPS). CUS aims to address safety concerns that employees might otherwise be reluctant to express. Along the same lines, Healthcare Performance Improvement developed ARCC, which stands for *ask* a question, *request* a change, voice a *concern*, and *chains* of command.

Every healthcare safety and quality leader faces—and might even be intimidated by—the same question: Where should I start in my efforts to create a culture of safety and high reliability? An organization's starting point is determined by the weaknesses of its system. Because healthcare delivery is not a single sociotechnical system but rather a collection of microsystems, a healthcare leader could conceivably have several starting points—one for each specific microsystem. Three starting points are shown in exhibit 10.5. They correspond with three phases or waves of system reliability improvement that were observed in aviation safety (Hudson 2007) and in nuclear power safety and are now being observed in healthcare safety and quality. (For further reading on this topic, see Ghaferi et al. 2016.)

The first phase or wave provides system reliability through process reliability and technology solutions, which correspond with the underlying assumptions of the descriptive theory for HRO (as noted earlier in the chapter). The second phase focuses on standardization of training and practices. The third phase provides error trapping through use of universal skills for critical thinking and thinking as a team. The third phase also includes error trapping by human factors integration. The human factors discipline of thinking deals with work systems in which people perform well and experience few human errors; human factors integration involves providing good factors on a large scale. When systems are developed using human factors integration, reliability

EXHIBIT 10.5
Three Waves of Reliability Improvement

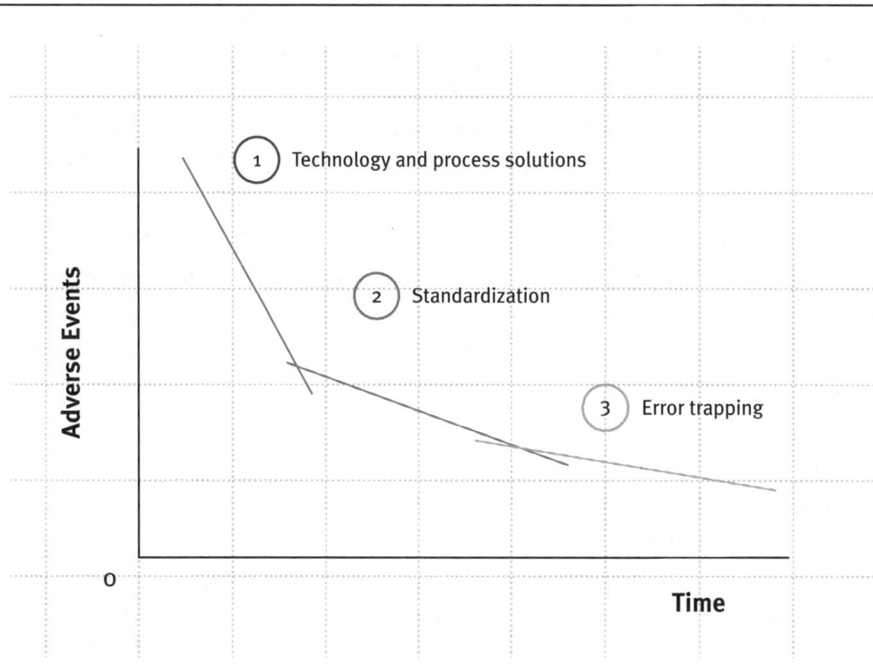

Source: Used with permission from Healthcare Performance Improvement. Copyright 2017 Healthcare Performance Improvement.

is high because the human errors are few in number and those few errors are trapped (i.e., identified and corrected before a loss event occurs). For each microsystem, leaders should identify the starting point and use the principles of safety science and HRO to push to the next level of reliability.

Important Topics in Safety and High Reliability

Because a just culture is so important to safety and high reliability, its principles should not be relegated to a single leader practice or tool in a leader bundle. James Reason (1997) first described just culture as critical to systems of safety, stressing the importance of maintaining strong accountability for safe practices while at the same time not punishing people who inadvertently cause human error. The concept of just culture was further developed by David Marx, who founded the Just Culture Community, and Sidney Dekker, who wrote a book titled *Just Culture*.

Safe systems—high reliability systems—need both strong accountability and a recognition of errors that does not punish the individuals deemed responsible for causing those errors. If accountability is not strong, then safe practices will not be implemented, and unsafe choices can and will be made.

However, if those individuals who are involved in system-caused human error are punished, those errors will go unreported and will not be discussed or corrected—and the systemic causes of those errors are likely to cause harm again.

Too often, just culture is reduced to an algorithm through which leaders try to distinguish "innocent" human error from negligent acts, where reasonable thought or attention were not applied, and from reckless acts, in which a conscious choice was made with knowledge that harm was likely to result. The algorithm may be the single largest piece of a just culture, but the algorithm is certainly not the *definition* of a just culture. Just culture is a subset of safety culture, deserving of its own safety management system. The safety management system for just culture includes the following:

1. Policy statements for just culture, including a safety-conscious work environment (i.e., an environment in which people can put forth safety concerns without fear) and mutual respect
2. A safety culture that protects those who have the courage to speak up for safety and in which caregivers and providers practice the universal skills of cross-checking
3. Safety promotion, whereby ideas and policies regarding just culture, safety culture, and HRO are continuously communicated to caregivers and providers
4. Learning systems in which the facts of each case are subjected to an algorithm in a well-defined process, such as progressive discipline for caregivers and peer review for individual credentialed providers; these learning systems should also look for causes of human error using a nonpunitive human factors approach

The algorithm component of just culture is most effective when included in a leader bundle for daily use, built directly into human resources processes for discipline, and built into peer-review processes. Healthcare safety and quality leaders have four algorithms from which to choose:

1. James Reason's (1997) Decision Tree for Determining the Culpability of Unsafe Acts, as well as derivative works such as the United Kingdom National Health Service's Incident Decision Tree (Meadows, Baker, and Butler 2005)
2. Patrick Hudson's (2004) refined Just Culture Model, from the Shell Oil Company's Hearts and Minds Project
3. David Marx's Just Culture Algorithm from Outcome Engenuity (2018)
4. Any of the several algorithms developed by healthcare delivery systems—in other words, "home-brew" algorithms

Although the concept has not been rigorously studied, the effectiveness of just culture appears to be more a function of the deployment of its safety management system—the policies, safety culture, promotion, and learning systems—than of the specific algorithm used. In this respect, the choice of an algorithm by an individual safety leader might be analogous to the choice of golf club by a golfer: The results depend more on how the golfer swings the club than on the design of the club selected.

Learning systems are equally important to safety and high reliability. They should include process improvement, performed by specialists, as well as local learning systems, which can be developed and implemented by teams of leaders, caregivers, and providers. Systems should incorporate lessons learned from both successes and failures, and they should consider learning opportunities that arise from both within and outside the organization:

1. *External success.* Learning systems geared toward external success study best practices and are often framed as benchmarking. Benchmarking can be accomplished by studying methods or outcomes.
2. *External failure.* These learning systems study failures in other organizations and are sometimes called *lessons-learned* or *operating experience programs.* The Joint Commission's sentinel event alert program is a good example of this type of learning. Many patient safety organizations (PSOs) offer this type of learning to regional or specialized learning communities.
3. *Internal failure.* These learning systems study failures within the organization and often use a type of cause analysis. Serious harm events are studied using root cause analysis. Significant near-miss events should also be studied with root cause analyses. Other events may be studied using apparent cause (or proximate cause) analysis. For example, a medication error resulting in patient death would be studied using root cause analysis, whereas a medication error with no harm and a small potential for harm would be studied using apparent cause analysis. All of the causal factors should be aggregated for study in a common cause analysis.
4. *Internal success.* These learning systems study success within the organization and tend to be underused in healthcare. Oddly, healthcare systems focus more on the study of failure, seeking to avoid repetition of a failure, than on the study of success and efforts to replicate that success. Recall that the goal of resilience engineering is to have as many things as possible go "right" (correctly), whereas the goal of traditional safety culture has been to have as few things as possible go wrong.

An important subculture in every learning system is the culture of problem reporting. Learning cannot occur unless opportunities from which to learn are reported. A just culture promotes a safe environment for reporters who might otherwise hesitate out of concerns about the consequences (either to themselves or their team) of reporting. The best practice for improving problem reporting is a three-pronged approach:

1. Promote a just culture so that reporters are not punished for human error and reporters are protected by leaders when they speak up.
2. Make improvements in reporting technology, so the timing of data entry for a report is not a burden for the reporter.
3. Make improvements in learning systems, so reporters see the benefits of their efforts in problem reporting.

The science of human factors is an engineering discipline that places people into sociotechnical systems to minimize human error and maximize efficiency. Human factors engineering is used to improve patient safety—specifically to reduce the frequency of harm events. Human factors engineering is also applied as part of HRO to improve safety (by reducing harm), quality (by improving outcomes), and the patient experience (by improving quality as perceived by the patient and family).

Educating leaders and quality/safety specialists about the principles of human factors provides for more effective improvement plans, both for proactive improvement and for cause analysis of harm events. The goals of education programs are to provide analysts with the ability to recognize problems with existing human factors; to correct those problems with reliable solutions; and to anticipate problems relating to human factors when making changes to systems, processes, protocols, and the use of devices.

Usability evaluation is a structured method for assessing new medical devices or new supplies, and it helps mitigate patient harm that could potentially result from poorly designed items. Participants learn the process and then perform a usability evaluation for either a device or a supply item. In this teach-and-do approach, a device is evaluated for use, and participants learn to perform evaluations for future devices. Even when the device has already been procured, it can still be evaluated to establish specific training requirements for safe and effective use. Another valuable tool is heuristic evaluation, which can be performed by human factors experts to confirm the consistent application of best practices.

Human factors integration solves human factors–related problems for an entire microsystem—a clinical protocol, a care team, an environment of care, and the medical devices used within the protocol. The science of human factors is about relationships among people and the sociotechnical system, the environment of care, the medical devices, the other caregivers, and so on.

Every healthcare delivery system has had some involvement with human factors—for instance, selecting a new endomechanical device or infusion pump. However, this example illustrates only one relationship—the relationship of a user to a device. Sociotechnical systems have many relationships. The provider has relationships to the care team, and the care team has relationships to the protocol. The provider also has relationships to the protocol, and the provider and caregivers both have relationships to the devices. Virtually all of the human factors integration work done today is performed by designers in the development of a medical device or a care setting—which is often too late for the users. Healthcare safety and quality leaders should also do human factors integration work for existing microsystems.

The process for human factors integration is simple:

1. Select a clinical protocol and an environment of care—for example, a protocol for postpartum hemorrhage during labor and delivery.
2. Apply human factors principles to the protocol, and ensure that the protocol is consistent with leading practices.
3. Train all the providers on the use of the new protocol in natural care teams (i.e., the team that normally works together performing the task) using in situ simulation.
4. Make improvements with each cycle of simulation, including practice habits, protocols, devices, and environment of care.

A summary of human factors methods, with illustrative examples, is provided in exhibit 10.6.

EXHIBIT 10.6
Summary of Human Factors Methods

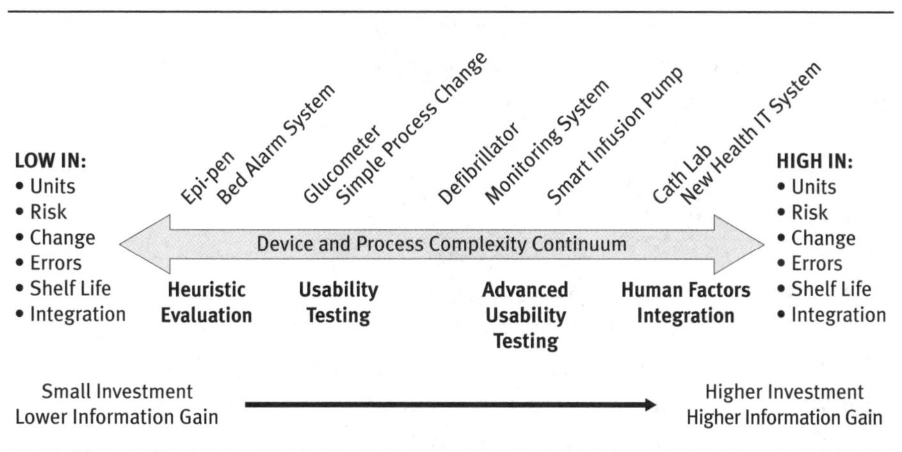

Source: Used with permission from Healthcare Performance Improvement. Copyright 2015 Healthcare Performance Improvement.

Sustaining Cultures of Safety and High Reliability

Admiral Hyman G. Rickover (1982), known as the "Father of the Nuclear Navy," once observed:

> Good ideas are not adopted automatically. They must be driven into practice with courageous impatience. Once implemented they can be easily overturned or subverted through apathy or lack of follow-up, so a continuous effort is required.

Creating cultures of safety and high reliability is difficult, but sustaining those cultures can be even more challenging. Healthcare appears to be particularly challenged by changes in executive leadership, with the attendant changing priorities; stresses of mergers, acquisitions, and reduced payments; and the competing priorities of improving quality, the patient experience, or efficiency.

The best way to sustain a culture of safety and high reliability is to advance that culture inch by inch and step by step. First, use the culture of safety to reduce serious preventable harm to patients. A logical next step, a small one, would be to use that very same culture of safety to reduce workforce injury. A next, larger step would be to use the culture of safety and high reliability to simultaneously reduce harm and improve quality to achieve both zero preventable harm and 100 percent appropriate care. Achieving best practice today requires applying the culture of safety and high reliability to the entirety of the patient experience—safety, quality, and the perception of quality (i.e., the way patients and family experience care). Soon, this same culture of safety and high reliability will become a single operating system for all of healthcare delivery—safety, quality, experience of care, engagement of caregivers and providers, and efficiency. In this model—in which all cultures are equally important—no other competing cultures or priorities exist, so the likelihood of sustainment is greatest.

Study Questions

1. Describe the characteristics of a high reliability organization. How do the characteristics of your own organization compare?
2. Describe your commitment to patient safety and workforce safety. Where do you stand currently on your journey to high reliability, and what do you need to do to move forward?
3. Explain the concept of competing commitments, and give examples of competing commitments in your organization.

4. Explain how high reliability organizing provides a common framework for meeting competing commitments.
5. Explain how leader tools can be used to create a culture of safety and high reliability. Which of the leader tools discussed in this chapter would be best for your organization?
6. Explain how universal skills can be used to create a culture of safety and high reliability. Which of the suggested universal skills would be best for your organization?
7. Describe the importance of just culture in a culture of safety and high reliability. Which elements of just culture—beyond a culpability algorithm—does your organization need?
8. Describe the challenges of sustaining a culture of safety and high reliability. Which of the available paths to advancement would be best for your organization?

References

Amalberti, R., Y. Auroy, D. Berwick, and P. Barach. 2005. "Five System Barriers to Achieving Ultrasafe Health Care." *Annals of Internal Medicine* 142 (9): 756–64.

Bureau of Labor Statistics. 2017. "Employer-Reported Workplace Injuries and Illnesses (Annual)." Modified November 9. www.bls.gov/web/osh.supp.toc.htm.

Ciavarelli, A. 2008. "Culture Counts." *Aerosafety World* 3 (2): 18–23.

Clapper, C., and K. Crea. 2010. "Common Cause Analysis." *Patient Safety & Quality Healthcare* 7: 30–35.

Cook, R. I. 2002. "How Complex Systems Fail." Cognitive Technologies Laboratory. Revised April 21. www.researchgate.net/publication/228797158_How_complex_systems_fail.

Donabedian, A. 1988. "The Quality of Care: How Can It Be Assessed?" *JAMA* 260 (12): 1743–48.

Ghaferi, A. G., C. G. Myers, K. M. Sutcliffe, and P. Pronovost. 2016. "The Next Wave of Hospital Innovation to Make Patients Safer." *Harvard Business Review*. Published August 8. https://hbr.org/2016/08/the-next-wave-of-hospital-innovation-to-make-patients-safer.

Hollnagel, E. 2013. "A Tale of Two Safeties." *Nuclear Safety and Simulation* 4 (1): 1–9.

Hudson, P. 2007. "Implementing a Safety Culture in a Major Multi-National." *Safety Science* 45 (6): 697–722.

———. 2004. "Refined Just Culture Model." Paper for Shell International Hearts and Minds project.

———. 1999. "Safety Culture—Theory and Practice." Paper presented at the Research and Technology Organization Human Factors and Medicine Panel Workshop, Siena, Italy, December 1–2.

Institute of Nuclear Power Operations (INPO). 2013. "INPO 12-012: Traits of a Healthy Nuclear Safety Culture." Published December. www.nrc.gov/docs/ML1303/ML13031A707.pdf.

James, J. T. 2013. "A New Evidence-Based Estimate of Patient Harms Associated with Hospital Care." *Journal of Patient Safety* 9 (3): 122–28.

Kohn, L. T., J. M. Corrigan, and M. S. Donaldson (eds.). 2000. *To Err Is Human: Building a Safer Health System.* Washington, DC: National Academies Press.

Makary, M. A., and M. Daniel. 2016. "Medical Error: The Third Leading Cause of Death in the US." *BMJ.* Published May 3. www.bmj.com/content/353/bmj.i2139.full.

Meadows, S., K. Baker, and J. Butler. 2005. "The Incident Decision Tree: Guidelines for Action Following Patient Safety Incidents." In *Advances in Patient Safety: Vol. 4*, edited by K. Henriksen, J. B. Battles, E. S. Marks, and D. I. Lewin, 387–99. Rockville, MD: Agency for Healthcare Research and Quality.

Outcome Engenuity. 2018. "The Just Culture Algorithm." Accessed November 1. www.outcome-eng.com/the-just-culture-algorithm/.

Reason, J. 1997. *Managing the Risks of Organizational Accidents.* Aldershot, UK: Ashgate.

Rickover, H. G. 1982. "Doing a Job." Speech at Columbia University, New York City. Accessed November 1. https://govleaders.org/rickover.htm.

Roberts, K. H. 1990. "Some Characteristics of High-Reliability Organizations." *Organization Science* 1 (2): 160–77.

Roberts, K. H., and C. Libuser. 1993. "From Bhopal to Banking: Organizational Design Can Mitigate Risk." *Organizational Dynamics* 21 (4): 15–26.

Sammer, C. E., K. Lykens, K. P. Singh, D. A. Mains, and N. A. Lackan. 2010. "What Is Patient Safety Culture? A Review of the Literature." *Journal of Nursing Scholarship* 42 (2): 156–65.

Stockmeier, C., and C. Clapper. 2011. "Daily Check-in for Safety: From Best Practice to Common Practice." *Patient Safety & Quality Healthcare* 8: 30–36.

Stolzer, A. J., C. D. Halford, and J. J. Goglia. 2011. *Implementing Safety Management Systems in Aviation.* Aldershot, UK: Ashgate.

Trist, E. L., and K. W. Bamforth. 1951. "Some Social and Psychological Consequences of the Longwall Method of Coal-Getting." *Human Relations* 4 (1): 3–38.

Weick, K. E., and K. M. Sutcliffe. 2007. *Managing the Unexpected: Resilient Performance in an Age of Uncertainty*, 2nd ed. San Francisco: Jossey-Bass.

Weick, K. E., K. M. Sutcliffe, and D. Obstfeld. 1999. "Organizing for High Reliability: Processes of Collective Mindfulness." *Research in Organizational Behavior* 21: 81–123.

Westrum, R. 1993. "Cultures with Requisite Imagination." In *Verification and Validation of Complex Systems: Human Factors Issues*, edited by J. A. Wise, V. D. Hopkin, and P. Stager, 401–16. Berlin, Germany: Springer-Verlag.

CHAPTER

11

EDUCATION FOR HEALTHCARE QUALITY AND SAFETY

David Mayer and Anne J. Gunderson

The ultimate purpose of a curriculum in medical education is to address a problem that affects the health of the public.

—David E. Kern, Patricia A. Thomas, Donna M. Howard, and Eric B. Bass (1998, 9)

Introduction

Without question, lapses in quality and safety of patient care are major problems that affect public health, not only in the United States but also around the world. Furthermore, growing research and data show that patients and families are not the only casualties of the problems with our current system. Caregivers—our friends and colleagues who come to work each day trying to help and heal—also feel the effects. Depression, a loss of empathy, career burnout, and suicide are far too prevalent in today's healthcare workforce. In the interest of patients, families, and caregivers, we need to acknowledge that our broken healthcare system needs a major overhaul.

Following the release of the Institute of Medicine's (IOM's) landmark *To Err Is Human* report (Kohn, Corrigan, and Donaldson 2000), the modification of health science education became the focus of much discussion in both the public and private sectors. Systematic safety and quality education for healthcare professionals was lacking, and the available literature provided no insight into how improvements could be accomplished. In addition, interprofessional team training—a necessary component of high-quality, safe care—was just beginning to attract attention. Dr. Jordan Cohen (1999), then president of the Association of American Medical Colleges, stated that there needed to be a "collaborative effort to ensure that the next generation of physicians is adequately prepared to recognize the sources of error in medical practice, to acknowledge their own vulnerability to error, and to engage fully in the process of continuous quality improvement."

A single chapter cannot possibly provide comprehensive coverage of the history and present state of clinical quality and patient safety education in the health sciences; indeed, it would take an entire book. Even as we write this chapter, a growing number of quality and safety curricular programs are being implemented for all disciplines and levels of experience across the healthcare landscape. Therefore, to contain the scope of this chapter, we have decided to focus on the central premise of *educate the young*. We will examine curricular activities that have targeted the next generation of healthcare leaders and caregivers, with the belief that the most effective way to truly change our culture to one of high-quality, safe care is to equip future professionals with the necessary knowledge, skills, and attitudes that past generations never were afforded.

We all know healthcare is a high-risk industry. Although we have made tremendous advances in the treatment of cancer, heart disease, and diabetes, just to name a few, too many patients are still not receiving high-quality care, and too many continue to die from preventable medical harm. To address its failures, healthcare has turned to other high-risk industries—such as aviation, nuclear energy, and military defense—for tools, techniques, behaviors, and educational models that have proved effective in reducing risk. Aviation, for instance, is the safest it has been since the invention of the jet engine, in part because of checklists, debriefs, team-based simulations, and new models of leadership that have been validated through resilience science.

In seeking to learn from these high-risk industries, healthcare leaders with the IOM met with aviation safety experts David Musson and Robert Helmreich, who placed a similar emphasis on educating the young to address the current state of healthcare. The key takeaway of the interaction was that, if healthcare is to truly change its culture to one of safety and optimal quality outcomes, education and experiential application should be introduced early in healthcare training—specifically, at the medical student level, which is generally the period of acculturation into the profession. Medical schools, therefore, must invest in curriculum development to address these safety issues at the earliest stages.

Despite all the discussion that followed the release of *To Err Is Human* and subsequent reports, action to drive educational change was still slow at best. As recently as 2014, medical journals routinely lamented our nation's lack of research investment in medical education, which stood in stark contrast to the large financial commitment to biomedical research provided by the pharmaceutical industry, philanthropic organizations, and the public. Even today, a formal, systematic clinical quality and patient safety curriculum at the health science student or graduate physician level still is lacking.

To begin to meet this requirement, education and training in quality and safety have to become part of the core foundation for every academic healthcare institution. Reforming medical education presents major challenges to educators, given that the shortcomings that need to be addressed are deeply entrenched in the tradition and culture of our institutions and organizations. Indeed, many of the traditions and curricular maps that need to be addressed have been in place for 100 years. Medical educators—many of whom themselves lack the quality and safety knowledge, skills, and attitudes needed for successful programs—have struggled to align existing learning competencies with newer quality care and patient safety competencies. Instead of continuing to teach to the content of national examinations, academic institutions will need to focus on developing effective curricula that meet the needs of today's healthcare systems, address our current problems, and, most importantly, provide the highest-quality, safest care possible to patients.

The training of young learners requires knowledge, skills, and competency in critical disciplines not traditionally taught in health science education. Quality and safety curricula require a qualitative culture shift in the way that learners, even educational experts, think about healthcare education. Healthcare education, as it currently exists, is still primarily focused on an individual's performance and the assessment of that performance. Not much attention is paid to the systems needed to link those functions into a coherent, integrated, and safe system. In addition, recognition of the system as a source of error is generally not part of the training of resident physicians and health science students. Instead, young learners are trained to individually meet their patients' immediate needs while working around recurrent system problems, ambiguities, and inefficiencies.

Much of the curricular reform applicable to quality and safety education involves what have been termed the *soft sciences* of medicine. Quality scientist David Eddy has estimated that about 19 percent of what is practiced in medicine is based on science and that the rest is based on soft science (Carnett 2002). The soft sciences of medical practice can include such areas as communication, leadership, teamwork, collaboration, personal clinical experience, and patient relationships, among other skills. Loeb (2004, 6) observes that "not all decision making in medicine is grounded in scientific fact and clinical evidence" and that "opinion plays a significant role."

Continuous improvement requires systematic problem solving, applications of systems engineering techniques, operational models that encourage and reward sustained quality and improved patient outcomes, transparency on cost and outcomes, and strong leadership with a vision devoted to improving processes. Future healthcare professionals have a tremendous need to develop expertise in healthcare quality and patient safety. These disciplines have emerged only relatively recently as central components of safe, patient-focused care, and they require knowledge and skills that have long been lacking in standard health sciences curricula.

Early Curricular Work in Clinical Quality and Patient Safety

The IOM report generated heightened interest in clinical quality and patient safety education, and great work in both quality and safety continued in such organizations as the Institute for Healthcare Improvement (IHI) and the

International Society for Quality in Health Care (ISQUA). Initially, health science student and graduate physician curricular change began to take root with more of a focus on the patient safety and risk reduction side. Between 2005 and 2008, however, things began to change, with a number of quality and safety educational activities implemented at both the health science student and resident physician levels.

A study by Wong and colleagues (2010) systematically reviewed published quality improvement (QI) and patient safety (PS) curricula for medical students and residents, and it identified 41 QI- or PS-focused curricula that specifically targeted medical students or residents between 2000 to 2009. Concepts of continuous quality improvement, systems thinking, and root cause analysis were among the most common topics covered. Specific projects often involved chart audits.

At this time, the work of three distinct task forces was particularly noteworthy. As detailed in the sections ahead, each group released a sentinel paper that provided recommendations for a curricular road map on the content domains, teaching methodologies, and curricular assessment and evaluation tools needed for health science and graduate resident training in quality and safety.

The Telluride Experience

In 2004, medical educators from the University of Illinois at Chicago began organizing what would become an annual invitational roundtable, with the goal of designing a patient safety and quality care curriculum for undergraduate medical education. Expert stakeholders from the fields of nursing, pharmacy, medicine, public health, law, healthcare administration, and patient and family advocacy were invited to discussions in Telluride, Colorado. The gathering also included students and residents. Content experts included representatives from medical education, curriculum innovation, quality care improvement, simulation science, and informatics.

The article "Designing a Patient Safety Undergraduate Medical Curriculum: The Telluride Interdisciplinary Roundtable Experience" by Mayer and colleagues (2009) describes the interactive deliberative inquiry and consensus building that occurred over the Telluride roundtables of 2005 and 2006. The key educational themes identified by the expert panel included students and faculty seeing healthcare through a different lens; the need for interprofessional team training; implementation of a longitudinal educational approach to quality and safety, as opposed to "one-off" courses that lack continuity; and a focus on case-based learning, using real patient stories and narratives. Roundtable members came to consensus on the following curricular domains for safety and quality education (Mayer et al. 2009):

1. The history of the safety and quality movement
2. Healthcare microsystems
3. Teamwork
4. Interprofessional communication
5. Time and stress management
6. Informatics
7. The electronic health record and its use for quality improvement and risk reduction
8. Disclosure
9. Root cause analyses
10. Human factors
11. Medication errors and reconciliation

Teaching methodologies identified by the group included plenaries, small-group learning sessions, experiential learning, simulation, standardized patient role plays, case-based learning, individual and team-based learning, and supportive audiovisual material. Recommended assessment strategies included the use of multiple-choice questions for patient safety knowledge, team-based assessment of interprofessional students as they work through clinical scenarios, standardized patient assessment of full disclosure skills, and evaluation of quality improvement projects undertaken in the third year of medical school (Mayer et al. 2009).

The World Health Organization Curriculum Guide

Around the same time as the Telluride roundtable meetings, another group was beginning to meet on the other side of the world to address similar curriculum issues. Under the leadership of Merilyn Walton and Bruce Barraclough, a team from the University of Sydney and Monash University, assisted by an Expert Consensus Working Group with international representation from the six World Health Organization (WHO) regions, collaborated to develop a patient safety curriculum guide. Using deliberative inquiry and discussions similar to those in Telluride, the group identified 11 topics or domains that would be included in the *WHO Patient Safety Curriculum Guide for Medical Schools* (Walton et al. 2010):

1. What is patient safety?
2. What is human factors engineering, and why is it important to patient safety?
3. Understanding systems and the impact of complexity on patient care
4. Being an effective team player

5. Understanding and learning from errors
6. Understanding and managing clinical risk
7. Introduction to quality improvement methods
8. Engaging with patients and carers
9. Minimizing infection through improved infection control
10. Patient safety and invasive procedures
11. Improving medication safety

One of the most valuable components of the WHO curriculum guide is its *Teacher's Guide*—a tool for faculty that had been badly missing in the literature up to that point. The *Teacher's Guide* provides "guidance on the structure of the curriculum, how to implement it, curriculum integration, curriculum development, use of narrative, assessment, evaluation, the hidden culture, available resources and activities to assist student learning" (Walton et al. 2010, 544). The WHO curriculum guide also includes rationale for each of the topics identified, and it follows a standard educational format—with learning objectives, assessment tools, and presentation slides—for each of the patient safety domains.

Lucian Leape Institute

Probably the most notable work related to patient safety and quality care education at the health science and resident physician level came from the Lucian Leape Institute (LLI), in collaboration with the National Patient Safety Foundation (NPSF). The group met in 2008 and again in 2009, with a roundtable format that included leaders in medical education, representatives from national organizations, experts from various quality and safety fields, students, and patients.

Based on in-depth deliberations, discussions, and consensus building, the LLI (2010) published *Unmet Needs: Teaching Physicians to Provide Safe Patient Care*, a report that shares the panel's view on "the current state of medical education, what medical education should ideally become, and what strategies should be used to leverage desired changes in medical education." The report calls for serious educational change:

> Substantive improvements in patient safety will be difficult to achieve without major medical education reform. . . . Medical schools must not only assure that future physicians have the requisite knowledge, skills, behaviors, and attitudes to practice competently, but also are prepared to play active roles in identifying and resolving patient safety problems.

Specifically, the LLI (2010) report provides the following recommendations:

- Recommendation 1. Medical school and teaching hospital leaders should place the highest priority on creating learning cultures that emphasize patient safety, model professionalism, enhance collaborative behavior, encourage transparency, and value the individual learner.
- Recommendation 2. Medical school deans and teaching hospital CEOs should launch a broad effort to emphasize and promote the development and display of interpersonal skills, leadership, teamwork, and collaboration among faculty and staff.
- Recommendation 3. As part of continuing education and ongoing performance improvement, medical school deans and teaching hospital CEOs should provide incentives and make available necessary resources to support the enhancement of faculty capabilities for teaching students how to diagnose patient safety problems, improve patient care processes, and deliver safe care.
- Recommendation 4. The selection process for admission to medical school should place greater emphasis on selecting for attributes that reflect the concepts of professionalism and an orientation to patient safety.
- Recommendation 5. Medical schools should conceptualize and treat patient safety as a science that encompasses knowledge of error causation and mitigation, human factors concepts, safety improvement science, systems theory and analysis, system design and re-design, teaming, and error disclosure and apology.
- Recommendation 6. The medical school experience should emphasize the shaping of desired skills, attitudes and behaviors in medical students that include, but are not limited to, the Institute of Medicine and Accreditation Council for Graduate Medical Education (ACGME)/American Board of Medical Specialties (ABMS) core competencies—such as professionalism, interpersonal skills and communication, provision of patient-centered care, and working in interdisciplinary teams.
- Recommendation 7. Medical schools, teaching hospitals, and residency training programs should ensure a coherent, continuing, and flexible educational experience that spans the four years of undergraduate medical education, residency and fellowship training, and life-long continuing education.
- Recommendation 8. The LCME [Liaison Committee on Medical Education] should modify its accreditation standards to articulate expectations for the creation of learning cultures having the characteristics described in Recommendation 1 above; to establish patient safety education—having the characteristics described herein—as a curricular requirement; and to define specific terminal competencies for graduating medical students.
- Recommendation 9. The ACGME should expand its Common Program Requirements to articulate expectations for the creation of learning cultures having the characteristics described in Recommendation 1; to emphasize the importance of patient safety-related behavioral traits in residency program faculty; and to set forth expected basic faculty patient safety competencies.

- Recommendation 10. The LCME and the ACGME should direct particular attention to the adequacy of the patient safety–related preparation of graduating medical students for entry into residency training.
- Recommendation 11. A survey of medical schools should be developed to evaluate school educational priorities for patient safety, the creation of school and teaching hospital cultures that support patient safety, and school effectiveness in shaping desired student skills, attitudes, and behaviors.
- Recommendation 12. Financial, academic, and other incentives should be utilized to leverage desired changes in medical schools and teaching hospitals that will improve medical education and make it more relevant to the real world of patient care.

With the first recommendation, the roundtable panelists target the current educational culture and suggest changes that will need to be made before any safety and quality curriculum can have any success. Noting that hierarchical systems in healthcare too often tolerate disrespectful or abusive behavior toward students, residents, and others, the report proclaims that "medical school deans and teaching hospital CEOs should declare and enforce a zero tolerance policy for confirmed egregious disrespectful and abusive behaviors." Such behaviors can take many forms—"as subtle as making a student feel foolish for asking a question or as overt as throwing surgical instruments in the operating room" (LLI 2010).

Current Curricular Work in Clinical Quality and Patient Safety

The Accreditation Council for Graduate Medical Education's Clinical Learning Environment Review Program

One of the more exciting and promising current programs focusing on quality and safety education was created by the Accreditation Council for Graduate Medical Education (ACGME), originally known as the Liaison Committee for Graduate Medical Education. Founded in 1981, the ACGME accredits residency and fellowship education programs in the United States. More than 120,000 resident and fellow physicians work in teaching hospitals and medical centers in the United States, and they frequently interact with and provide much of the care for patients (ACGME 2017). Thus, the ACGME seeks to ensure that every resident and fellow physician—the next generation of US physicians—has the knowledge, skills, and attitudes necessary for providing safe, high-quality patient care.

In 2009, the ACGME established a Task Force on Quality Care and Professionalism to raise awareness of the need to educate residents and fellows on patient safety and quality improvement. Soon after, it launched the Clinical Learning Environment Review (CLER) program, with formal site-visit reviews of academic medical centers starting in September 2012. In its original model, the CLER program sought to shift from a focus on resident duty hours to a focus that better encompassed the learning environment within US graduate teaching institutions and ways of delivering higher-quality and safer patient care.

As part of the CLER program, ACGME-accredited institutions would be provided with periodic feedback through scheduled site visits that addressed six specific areas (ACGME 2013):

- *Patient Safety*—including opportunities for residents to report errors, unsafe conditions, and near misses, and to participate in interprofessional teams to promote and enhance safe care.
- *Quality Improvement*—including how sponsoring institutions engage residents in the use of data to improve systems of care, reduce health care disparities, and improve patient outcomes.
- *Transitions in Care*—including how sponsoring institutions demonstrate effective standardization and oversight of transitions of care.
- *Supervision*—including how sponsoring institutions maintain and oversee policies of supervision concordant with ACGME requirements in an environment at both the institutional and program level that ensures the absence of retribution.
- *Duty Hours Oversight, Fatigue Management, and Mitigation*—including how sponsoring institutions: (1) demonstrate effective and meaningful oversight of duty hours across all residency programs institution-wide; (2) design systems and provide settings that facilitate fatigue management and mitigation; and (3) provide effective education of faculty members and residents in sleep, fatigue recognition, and fatigue mitigation.
- *Professionalism*—with regard to how sponsoring institutions educate and monitor professionalism of their residents and faculty members.

During the site visits, CLER representatives meet with individuals who oversee and influence resident physician education, including executive leadership, quality and safety leadership, and graduate medical education leadership. In addition, they conduct interviews with residents and fellows, faculty members, and program directors. Similar to the site visits conducted by The Joint Commission, the CLER site visits incorporate tracer methodologies, in which representatives follow residents or fellows through their daily patient care activities in an attempt to assess the quality and safety learning environment. At the conclusion of each visit, the CLER team shares its observations in each of the six key areas.

In 2017, the ACGME released a newer version of the CLER guidelines, in which the focus area formerly called "Duty Hours, Fatigue Management, and Mitigation" was renamed "Well-Being" and has evolved to address four interrelated topics (ACGME 2017):

1. Work–life balance
2. Fatigue
3. Burnout
4. Support of those at risk of or demonstrating self-harm

Quality and Safety Education for Nurses

The Quality and Safety Education for Nurses (QSEN) project, launched in 2005, has led the transformation of nursing education and practice to improve quality and safety (Cronenwett et al. 2007, 2009; QSEN 2018). With four phases of funding from the Robert Wood Johnson Foundation through 2012, the QSEN Expert Panel identified a collection of knowledge, skills, and attitudes (KSAs)—numbering 162 overall—across the six competency areas outlined by a 2003 IOM think tank: (1) patient-centered care, (2) teamwork and collaboration, (3) evidence-based practice, (4) quality improvement, (5) safety, and (6) informatics (QSEN 2018). The project seeks to build on past improvements in quality and safety and integrate them into nursing education standards and professional practice models for hospitals.

The original two dozen pioneers who launched QSEN established a robust website, led a Pilot Schools Learning Collaborative to provide demonstration models, and established the annual QSEN Forum as an idea-sharing platform. Transformation has been swift and pervasive in many settings, though some gaps remain. The six quality and safety competencies from QSEN are firmly embedded in the essential standards and accreditation criteria of the National League for Nurses and the American Association for Colleges of Nursing, and they are spreading globally across educational and clinical settings.

Based on the fundamental premise that quality and safety are universal values in healthcare, QSEN considers *will*, *ideas*, and *execution* as the building blocks for transforming systems. When nurses in any setting have the *will* through a common value system, are helped to develop *ideas* for leading change, and work with leaders willing to *execute* the change needed, we can work across healthcare disciples to coordinate system change. The IOM competencies apply to all of healthcare, and by working together we can redefine healthcare as a high reliability system focused on safety and quality.

The Institute for Healthcare Improvement Open School

Another contemporary initiative for quality and safety education in healthcare is the IHI Open School, which offers more than 30 online courses, more than 900 Chapters, and a growing array of experiential learning opportunities for students, residents, and health professionals (IHI 2017, 2018b). The Open School's three pillars—online courses, community, and project-based learning—are displayed in exhibit 11.1.

EXHIBIT 11.1
Three Pillars of the Institute for Healthcare Improvement Open School

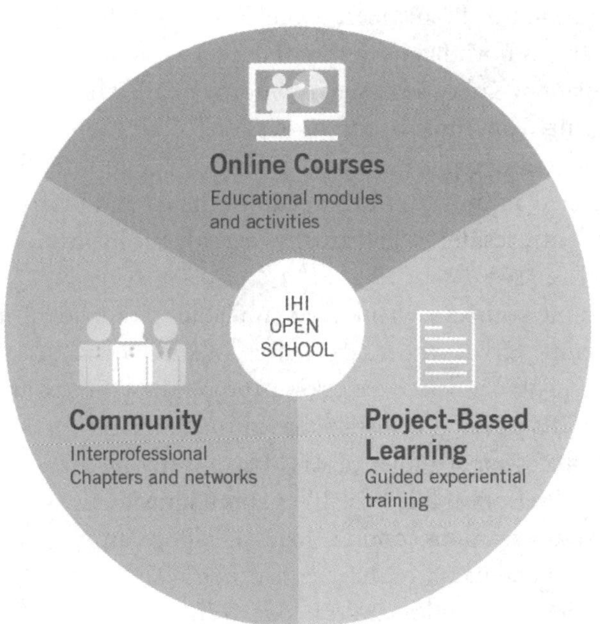

Source: Reproduced with permission from IHI (2018b).

IHI (2018a) has identified eight knowledge domains as essential core content for all students in the health professions:

1. Healthcare as a process and system
2. Variation and measurement
3. Customer/beneficiary knowledge
4. Leading, following, and making changes in healthcare
5. Collaboration (i.e., working effectively in teams)
6. Social context and accountability (including an understanding of the financial impact and costs of care)
7. Developing new, locally useful knowledge
8. Knowledge of one's specific discipline, along with the ability to connect it to the other domains

Examples of Open School courses include "Introduction to Patient Safety," "Introduction to Healthcare Leadership," and "How to Improve with the Model of Improvement." Students and residents access the courses via the IHI website.

The IHI Open School started in 2008, with seed funding from the Rx Foundation, Kaiser Permanente Community Benefit, and the MacArthur Foundation. It was born from a sense of urgency to equip new health professionals with patient safety and quality improvement knowledge, which was generally missing from most health professions' educational curricula, and to support learning and application of that knowledge in interprofessional settings. IHI created an initial set of six online courses and offered them free of charge to students, residents, and faculty in academic institutions throughout the world (IHI 2017).

The online courses remain freely available to individual students, residents, and faculty. However, in 2010, after looking at two years of data, IHI observed that professionals were taking the online courses just as much as students were. To develop a sustainable business model for expanded availability to the professional audience, IHI began offering access to the courses for an annual subscription fee, available to both individuals and organizations. Organizational subscriptions continue to grow in popularity, with health systems recognizing the benefits of the courses for their teams and staff (IHI 2017).

Observers, both inside and outside IHI, point to the Open School's growth as a major success. As of November 2018, IHI (2018b) reported the following figures:

- 740,680 students and residents have registered on IHI's website.
- 601,804 learners have completed an online course.
- 147,298 learners have earned the IHI Open School Basic Certificate in Quality and Safety.
- 924 chapters have been started in 94 countries.

More than 1,000 organizations (academic and professional) around the world use the Open School as part of their training programs. Some use the full course catalog, whereas others choose specific courses to meet their immediate needs. The Open School is also looking to expand its reach beyond English-speaking audiences. Thus far, courses have been translated into Spanish, Portuguese, and French. Carly Strang, the Open School's executive director, says, "The Open School is considering new ways to activate our audience and catalyze action around urgent health challenges, such as campaigns that tackle the opioid crisis, focus on obesity, or improve health equity for all" (IHI 2017).

The Open School is also looking into new ways to teach content beyond asynchronous and semisynchronous online courses. It engages in continuous conversation with the students and professionals it serves, and it experiments to find the best ways to deliver practical, useful content while accommodating exceedingly busy health professional schedules (IHI 2017).

The Academy for Emerging Leaders in Patient Safety: The Telluride Experience

In 2010, the Academy for Emerging Leaders in Patient Safety (AELPS) was officially launched in Telluride, Colorado, as a spin-off of the Telluride Interdisciplinary Roundtables discussed earlier in the chapter. With funding from the Agency for Healthcare Research and Quality, an inaugural class of 20 health science students and resident physicians was selected to attend a weeklong educational immersion in quality and safety (AELPS 2018).

The curriculum for the annual AELPS programs grew out of the interactive deliberative inquiry and consensus building from the roundtables of 2005 and 2006—including the 11 core quality and safety domains listed earlier in the chapter. (For the full curriculum and a list of national expert panelists involved in its development, see Mayer and colleagues 2009.) The deliberative inquiry process was chosen to ensure that the educational content was representative of all health science disciplines and included multiple expert perspectives, including those of patients and families, on the educational experience and learning needed in a comprehensive clinical quality and safety training program.

With continued support from the Doctors Company Foundation, COPIC insurance company, and other organizations, AELPS has expanded significantly since its inception (AELPS 2018). It now offers its weeklong quality and safety educational programs to close to hundreds of future healthcare leaders each year in Telluride; Washington, DC; Napa, California; Doha, Qatar; and Sydney, Australia. More than 1,200 nursing students, medical students, and graduate resident physicians have gone through the program since 2010.

Key educational themes for the AELPS programs include the need for interprofessional team training; a focus on case-based learning, using real patient stories and narratives; and the use of gaming and simulation models. Although instructional methodologies in health science schools and residency programs have somewhat shifted from a teacher-centered pedagogical approach to a more student-centered approach, major gaps still exist in undergraduate and graduate medical education. The AELPS programs aim to address these gaps through the use of small group breakouts, multiple active gaming and simulaton role plays, and reflective practice, and by having faculty members serve more as facilitors than as slide-show lecturers. Through these forms of instruction, students and residents become active constructors of knowledge, as opposed to passive learners.

The AELPS weeklong curriculum includes in-depth training in the following quality and safety domains:

1. Error science
2. Quality improvement tools and techniques

3. Interdisciplinary teamwork and peer–peer communication skills
4. Leadership and professionalism
5. Mindfulness
6. Patient and family partnerships
7. Effective communication skills related to unanticipated patient care outcomes, transparency, disclosure, apology, and early resolution models
8. Informed consent / shared decision making
9. Resilience science
10. System error and human factors engineering
11. Event review (root cause analysis) methodologies
12. Just culture within the framework of personal accountability
13. "Care for the caregiver" programs, caregiver burnout

As a condition of acceptance into the program, all students and residents must commit to completing one clinical quality improvement or patient safety project that will lead to improved quality or reduced medical risk back at their home institution. During the weeklong immersion, participants work with faculty to develop their project. The projects can be as basic as implementing a safety moment (a resilience science tool) into resident morning reviews or starting a quality and safety journal club, or they can be larger, more complicated initiatives to address specific challenges in their work environments. After finishing the weeklong program, AELPS graduates are prepared to lead real change at their home institutions. Alumni provide faculty leaders with updates on their projects and continue networking through the AELPS website and blog, which support participants long after they graduate.

A number of factors make the AELPS experience unique relative to other quality and safety educational programs. Because each program is limited to 25 to 30 young learners, the format allows for a greater focus on student-directed learning through such methods as role playing, trust-building exercises, and small group activities that foster honest discussion and the sharing of personal stories. Significant portions of the program are taught by patients and family members, alongside quality and safety content experts. The patients and family members share their personal experiences with the learners, helping foster discussion about why healthcare professionals need to talk about medical mistakes, admit errors to patients and families, and learn from those errors so that clinical care models can be improved.

Although plenaries and small group breakout discussion sessions are used to deliver aspects of the quality and safety educational content, the three methodologies that form the true learning foundation of the weeklong program are stories and narratives, gaming and simulation, and reflective practice.

The Use of Stories, Narratives, and Reflective Practice

Anyone who has ever sat in a movie theater knows the power of stories and narratives. They can be a call to action while at the same time providing a true foundation for deep-rooted learning. A growing movement in healthcare emphasizes the honoring of stories within the process of delivering care. Stories that connect the heart with the head serve as a reminder to healthcare professionals of why they chose to dedicate their lives to caring for others. Stories and narratives can also serve as vehicles for culture change, introducing difficult topics into conversations and enabling healthcare professionals to learn from a safe distance.

Teaching through real stories can bring out the natural ability of a narrative to deliver an educational message that data, facts, and presentation slides often cannot. Hollywood writers and film producers have known of this capacity for years. To help drive this manner of learning, the AELPS curriculum incorporates two award-winning films—*The Story of Lewis Blackman* and *The Story of Michael Skolnik*—from the series *The Faces of Medical Error: From Tears to Transparency*. When these special stories and narratives are reinforced with interactive group discussion and personal reflection, the transferred knowledge remains, and the underlying facts can be encoded at a deeper level through the emotions that have been triggered.

Stories and narratives can also be effective as a way of breaking down long-held beliefs. Anecdotal evidence suggests that, when healthcare professionals, learners, and patients authentically share stories and personal experiences, the learning through collaboration not only becomes contagious; it can also start breaking down the well-ensconced walls of our traditional medical culture.

Learners in AELPS programs have the opportunity to work closely with patients and families who have personally experienced preventable medical harm. These experiences provide opportunities for learners to discuss real medical errors with people who have lost loved ones from such errors, enabling better understanding of the multiple breakdowns in care that can lead to unintentional but preventable harm. During these emotional learning sessions, student and resident concerns and fears are brought to the forefront, providing for open and honest discussion—and sometimes even resolution. The involvement of patients and family members in the learning process enhances the discussions and ultimately transforms the learning experience into something powerful and memorable. Many young learners have developed long-standing relationships with these patients and family members.

Learners in the AELPS programs also benefit from stories told by practicing healthcare professionals. Many professionals can eloquently recount their own personal experiences in learning sessions, and many others have become valued storytellers through blogging and other social media venues.

Narrative and personal reflection can generate both positive and negative emotions. The intention of caregivers is to serve their patients, to do no harm, and to improve the health of the people they care for. When care does not go as planned, everyone is devastated—especially the people directly involved in that care. A growing body of literature has called to light the anxiety, depression, and even suicide attempts experienced by caregivers who have been involved in a preventable medical harm event. The sharing of stories can be a source of comfort and route to healing for those caregivers, while at the same time promoting learning and the development of new insights into system processes.

Aligned with teaching through stories and narratives, another major focus of the AELPS programs is to teach learners the value of their own stories and the importance of reflective practice. Every experience that health science students and resident physicians have in caring for others should be considered both a valuable learning tool and a gift. As students and residents deal with emotionally charged content, they engage in critical thinking, frame the stories in a way that makes sense within their current worldview, and learn through reflection.

Gaming and Low-Fidelity Simulation

Another key educational strategy used in the AELPS programs is the use of games and low-fidelity simulation to drive retention of learning. Learners of the "millennials" generational cohort are radically different from those of prior generations, in large part because of their high degree of technological literacy. Millennials enjoy learning about new technology through discovery—by experiencing and experimenting with it. They read less and are more comfortable in image-rich environments. Their clear preference is for active, first-person, experiential learning and a high level of interactivity. This interactivity is largely absent from traditional lectures but vibrantly present in new media technologies.

Digital games can be effective in teaching and reinforcing such essential job skills as teamwork, collaboration, problem solving, and communication, as well as in introducing new concepts (McClarty et al. 2012). The importance of game-based learning was highlighted in the US Department of Education's 2010 National Education Technology Plan, with a call for research in how "assessment technologies, such as simulations, collaboration environments, virtual worlds, games, and cognitive tutors, can be used to engage and motivate learners while assessing complex skills" (US Department of Education 2010).

Games can be useful for guiding learners in acquiring knowledge and skills according to a learning progression—often, for instance, games require the learner to show mastery of one skill or concept before advancing to other levels (McClarty et al. 2012). One attractive element of learning through gaming is that failure is not typically linked with negative consequences; rather, it serves as an integral part of the learning experience, encouraging learners to improve through repeated practice. Learners can take risks and learn quickly from their mistakes (McClarty et al. 2012).

Well-designed educational games challenge the learner while also providing an obvious learning message. McClarty and colleagues (2012) point out that games "do not provide the entire learning experience"; rather, they "work best when coupled with effective pedagogy." Steinkuehler and Chmiel (2006) suggest that games are likely to serve as an alternative to textbooks and laboratory activities, but not as a replacement for teachers and classrooms.

Games should be designed with clear goals and should provide immediate feedback to the learners. Learning does not end with the game; debriefing is critical (McClarty et al. 2012). Feedback should be clear, unobtrusive, and immediately responsive to the learner's actions, and the debriefing process should help learners apply what they learned in the gaming session to other contexts. Educators can facilitate learning through both pre- and postgame discussions, in which students link the game experience with class concepts and share their own ways of developing strategies and approaching problems (McClarty et al. 2012).

The AELPS program uses multiple games to engage participants in interactive learning and to reinforce the content learned via traditional education. Many learners find the games to be the highlight of the week. One of the more popular games for teaching concepts related to teamwork, communication, and leadership skills is the teeter-totter game, described in exhibit 11.2. It is relatively quick, inexpensive, and easy to administer, but it can deliver a lasting impact.

Graduate-Level Educational Programs in Quality Improvement and Patient Safety

A number of universities have begun offering master's programs specifically focused on quality improvement and patient safety. In the early 2000s, Northwestern University became the first academic medical center with a master of science program in this domain. In 2007, the University of Illinois followed suit by launching an online master of science in patient safety leadership (PSL) program. Similarly, Thomas Jefferson University's School of Population Health, established in 2008, has a master of science in healthcare quality and safety (HQS) program. The purpose of these programs is to prepare students with the analytic, evaluative, and change management skills necessary to guide and enhance quality improvement efforts across a variety of healthcare delivery settings. In addition to these new programs, many existing healthcare management graduate programs have begun adding courses dedicated to patient safety and healthcare quality.

EXHIBIT 11.2
Teeter-Totter Game

Equipment
One treated board, 12 feet × 10 inches × 2 inches
One cinder block, 12 inches × 6 inches × 6 inches
One dozen eggs

Basics

1. Imagine that the teeter-totter is a new piece of equipment that performs a medical procedure.
2. The care team consists of nine people: one leader, one observer, and seven others who will complete the procedure.
3. The board is centered on top of the cinder block to create the teeter-totter effect; one egg (representing a patient) is placed under each end of the board.
4. The goal is to successfully move all seven people onto the board, entering one at a time, and then move all seven people off of the board without harming the eggs under each end.
5. The team has ten minutes to complete the task (the medical procedure) without crushing the eggs (patients).

Instructions

1. The team first has five minutes to discuss the plan for performing the procedure.
2. The team decides which members will serve as leader, as observer, and as people on the teeter-totter.
3. The seven members must step onto the board one at a time.
4. Each of the seven members must step onto the board at the center and move along the board until all seven are successfully on the board.
5. All seven members must stay on the board, together, for ten seconds before starting to get off of the board.
6. Members must step off the board the same way they entered (at the center) until all are off.
7. The team members on the board can touch each other, but no one else can touch those on the board.
8. The task ends after all seven people are off the board and the patients (eggs) are safely moved from under each side of the board.

Several associations now offer certifications in the field of quality and safety. For instance, the National Patient Safety Foundation has a Certified Professional in Patient Safety (CPPS) certification, and the National Association for Healthcare Quality has a Certified Professional in Healthcare Quality (CPHQ) certification.

Some universities, including Georgetown University, have begun offering graduate-level programs in quality and safety to meet the growing demands of healthcare professionals seeking higher-level education in these areas. Significant interest and enrollment have been seen among physicians, nurses, pharmacists, and health administrators.

Additional Examples of Health Sciences Student and Resident Physician Quality and Safety Programs

Quality Reports for Residents at Thomas Jefferson University

Healthcare leaders at Thomas Jefferson University, in partnership with the performance improvement department, aimed to design a resident quality and safety report for all core programs, with the following criteria for success (Jaffe et al. 2017):

1. Each residency program must be able to define its own attribution strategy so that subsequent review will be meaningful to learners.
2. Reports must include individual performance for each metric, as well as patient identifiers so that learners can review their performance at the case level.
3. Existing performance analysis infrastructure should be used to make the process resource neutral.
4. Metrics must align with institutional and educational priorities.

The university created a mandatory field in its electronic health record's discharge order in which a "discharge resident" is specified by a unique identifier, tying the selected individual to the administrative data for a particular patient case. Jaffe and colleagues (2017) explain:

> An attribution strategy was defined by each program director, and residents were educated at the program level. Using the same process that our institution employs for the preparation of faculty Ongoing Professional Practice Evaluations (OPPEs), . . . our performance improvement department abstracted inpatient provider-level quality data for residents.

Resident Engagement in Quality Improvement at Detroit Medical Center

In 2014, the Detroit Medical Center launched a program to engage residents and fellows to deliver optimal care. It sought to establish a focus on quality at an early stage in people's careers and prepare them for future work (Hussain et al. 2016). Hussain and colleagues (2016, 214) explain:

> Residents from clinically relevant residency and fellowship programs were selected to be Resident Quality Directors. The project involved development of an interactive electronic health record (EHR) checklist to visually depict real time gaps in 40 process measures, while focusing on 14 areas related to stroke and venous thromboembolism (VTE) prophylaxis.

The Family Medicine Resident Curriculum in Colorado

In 2009 and 2010, a comprehensive patient safety program at three sites in Colorado provided safety-oriented learning for 36 transitional-year interns and

36 family medicine residents (Winslow et al. 2011). Winslow and colleagues (2011) describe the program:

> The curriculum requires each resident to report adverse events, report near misses or unsafe conditions, attend 12 patient safety lectures per year, and disclose a medical error to standardized patients in 2 separate exercises. Residents' communication skills during the disclosure are rated by the standardized patients, and residents receive feedback from attending physicians who observe the exercise. Events reported by the residents are collected, deidentified, and analyzed, and education is provided to all residents in the program. Residents are surveyed before and after the intervention regarding their attitudes and assumptions about patient safety.

The curriculum is patterned after the University of Illinois at Chicago Full Disclosure and Transparency Program.

Conclusion

Almost 20 years after the release of IOM's *To Err Is Human* report, true progress in educational reform is still slow. Despite continued reports of overwhelming numbers of preventable patient deaths and poor-quality care, formal, systematic quality and patient safety curricula remain lacking in many healthcare educational programs across the country. Reforming medical education to adequately address quality and safety issues presents a major challenge to medical educators, given that the shortcomings that need to be addressed have been so deeply entrenched in the tradition and culture of medical education. Because of this culture, much of health science education remains stuck in the 1980s. Despite these cultural barriers, innovative healthcare educators have developed unique program offerings to empower young learners and provide them with best practices related to quality and safety for their patients as well as their colleagues.

The authors would like to acknowledge Gwen Sherwood, Wendy Madigosky, and Tracy Granzyk for their contributions to this chapter.

Study Questions

1. How have lessons from such industries as aviation and military defense been applied to education for healthcare quality and safety?
2. Compare and contrast the Telluride roundtables, the World Health Organization curriculum guide, and the work of the Lucian Leape

Institute with regard to health science and graduate resident training in quality and safety. Which do you consider most useful, and why?
3. What are some of the benefits and limitations of game-based learning?
4. What future steps do you consider necessary to bring about meaningful reform in quality and safety education?

References

Academy for Emerging Leaders in Patient Safety (AELPS). 2018. "About." Accessed November 7. http://telluridesummercamp.com/about/.

Accreditation Council for Graduate Medical Education (ACGME). 2017. *CLER Pathways to Excellence: Expectations for an Optimal Clinical Learning Environment to Achieve Safe and High Quality Patient Care, Version 1.1.* Accessed November 6, 2018. www.acgme.org/Portals/0/PDFs/CLER/CLER_Pathways_V1.1_Digital_Final.pdf.

———. 2013. *Encouraging Excellence: Accreditation Council for Graduate Medical Education 2012 Annual Report.* Accessed November 7. www.acgme.org/Portals/0/84938_ACGME_full.pdf.

Carnett, W. G. 2002. "Clinical Practice Guidelines: A Tool to Improve Care." *Journal of Nursing Care Quality* 16 (3): 60–70.

Cohen, J. 1999. Letter to medical school deans, Association of American Medical Colleges, December.

Cronenwett, L., G. Sherwood, J. Barnsteiner, J. Disch, J. Johnson, P. Mitchell, D. T. Sullivan, and J. Warren. 2007. "Quality and Safety Education for Nurses." *Nursing Outlook* 55 (3): 122–31.

Cronenwett, L., G. Sherwood, J. Pohl, J. Barnsteiner, S. Moore, D. T. Sullivan, D. Ward, and J. Warren. 2009. "Quality and Safety Education for Advanced Nursing Practice." *Nursing Outlook* 57 (6): 338–48.

Hussain, S. A., C. Arsene, C. Hamstra, T. H. Woehrlen, W. Wiese-Rometsch, and S. R. White. 2016. "Successful Resident Engagement in Quality Improvement." *Journal of Graduate Medical Education* 8 (2): 214–18.

Institute for Healthcare Improvement (IHI). 2018a. "Eight Knowledge Domains for Health Professional Students." Accessed November 7. www.ihi.org/education/IHIOpenSchool/resources/Pages/Publications/EightKnowledgeDomainsForHealthProfessionStudents.aspx.

———. 2018b. "IHI Open School: Overview." Accessed November 7. www.ihi.org/education/ihiopenschool/overview/Pages/default.aspx.

———. 2017. *10 IHI Innovations to Improve Health and Health Care.* Cambridge, MA: Institute for Healthcare Improvement.

Jaffe, R., G. Diemer, J. Caruso, and M. Metzinger. 2017. "Creating Provider-Level Quality Reports for Residents to Improve the Clinical Learning Environment."

Journal of Graduate Medical Education. Published June. www.jgme.org/doi/full/10.4300/JGME-D-16-00752.1.

Kern, D. E., P. A. Thomas, D. M. Howard, and E. B. Bass. 1998. *Curriculum Development for Medical Education: A Six-Step Approach*. Baltimore, MD: Johns Hopkins University Press.

Kohn, L. T., J. M. Corrigan, and M. S. Donaldson (eds.). 2000. *To Err Is Human: Building a Safer Health System*. Washington, DC: National Academies Press.

Loeb, J. M. 2004. "The Current State of Performance Measurement in Health Care." *International Journal for Quality in Health Care* 16 (Suppl. 1): 5–9.

Lucian Leape Institute (LLI). 2010. *Unmet Needs: Teaching Physicians to Provide Safe Patient Care*. Accessed November 6, 2018. www.npsf.org/resource/resmgr/LLI/LLI-Unmet-Needs-Report.pdf.

Mayer, D. M., D. L. Klamen, A. Gunderson, and P. Barash. 2009. "Designing a Patient Safety Undergraduate Medical Curriculum: The Telluride Interdisciplinary Roundtable Experience." *Teaching and Learning in Medicine* 21 (1): 52–58.

McClarty, K. L., A. Orr, P. M. Frey, R. P. Dolan, V. Vassileva, and A. McVay. 2012. "A Literature Review of Gaming in Education: Research Report." Pearson. Published June. https://images.pearsonassessments.com/images/tmrs/Lit_Review_of_Gaming_in_Education.pdf.

Quality and Safety Education for Nurses (QSEN). 2018. "QSEN Competencies." Accessed November 7. http://qsen.org/competencies/pre-licensure-ksas/.

Steinkuehler, C., and M. Chmiel. 2006. "Fostering Scientific Habits of Mind in the Context of Online Play." In *Proceedings of the International Conference of the Learning Sciences*, edited by S. A. Barab, K. E. Hay, N. B. Songer, and D. T. Hickey, 723–29. Mahwah, NJ: Erlbaum.

US Department of Education. 2010. *Transforming American Education: Learning Powered by Technology*. Published November. www.ed.gov/sites/default/files/netp2010-execsumm.pdf.

Walton, M., H. Woodward, S. Van Staalduinen, C. Lemer, F. Greaves, D. Noble, B. Ellis, L. Donaldson, and B. Barraclough. 2010. "The WHO Patient Safety Curriculum Guide for Medical Schools." *Quality & Safety in Health Care* 19 (6): 542–46.

Winslow, B., B. S. Bacak, B. G. Dwinnell, and S. Dierking. 2011. "Patient Safety Education for Residents—A Colorado Story." *Journal of Graduate Medical Education*. Published June. http://jgme.org/doi/full/10.4300/JGME-D-11-00076.1.

Wong, B. M., E. E. Etchells, A. Kuper, W. Levinson, and K. G. Shojania. 2010. "Teaching Quality Improvement and Patient Safety to Trainees: A Systematic Review." *Academic Medicine* 85 (9): 1425–39.

CHAPTER

12

CREATING ALIGNMENT: QUALITY MEASURES AND LEADERSHIP

Michael D. Pugh

Introduction

Creating alignment around strategic quality and operational objectives is a critical leadership function. When organizational quality strategy fails to deliver, the question is often presented as a binomial choice of whether the failure was the result of a poorly conceived strategy or poor execution. Usually, it is a combination of both: Poorly articulated, nonmeasurable quality aims generally lead to poor execution. Organizational efforts to improve quality, patient safety, patient experience, and clinical care begin with clearly articulated and measurable quality aims, with measures that then can be cascaded down the organization to create alignment of efforts at all levels. This chapter will explore some of the measurement tools and approaches that organizational leadership can use to create alignment and deliver results.

Quality Measures and Metrics

The past decade has witnessed an explosion of quality metrics and quality measurement across healthcare, not only to support organizations' internal quality improvement efforts, but also to meet the demands of external accreditation agencies (e.g., The Joint Commission), health insurance companies, and government payment programs.

The Centers for Medicare & Medicaid Services (CMS) requires hospitals to submit more than 60 measures—in addition to Hospital Consumer Assessment of Healthcare Providers and Systems (HCAHPS) survey results—as a condition of participation in the Medicare and Medicaid programs. These measures are used by CMS both for payment programs and for efforts to inform the public about comparative hospital performance (including published star ratings). CMS also requires submission of quality measures for long-term care (e.g., nursing homes), physician services, dialysis centers, and some ambulatory care settings.

Payment systems continue to evolve from the traditional fee-for-service models to value-based payment models in which payments are modified based on the achievement of measure-based quality goals. Accountable care organizations (ACOs) must submit quality metrics and achieve certain measurable goals to qualify for risk-sharing payments. Hospitals that participate in the Medicare Value-Based Purchasing Program have a percentage of their Medicare payment at risk, depending on comparative quality performance.

Physician payment for professional services is increasingly being tied to achievement of quality goals and submission of quality metrics in the physician office setting. The Medicare Access and CHIP Reauthorization Act of 2015 (MACRA), for instance, made significant changes in the way that physicians are paid for their services.[1] These changes are not limited to government programs. Private health insurance payment systems, too, are moving toward value-based payment programs that require the submission of performance and quality measures.

The collection and publication of quality measures have become big business for a number of organizations and a major cost for healthcare providers. Kevin Sower, former CEO of Duke University Hospital in Durham, North Carolina, noted in 2016 that Duke spent approximately $11,000,000 per year collecting, analyzing, and reporting healthcare quality measures to various external agencies.[2]

CMS uses quality measures submitted by hospitals, nursing homes, rehabilitation centers, and other provider types, as well as quality measures collected from Medicare Advantage health plans, to present consumer-facing comparative information. This information is available via the Nursing Home Compare (www.medicare.gov/nursinghomecompare/) and Hospital Compare (www.medicare.gov/hospitalcompare/) websites, which use five-star quality rating systems, as well as through the Medicare Advantage star ratings for health plans.

Beyond CMS, a variety of online systems use both the publicly available Medicare database of submitted measures and proprietary databases to present ratings and rankings. Multiple states, state hospital associations, hospital trade groups, commercial websites (e.g., Healthgrades.com), and business coalitions (e.g., the Leapfrog Group) also publish sets of quality measures.

Transparency about quality and performance is intended to spur healthcare organizations to pay closer attention to important indicators and to provide consumers with the information they need to make better healthcare purchasing decisions. However, many people in the healthcare field consider the public reporting of performance data as a questionable regulatory process that does not necessarily provide a meaningful reflection of an organization's performance. Complying with regulatory reporting requirements, they note, is different from focusing on a set of key performance indicators that organizational leaders use to guide improvement efforts.

Commonly Used Quality-Measurement Sets

Hospitals routinely collect and review patient satisfaction and financial indicators and monitor a large, diverse set of quality indicators. The Joint Commission requires organizations to collect, monitor, and report specific sets of indicators as a condition of accreditation. Currently, CMS requires both hospitals and long-term care facilities to collect a broad set of quality and clinical indicators that are then made publicly available through CMS websites.

The National Committee for Quality Assurance (NCQA) sponsors the Healthcare Effectiveness Data and Information Set (HEDIS), which is used by more than 90 percent of US health plans and managed care organizations to measure performance across important dimensions of care and service. To demonstrate effectiveness of care for their members, health plans collect data on the percentage of eligible members who receive screening for breast cancer and colorectal cancer, among other measures. They also collect information on whether members receive appropriate treatment for diabetes, cholesterol management in heart disease, and upper respiratory infections in children.

HEDIS measures extend to individual physician practices and organized medical groups, which are measured on patient satisfaction as well as on the HEDIS clinical data set. Medical groups and outpatient care systems may also collect and track workflow and process indicators, such as the average waiting time to the next open appointment, the number of clinic visits per day, and the waiting time before patients are seen by a clinician.

Background and Terminology

Robert S. Kaplan and David P. Norton first used the term *balanced scorecard* in their 1992 *Harvard Business Review* article "The Balanced Scorecard: Measures That Drive Performance." Based on a study of multiple companies, the authors examined approaches to organizational performance management beyond the use of standard financial and accounting measures. Kaplan and Norton's theory is that reliance on traditional financial measures alone limits a company's ability to increase shareholder value. This investigational premise is consistent with the position of quality guru Dr. W. Edwards Deming, who maintained that companies cannot be run by visible numbers alone (Aguayo 1991). To overcome this limitation, successful organizations use a broader index of performance metrics to create a balance between financial results and other important dimensions of performance.

Kaplan and Norton's 1996 follow-up book, *The Balanced Scorecard: Translating Strategy into Action,* further examined the development of performance measures linked to organizational strategy. They advised that, for an organization to achieve results, the balanced scorecard should be central to the leadership system—not merely a balanced set of outcome measures for the organization. Kaplan and Norton (1996) observed that most organizations collect performance measures for important nonfinancial dimensions, such as customer service and product quality, but that those measures are usually reviewed separately from the financial results and with less emphasis by senior leadership. Kaplan and Norton also noted that leaders can increase organizational alignment by simultaneously reviewing and monitoring critical measures across multiple dimensions of performance, not just financial dimensions. According to Kaplan and Norton, the balanced scorecard is more than a way to monitor a broad set of outcome or process measures—it is central to deploying organizational strategy.

Dashboards

Although the terms *dashboard* and *scorecard* are often used interchangeably, they actually refer to two different things.[3] The term *dashboard* brings to mind the instrument panel on an automobile, which, when the car is moving, enables the driver to monitor key performance metrics such as speed, fuel level, and direction. The driver may also have access to such metrics as tire pressure, revolutions per minute, engine temperature, and oil pressure. Many of the more detailed engine and car performance measures may be important to a professional driver in a high-performance race car but are generally not critical to the average driver's journey from point A to point B. Instead, casual drivers rely on a dashboard that presents a core set of high-level measures to track the real-time process of driving the car. The pilot of an airplane, meanwhile, depends on a dashboard with a much more complex collection of instruments to track critical operating information.

Both the driver of a car and the pilot of an airplane monitor multiple performance indicators simultaneously to arrive at the intended destination successfully. At any given point in the journey, the driver or the pilot might focus on a particular indicator, but overall success depends on the collective performance of the systems represented by the various indicators on the dashboard. Similarly, in the business world, dashboards are tools that report on the ongoing performance of the critical processes that lead to organizational success rather than on the success itself.

Scorecards

The term *scorecard* brings to mind a different image. Scorecards are used to record and report on periods of past performance, rather than on real-time performance. Generally, scorecards reflect outcome measures rather than process measures. They are analogous to school report cards, which are issued after all work has been completed and use a specific grading standard to indicate how an individual student performed.

Although a lag time exists between the performance and the reporting, the information in a report card can still be used to make changes to influence future outcomes—for instance, improvements in the student's study habits or class attendance, allocation of additional study time to specific subject matter, outside tutoring, or help with homework preparation. However, the possible changes result from the investigation of the current process rather than the review of past performance information presented in the report card.

The differences between scorecards as measures of outcomes or results and dashboards as measures of process may be logical, but in terms of practical application in healthcare, they are rarely distinct. Healthcare organizations are complex, and a metric often may serve as a process measure and the proxy for an outcome measure at the same time. As a result, many organizational scorecards and dashboards contain a mix of outcome-, strategy-, and process-related measures. The key issue is how leadership uses individual measures and measurement sets to align priorities and achieve desired organizational results.

FUNCTIONALLY VERY SIMILAR

Quality Assurance, Quality Control, and Quality Improvement

Quality assurance, quality control, and quality improvement are related but distinct concepts that represent different mental models and different uses of quality measures and data in healthcare delivery organizations. Exhibit 12.1 illustrates some of the key characteristics of each.

EXHIBIT 12.1 Quality Control, Assurance, and Improvement

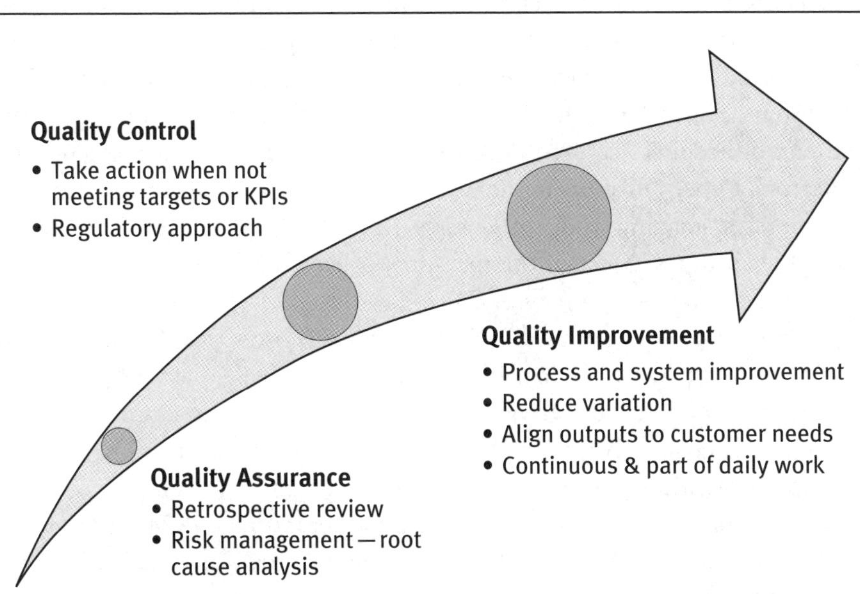
Quality Control
• Take action when not meeting targets or KPIs
• Regulatory approach
Quality Improvement
• Process and system improvement
• Reduce variation
• Align outputs to customer needs
• Continuous & part of daily work
Quality Assurance
• Retrospective review
• Risk management—root cause analysis

Source: MdP Associates, LLC. Used with permission.

Quality Assurance

Quality assurance (QA) can generally be described as the process of retrospective review or study to identify problems or patterns of problems. The collection of patient incident data can be categorized as a QA risk management function, as can the routine or special retrospective audit of patient medical records. Audit processes are routinely used by researchers, clinical staff committees, and others to compile retrospective performance data or investigate incidents or other questions about clinical care. The data produced may be useful for finding areas that need improvement or identifying incidents of patient harm that may need further investigation.

Quality Control

Quality control (QC) can generally be described as the collection and ongoing monitoring of process and clinical measures that have been identified by the organization or are required for submission to an external payer or regulatory agency. It is essentially a management function, and the data monitored should be important to the managers and clinicians in the care delivery system as a means of spotting problems and issues that need to be addressed.

One way to think about QC is to imagine a common scene from old science fiction movies. A control room is full of people in white coats staring at monitors and dials when, suddenly, something dramatic happens. Red lights flash, dials spin, and warning sirens go off, signaling an emergency and causing people to quickly react. Quality control in healthcare is often similar. Measures are collected and monitored, and when a measure is not meeting expected levels of performance, management is expected to take prompt corrective action.

Hundreds of QC measures are collected throughout the healthcare delivery system. For instance, hospitals routinely collect and monitor the number and rate of hospital-acquired infections, patient falls, and other patient safety indicators. Other QC measures may include appointment no-show rates, readmission rates, imaging study retake rates, clinical care guideline adherence, and average wait times. Most of the measures collected and reported to external agencies fall into the category of QC.

Sometimes, organizations select certain subsets of QC measures and label them as *key performance indicators* (KPIs), with assigned targets for performance. The KPIs are then used for a variety of management incentive and performance review programs. Organizations may also use their QC measures to help set organizational priorities for improvement.

One of the early quality pioneers, Dr. Joseph Juran (1974), is known for the "Juran Trilogy" of quality planning, quality control, and quality improvement. Quality planning involves understanding what is important, needs to be measured, and needs to be "controlled." Quality control involves monitoring key performance metrics to ensure that performance is within expected standards, or the "zone of control." When leaders determine that a metric needs to operate at a different level of performance or with a different set of standards, they pursue quality improvement to move the performance of the system into a new "zone of control."

Quality Improvement

An old adage states that "you do not fatten a cow by weighing it." Moving beyond simply collecting and reporting measures for QC, quality improvement (QI) in healthcare can be described as the active effort to improve clinical, experience, safety, and cost outcomes by focusing on the processes and systems that produce those outcomes.

Hospital mortality rates, patient satisfaction scores, readmission rates, inpatient length of stay, glycemic control in diabetic patients, blood pressure control, patient functional outcome measures, cost per discharge or procedure, and cost per member per month in health plans are all examples of outcome measures of complex clinical and administrative processes. In recent years, the Institute for Healthcare Improvement's (IHI's) Triple Aim, shown in exhibit 12.2, has sought to move the discussion about outcomes from delivery system outcomes to the population-based outcomes of population health, patient experience, and cost per capita (IHI 2018; Stiefel and Nolan 2012).

In developing and deploying a QI strategy, organizational leadership might focus on one or two high-level outcome measures—such as hospital mortality, patient harm index, or patient satisfaction scores—and then seek to focus improvement efforts on the processes and care systems that contribute to the outcomes being measured. For example, improving hospital mortality

EXHIBIT 12.2
The Triple Aim

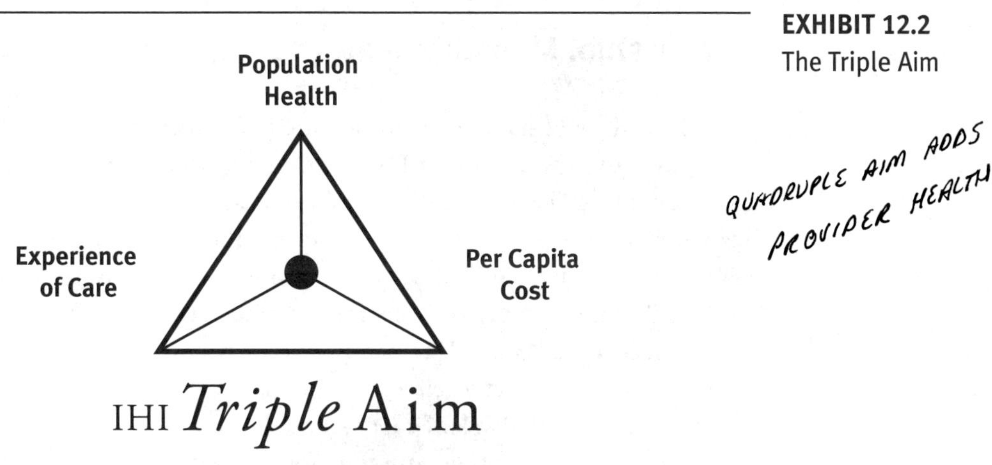

Source: The IHI Triple Aim framework was developed by the Institute for Healthcare Improvement in Boston, Massachusetts (www.ihi.org).

generally requires an organization to focus on reducing device-related infections from central line insertion and ventilators; ensuring the early identification and aggressive treatment of sepsis; working to prevent medication errors, patient falls, and other patient harm events; and reducing delays in treatment. Rather than simply monitoring measures and levels, organizations apply QI tools and methods to find ways to dramatically reduce or eliminate events that contribute to hospital mortality.

The description of QI presented in this section is intentionally narrow to enable comparison with the functions of QA and QC. However, for some healthcare organizations and leaders, QI is not just a set of projects or activities but rather a philosophy that shapes leadership and management systems. Organizations such as Virginia Mason (Seattle, Washington), Park Nicolett (Minneapolis, Minnesota), ThedaCare (Appleton, Wisconsin), and McLeod Health (Florence, South Carolina) treat QI as a specific management philosophy and corresponding set of mental models that leaders adopt and use to organize their leadership and management systems.

Leaders in these organizations, building largely on the work of Deming (2000) and his System of Profound Knowledge, have sought to transform the way healthcare work is designed, organized, and performed to reduce cost, remove waste, and improve the patient experience and clinical outcomes. The branding of these efforts, with specific sets of tools, activities, and methods, has led to popular approaches such as Lean, the Toyota Production System (TPS), Robust Process Improvement (RPI), and Continuous Quality Improvement (CQI). The leadership effort involved in transforming an organization based on the principles of a management philosophy is significantly broader than simply using QI or Lean tools for certain projects or initiatives.

Leadership, Measurement, and Improvement

In 2013, IHI published a white paper titled "High-Impact Leadership: Improve Care, Improve the Health of Populations, and Reduce Costs." In that paper, Swensen and colleagues (2013) propose that, to achieve Triple Aim results, leaders need to adopt new mental models about quality and value, practice high-impact leadership behaviors, and create a deployment strategy around the IHI High-Impact Leadership Framework (see exhibit 12.3).

According to the IHI paper, one of the five high-impact leadership behaviors that is directly related to the measures and measurement is transparency (see exhibit 12.4). Leaders model transparency by being open about organizational progress against strategic quality aims and by promoting the

EXHIBIT 12.3
IHI High-Impact Leadership: Improve Care, Improve the Health of Populations, and Reduce Costs

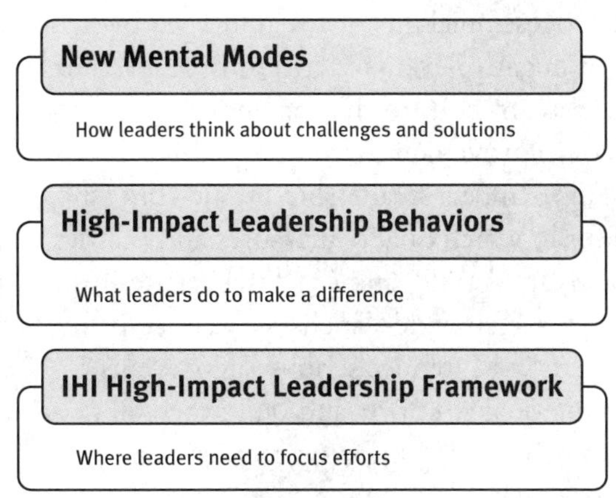

Source: Swensen S, Pugh M, McMullan C, Kabcenell A. *High-Impact Leadership: Improve Care, Improve the Health of Populations, and Reduce Costs.* IHI White Paper. Cambridge, MA: Institute for Healthcare Improvement; 2013. (Available at ihi.org.)

EXHIBIT 12.4
High-Impact Leadership Behaviors

1. Person-centeredness	Be consistently person-centered in word and deed
2. Front Line Engagement	Be a regular authentic presence at the front line and a visible champion of improvement
3. Relentless Focus	Remain focused on the vision and strategy
4. Transparency	Require transparency about results, progress, aims, and defects
5. Boundarilessness	Encourage and practice systems thinking and collaboration across boundaries

Source: Swensen S, Pugh M, McMullan C, Kabcenell A. *High-Impact Leadership: Improve Care, Improve the Health of Populations, and Reduce Costs.* IHI White Paper. Cambridge, MA: Institute for Healthcare Improvement; 2013. (Available at ihi.org.)

use of visual boards and the posting of quality and safety data about harm, satisfaction, and process reliability at the unit level by frontline workers. The open discussion of negative events is critical to leadership efforts to shape an organizational and team culture that promotes patient safety and supports accelerated rates of improvement.

The IHI High-Impact Leadership Framework (shown in exhibit 12.5) has two dimensions in which quality measures and metrics play a key role: (1) "Create Vision and Build Will" and (2) "Deliver Results." Establishing measurable quality aims systemwide—such as "Reduce hospital mortality by 50 percent over five years" or "Reduce serious safety events by 70 percent"—helps create a vision of the quality efforts and build the will to achieve that vision.

The "Deliver Results" dimension requires leaders to have a plan to use proven QI methods that are dependent on quality and process metrics and deliver measurable outcomes that correspond to the three elements of the Triple Aim.

EXHIBIT 12.5
IHI High-Impact Leadership Framework

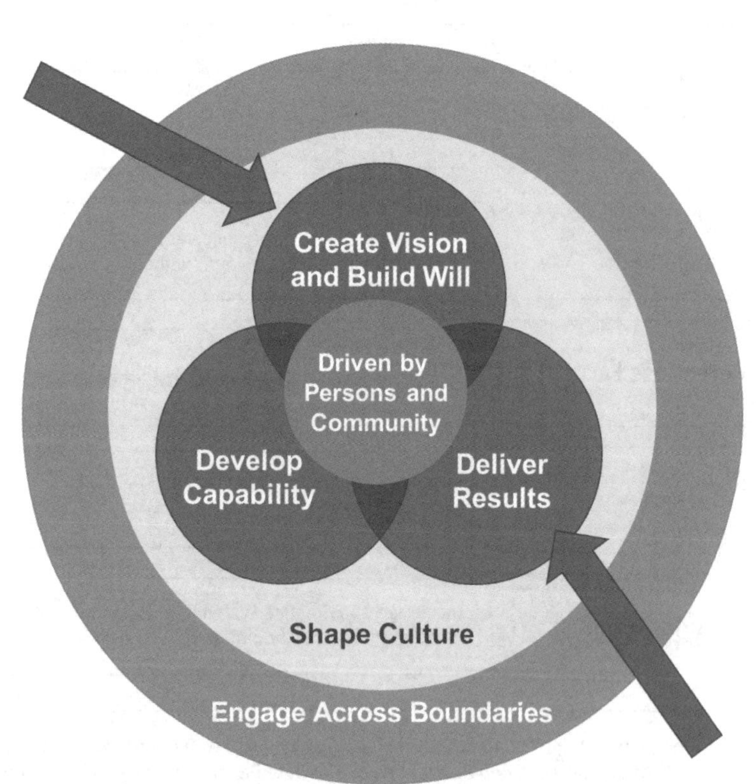

Source: Swensen S, Pugh M, McMullan C, Kabcenell A. *High-Impact Leadership: Improve Care, Improve the Health of Populations, and Reduce Costs.* IHI White Paper. Cambridge, MA: Institute for Healthcare Improvement; 2013. (Available at ihi.org.)

Dashboards and Scorecards in a Strategic Leadership System

Leadership in a healthcare organization is a complex system that incorporates beliefs, values, and behaviors, as well as a series of complex processes. Although the term *leadership* is commonly defined or associated with individual behaviors or characteristics, every organization has a *system* of leadership that is defined by the values, behaviors, and actions of leaders—in particular, where and how they spend their time, energy, and attention.

Exhibit 12.6 presents one depiction of a leadership system in a healthcare delivery organization. The system drives both organizational culture and the design and alignment of daily work, ensuring consistency with the mission and vision of the organization. One of the key elements of the leadership system is the measurement process, which includes dashboards and scorecards.

The challenge for healthcare leaders is to make sense of the multitude of measures and metrics that are routinely available. Scorecards and dashboards are useful for organizing important metrics, but healthcare leaders struggle with the question: What should we measure? That answer is tied to the answer to another question: For what purpose? Form should follow function.

Scorecards and dashboards should drive leadership behavior and be used to create alignment in organizations. Financial and volume measures have traditionally driven management behavior in healthcare. Governing boards of healthcare organizations have spent considerably more time reviewing and discussing financial reports than quality or patient satisfaction reports. Financial review still tends to dominate governance assessments of organizational performance, but

EXHIBIT 12.6
Healthcare Leadership System

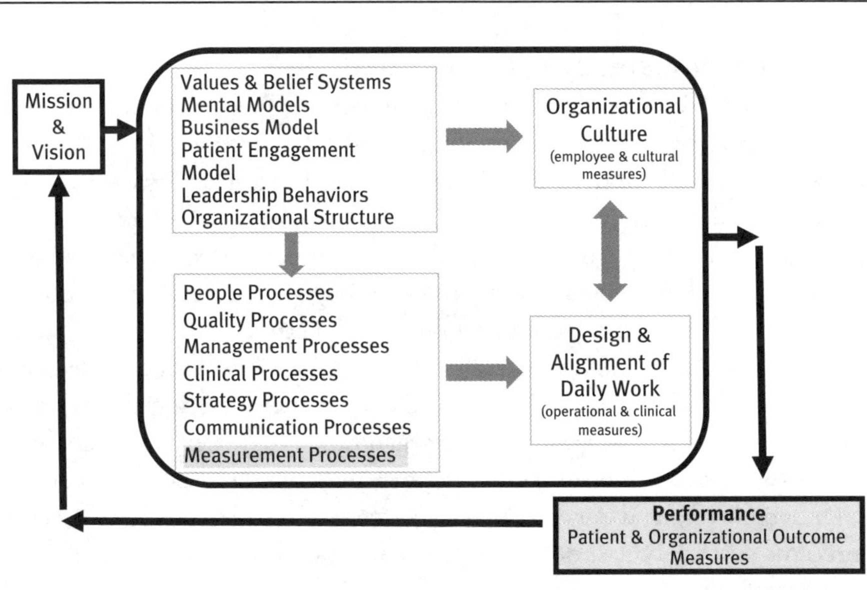

Source: MdP Associates, LLC. Used with permission.

an important shift has occurred over the past decade. Increasing numbers of hospital boards and senior leadership teams are recognizing that performance in healthcare involves much more than the financial bottom line and are now devoting equal or more time to reviewing clinical quality, workplace culture, and patient experience data. However, despite the increased global emphasis on patient safety and harm prevention, patient safety indicators still tend to be underrepresented on many organizational performance scorecards, relative to other measures of performance.

A typical hospital routinely collects hundreds of quality and performance measures for external reporting to regulatory agencies and for internal quality monitoring. Reports generated by the quality department are often voluminous, populated with hundreds of process-based measures and some outcome measures, and they tend to be reports of past performance rather than drivers of future efforts. It is up to leadership to create a focus around a core set of measures to drive the quality strategy.

For example, a quality control measure such as the hospital infection rate or the hospital inpatient mortality rate is commonly included in a leadership report, even absent an active improvement effort or link to organizational strategy. Healthcare organizations have monitored infection rates and mortality rates for years but have tended to act only when an infectious outbreak has occurred or when an incident report or the medical staff peer review process has revealed known instances of avoidable patient harm or death. Simply tracking an indicator is not enough. Often, a wide gap exists between the measurement set that is considered to be a scorecard or dashboard and leadership's actual use of the tool to drive improvement and change.

Organizing Measures by Category

Creating useful information out of the myriad measures and data routinely collected for internal improvement efforts and external reporting to CMS or others is a challenge for healthcare organizations. The availability of electronic medical record and billing systems in the United States is making it easier for healthcare delivery organizations to collect some quality and performance measures, but taking full advantage of technology to track and report quality measures remains, for many organizations, a significant challenge and expense.

Healthcare organizations traditionally sort the measures they collect into categories such as financial, volume, satisfaction, patient safety, clinical quality, and population health. Some healthcare organizations have developed summary dashboards of key indicators, organized by category, to sharpen focus and to facilitate reporting and day-to-day management of various functions. Quality scorecards and safety dashboards have become popular ways of reporting on clinical quality to medical staff committees and to the board.

Dashboards and scorecards may be organized in formats ranging from simple tables to web-based graphical reports embedded in computerized decision-support systems. Data report formats include tables, radar charts, bar graphs, run or control charts, and color-coded indicators designed to highlight metrics that do not meet targets or expectations.[4] In some organizations, each operating unit has a scorecard of key indicators that mirrors the organizational scorecard.

Formatting available measures into a summary dashboard—whether departmental, category specific, or cross-dimensional—is a start. However, senior leaders can harness the real power of measures by organizing their leadership systems to achieve results.

Measures for Governance and Leadership

Healthcare organizations should consider the use of three basic sets of measures when designing a scorecard or dashboard: those of governance function, leadership function, and management function. These three basic types are summarized in exhibit 12.7.

At the governance level, a set of organizational performance measures should be defined and monitored, and the organization should link those measures to how it defines performance within the context of its mission, vision, and values. A governance-level scorecard of performance measures should be a basic tool for all healthcare governing boards.

At the senior leadership level, an additional set of measures should be used to align priorities, lead the organization, and embody the concept of a balanced scorecard. The organization should link these measures to its critical strategies, or "vital few" initiatives, and use them to drive desired results. As Kaplan and

EXHIBIT 12.7
Measures Aligned to Function

Governance Function	Leadership Function	Management Function
• Link to mission and vision • Outcome measures used to judge overall organizational performance • Comparative performance measures	• Measures related to strategy execution • Focal point of leadership system • Used to create alignment and focus	• Process measures important to daily work • Key financial & operational measures • Quality control • Quality improvement

Source: MdP Associates, LLC. Used with permission.

Norton (1992, 1996) suggest, strategic measures should be at the center of the organization's leadership system. Although leadership's main role is to deploy strategy, monitoring deployment is also its responsibility. A dashboard of strategic measures is a tool that leaders can use to set priorities and drive change.

The board may use the same dashboard as a scorecard to monitor the deployment of strategy and assess leadership effectiveness. An important relationship exists between the overall organizational performance measures and the strategic measures. Strategy should focus on what drives desired results. The test of good strategy and strategic measures is whether successful deployment of the strategies results in improved performance as measured by the scorecard.

Dimensions of Performance in Healthcare

What is good performance in healthcare? How do we know whether we are doing a good job? How should we organize our important measures to have the greatest effect? What should be on our organizational scorecard?

These questions are critical for healthcare leaders. Exhibit 12.6 indicates that performance is an outcome of the leadership process and ultimately should be measured in terms of the organization's ability to achieve its mission and vision. Another way to think about performance is by important dimensions. Healthcare is about more than the bottom line. In exhibit 12.8, use of the word *performance* instead of *quality* emphasizes that performance is a broader concept that encompasses quality—although some advocates of QI theory may disagree. The point is that performance and quality in healthcare should be considered broadly; therefore, leaders and managers should identify the multiple important dimensions of performance for their organization, department, or function.

One method of defining performance is in terms of traditional financial, satisfaction, human resource, and clinical dimensions. However, many organizations have benefited from a broader view of the critical dimensions of performance, as shown in exhibit 12.8.

EXHIBIT 12.8
Critical Dimensions of Performance in Healthcare Organizations

- Patient Engagement
- Patient Satisfaction
- Effectiveness (clinical outcomes)
- Appropriateness (evidence and process)
- Safety (patient and staff)
- Equity
- Employee and Staff Satisfaction (culture)
- Efficiency (cost)
- Financial
- Flow (wait times, cycle times, and throughput)
- Access
- Population Health

Source: MdP Associates, LLC. Used with permission.

In its *Crossing the Quality Chasm* report, the Institute of Medicine (IOM) suggested a different way of thinking about performance in healthcare. It recommended that patient care be reorganized and redesigned to focus on six specific aims (IOM 2001):

- Safety
- Effectiveness
- Patient centeredness
- Timeliness
- Efficiency
- Equity

Some organizations have found these six aims useful in defining organizational performance and the metrics that should be included on their scorecards.

Organizations can use a variety of approaches to develop and define the important dimensions of performance. Traditional financial, human resource, satisfaction, and clinical dimensions provide the foundation for most methods. In addition, religiously affiliated healthcare organizations often include dimensions of performance related to the mission of their sponsoring organization.

Creating an Organizational Scorecard

The development of an organizational scorecard should involve more than a simple transfer of existing measures into a new format or framework. The first step is to decide on an appropriate framework. Next, senior leadership and the governing body should define the dimensions of performance that are relevant to the organization's mission and the results they wish to achieve. Once they have agreed on these dimensions, they should select appropriate outcome measures for each of the chosen dimensions.

At the organizational level, the ideal cycle time for performance measurement is quarterly. However, some metrics may be too difficult or expensive to obtain every quarter, so the organization may be forced to make exceptions and settle for one or more annual measures. Sometimes, the preferred outcome measure for a dimension does not exist, in which case the organization must use a proxy measure or invest in the development of new metrics.

Healthcare leaders and trustees should include enough measures in the organizational scorecard to define the desired results for each of the important dimensions. Initially, in their enthusiasm for the new approach and their desire to include great detail, organizations may identify more measures than are practical to track and focus on process measures rather than outcome measures. Additional measures may be interesting, but the focus should remain on results. Organizations can maintain this focus by concentrating on the results they want to achieve rather than on potentially good measures. In the for-profit corporate world, the aim is fairly straightforward—increased shareholder value (which extends beyond ever-changing stock prices). In the not-for-profit healthcare world, the aims may be more numerous, but they are just as measurable.

The governing body and senior leadership of a healthcare organization should use a scorecard to monitor overall performance and balance. They also should use it to assess CEO and leadership performance. Although boards and senior leadership will continue to look at supporting reports of financial performance, clinical quality, and other areas, they should focus on the results they wish to achieve as defined by the scorecard of organizational performance measures.

When possible, organizations should compare their performance results to the best levels of performance, or benchmarks, reported by similar types of organizations. They should then deploy strategies to close the gaps between their current performance scores and the benchmarks.

Benchmarking in healthcare is a challenge, but it is becoming easier in some areas. Benchmarks for patient and employee satisfaction are available through proprietary databases maintained by survey companies and by CMS. Comparative financial and workforce information is available through multiple sources—some free and some subscription based. Comparative clinical outcome metrics are becoming more widely available as well. Setting best-in-class targets and high expectations on performance scorecards will help organizations achieve their desired results and thus increase healthcare reliability in key areas.

For some clinical and safety measures, the organizational goal or target should be 100 percent or 0 percent. For instance, for the patient, there is no "right rate" of patient harm other than 0. Many healthcare organizations and leaders, however, struggle with the concept of 100 percent or 0 percent as a goal or target on a scorecard or a unit's visual board. One common approach is to acknowledge that the goal is "no harm" or "should always happen" but that current systems are incapable of producing that result. So, as an interim target, the organization might count the number of incidents (e.g., 20 patient falls with injury last quarter) and then set a target of reducing that number by 50 percent (or more) over a specified period to focus efforts on reduction of patient harm. Once that target has been achieved, the organization might then repeat the "cut in half" approach or switch to a measurement system that counts the "days since the last occurrence" method of measuring and informing staff about progress.

A healthcare organization could begin to create a scorecard by identifying potential measures for each of the six IOM aims. For example:

- Safety: Number of patient harm or serious safety events (SSEs)

- Effectiveness: Functional outcomes as defined by SF-12 health surveys,[5] hospital mortality rates, compliance with best-practice guidelines, and disease-specific measures
- Patient centeredness: Satisfaction levels reported on patient discharge survey
- Timeliness: Number of days until the third next available appointment
- Efficiency: Hospital or clinic costs per discharge
- Equity: Access to care and clinical outcomes compared by race/ethnicity and gender

The sample performance scorecard in exhibit 12.9 organizes the key metrics by culture, preventing harm (patient safety), clinical quality, and financial health, demonstrating the balance between the various dimensions. The scorecard then shows the ultimate level of performance to be achieved in three years, the performance target for the current year, and the prior year's performance. The quarterly performance is color-coded to indicate whether it exceeded, met, or fell below the target for that quarter.

EXHIBIT 12.9 Sample Performance Scorecard for a Hospital Board

Main Street Hospital FY 2018 Board Performance Scorecard		Exceeds Target	Meeting Target	Below Target			
CULTURE	**3 Year Goal**	**FY Target Range**	**Prior Year**	**FY 18 QTR 1**	**FY 18 QTR 2**	**FY 18 QTR 3**	**FY 18 QTR 4**
Employee Turnover Rate (Unplanned)	3% per quarter	5.5-6% per quarter	7.50%	2.41%	2.84%	4.00%	2.80%
Employee Satisfaction (% Recommend as Place to Work)	90%	60-70%	47%	75%	78%	80%	73%
PREVENTING HARM (Safety)	**3 Year Goal**	**FY Target Range**					
Falls with injury **(Quarterly)**	0	2-4 per Quarter	22 (FY)	5	5	3	5
Number of Patients Harmed from ADE	0	5-10 per Quarter	102 (FY)	12	13	7	3
# of Central Line Infections	0	0	9 (FY)	0	0	0	0
# of Ventilator Associated Pneumonia	0	0	6 (FY)	4	3	0	1
# of Pressure Ulcers	0	8-12 per Quarter	72 (FY)	20	26	10	12
CLINICAL QUALITY	**3 Year Goal**	**FY Target Range**					
EVIDENCE-BASED CARE % OF PATIENTS RECEIVING ALL REQUIRED ELEMENTS							
Acute MI	100%	90-95%	88%	98%	98%	96	97
Pneumonia	100%	80-90%	75%	69%	48%	59%	70%
Congestive Heart Failure	100%	90-95%	85%	90%	98%	95	92
Hospital Infection Rate (Per State Reporting Criteria)	5%	9-11%	14%	13.0%	14.5%	12.0%	10.5%
Unplanned Readmission Rate	0%	4-6.5%	8%	9.0%	5.0%	8.6	7.5
# of Inpatient Deaths (unplanned, non-comfort care mortality)	0	3-5 quarter	28 (FY)	6	8	5	5
FINANCIAL HEALTH	**3 Year Goal**	**FY Target Range**					
Contribution Margin %	8%	2.5 to 4%	1.50%	2.50%	-2%	3%	2.5%
Days Cash On Hand	180 days	80-90	65	89	80	67	81

Source: MdP Associates, LLC. Used with permission.

Case Study: Board-Adopted Quality Aims

In 2010, the board of a regional multihospital healthcare system in the southern United States was concerned about its governance oversight of quality performance. After several months of data review and the investigation of a series of patient harm events, the board adopted a set of high-level quality aims to be achieved over a five-year time frame. The aims included the following:

- Reduce overall mortality (excluding inevitable mortality) by 50 percent.
- Reduce all cases of patient harm by 80 percent.
- Provide the "right care" to 100 percent of patients.
- Reduce unplanned readmissions by 80 percent.
- Achieve patient satisfaction scores in the top 10 percent.

Exhibit 12.10 provides a simple but powerful one-page display of how the board set interim targets and tracked the key quality aims.

EXHIBIT 12.10 Dashboard of Quality Aims Tracked by the Board

	FY 2010	20%	FY 2011	Trend
Inpatient Mortalities	1,254	251	1,003	
Inpatient All-Cause Readmissions	10,392	2,078	8,314	
Harm				
Related to Medical Management	679	136	543	
Hospital Acquired Infections	1,549	310	1,239	
Related to Patient Care	905	181	724	
Other	14	3	11	
Total	3,147	629	2,518	
Sentinel Events	162	32	130	
with harm	75	15	60	
Perfect Care	81%	16	97%	

Source: MdP Associates, LLC. Used with permission.

The board-adopted aims provided a framework for the organizational quality and improvement strategy. In addition to using the high-level dashboard, the board routinely received reports from leadership on specific initiatives and measures linked to the aims. For example, leadership conducted an in-depth analysis of hospital mortality using a variety of tools and methods, which revealed that contributors to hospital mortality included sepsis recognition and management, device-related infections, delays in recognition and response to deteriorating patient conditions, delays in diagnosis and initiation of treatment, and incidences of falls and other patient harm events. Reducing mortality required multiple strategies and initiatives across the organization to reduce patient harm events and infections and to improve response times to critical patient needs.

Five years later, hospital mortality had been reduced by approximately 48 percent. The system calculated that more than 1,000 lives had been saved by the efforts to improve quality and performance.

Keys to Success

The successful use of measures and measurement to drive change and improve performance depends on a variety of factors. This section describes some of the critical steps that organizations can take to maximize their effectiveness.

Develop a Clear Understanding of the Intended Use

The CEO, senior leadership team, and board must have a clear understanding of why a scorecard or dashboard is being created and how the measures will be used to drive execution and improvement.

Engage the Governing Board in Development of Organizational Performance Measures

Ultimately, the governing body is responsible for the performance of the organization. This responsibility extends beyond simple fiduciary duties and includes clinical and service performance. Because scorecards should reflect desired performance results, governing bodies must be involved in defining the important dimensions, choosing the relevant measures, and setting the desired levels of performance. Much of the development work may be assigned to leadership and clinical teams, but the final determination of the important dimensions, the measures, and the targets is the board's responsibility.

Use the Scorecard to Evaluate Organizational and Leadership Performance

Once developed, the performance scorecard should be central to the organization's governance system. The scorecard should reflect the mission of the organization and be used by the board and leadership to evaluate progress toward achieving that mission. The governing board should review the scorecard at least quarterly. Because scorecards are about results, they can be useful in evaluating CEO performance and serve as a balanced set of objective measures that can be tied to compensation plans and performance criteria.

Be Prepared to Change the Measures

Developing a good organizational performance scorecard may sound like a simple idea, but it is difficult to do. An organization is unlikely to achieve a perfect set of measures the first time. Often, measures of desired results for a performance dimension do not exist and must be developed. Other times, organizations realize after a couple of review cycles that they want better measures than those they currently use. Scorecard development is usually an iterative process rather than a single-shot job. Organizations should continue to improve their scorecards as they gain an understanding of the desired results linked to each dimension and as better metrics are developed. Nevertheless, to borrow a phrase from the philosopher Voltaire and others, "Perfect is the enemy of good." Organizations should work toward creating a good scorecard, not a perfect one.

Make the Data Useful, Not Pretty

Scorecard formats should be useful and understandable. Many organizations struggle with fancy formats and attempts to create online versions. A good starting point is to construct simple run charts that display the measures over time and the desired target for each measure. Simple spreadsheet graphs can be dropped into a text document, four or six per page. The information conveyed, not the format, is what matters. Organizations have had mixed success with more sophisticated formats, such as radar charts. Some boards find radar charts invaluable because they display all the metrics and targets on a single page; other boards have difficulty interpreting the charts. The admonition to start simple does not imply that other approaches will not work. One innovative computer-based display, for instance, used a radar chart backed by hotlinked run and control charts for each performance metric.

Integrate the Measures to Achieve a Balanced View

Although some organizations like to use scorecard and dashboard formats for financial and quality reports, the routine display of metrics in separate, category-driven reports may reflect a lack of integration. Organizations that compile separate, detailed scorecards of financial, quality, and service metrics and review each independently, as tradition dictates, will probably place more emphasis on financial results and pay less attention to clinical, satisfaction, and other dimensions, except when a crisis erupts in one or more of these areas.

However, if an organization has developed a broader set of high-level measures and the category-based reports support those measures, the use of detailed, separate scorecards can be useful.

Develop Clear and Measurable Strategies

Kaplan and Norton (1992, 1996) contend that strategic measures should be central to the leadership system. Strategic dashboards and balanced scorecards are key tools that leaders can use to align strategies and actions. Unfortunately, in healthcare, strategy and strategic planning are generally underdeveloped. Many organizations engage in a superficial annual process that results in a set of vague objectives that are task oriented rather than strategic. Often, the strategic plan is then set aside until the time comes to prepare for the next board retreat. Organizations will have difficulty developing a balanced scorecard as envisioned by Kaplan and Norton if their strategies are not clear, measurable, and truly strategic. Most organizations do, in fact, have a simple set of critical strategies that, if successfully deployed, will accelerate progress toward their mission and vision. Organizations should clearly identify those critical strategies and develop a set of specific measures for each strategy.

Tracking progress on a specifically designed strategic dashboard can be highly effective. The choice of measures is important because they reflect what the strategy is intended to accomplish. Most critical strategies inspire innumerable ideas and potential approaches. All proposed tactics, initiatives, and projects should directly affect one or more strategic measures. If not, leadership should invest its resources elsewhere.

Use Organizational Performance Dimensions to Align Efforts

One approach for using scorecards and dashboards to create alignment is to build cascading sets of metrics that correspond to the key dimensions of performance on the scorecard. Under this approach, each operating unit or department is required to develop a set of metrics for each of the key dimensions. For example, if patient safety is a key dimension, each nursing unit could track and seek to improve its fall rate or rate of adverse drug events. If employee well-being is a key performance dimension, each department could track voluntary turnover rates. Executive review of departmental performance should include the entire set of clinical, process, financial service, and safety measures, rather than focusing on the financial dimension one month and a service or clinical quality dimension the next month.

Avoid Using Indicators Based on Averages

Because averages mask variation and tend to be misleading, they should be avoided when developing scorecards and dashboards. For example, the average time from door to drug in the emergency department may be lower than the preset operating standard; however, examination of the data may reveal that a significant percentage of patients do not receive treatment within the prescribed amount of time. A better approach is to measure the percentage of patients who receive treatment within the amount of time specified in the standard. Average waiting times, average length of stay, average satisfaction scores, and average cost are all suspect indicators.

Develop Composite Clinical Indicators for Processes and Outcome Indicators for Results

Approaches to clinical indicators continue to evolve. Healthcare organizations are complex and generally provide care across a wide spectrum of conditions and treatment regimens, and they often have difficulty determining which clinical indicators are truly important and representative of the processes of care provided. One approach is to develop composite indicators for high-volume, high-profile conditions. For example, the CMS review set for heart attack contains six cardiac indicators. Most hospital organizations track their performance against each of the indicators, which is appropriate at the operational level. However, at the senior leadership level, tracking the percentage of cardiac patients who received all six required elements may be more useful. This tracking accomplishes two things. First, it limits the number of metrics on a senior leadership or governing board scorecard. Second, it emphasizes that all patients should receive all required aspects of care in the bundle, not just four out of six.

Organizations can use the same approach to track performance for chronic diseases such as diabetes. They can establish the critical aspects of care that should always be performed (e.g., timely hemoglobin testing, referral to the diabetes educator, eye and foot exams) and develop a composite measure that reflects the percentage of patients who receive complete care.

Another approach to developing clinical performance metrics is to consider the results rather than the process. Mortality and readmission rates are obvious results. Some organizations are beginning to look beyond such measures and are considering clinical results from the perspective of the patient. Development of experimental questionnaires and new approaches to assessing patient function are under way and may include the following types of patient-centered questions:

- Was pain controlled to my expectations?
- Am I better today as a result of the treatment I received?
- Am I able to function today at the level I expected?
- Is my function restored to the level it was at before I became ill or was injured?
- Did I receive the help I need to manage my ongoing condition?

- Am I aware of anything that went wrong in the course of my treatment that delayed my recovery or compromised my condition?

Use Comparative Data and External Benchmarks

When possible, use external benchmark data to establish standards and targets. Many organizations track mortality and readmission rates on their scorecards. Mortality is a much stronger performance measure when it is risk adjusted and compared to other organizations' performance to establish a frame of reference. Without that frame of reference, mortality tracking provides little useful information other than directional trends.

Beyond establishing a frame of reference, however, organizations should set targets based on best performance in class, rather than peer group averages. Comparison to a peer group mean tends to reinforce mediocrity and deflects attention from the importance of the desired result monitored by the performance measure. Consider, for instance, the peer averages and percentiles that most vendors of national patient satisfaction surveys provide. Being above average or in the top quartile does not necessarily equate to high patient satisfaction. A significant percentage of patients may be indifferent about or dissatisfied with the care they received. Instead of percentile-based targets (targets based on ranking), average raw score or the percentage of patients who express dissatisfaction may be better indicators.

Change Your Leadership System

One mistake that some organizations have made is to roll out an elaborate set of cascading dashboards and scorecards and then fail to change the way the leadership system functions. Scorecards and dashboards can quickly become another compliance effort, or something done for The Joint Commission outside of the organization's "real work." Leadership must make the review of measurement sets an integral part of its function. When senior leaders review departments or operating units, the unit scorecard or dashboard should be their primary focus. If a strategic dashboard is developed, progress review should occur at least monthly or be coordinated with the measurement cycles of the indicators. Governing boards should review the organizational performance measures at least quarterly. Reviews should not be done solely for the sake of reviewing but for the purposes of driving change and setting priorities.

Focus on Results, Not on Activities

A well-developed system of dashboards and scorecards allows leadership to focus on results instead of activities. Many results-oriented, high-performing organizations work from a leadership philosophy of tight-loose-tight. Senior leaders are very clear and "tight" about the results they wish to achieve and measure them through the use of strategic and operational dashboards. At the same time, they are "loose" in their direct control of those doing the work, creating a sense of empowerment in those charged with achieving the results. In the absence of clear measures, leaders tend to control activities, micromanage, and disempower others in the organization. When desired results are clear, senior leaders can be "tight" about holding individuals and teams accountable for achieving them.

Cultivate Transparency

One characteristic of high-performing organizations, such as Baldrige Award winners, is that every employee knows how her individual efforts fit into the bigger picture. Healthcare has a long tradition of secrecy about results—in part a reflection of the historical view that quality is about physician peer review and in part a reaction to the malpractice environment. Transparency is a big step for some organizations, but the results gathered on the organizational scorecard should be discussed openly and shared with employees and clinical staff. Ideally, the results should also be shared with the community served.

Employees and clinical staff need to know what dimensions of performance are important to the organization, what process and management indicators are used for evaluation, what dashboards are related to their daily work, what the quarterly performance results are, and what those results mean. The same is true for strategic measures. Many organizations seek to keep their strategic measures confidential and do not routinely share them with employees. That approach is usually counterproductive. After all, successful deployment of strategy depends on what an organization itself does, not on what its competitors may do. Sometimes, a specific tactic, such as building a new clinic in a competitive part of town, may need to be kept confidential because of market issues, but the critical strategy relating to growth of the enterprise should not be a secret. Creating awareness and improving key processes can be difficult if the underlying strategy and strategic measures are not widely known.

Conclusion

Healthcare organizations are complex service-delivery systems, and they are increasingly dependent on quality and performance measures for regulatory and payment purposes. Performance is measured across multiple dimensions, including financial performance, patient experience, clinical outcomes, employee engagement, and patient safety. Scorecards and dashboards are useful leadership and governance tools for creating focus and alignment within the organization on areas that need to be improved, and they are critical to tracking progress on strategic objectives. A direct link should exist between an organization's strategy and quality improvement efforts, so that resources are committed to improvements that move the organizational and governance performance measures in the desired direction.

Notes

1. The Medicare Access and CHIP Reauthorization Act of 2015 (MACRA) was passed with bipartisan support and signed into law on April 16, 2015. MACRA created the Quality Payment Program that repeals the Sustainable Growth Rate formula, changes the way that Medicare rewards clinicians for value over volume, streamlines quality programs under the Merit-Based Incentive Payments System (MIPS), and provides bonus payments for participation in eligible alternative payment models (CMS 2018).
2. Kevin Sower shared this information during a panel discussion at the 2016 Institute for Healthcare Improvement (IHI) Change Conference. The chapter author was a member of the IHI Expert faculty supporting the conference and verified the statements with Mr. Sower.
3. In deference to the work of Kaplan and Norton (1992, 1996) and the specific idea of leaders using balanced scorecards of strategic measures, this chapter does not use the term *balanced scorecard* except in direct reference to Kaplan and Norton's concept. Instead, it discusses the use of dashboards and scorecards in broader, generic terms, exploring a variety of applications that create focus and alignment in healthcare organizations.
4. A popular approach has been to use the "stoplight" color scheme of red, yellow, and green to highlight indicators when performance is judged against a predetermined standard. Indicators that reflect negative performance are highlighted in red, and indicators judged to be satisfactory or above expectations are highlighted in green. Yellow can signify caution or need for further review. Although useful for identifying problems or failure to meet a target, this format does not provide trended information useful for assessing progress or decline and, depending on the standard chosen, may reinforce poor actual results.
5. The 12-Item Short Form Health Survey (SF-12) was developed for the Medical Outcomes Study, a multiyear study of patients with chronic conditions (RAND Corporation 2018). The short-form survey instrument provides a solution to the problem faced by many investigators who have needed to restrict survey length. The instrument was designed to reduce respondent burden while still achieving minimum standards of precision for purposes of group comparisons across multiple health dimensions.

Study Questions

1. Based on your experience with healthcare, what do you consider the important dimensions of performance? How would you know whether an organization is performing well? What indicators do you think are important for a hospital to track? For a physician practice? A home care agency? A long-term care facility? A managed care organization?
2. What might be good indicators of patient centeredness as recommended by the Institute of Medicine?
3. What are some of the pitfalls of overmeasurement? How do you determine what is important to measure in an organization?
4. Why is creating alignment an important leadership function? What are some methods of creating alignment, and how can the use of measurement support their deployment?

References

Aguayo, R. 1991. *Dr. Deming: The American Who Taught the Japanese About Quality.* New York: Simon & Schuster.

Centers for Medicare & Medicaid Services (CMS). 2018. "MACRA." Modified September 21. www.cms.gov/Medicare/Quality-Initiatives-Patient-Assessment-Instruments/Value-Based-Programs/MACRA-MIPS-and-APMs/MACRA-MIPS-and-APMs.html.

Deming, W. E. 2000. *The New Economics for Industry, Government, Education*, 2nd ed. Cambridge, MA: MIT Press.

Institute for Healthcare Improvement (IHI). 2018. "IHI Triple Aim Initiative." Accessed November 9. www.ihi.org/Engage/Initiatives/TripleAim/Pages/default.aspx.

Institute of Medicine (IOM). 2001. *Crossing the Quality Chasm: A New Health System for the 21st Century.* Washington, DC: National Academies Press.

Juran, J. M. 1974. *Quality Control Handbook*, 3rd ed. New York: McGraw-Hill.

Kaplan, R. S., and D. P. Norton. 1996. *The Balanced Scorecard: Translating Strategy into Action.* Boston: HBS Press.

———. 1992. "The Balanced Scorecard: Measures That Drive Performance." *Harvard Business Review* 70 (1): 71–79.

RAND Corporation. 2018. "12-Item Short Form Survey (SF-12)." Accessed November 9. www.rand.org/health/surveys_tools/mos/12-item-short-form.html.

Stiefel, M., and K. Nolan. 2012. "A Guide to Measuring the Triple Aim: Population Health, Experience of Care, and Per Capita Cost." Institute for Healthcare Improvement. Accessed November 9, 2018. www.ihi.org/resources/Pages/IHIWhitePapers/AGuidetoMeasuringTripleAim.aspx.

Swensen, S., M. Pugh, C. McMullan, and A. Kabcenell. 2013. "High-Impact Leadership: Improve Care, Improve the Health of Populations, and Reduce Costs." Institute for Healthcare Improvement. Accessed November 9, 2018. www.ihi.org/resources/Pages/IHIWhitePapers/HighImpactLeadership.aspx.

CHAPTER

13

GOVERNANCE FOR QUALITY

Kathryn C. Peisert

Background: Why Is Quality the Board's Responsibility?

When we think about "governance" in relation to healthcare quality, what does it really mean? Why do healthcare provider institutions require governance in addition to healthcare leadership? This chapter explores the need for governance of healthcare quality, discusses who the "governors" are and in which care settings governance applies, defines and demonstrates how boards ensure high-quality care, and examines the differing roles of boards versus healthcare leadership in overseeing and ensuring quality.

What Is Governance?

Governance is "the process through which the representatives of the owners of an organization oversee the mission, strategy, executive leadership, quality performance, and financial stewardship of the institution. The owner's representatives usually are structured into a board of directors or board of trustees. (In the case of not-for-profit institutions, the owner is the community—usually through a state-chartered process monitored by the state's attorney general.)" (Reinertsen 2014, 358)

An Ethical and Legal Obligation

Although individual physicians and other clinicians are directly responsible for the care provided to their patients, countless systemic issues can arise in complex healthcare settings, and patients, especially in hospitals, are "touched" by many care providers other than their personal physician. Thus, all not-for-profit hospitals and health systems in the United States are overseen by a board of directors or board of trustees that serves as the ultimate body responsible for the quality of care provided. Not-for-profit physician groups and accountable care organizations also are usually overseen by a board. As an increasing number of physicians become employed by hospitals and health systems, these boards also are responsible for the quality of care provided in doctors' offices and outpatient clinics owned by hospitals and systems. In short, there are very few care settings in which a board does not exist to oversee quality of care.

The board is primarily made up of unpaid volunteers from various business backgrounds and prominent members of the community, and it holds legally binding fiduciary duties to ensure that the organization fulfills its mission of providing safe, high-quality care to patients. The board is also legally required to ensure strong financial stability and to set the organization's vision and strategic direction.

The responsibility for quality is central to healthcare organizations' mission—it is essentially their very purpose. Quality of care is intricately related to a healthcare organization's brand reputation, success, and—as the industry moves away from fee-for-service to value-based payments—financial well-being. As such, the board needs to set strategic direction for the organization with regard to quality and include quality goals in the strategic plan.

Two Fiduciary Duties

The term *fiduciary* suggests a duty that is "held in trust," and a board's fiduciary concerns go beyond a simple responsibility for a corporation's financial health. The responsibility for quality in healthcare falls under two fiduciary duties: the *duty of care* and the *duty of obedience to the mission*.

The duty of care requires directors to act in "good faith," with the same level of care that an ordinarily prudent person would exercise in similar circumstances, and in a manner that they reasonably believe to be in the best interest of the organization and its stakeholders. In a not-for-profit hospital, stakeholders include employees, physicians, the community, and, most importantly, patients.

The duty of obedience requires that directors be faithful to the underlying charitable purposes and goals of the nonprofit organization they serve, as set forth in the organization's governing documents. It presumes that the mission of the organization and the means to achieve it are inseparable (Peregrine 2005).

The board's ultimate responsibility for quality was affirmed in the landmark 1965 court case *Darling v. Charleston Community Memorial Hospital*. The plaintiff in the case, Dorrence Darling II, had been taken to the emergency room at Charleston Community Memorial Hospital, in Illinois, after breaking his leg, and the attending physician, Dr. Alexander, set the break and put Darling's leg in a cast. The next day, however, Darling's toes turned dark and cold. Much of the tissue in the leg had become necrotic from constriction caused by the cast, and eventually the lower leg had to be amputated. Darling brought suit against Alexander and the hospital. After settling with Alexander, he tried the case against Charleston, and the jury returned a verdict of $150,000. The court of appeals affirmed the ruling, and the Supreme Court of Illinois granted review on the question of whether a hospital could be held liable for the negligence of its staff (CaseBriefs 2018). The answer to the question was yes, and the ruling thereby placed responsibility for quality of care directly on the hospital board.[1] This decision is reflected in the standards set by The Joint Commission (2016), the primary accrediting institution for US hospitals, which say that a hospital's governing body is ultimately responsible for the quality of care provided by the hospital.[2]

Another important reason for board oversight of quality of care is that successfully addressing quality involves more than just singling out individual care providers who might have made mistakes; rather, it requires a "systemic" approach—one that takes into account every action in the course of a patient's experience, from the doctor's office to the hospital and even after leaving the hospital. Over the past 20 years, healthcare leaders and boards have learned that, given the complexity of our healthcare system, opportunities for errors are many. Most errors occur not because a clinician is careless or lacks proper knowledge but because the complexity of the system allows for such errors to occur. What needs to be addressed are the processes, procedures, and culture of the organization (Reinertsen and Resar 2006).

The Institute for Healthcare Improvement (IHI), which has done much of the legwork to demonstrate systemic quality improvements, posits the following (IHI 2018):

> The board's responsibility for ensuring and improving care cannot be delegated to the medical staff and executive leadership; ensuring safe and harm-free care to the patients is the board's job, at the very core of their fiduciary responsibility. An activated board, in partnership with executive leadership, can set system-level expectations and accountability for high performance and the elimination of harm, and, properly conducted, this leadership work can dramatically and continually improve the quality of care in the hospital.[3]

When the board sets the tone from the top, changes can be made throughout the entire organization. Without emphasis and support from the board, quality improvements can be extremely difficult to implement and sustain.

The Relationship Between the Board and Hospital Management for Ensuring Quality

Hospitals and health systems employ high-level senior executives and physician leaders who are responsible for quality, including the chief executive officer

(CEO), chief medical officer (CMO), and chief quality officer, among others. So why do they also need a board to oversee quality?

The board has the ultimate responsibility for quality because it is at the top of the leadership hierarchy. It is responsible for overseeing management and holding senior leaders accountable. It hires—and, when necessary, fires—the chief executive.

The role of the board and the role of management in ensuring quality have important distinctions. Other chapters in this book cover the role of management in greater detail, but for the purposes of this chapter, the board's role differs from that of management in the following ways:

- The board charges management with making recommendations on which metrics to monitor, and it holds management accountable for meeting quality targets. The board relies on management to provide information about quality metrics so that the board can ensure that the metrics being used are those necessary for accreditation, compliance, and reimbursement requirements, as well as for providing a true picture of how the organization is doing with regard to quality and patient safety. The board makes the final decisions on which metrics to use. (Further information will be provided in the section on measuring quality at the board level.)
- The board sets strategies and policies around quality and related goals, and it charges management with implementing such strategies and policies and developing plans to achieve goals for board approval and monitoring.
- Although the board needs to have a detailed enough picture of how the hospital or health system is doing with regard to quality and patient safety, with very few exceptions, the board should not drill down to such a level of detail that it becomes involved in advising managers and quality improvement staff on how they should be accomplishing their goals. Essentially, in governance, the board determines the "what," and management figures out "how."
- The best way for board members to hold management accountable for quality is to ask deep, probing questions that get at the root causes of quality problems. Board members need not have healthcare expertise to successfully monitor quality, as long as they have a strong understanding of their role versus the role of management and physician leaders.

Research Connecting Board Practices with Quality

Proving quantitatively that board oversight affects quality is nearly impossible, given the layers and uncontrolled variables between the board and frontline patient care. Nonetheless, it is well known and understood, generally speaking, that governance affects quality of care and, more specifically, that effective boards help to improve quality. Several studies over the past decade have found statistically significant correlations between board practices and care outcomes. Some of that research has been limited to board practices specifically related to quality oversight, whereas other research has looked at board practices in other areas of oversight as well.

In one of the first studies looking at the board's oversight of quality, Joshi and Hines (2006) sought to determine the extent to which hospital leaders understand safety and quality issues, which actions boards and CEOs were taking to drive quality improvement, and whether board knowledge and daily activities were associated with different outcomes. The researchers conducted interviews with board chairs and CEOs at 30 hospitals in 14 states and also used a survey instrument to measure expertise and knowledge in quality improvement. Results showed significant differences between the CEO's perception of the level of knowledge of the board chairs and the board chairs' self-perception. A mild association was found between board engagement in quality and hospital performance as defined by rates in a composite measure of heart failure, heart attack, and pneumonia. Joshi and Hines (2006) identified the following areas of opportunity for engaging hospital boards to improve overall hospital performance:

1. Increasing education on quality to increase the board's quality literacy
2. Improving the framing of an agenda for quality
3. More planning, focus, and incentives for leadership and governance for quality improvement
4. Greater focus on patients

Prybil and colleagues (2012) conducted a four-phase, in-depth study of governance in the nation's largest health systems in 2012. The study was not focused specifically on quality oversight, but it identified a composite listing of nine "contemporary benchmarks of effective governance," with several indicators for each benchmark. All of these benchmarks likely have an effect on quality oversight, due to their being considered characteristics of an effective board overall. However, for the purposes of this chapter, the following four benchmarks from the study are most closely related to quality of care (Prybil et al. 2012):

- Effective boards insist on governance policies and structures that facilitate efforts to perform the board's functions and fulfill its responsibilities.
- Effective boards are made up of highly dedicated people who collectively have the competencies, diversity, and independence

that produce constructive, well-informed deliberations. (Clinician engagement in governance is included as an indicator for this benchmark.)

- Effective boards insist on meetings that are well organized; focus principally on systemwide strategy and key priorities, such as patient care quality and community benefit; and use board members' time and energy wisely.
- Effective boards purposefully create a culture that nurtures enlivened engagement, mutual trust, willingness to act, and high standards of performance.

Prybil, Bardach, and Fardo (2014) conducted a follow-up study of board oversight of patient care quality in 14 of the largest nonprofit US health systems. They identified the following common characteristics of quality-focused board actions that are supported by the benchmarks of effective governance identified in the 2012 study (Prybil, Bardach, and Fardo 2014):

1. A standing committee with oversight responsibility for patient quality and safety
2. Formal adoption of systemwide quality measures and standards
3. Regular written reports on systemwide and hospital quality performance
4. Adoption of action plans directed at improving systemwide performance with respect to patient care quality

In 2008 and 2009, Jiang and colleagues conducted analyses that compared board practices related to quality—using data from The Governance Institute's 2006 quality survey of all US not-for-profit hospitals and health systems (Lockee et al. 2006)—against hospital outcome measures reported to the Centers for Medicare & Medicaid Services (CMS). The analyses identified the following board practices that had a statistically significant positive correlation with patient outcomes (Jiang et al. 2008, 2009):

- Establishing a board-level quality committee
- Reviewing quality performance measures using dashboards or balanced scorecards at least quarterly to identify needs for corrective action
- Basing hospital quality goals on the theoretical ideal (e.g., reducing sepsis cases to zero)
- Reporting quality and safety performance to the public
- Requiring new clinical programs and services to meet quality-related performance criteria

- Devoting a significant amount of time to quality issues and related discussion at most board meetings
- Involving the board and medical staff in setting the organization's quality goals
- Having the board participate in the development and approval of explicit criteria to guide medical staff appointments, reappointments, and clinical privileges

In a survey of almost 1,000 hospital board chairs, Jha and Epstein (2010) revealed differences in board activities between high-performing and low-performing hospitals. Their key findings included the following:

- 87 percent of high-performing hospitals have moderate or substantial expertise in quality of care on their boards, compared with only 66 percent of low-performing hospitals.
- 49 percent of high-performing hospitals provide formal training in clinical quality to their boards, as opposed to 21 percent of low-performing hospitals.
- Board chairs of high-performing hospitals were twice as likely as those of low-performing hospitals to choose clinical quality as one of the top two priorities for board oversight.
- Quality performance was on the agenda at every board meeting for 74 percent of the high-performing hospitals, as opposed to 57 percent of the low-performing hospitals.
- 91 percent of boards at high-performing hospitals regularly review quality dashboards, as opposed to 62 percent at low-performing hospitals.

In another study, The Governance Institute compared adoption and performance of board practices in all oversight areas from its 2013 biennial survey of hospitals and healthcare systems (Peisert 2013) against process-of-care and clinical outcomes scores from the CMS Value-Based Purchasing (VBP) data set for fiscal year (FY) 2014 (Stepnick 2014). The methodology was to match, where possible, hospital-specific responses from the 2013 survey to the publicly reported performance on measures included within the FY 2014 CMS VBP program. The VBP program calculates four separate scores (Stepnick 2014):

- The *process-of-care (POC)* score is determined by performance on a standard set of measures in four different areas of care: (1) acute myocardial infarction (two measures), (2) pneumonia (two measures), (3) heart failure (one measure), and (4) hospital-associated infections (seven measures).

- The *patient experience of care* score is based on performance in eight areas measured by the Hospital Consumer Assessment of Healthcare Providers and Systems (HCAHPS) survey: communication with doctors, communication with nurses, responsiveness of hospital staff, pain management, communication about medicines, hospital cleanliness and quietness, discharge information, and overall hospital rating.
- The *clinical outcomes* score is based on performance on mortality rates within 30 days of patient discharge for heart attack, heart failure, and pneumonia.
- The *total VBP* composite score is calculated by giving a 45 percent weighting to the POC scores, 30 percent to patient experience scores, and 25 percent to clinical outcomes scores.

Exhibit 13.1 lists 27 distinct board practices that showed a significant correlation with better performance on the overall VBP score and/or the POC and clinical outcomes components of that score. Practices with markings in more than one column were found to be correlated with better performance on multiple components, suggesting broad value in promoting quality (Stepnick 2014). The practices in the list that are not directly related to quality oversight are considered practices of boards that are high-performing in all areas of oversight; thus, we can infer that such practices are likely to reflect strong performance in quality oversight duties.

EXHIBIT 13.1
Board Practices Associated with Higher Value-Based Purchasing Scores

Board Practice	Total Score	Process of Care Score	Clinical Outcomes Score
PRACTICES RELATED TO QUALITY OVERSIGHT			
The board requires major hospital clinical programs and services to meet quality-related performance criteria.	X		
The board includes objective measures for the achievement of clinical improvement and/or patient safety goals as part of the CEO's performance evaluation.	X	X	
The board requires that major strategic projects specify both measurable criteria for success and who has responsibility for implementation of the projects.	X	X	
The board requires management to base at least some of the organization's quality goals on the "theoretical ideal" (e.g., no central line infections, no sepsis).		X	
The board is willing to challenge recommendations of the medical executive committee(s) regarding physician appointment or reappointment to the medical staff.		X	X

EXHIBIT 13.1
Board Practices Associated with Higher Value-Based Purchasing Scores *(continued)*

PRACTICES RELATED TO COMMUNITY HEALTH			
The board provides oversight with respect to organizational compliance with IRS requirements to maintain its tax-exempt status that pertain to community benefit and other related issues.	X	X	X
The board considers how the organization's strategic plan addresses community health status and needs before approving the plan.	X	X	
The board has adopted a policy or policies on community benefit that include all of the following: a statement of its commitment, a process for board oversight, a definition of community benefit, a methodology for measuring community benefit, measurable goals for the organization, a financial assistance policy, and a commitment to communicate transparently with the public.	X	X	
The board ensures the adoption and implementation of strategies to meet the needs identified in the community health assessment.		X	
The board requires that management report each year on the community benefit value provided by the organization to the general public (i.e., the community).		X	
The board ensures that a community health needs assessment is conducted at least every three years to understand the health issues of the communities being served.	X	X	
PRACTICES RELATED TO AUDIT AND COMPLIANCE			
The board has established a direct reporting relationship with the compliance officer.		X	
The board has a written external audit policy that makes the board responsible for approving the auditor and the audit oversight process.			X
The board has adopted a policy that specifies that the audit committee (or other committee/subcommittee with primary responsibility for audit oversight) must be composed entirely of independent persons who have appropriate qualifications to serve in such a role.			X
The board seeks expert advice and information on industry comparables from independent (i.e., third party) sources before approving executive compensation.	X	X	X
Board members responsible for audit oversight meet with external auditors, without management, at least annually.	X		X
The board delegates its executive compensation oversight function to a group (committee, ad hoc group, task force, etc.) composed solely of independent directors of the board.	X		X
The board (directly or through a dedicated committee) ensures that the compliance plan is properly implemented and effective.		X	
The board has created a separate audit committee, audit/compliance committee, or another specific committee/subcommittee to oversee the external and internal audit functions.			X
The board works closely with legal counsel to assure all advocacy efforts are consistent with tax-exempt status requirements.	X		

(continued)

EXHIBIT 13.1 Board Practices Associated with Higher Value-Based Purchasing Scores *(continued)*

OTHER "GOOD GOVERNANCE" PRACTICES			
The board uses competency-based criteria when selecting new members.	X	X	
The board reviews the sufficiency of the organizational structure every five years.	X		
The board assists the organization in communicating with key external stakeholders (e.g., community leaders, potential donors).	X		
The board has a written policy establishing its role in fund development and/or philanthropy.			X
The board assesses its own bylaws/structure at least every three years.	X		
Board members complete a full conflict-of-interest disclosure statement annually.			X
The board receives important background materials within sufficient time to prepare for meetings.	X		

Source: Reprinted with permission from The Governance Institute (Stepnick 2014).

Finally, a more recent US study reviewed data from surveys of nationally representative groups of hospitals in the United States and England to examine the relationships among hospital boards, management practices of frontline managers, and the quality of care delivered (Tsai et al. 2015). The researchers found that (1) hospitals with more effective management practices provided higher-quality care and (2) higher-rated hospital boards had superior performance by hospital management staff. They also identified two signatures of high-performing hospital boards and management practice. First, "hospitals with boards that paid greater attention to clinical quality had management that better monitored quality performance." Second, "hospitals with boards that used clinical quality metrics more effectively had higher performance by hospital management staff on target setting and operations" (Tsai et al. 2015, 1304).

The studies discussed in this section used different methodologies and presented different results, but they share a common theme: They make meaningful connections between board activities and quality of care. To achieve desired results, effective boards rely on a framework for fulfilling their quality oversight responsibilities. The framework is a compilation of information from the research described in this section; lessons learned in the field from such groups as IHI, the Agency for Healthcare Research and Quality (AHRQ), and The Joint Commission; and work from The Governance Institute, with quantitative data and supporting information from healthcare consultants, attorneys, hospital executives, and academic experts.

Best Practices for Quality Oversight

The Governance Institute has developed a list of board "best practices" (those practices that are applicable for most boards at most types of not-for-profit hospitals and health systems) related to quality oversight. The list is the product of 20 years of surveying hospital and health system boards on how they spend their time, as well as consulting with healthcare experts and attorneys on how boards need to fulfill their fiduciary obligations with respect to quality (Peisert 2013, 2017):

- The board reviews quality performance measures (using dashboards, balanced scorecards, run charts, or other standard mechanisms for board-level reporting) at least quarterly to identify needs for corrective action.
- The board requires all hospital clinical programs or services to meet quality-related performance criteria.
- The board includes objective measures for the achievement of clinical improvement and/or patient safety goals as part of the CEO's performance evaluation.
- The board participates in the development and/or approval of explicit criteria to guide medical staff recommendations for physician appointments, reappointments, and clinical privileges.
- The board works with medical staff and management to set the organization's quality goals.
- The board devotes a significant amount of time in its board meeting agendas to quality issues/discussion.
- The board requires management to base *at least some* of the organization's quality goals on the "theoretical ideal" (e.g., zero central line infections, zero sepsis).
- The board reviews its quality performance by comparing its current performance to its own historical performance, as well as industry benchmarks.
- The board has a standing quality committee.
- The board reviews patient satisfaction / patient experience scores at least annually (including information publicly reported by CMS).
- The board participates at least annually in education related to its responsibility for quality of care.
- The board has adopted a policy for the reporting of the organization's quality/safety performance to the general public.
- The board is willing to challenge recommendations of the medical executive committee regarding physician appointment or reappointment to the medical staff.

What Are the Board's Quality Oversight Duties?

As part of its leadership role, the board establishes an organizational definition of *quality* and a formal policy or statement that puts quality of care and patient safety at the forefront of the organization's priorities. The board provides affirmation that quality care is the primary purpose of the organization. A framework for the board's leadership of quality is shown in exhibit 13.2.

Ensuring Quality and Patient Safety

The board needs to ensure that an efficient and effective quality program is in place and operating as expected in all settings where the organization's patients receive care. The board must ensure that working mechanisms are in place to measure, maintain, and improve quality, safety, and patient experience. The board approves quality improvement plans and goals, monitors performance in relation to those goals, and exercises accountability in seeing that the goals are met. It sets the quality agenda for the organization, weighs issues and concerns, and establishes priorities, such as top goals for the coming year and key targets to achieve in three to five years.

Measuring Quality and Setting Performance Targets

The board cannot set the quality agenda without knowing the organization's key issues and concerns. The best way to gain that knowledge is to have a robust measuring system in place that shows hospital quality performance over time and also compares the organization to other similar organizations in the region and across the nation. This comparison is known as *benchmarking*, and

EXHIBIT 13.2 Framework: Board Leadership of Quality

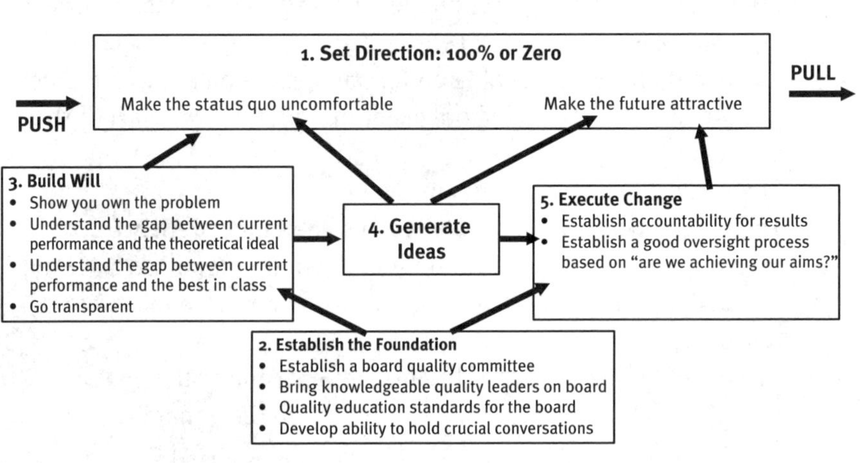

Source: James Reinertsen and Roger Resar, VHA Georgia, October 2006. Reprinted with permission from Reinertsen and Resar (2006).

the goal of benchmarking is to identify a minimum acceptable performance standard and work to exceed it.

Hospitals should benchmark themselves against "the best" rather than an average. In today's healthcare industry, performing "above average" is not a strong enough target to set. Rigorous quality improvement processes and applications of reliability science have helped many organizations achieve significantly higher quality of care and dramatic reductions in certain medical errors and patient safety concerns—for instance, reducing sepsis or ventilator-associated pneumonia to zero (Reinertsen and Resar 2006). Thus, boards should be setting both aggressive targets that are achievable and "theoretical ideals" that stretch the organization to make bigger improvements faster.

Gathering and reporting quality data are key parts of this process, and the data need to be organized in a way that is meaningful and useful to those who are interpreting them. Hospitals and health systems thus need to invest in not only a strong electronic medical record used by all physicians but also data reporting technology.

The items measured should result from strategic board-level decisions about where to focus quality improvement efforts. Management and the quality improvement staff assist the board in determining what to measure and how to set targets. Quality of care needs to be measured in many different ways, and targets should be set based on certain time frames (i.e., how much, by when).

The board and board quality committee should regularly review quality dashboard reports showing metrics that are considered to be indicators of quality and patient safety. Over time, other areas will be chosen for emphasis, depending on the board's decisions about where to shift improvement efforts. The improvement processes—their design, implementation, measurement, analysis, reporting, and corrective actions—are then carried out by hospital and health system staff under the direction of management and physician leadership.

Metrics commonly used to measure quality come from CMS, The Joint Commission, the National Quality Forum (NQF), AHRQ, and other groups. Organizations participating in any type of value-based payment model measure quality according to metrics agreed upon between the payer and the organization. For instance, participants in the Medicare Shared Savings Program have a specific set of metrics on which to focus and are paid based on whether targets are met. Some typical quality indicators include the following:

- NQF "never events" and sentinel events defined by The Joint Commission
- Hospital-acquired conditions (e.g., pressure ulcers, device-associated infections)
- Surgical wound infections
- Overall hospital/system mortality
- Neonatal mortality

- Perioperative mortality
- Cesarean section rate
- Heart failure "appropriate care" measures
- Pneumonia "appropriate care" measures
- Inpatient fall rate per 1,000 inpatient days
- Bundled payment metrics, such as complete joint replacement protocols
- Unplanned readmissions to the hospital (or overall hospital readmissions)
- Unplanned transfers to a special care unit
- Unplanned returns to the operating room
- Patient experience measures (e.g., doctor/nurse communication, hospital environment, staff responsiveness)

Measuring outcomes alone is not sufficient. Some adverse outcomes are very rare, and others develop over long periods of time. In addition, many significant intermediate steps ultimately affect outcomes. Incidents of "almost harm" are also of concern and should be reported. Given that quality improvement involves efforts by the hospital or health system to improve its care processes, the board needs to monitor and measure these processes as well.

Another way to evaluate quality of care is to focus on service outcomes, which assess patients' experience while in the hospital. Many of these experience measures are included in the HCAHPS surveys, which hospitals are required to conduct and report to CMS (with a portion of hospital reimbursement for Medicare patients being tied to these scores). Examples of such measures include length of wait in the emergency room, ease of preadmission procedures, staff responsiveness, doctor communication, nurse communication, and hospital environment. Organizations using a population health model need to measure population health–related metrics such as indicators for diabetes risk, detection, and management; obesity reduction; behaviors such as exercise, diet, and tobacco use; and preventable hospitalizations.

The Quality Dashboard Report for the Board

As part of the measurement process, management and quality improvement staff prepare an in-depth report for the board-level quality committee. Staff members also prepare another, shorter report for the board that provides essential information at a glance, with key, high-level indicators related to quality, patient safety, and patient experience. Dashboards typically report 12 months of performance and are trended over time to reveal the effect of improvement efforts on each of the measures they present.

The board dashboard conveys the most important information on a single page, with backup dashboards for more detail, and it uses color coding to make key changes instantly visible. The dashboard includes benchmarks and trended data to offer context, and it summarizes the big picture for the board; operational details are not included. It should be concise yet, at the same time, provide information on the major clinical services the hospital provides. The dashboard report needs to be connected to the information systems currently used to measure quality within the organization, and it needs to summarize the important aspects of quality, safety, and patient experience.

Both the dashboard report and an accompanying presentation (by a member of management or a clinical leader) should highlight problem areas and significant variations for the board or the board quality committee. Directors, in particular, will want to look at persistent trends that are below targets. They should seek information that assures them that the staff is working to understand why the hospital or health system is not performing as it should and that immediate steps are being taken to improve.

Dashboards are often distributed to management, the medical executive committee, and supervisory staff to improve communication among these groups. The quality indicators featured on the dashboard can be affected by many levels of the organization, and hospital staff need to be aware of which indicators need improvement and which changes will be put in place to meet targets. Sample dashboards are shown in exhibits 13.3 and 13.4 (Byrnes 2012; Byrnes and Fifer 2010b).

EXHIBIT 13.3 Sample Board and Executive Quality Dashboard

Composite Measures	FY13 Target	FY16 Target	Ending September 2013	Comments or Notes
Core Measures and HCAHPS				
1. Appropriate Care Score (24-month mean)	95%	100%	96%	Meeting 2013 target
2. HCAHPS (24-month mean)	80%	85%	78%	May miss 2013 target
3. VBP Estimate (% payment and amount)	125%/ $1.9 M	200%/ $3.5 M	97%/$1.6 M	Estimating a partial loss of withhold
Readmissions and Mortality				
1. Overall Readmission Rate (24-month mean)	12.5%	10.0%	12.2%	Statistically significant decrease in January 2013
2. Overall Mortality Rate (24-month mean)	1.9%	1.7%	2.3%	No improvement
Safety				
1. AHRQ Patient Safety Measures (%>AHRQ benchmark, rolling 12 month)	<20%	0%	13.3% (2/15)	Meeting 2013 target
2. Serious Safety Event Rate (rolling 12 months)	0.50	0.20	0.88	Meeting 2013 target

(continued)

EXHIBIT 13.3 Sample Board and Executive Quality Dashboard *(continued)*

3. Infection Prevention (composite score FYTD)	85%	100%	95%	Meeting 2013 target
4. Medication Safety (composite score FYTD)	85%	100%	63%	May miss 2013 target
Improvement and Savings—All Clinical Dashboards				
1. No. Statistically Improved EBM Measures (FYTD)	15	15	17	Meeting 2013 target
2. No. Statistically Improved Complication Rates (FYTD)	15	15	12	May miss 2013 target
3. No. Statistically Improved Mortality Rates (FYTD)	5	5	7	Meeting 2013 target
4. No. Statistically Improved Readmission Rates (FYTD)	5	5	8	Meeting 2013 target
5. Cost Savings from Outcome Improvements	$20 M	$20 M	$17.25 M	On track to meet year-end goal
Pay-for-Performance				
1. Health Plan A (composite score, FYTD)	100%	100%	100%	100% performance =$6.3 million
2. Health Plan B (composite score, FYTD)	100%	100%	90%	90% performance=loss of $300,000
3. Quality ICP Score (January–March 2012)	90%	100%	93%	Meeting 2013 goal
Other				
1. HAC (occurrences reported by CMS)			12	
2. Readmission Calculator (% payment and amount)			–0.15%/ $23,499	

Note: This dashboard streamlines oversight and review by highlighting a series of measures that blend similar items of data into composite representations of key performance indicators taken from scores of more detailed reports for frontline staff. The dashboard is accompanied by supporting documents, including detailed dashboards or process control charts.

Source: Byrnes, J., "Driving Value: Solving the Issue of Data Overload with an Executive Dashboard," *hfm*, October 2012. Copyright 2012, Healthcare Financial Management Association. Reprinted with permission.

Measuring quality is only the beginning of effective quality oversight at the board level. Ideally, the board's expectation will be that the hospital is performing at the very top of the scale on all metrics; if it is not, the board will probe whether the failure to perform at a particular level of excellence is indicative of larger quality issues that need to be addressed.

Going Beyond Measuring to Dig Deeper

Sometimes, board members need to look more closely at the "green" targets on the dashboard and ask probing questions to ensure that those targets

Overseeing Quality in Multiple-Board Health Systems

In health systems with multiple boards, the local or "subsidiary" boards are usually charged with monitoring quality using standards and metrics set at the system level. Depending upon the other duties of the subsidiary board, quality may be overseen by the full board or by a committee of the board. At the system level, the board sets goals and standards for the entire system and works to ensure that all hospitals and boards within the system are meeting those quality goals and adhering to standards. The system board also sets standardized criteria and processes for physician credentialing.

Health system boards need to look at dashboards showing standardized metrics for each of their hospitals so they can make comparisons systemwide. The metrics shown on the first page of the system board dashboard should be high-level, big-picture metrics, such as overall mortality, overall system score for hospital-acquired conditions, bundled payment metrics for the whole system, and overall error rate. Subsequent pages can show comparisons by hospital, so the system knows where the weak areas are. Organizations can also measure population health in this way, in collaboration with cross-continuum partners like post-acute care.

represent an acceptable level of error, if the goal is not 100 percent or zero. For example, a common metric is surgical site infections for cardiac surgery. Perhaps an organization sets the target as anything better than 50 percent on the national nosocomial infection survey, which results in a green dot on the dashboard; however, this level is barely above average. In a given year, it could represent 11 deep sternal wound infections—highly devastating complications that double or triple the patient's risk of dying. Instead, the target for this metric should be set at the theoretical ideal of zero or close to zero, and boards should be asking their management teams to bring them information showing how other hospitals are achieving zero on this metric. Board members are free to ask for more information on the green targets and to ask management how they decide when "green" is acceptable (Reinertsen and Resar 2006).

Gaining an overall sense of the organization's quality status often requires board members to ask big-picture questions such as the following:

- How much variation is there in what we do?
- Is there evidence to support what we do?
- Even if a target is green on our dashboard, how much harm is still occurring?

- In situations where the best practice is well defined, how often do we actually follow best practices?
- If we are showing improvement, do we fully understand why a score is improving and what changes are responsible for that improvement?
- Are we as efficient as we can be? Where are opportunities to eliminate inefficiencies?

Effective boards make quality a strategic focus of their fiduciary oversight activities, and they dedicate a significant amount of time to discussion of quality at most board meetings. Making quality a priority also requires integrating into the board decision-making process questions about how decisions will positively affect quality, what steps are being taken to maximize the positive quality impact, and how the positive quality impact will be measured and evaluated as part of assessing the overall success of the hospital or health system's strategic plan.

Credentialing

Physician credentialing—an important component of the board's role in ensuring quality and patient safety—involves granting privileges to physicians to practice medicine in the hospital. The credentialing process determines whether a practitioner is competent and meets the hospital's high standards of clinical skill and professional conduct. Credentialing determines which doctors are qualified to join the medical staff, which procedures they are qualified to perform, and which conditions they may treat (Sagin 2007).

Those involved in the credentialing process include the board and its quality committee, the management team, the medical executive committee (MEC), clinical department chairs, and other medical staff leaders. The board is ultimately responsible for both the process and the outcome. Both medical staff and board participants in the credentialing process must be educated carefully in best credentialing practices (Sagin 2007).

The board begins by establishing credentialing policies and criteria for physicians to hold particular privileges, with the assistance of the MEC. These criteria are developed to ensure that practitioners have current competence to perform clinical tasks. The criteria may differ from organization to organization or be modified from time to time within the organization. Criteria for specific privileges will be recommended by the medical staff but must be approved by the board. Once the criteria have been established, they need to be periodically reassessed. The credentialing process ensures that practitioners are only assigned privileges for which they are currently competent and for which they meet the established criteria. Typically, privileging criteria should enumerate the requirements for education, training, and evidence of current competence to perform a specific task or procedure (Sagin 2007).

Medical staff leaders collect and summarize information about applicants for medical staff membership and privileges. Department chairs, the quality committee or credentials committee, and the MEC evaluate applicants and make formal recommendations to the board regarding requests for medical staff membership, the assignment of specific privileges to practitioners, and the appropriateness of any policies and procedures that should be adopted. The board reviews and then grants, denies, or restricts those privileges. In general, board members will give the greatest scrutiny to the 5 to 10 percent of practitioners who have some type of unusual event in their past (Sagin 2007).

The board is directly involved in the first and last of the credentialing steps (i.e., setting policies and assigning membership and/or privileges), but it has oversight over the entire process. It must ensure that all steps are carried out diligently, in compliance with the requirements of medical staff bylaws and policies, and in a manner consistent with hospital accreditation requirements (Sagin 2007).

Governing boards will sometimes adopt policies to "close" the medical staff in particular specialties. Policies can also be adopted that require applicants to show how they will advance the mission of the hospital. Sometimes, boards adopt physician conflict-of-interest policies, which might restrict access to the medical staff under well-defined circumstances (Sagin 2007).

Linking Quality and Finance

The traditional fee-for-service payment system in healthcare is slowly giving way to value-based payment models. In healthcare, *value* is defined by measuring quality outcomes against costs. Hospitals are changing care delivery methods to improve quality and reduce cost at the same time, looking more critically at whether procedures are necessary and whether lower-cost options are available that can achieve the same or better outcomes for patients. Hospitals can be paid based on value through a variety of methods, and most US hospitals and health systems have some percentage of their payment contracts under value-based formats. This percentage will likely continue to increase in the coming years. As such, hospital and health system boards are responsible for ensuring that quality and cost are appropriately related and that the organization's culture and strategy support the need for all staff and physicians to understand and focus on efforts related to increasing quality and reducing cost.

Countless cases have shown that providing higher-quality care is not more expensive than providing lower-quality care; in fact, it can lower costs in a variety of ways—for instance, by shortening hospital length of stay or reducing the need to provide additional care services related to medical errors, infections, and other complications. These cases and the research supporting them often result in evidence-based care protocols, which essentially are care process maps outlining what steps need to be taken and when, to ensure that the patient receives the necessary care for the optimum outcome. In the existence of evidence-based care protocols, hospitals should implement processes to ensure that the protocol is followed for every patient with a particular condition, every time.

In one case example, a health system evaluated the results of process changes to reduce the time from arrival in the emergency department to balloon catheterization for patients with acute myocardial infarction. By increasing the percentage of patients who were catheterized within 90 minutes of arrival from 37 percent to 97 percent, the system decreased the incidence of complications, readmissions within 30 days, and length of stay. The improvement in these quality metrics resulted in a savings of $1.37 million (Byrnes and Fifer 2010a). The health system in this case applied the same model that is used for financial reporting as the basis for measuring quality, safety, and value. With this approach, board finance and quality committees can view performance improvement from the same structured vantage point and analyze financial and quality metrics in the same rigorous manner (Fifer 2014).

Hospitals today are well aware that cost reduction and overall financial growth depend on quality and safety, and boards are responsible for ensuring that quality and finance are appropriately linked. They can do so in a variety of ways. The chief financial officer (CFO) needs to be a strong leader and advocate for quality and safety improvement. Boards that are particularly engaged in the quality/cost issue require that the CFO partner with the CMO and chief quality officer to approach projects from both quality and cost perspectives. CFOs who sit on the board-level quality committee can provide valuable insight into healthcare costs and also learn important information about care processes. Conversely, having the CMO and chief quality officer sit on the board-level finance committee can have similar advantages. These two committees can meet together periodically to further enhance communication and teamwork. Board member education on how quality and finance interact with each other is important. Finally, linking financial and quality metrics on the board dashboard provides board members with a more complete picture of how the organization is doing, enabling them to make more informed decisions and set the right strategic goals.

Ensuring Clinician Engagement and Leadership to Promote Quality

Another common issue faced by hospitals and health systems involves the quality and financial effects of variation in physician practice, which can account for up to 80 percent of a hospital's resource utilization (Fifer 2014). Reducing this variation can significantly cut costs, but beyond the cost issue, boards need to know that physicians are providing appropriate care for patients.

Physicians are the end point of the care/cost decision-making process. A hospital or health system cannot change the value equation without changing

EXHIBIT 13.4
Sample Strategic Quality and Safety Plan Dashboard

Focus Area	Goal	Five-Year Target	Fiscal-Year Target	Accountable Executive
Clinical Improvement				
	Maintain core measures in top 10 percentile nationally.	100%	+90%	CMO, CQO, CNO
	Implement evidence based care in high volume, high-cost conditions (representing ⇢50 percent of inpatient volume).	20 high-volume, high-cost conditions	Five high-volume, high-cost conditions	CMO, CQO, CNO
	Decrease complications in high-volume, high-cost conditions.	20%	5%	CMO, CQO, CNO
	Decrease cost of treatment for high volume, high-cost conditions.	5%	2%	CMO, CQO, CNO
Safety				
	Create a culture of safety and high reliability by decreasing the rate of serious safety events (events causing harm).	0.20	0.50	CMO, CQO, CNO
	Improve medication safety.	100%	85%	VP Pharmacy
		Implement computerized provider order entry and bar code administration for medications.	Conduct Institute for Safe Medication Practices survey and correct all deficiencies.	VP Pharmacy
Patient Satisfaction				
	Maintain top satisfaction scores with patients, staff, and physicians.	+90%	90%	CMO, CQO, CNO
	Increase market share as a result of improved satisfaction.	2%	0.5%	CEO, CFO
Operational Improvement				
	Reengineer high volume processes to improve efficiency.	20%	5%	CEO, CFO, CQO, CMO, CNO
	Reduce errors as a result of reengineering high-volume processes.	50%	15%	CEO, CFO, CQO, CMO, CNO
	Achieve cost savings as a result of reengineering high-volume processes.	$1 million	$250,000	CEO, CFO

Note: This sample Strategic Quality and Safety Plan Dashboard categorizes strategic planning initiatives by the area that is being targeted for improvement, sets goals that can be measured consistently in and across departments, establishes long- and short-term targets, and assigns executive responsibility for performance improvement.

Source: Byrnes, J., and Fifer, J., "Moving Quality and Cost to the Top of the Hospital Agenda," *hfm*, August 2010.

physician behavior. Standardizing care protocols and encouraging physicians (and nurses) to follow the same protocols, as much as possible, are considered best practices for improving quality and safety. Hospital and health system boards therefore need to charge physician and nurse leaders as champions for promoting these efforts to all medical staff physicians and nurses.

In a value-based health system model, physician leaders are needed to help redesign the care delivery system for optimum value, and they share responsibility for cost-effectiveness as well as for quality and safety. Sometimes, this responsibility involves managing care that takes place outside the hospital, managing risk for large populations of patients, or leading multidisciplinary teams. Physician and nurse leaders promote the quality culture and agenda, and they help remind staff that quality and cost are everyone's responsibility. This effort may require physician and nurse leadership positions that might not have existed previously, as well as new skills for physicians and nurses that may not have been a part of their training.

What is the board's role in this regard? The board needs to ensure that a leadership development program or process of some kind is available for physicians and nurses, either in-house or via recognized third-party institutions. Physicians and nurses need to be involved at the board level—whether as board members, members of the finance and quality committees, or part of a physician leadership advisory council to the board—to help develop strategic goals around quality and cost improvement efforts. The board, with the help of the management team, needs to put in place a physician and nurse leadership structure to enable changes in practice throughout all levels of the organization and to achieve quality and financial targets. Finally, just as the board connects a portion of the chief executive's compensation incentive to quality and finance targets, when appropriate, boards can do the same with employed physician leaders.

The Board-Level Quality Committee

Boards generally are not able to devote sufficient time during board meetings to the work needed to measure and monitor quality. Thus, to ensure high-quality performance, a robust board quality committee is essential. Effective quality committees can drive continuous improvement in quality and safety throughout the organization. Elements that the board must consider include how the committee is structured, how it operates, and how it spends its time. Ideally, the quality committee meets frequently, such as on a monthly basis, to provide opportunities for improving the metrics and to prepare for board meetings. The committee delves more deeply than the board can into metrics and quality issues, so committee members will have additional context and insight to share with the board during board meetings.

Quality committee responsibilities vary, depending upon whether the board oversees an independent hospital, a health system, or a subsidiary hospital of a health system. The following list of responsibilities are for the quality committee of an independent hospital board:

- Develop board-level policies regarding patient care and quality.
- Make recommendations to the full board for setting quality goals, parameters, and metrics.
- Oversee quality improvement systems, priorities, and plans.
- Work with medical staff to set criteria and processes for credentialing and ongoing quality monitoring of clinicians, and ensure that the credentialing procedure is disciplined, consistent, and effective.
- Make recommendations to the board about medical staff appointments, reappointments, and privileges.
- Monitor performance against policies, goals, systems, and plans.
- Review sentinel events, and recommend corrective action as appropriate.
- Review management's plans to address negative performance and serious errors.
- Oversee compliance with quality and safety accreditation standards.

A health system board quality committee would typically have the following responsibilities:

- Develop board-level policies regarding patient care and quality standards systemwide.
- Set systemwide quality goals, parameters, and metrics.
- Work with system medical staff leaders to set systemwide criteria and processes for credentialing and ongoing quality monitoring of clinicians by the subsidiary boards.
- Monitor systemwide performance against policies, goals, systems, and plans by requiring the proper level of reporting from subsidiary boards and quality improvement staff.
- Hold subsidiaries accountable for meeting goals and following processes set by the system.

A subsidiary board quality committee would have the following responsibilities regarding oversight of its own hospital:

- Oversee quality improvement systems, priorities, and plans.
- Make recommendations to the subsidiary board on medical staff appointments, reappointments, and privileges (or, in the case of a consolidated, systemwide medical staff, the recommendations would be made to the system board quality committee), and ensure that the credentialing procedure is disciplined, consistent, and effective.
- Monitor hospital performance against policies, goals, systems, and plans, and report up to the system-level quality committee.
- Review sentinel events, and recommend corrective action as appropriate.
- Review management's plans to address negative performance and serious errors.
- Oversee compliance with quality and safety accreditation standards.

Individuals who can bring intellectual interest and energy to clinical quality issues are selected for the committee. Some boards have recruited people with expertise in quality improvement methodologies (e.g., Lean, Six Sigma), safety, statistical process analysis, patient experience, risk and legal issues, and finance. Along with board members, the committee also includes physicians, the chief of staff, the chief nursing officer, and the senior-most quality executive, such as the chief quality officer or CMO. Some organizations even include former patients, family members of patients, and representatives of the community on the committee, which helps the group retain a patient-focused perspective.

Building a Culture of Quality and Safety

In complex environments, significant changes require a thoughtful, methodological approach. The changes implemented need to start with the mind-set of those involved in the change process. Hospitals and health systems have their own culture, and to be successful in quality efforts, boards will have to develop and nurture a strong culture of quality in their organizations. The starting place, as described earlier, is to position the commitment to quality centrally in the organization's mission statement and in its strategic planning, and then place it as a prominent topic at each and every board meeting. Putting quality toward the top of the agenda sends a strong message about its importance to the organization. An even more powerful way to nurture this culture is to regularly bring patients and their families into the boardroom to share their experiences, both good and bad, and provide better understanding of systemic problems that can be addressed at the board level.

Some other ways that boards build a strong cultural commitment to quality and safety include the following:

- Linking quality and safety with executive and physician compensation
- Transparently reporting quality and safety performance to the general public, including information on organizational performance, errors, and adverse events
- Building internal structures, policies, and technology to support quality and safety initiatives
- Providing quality improvement training for staff and leadership
- Demonstrating a commitment to accountability and responsibility for the safety of each patient

Case Example: Governing for Quality

BayCare Health System is a 15-hospital system in Clearwater, Florida, that serves approximately 4 million people. In 2009, it embarked on a far-reaching effort to gather quality data about every aspect of the system, not just the events that take place within hospital walls. The following is a summary of a 2014 case study, focusing in particular on how BayCare made changes at the governance level to address quality across the system's various care settings (Zablocki 2014).

BayCare is organized into three community health alliances, each with several hospitals. It has a clinically integrated network, called BayCare Physician Partners, which includes about 1,200 physicians. Although some of the physicians are employed by the system, the majority are in independent practice (Zablocki 2014). BayCare's board of directors consists of more than 20 community members and meets every other month. In addition, each community health alliance has a local board of directors.

All senior leaders receive quality training, and all employees are trained in quality and the system's quality model, which "builds from the ground up with a focus on customer needs, processes, and continuous improvement of those processes" (Zablocki 2014, 1). The model incorporates quality planning, quality improvement, quality assessment, and reporting. The process improvement department looks at workflows and identifies opportunities for improvement using Lean Six Sigma, a methodology based on continuous improvement and elimination of waste. More than 20 Lean Six Sigma Black Belt staff have been trained to facilitate and assist various departments and team members in quality improvement. The quality committee of the system board consists of the chairs of subregional quality committees, board members, the system CEO, community members, and others. The system quality committee reports at every board meeting.

Each year, BayCare holds a "Quality Sharing Day," attended by board members, hospital leaders, and staff, to celebrate initiatives that various

(continued)

team members have developed and to offer recognition for best achievements in various categories of service, outcome, cost, and overall quality (Zablocki 2014). All staff members have an opportunity to define key metrics for which they are personally accountable; these metrics are aligned with their yearly goals, as well as with organizational goals.

In 2009, the system began a three-phase, multiyear initiative to develop enterprisewide scorecard reporting in an effort to become more fully aware of the quality of care delivered by each division. The board decided that the enterprise-level quality committee would oversee the quality of all the care the system delivers, not just inpatient hospital care, and it worked with staff, physicians, and committees to develop quality scorecards for each area. Over time, these scorecards dovetailed into the acute-care scorecard and, together, provided a broad look at the entire organization. According to Dr. Bruce Flareau, executive vice president and CMO, this kind of quality reporting system is what healthcare organizations need in order to succeed in a population health model (Zablocki 2014).

Around this same time, BayCare began looking more closely at the relationship between the system board and its subsidiary advisory boards. It found that quality committees were examining the acute-care hospital space in a heavily focused way, with somewhat duplicative efforts, but that a broader view was necessary. For example, the system was offering a range of post-acute services, but it had no forum where all the team members who provide and manage post-acute care could transfer knowledge and best practices consistently to acute-care teams, and vice versa (Zablocki 2014).

To address this problem, the system board instituted a clinical leadership council that included all of the system's clinical leadership. Various leaders reviewed all of the system's service lines, including home care, ambulatory surgical centers, outpatient imaging, employed physician practices, behavioral health services based outside the hospital, rehab centers, and skilled nursing facilities. The system determined that five categories of care delivered outside the hospital warranted their own quality reports (Zablocki 2014):

- Ambulatory care
- Home care
- Physician services
- Behavioral health
- Post-acute care

The BayCare initiative consisted of three phases. The first phase was an internal assessment to review the current quality structure and currently used internal quality metrics. The second phase was an assessment of externally developed, standardized, evidence-based quality metrics. The third phase involved the development of performance improvement processes and a mature quality report card for each of the areas.

One of the members of the clinical leadership council serves as a sponsor for each area and meets regularly with that area's team, working to monitor performance, identify opportunities, and set internal goals. That team reports to the clinical leadership council, which reports to the system-level board quality committee.

Zablocki (2014, 4) explains:

> Selecting and defining the most appropriate quality measures in post-acute care . . . unleashed a flood of creative effort at improving care processes and outcomes. Throughout 2012, the post-acute team focused on these areas and saw significant improvements in several measures. For example, there was a 20 percent reduction on pressure ulcers per 1,000 patient days, compared to 2011. The likelihood that patients would recommend the hospital to friends and family, as measured by the HCAHPS survey, improved by 10 percent compared to 2011.

Achieving these results required numerous small changes, improved communication and collaboration between acute and post-acute care teams, and considerable attention to detail.

Another area for which BayCare worked to develop improved quality reporting is physician services. The system had seven different companies that employ physicians and was in the process of bringing them together under a single umbrella. The physicians found that developing common definitions of key measures—even for common events one might expect to be simple to define—took a great deal of work. For example, some offices were monitoring same-day appointment availability, whereas others were looking at available appointments by the third day, or missed appointments. A similar example involves efforts to gain information about smoking habits. One clinic asked whether the patient currently smokes and, if so, how much; a second clinic asked if the patient ever smoked in the past and if they smoke now; and a third clinic asked whether a patient is exposed to other smokers at home. The system needed several months to determine what items were most important to track and how exactly to define and measure those items to ensure consistency from one site to another (Zablocki 2014).

Zablocki (2014, 5) explains: "The physicians . . . developed a consolidated scorecard report that includes measures such as childhood immunization rates, HbA1c testing, colorectal cancer screening rates, 30-day

(continued)

readmission rates, and the patient's experience of care." The scorecard demonstrates trends over time, and the system makes the information available to physicians so they can see their own scorecard report.

According to Dr. Flareau, one of the most important things the board and senior leaders learned through this process is that data definitions really matter (Zablocki 2014). Organizations need to invest time in establishing precise data definitions, determining what to measure, agreeing on measuring it in a certain way, and fully integrating that definition into cultural understandings and agreements throughout the organization.

Furthermore, developing the competencies to deliver population health requires boards and executives to look beyond the hospital and think about how to manage quality in other care settings. When boards receive presentations from management regarding quality dashboards, they need to understand *why* things improved and whether such improvement can be replicated (Zablocki 2014). When an indicator shows improvement, what is being done differently? Are staff members learning from these occurrences? A level of transparency enables management to openly discuss the results with the board and understand what the results really mean, thereby facilitating quality improvement throughout the system.

Conclusion

Providing the highest-quality care is an essential component of the organizational purpose and charitable mission of any not-for-profit hospital or health system. Every decision made at the highest level of a hospital or health system should hold in mind how quality of care will be affected. The way a board of directors governs its organization and oversees quality has a significant impact on patient outcomes. Boards fulfill their fiduciary duties by instituting a robust quality measurement and improvement process; setting high-level policies and strategic goals regarding quality of care, safety, patient experience, and physician credentialing; engaging physician and nurse leaders in quality efforts; holding management accountable for meeting quality goals; and nurturing an organization-wide culture that supports sustained and ongoing quality improvement.

Notes

1. For more information about *Darling v. Charleston Community Memorial Hospital*, see www.casebriefs.com/blog/law/health-law/

health-law-keyed-to-furrow/liability-of-health-care-institutions/darling-v-charleston-community-memorial-hospital/.

2. Standard LD.01.03.01 of The Joint Commission's (2006) *Comprehensive Accreditation Manual for Hospitals* states, "The governing body is ultimately accountable for the safety and quality of care, treatment, and services," and the rationale for this standard is that the governing body's "ultimate responsibility for safety and quality derives from its legal responsibility and operational authority for hospital performance." For more information, see www.jcrinc.com/2018-comprehensive-accreditation-manuals/.
3. For more information, see the IHI resources available at www.ihi.org/Topics/GovernanceLeadership/Pages/default.aspx.

Study Questions

1. Why is the board of directors the body with ultimate responsibility for quality? Why isn't this responsibility limited to individual physicians?
2. What are the main differences between the role of the board and the role of the management team in ensuring quality and safety?

References

Byrnes, J. 2012. "Driving Value: Solving the Issue of Data Overload with an Executive Dashboard." *hfm* 66 (10): 116–18.

Byrnes, J., and J. Fifer. 2010a. "Case Study—Process and Structure for Quality and Cost Improvement." *Physician Executive Journal* 36 (2): 38–43.

———. 2010b. "Moving Quality and Cost to the Top of the Hospital Agenda." *hfm* 64 (8): 64–69.

CaseBriefs. 2018. "Darling v. Charleston Community Memorial Hospital." Accessed November 14. www.casebriefs.com/blog/law/health-law/health-law-keyed-to-furrow/liability-of-health-care-institutions/darling-v-charleston-community-memorial-hospital/.

Fifer, J. J. 2014. "How to Increase Board Engagement in Quality and Finance." *BoardRoom Press* 25 (1): 5–12.

Institute for Healthcare Improvement (IHI). 2018. "Governance Leadership of Safety and Improvement." Accessed November 13. www.ihi.org/Topics/GovernanceLeadership/Pages/default.aspx.

Jha, A., and A. Epstein. 2010. "Hospital Governance and the Quality of Care." *Health Affairs* 29 (1): 182–87.

Jiang, H. J., C. Lockee, K. Bass, and I. Fraser. 2009. "Board Oversight of Quality: Any Differences in Process of Care and Mortality?" *Journal of Healthcare Management* 54 (1): 15–30.

———. 2008. "Board Engagement in Quality: Findings of a Survey of Hospital and System Leaders." *Journal of Healthcare Management* 53 (2): 121–34.

Joint Commission. 2016. *Comprehensive Accreditation Manual for Hospitals.* Chicago: Joint Commission.

Joshi, M. S., and S. C. Hines. 2006. "Getting the Board on Board: Engaging Hospital Boards in Quality and Patient Safety." *Joint Commission Journal on Quality and Patient Safety* 32 (4): 179–87.

Lockee, C., K. Peisert (Croom), E. Zablocki, and B. S. Bader. 2006. *Quality.* San Diego, CA: The Governance Institute.

Peisert, K. 2017. *The Governance Evolution: Meeting New Industry Demands. 2017 Biennial Survey of Hospitals and Healthcare Systems.* San Diego, CA: The Governance Institute.

———. 2013. *Governing the Value Journey: A Profile of Structure, Culture, and Practices of Boards in Transition. 2013 Biennial Survey of Hospitals and Healthcare Systems.* San Diego, CA: The Governance Institute.

Peregrine, M. 2005. *Fundamental Fiduciary Duties of the Non-Profit Healthcare Director.* Elements of Governance series. San Diego, CA: The Governance Institute.

Prybil, L., D. R. Bardach, and D. W. Fardo. 2014. "Board Oversight of Patient Care Quality in Large Nonprofit Health Systems." *American Journal of Medical Quality* 29 (1): 39–43.

Prybil, L., S. Levey, R. Killian, D. Fardo, R. Chait, D. R. Bardach, and W. Roach. 2012. *Governance in Large Nonprofit Health Systems: Current Profile and Emerging Patterns.* Lexington, KY: Commonwealth Center for Governance Studies.

Reinertsen, J. L. 2014. "Leadership for Quality." In *The Healthcare Quality Book: Vision, Strategy, and Tools,* 3rd ed., edited by M. S. Joshi, E. R. Ransom, D. B. Nash, and S. B. Ransom, 355–74. Chicago: Health Administration Press.

Reinertsen, J., and R. Resar. 2006. *CEO Summit 2: Taking the Reliability of Care to the Next Level: The Second Stage.* VHA Georgia conference proceedings, October 26–27.

Sagin, T. 2007. *Physician Credentialing: An Orientation Manual for Board Members.* Elements of Governance series. San Diego, CA: The Governance Institute.

Stepnick, L. 2014. *Making a Difference in the Boardroom: Updated Research Findings on Best Practices to Promote Quality at Top Hospitals and Health Systems.* San Diego, CA: The Governance Institute.

Tsai, T. C., A. K. Jha, A. A. Gawande, R. S. Huckman, N. Bloom, and R. Sadun. 2015. "Hospital Board and Management Practices Are Strongly Related to Hospital Performance on Clinical Quality Metrics." *Health Affairs* 34 (8): 1304–11.

Zablocki, E. 2014. *Quality Reporting Expands Beyond Hospital Walls.* San Diego, CA: The Governance Institute.

PART

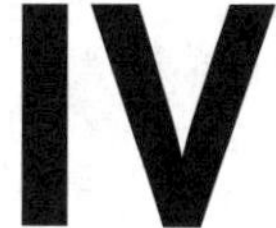

EMERGING TRENDS

Scott B. Ransom

For many years, discussions of healthcare quality have focused on improving hospital care with an implicit understanding that financial incentives generally support a fee-for-volume approach. However, the past decade has seen a transition away from this almost purely volume-driven paradigm, and providers are now starting to be compensated for generating greater *value*—defined as improving quality while maintaining or reducing cost. Moreover, many "hospital systems" have started transitioning into "health systems" by developing interventions to reduce hospital length of stay, shift care to lower-cost settings (e.g., ambulatory sites) or providers (e.g., advanced practice providers, pharmacists), reduce unnecessary testing and interventions, avoid readmissions, and encourage prevention and wellness. This part of the book will investigate many of these more contemporary, often disruptive, approaches and trends that are transforming the long-standing hospital-centric paradigm.

We begin our "Emerging Trends" section with chapter 14, which considers approaches for improving quality and safety in the ambulatory setting. Lawrence Ward and Rhea E. Powell provide contemporary insights for driving improvements in primary care and specialty offices, ambulatory surgery centers, urgent care centers, retail clinics, freestanding emergency departments, and work-based clinics. The chapter highlights the challenges in improving quality and patient safety throughout systems that are largely disjointed, often with multiple care transitions among various caregivers, laboratory testing and imaging facilities, and primary and specialty care providers—many of whom are part of different practices and companies that do not easily communicate. In the face of this complexity, key challenges may involve tracking and managing tests and referrals, ensuring appropriate medication administration, and sharing important patient information between providers. The chapter also promotes several strategies for improving care in the ambulatory setting, such as aligning provider incentives, creating better measurement systems, and developing interconnected computer systems to support better communication between providers and with the patient.

In chapter 15, Michael S. Barr and Frank Micciche provide an overview of the National Committee for Quality Assurance (NCQA), from its beginnings supporting employers and health plans in developing quality standards to its later efforts to create systems to measure those standards. The authors chronicle various incremental improvements, such as the Healthcare Effectiveness Data and Information Set (HEDIS) measures, health plan accreditation guidelines, the patient-centered medical home model, and recognition programs. The chapter then transitions to more contemporary influences on care delivery, such as electronic health record adoption; health plan expansions such as the Medicaid section 1115 waiver and Affordable Care Act (ACA) initiatives; and value-driven innovations, including those under the Medicare Access and CHIP Reauthorization Act (MACRA).

A. Mark Fendrick and Susan Lynne Oesterle present the fundamentals of value-based insurance design (V-BID) in chapter 16. They outline various strategies, tactics, and financial models (such as consumer cost sharing) to help with the transition from a volume-driven to value-driven design. They also highlight various policy implications of the transition, with discussions of the ACA, Medicare Advantage, high-deductible health plans, and the vision of high-value health plans. The authors provide several illustrative examples involving programs such as TRICARE, state Medicaid reforms, and state employee health plans. They conclude with some thoughts on the elimination of low-value care and the potential benefits of precision medicine.

In chapter 17, Neil Goldfarb looks at the ways in which purchasers can select and pay for healthcare services with a greater focus on value. Many employers—finding their business competitiveness threatened by the extremely high costs of the US healthcare system—have sought to lower their healthcare costs and create a healthier workforce by collecting information on quality and fostering transparency; taking a V-BID approach to plan design; selectively contracting with higher-value health plans and providers; pursuing payment reform to promote value; engaging consumers and employees in seeking higher-value care; and supporting wellness, disease prevention, and disease management. The chapter concludes with several examples of how employers are driving greater value, such as the Leapfrog value-based purchasing platform, the Bridges to Excellence program, the Purchaser Value Network, and Choosing Wisely.

In chapter 18, Laura Cranston, Matthew K. Pickering, Hannah M. Fish, and Mel L. Nelson present a summary of how to drive greater quality and lower cost through effective medication use. They outline strategies to more effectively utilize pharmacists in driving improvements in both patient safety and quality while reducing unnecessary costs. The authors then present approaches to measure and influence appropriate medication use, such as by incorporating the Centers for Medicare & Medicaid Services medication therapy management completion rate measures and by optimizing the use of pharmacists in improving Medicare Part D. The chapter concludes by discussing the future impact of comparative effectiveness research (CER) and patient-centered outcomes research (PCOR) in better understanding optimal medication use.

In our final chapter, Keith Kosel presents current thinking on population health quality and safety. He begins by providing a framework for defining various populations using such categories as geography, employee groups, type of illness, and covered health plan participants. He discusses the need to consider specific population health challenges while pursuing the targets of the Healthy People 2020 program, with interventions focusing on health status, health equity, racial and ethnic disparities, culturally competent care interventions, and social determinants of health. The chapter describes the benefits of a multidisciplinary team orientation—including providers, public health agencies, and community groups—in achieving population health goals. Kosel concludes with a vision for developing and implementing a comprehensive approach to attaining population health goals (e.g., the aims of safe, timely, effective, efficient, equitable, and patient-centered care), incorporating appropriate data collection as well as individual, community, and patient–clinician contributions and interventions.

This "Emerging Trends" section highlights a number of current approaches driving improvements in quality and patient safety; however, countless other approaches are being developed and tested by individuals, companies, universities, and policy experts. In the years ahead, the continued emergence of new value-enhancing technologies and practices will be exciting to watch. I can hardly imagine the possibilities for driving greater value and improved health outcomes through the use of avatars; future iterations of Fitbits; personal diagnostic testing devices; healthy living reminders; and personalized medicine backed by a better understanding of the relationships among genetics, the environment, and disease subtypes. I look forward to seeing the impact of new start-up companies and watching as innovative groups seek to enhance value through collaborations between payers and providers (e.g., the CVS/Aetna merger, Optum) and new potential healthcare disrupters (e.g., the collaboration between Berkshire Hathaway, Amazon, and Chase). Stay tuned—the next decade will be an exciting time for innovations aimed at achieving the goal of greater healthcare value for all.

CHAPTER

14

AMBULATORY QUALITY AND SAFETY

Lawrence Ward and Rhea E. Powell

The healthcare landscape in the United States is dynamic—continuously evolving as the transition from *volume* to *value* takes hold under pressure from increasing healthcare costs and a need to deliver better care. This foundational change in the way care is financed has greatly influenced the way care delivery is measured. Although the most acutely ill patients are managed in an acute (inpatient hospital) setting, the vast majority of patients are managed in ambulatory (outpatient) offices. The ambulatory setting is where most people, both those in good health and those with acute or chronic illnesses, have frequent contact with the healthcare system; likewise, it is where healthcare providers have the best opportunity to influence healthy behaviors and to prevent future illness. Providers, insurers, and regulatory agencies expect—and are increasingly demanding—to know more about the quality of care delivered in the ambulatory setting, raising the urgency of the need to develop appropriate methods and metrics. This chapter specifically examines the ambulatory-based quality and safety landscape, details important trends in this area, and provides an overview of the directions expected in the future.

The Ambulatory Care Setting

Ambulatory care refers to medical services performed on an outpatient basis, without admission to a hospital or other facility. Although the definition is evolving as a result of advances in technology, traditional sites of ambulatory care include primary care and specialty offices, as well as ambulatory surgery centers, urgent care centers, retail clinics, freestanding emergency departments, and work-based clinics (Medicare Payment Advisory Commission 2017). For the purposes of this chapter, we will focus on ambulatory-based providers in both primary care and subspecialist offices.

For many years, inpatient settings—such as acute care hospitals, surgical facilities, emergency departments, and other facilities with more acutely ill patients—have been subject to regulation, standards, and inspection by groups such as The Joint Commission, and metrics for performance in such settings have been clearly developed and defined. In addition, payers—notably, the Centers for Medicare & Medicare Services (CMS)—have linked financial payments and penalties to providers' performance on the metrics, and these financial incentives have provided motivation for a number of highly developed performance improvement infrastructures, often employing tools from Lean, Six Sigma, and other formal strategies.

Historically, ambulatory settings have not been subject to the same level of scrutiny and regulation that inpatient settings have seen, and they have not had the same incentives for improvement. However, given the large volume of patients seen in ambulatory settings and the significant potential for harm that exists, ambulatory settings need to develop a similar infrastructure to spur improvement.

Ambulatory settings present unique challenges related to the complexity of practice settings and issues with communication and flow of information. Furthermore, they often have difficulty obtaining critical quality data for such areas as medication errors, adverse drug events, missed/incorrect/delayed diagnoses, and delay of proper treatment or preventive services. Additional challenges involve the ambulatory setting's focus on population-based management—a key difference between ambulatory and inpatient care.

Hospitalized patients are tracked for the duration of their admission—and perhaps for some time afterward to reduce the likelihood of readmission—but they are not actively managed for long beyond a single episode of care. Therefore, inpatient quality and safety metrics are often one-time measures—for instance, a measure of whether patients develop a catheter-associated urinary tract infection over the course of a hospital stay. In the ambulatory setting, however, most measures focus on a population of patients seen over a certain period of time. For instance, an ambulatory practice might be responsible for ensuring appropriate colon cancer screening for every patient seen within the previous two years. An individual patient might have been seen only once, 15 months earlier, but if the data suggest that a gap in screening care has occurred, the practice is responsible for arranging for the proper screening to occur (or for correcting the data, if the screening has in fact occurred). Thus, an ambulatory practice needs to be able to identify gaps in care when patients arrive in the office, educate patients about the need for care, and arrange for appropriate follow-up. In cases where a patient chooses not to receive the recommended care, the practice needs to implement an efficient mechanism for identification, monitoring, and outreach.

Ambulatory Quality Improvement

Historical Development

Donabedian's (1966) seminal paper "Evaluating the Quality of Medical Care" created a framework that is still used to measure healthcare quality today. It divides measures into three categories: structure, processes, and outcomes.

This framework was instrumental in the establishment in 1970 of the Institute of Medicine (IOM), which has since launched numerous efforts focused on evaluating, informing, and improving the quality of healthcare delivered (National Academies of Sciences, Engineering, and Medicine 2018). Most influential among these IOM efforts were the reports *To Err Is Human* (Kohn, Corrigan, and Donaldson 2000) and *Crossing the Quality Chasm* (IOM 2001).

The organization currently known as the Agency for Healthcare Research and Quality (AHRQ) was founded in 1989, in response to data that revealed wide geographic variations in practice patterns without supporting clinical evidence (Steinwachs and Hughes 2008). Tasked with supporting a research program focused on clinical effectiveness, treatment outcomes, and practice guidelines, AHRQ has been instrumental in driving the quality agenda, especially in the form of researching and defining best practices (Hospital Consumer Assessment of Healthcare Providers and Systems 2017).

AHRQ and other quality-oriented entities were established in part because healthcare organizations were seeing a rise in costs and looking for practical methods to reduce waste and disseminate best practices. Promoting ambulatory quality by providing financial incentives for high-quality care was seen as one mechanism for accomplishing these goals (American College of Physicians 2009). Traditionally, insurance companies have paid ambulatory-based physicians according to a fee-for-service model, in which the primary financial incentive for the physicians has been to see a higher volume of patients and to perform more procedures—essentially, the more they did, the more they were paid. However, as insurance companies began recognizing the need to control rising healthcare costs, they implemented methods to diversify the incentives for physicians, especially those practicing primary care.

The movement to change financial incentives for physicians began in earnest during the late 1980s and into the 1990s, through the broad development of health maintenance organizations (HMOs). Having originated in the 1940s with Kaiser Permanente, HMOs became much more widespread during this period (Markovich 2003). HMOs were among the first large-scale examples of a nongovernmental (private) insurance company asking physicians to recognize that they were responsible for the care of a population of patients. Under the HMO structure, physicians were assigned a set of patients who chose the HMO as their primary care provider. The insurance company then paid each physician a set amount each month to care for this group of patients. The physician would receive this "capitated" payment whether the patient received care at the office or not; however, the physician would also be responsible for care provided to the patient by other physicians. If a patient saw subspecialty physicians or went to the emergency department too often, the primary care physician would be held ultimately responsible and could face a financial penalty from the insurance company (Markovich 2003).

Despite its many limitations, the HMO model successfully introduced primary care physicians to the concept of population health, which was central to an HMO's success. Beginning in the mid-1990s, insurance companies began to relax the restrictions of the HMO model. While continuing the practice of capitated payments, they modestly eased the rules on referral management and the penalties toward primary care physicians for high costs of care (Marquis, Rogowski, and Escarce 2004). However, the insurance companies needed some mechanism to incentivize physicians to provide care, so they turned toward paying providers for successfully meeting goals on quality-of-care measures. In this era, before widespread use of electronic health records (EHRs), the most easily agreed-upon and trackable measures focused on such elements as successful cancer screening, care for patients with diabetes, and the prescription of generic medications. These measures were generally accepted by everyone involved as evidence-based elements of good care (Rosenthal et al. 2004).

Expansion of Quality Improvement Through Pay for Performance

The National Committee for Quality Assurance (NCQA) was established in 1990, and it is tasked with managing accreditation programs for individual physicians, health plans, and medical groups, with the objective of improving healthcare quality (Sennett 1998). The organization measures accreditation performance through the administration and submission of the Healthcare Effectiveness Data and Information Set (HEDIS) and the Consumer Assessment of Healthcare Providers and Systems (CAHPS) survey (Marjoua and Bozic 2012).

Today, NCQA (2018) continues to have a significant influence on the selection and development of quality measures through their industry-leading recognition programs, including those for patient-centered medical homes (PCMHs) and patient-centered specialty practices (PCSPs). The PCMH, initially created for pediatrics in 1967 but now widespread among all primary care specialties, is a model of care that has, more than any other before it, influenced the transition of ambulatory medicine to a patient-centered, population-based construct that places an emphasis on quality improvement (Robert Graham Center 2007).

As policymakers, purchasers, and payers looked for ways to create efficiencies, a strong primary care system was identified as a vital aspect of managing cost and quality (Future of Family Medicine Project Leadership Committee 2004). The NCQA PCMH program asked primary care offices to commit to performance measurement and accept accountability for continuous quality improvement, and it required recognition on a continuous basis. In doing so, the program succeeded in providing financial incentives to implement permanent quality improvement elements that had rarely been seen before in ambulatory settings. Although early studies were mixed on the effectiveness of the PCMH model, more recent data have demonstrated a variety of benefits, including reduced hospitalizations and readmissions, better management of chronic illnesses, and improved patient satisfaction (Jackson et al. 2013; Friedberg et al. 2014; Friedberg, Rosenthal, and Werner 2015; NCQA 2017).

The drive toward increased emphasis on ambulatory quality continued with the establishment of the National Quality Forum (NQF) in 1999 (NQF 2017a). The NQF defined national goals and priorities for healthcare quality improvement, and it built a national consensus around standardized performance metrics for quantifying and reporting on national healthcare quality efforts. NQF endorsement has thus become the "gold standard" for healthcare performance measures, relied upon by healthcare purchasers such as CMS and, by extension, private insurers as well (Marjoua and Bozic 2012).

Influenced by the NQF's work, CMS implemented a new Physician Quality Reporting System (PQRS) in 2006 (CMS 2017e). Established under the Tax Relief and Health Care Act, PQRS was noteworthy as the first nationwide "pay-for-reporting" program, and it focused on the physician as the target of feedback and incentives. It provided a bonus on the total allowed Medicare Part B fee-for-service charges to incentivize successful reporting on a series of ambulatory quality measures (CMS 2017e). Initially voluntary in nature, reporting soon became mandatory. Financial incentives were removed, and penalties for practices that failed to achieve the desired results were instituted in their place (CMS 2015).

The Affordable Care Act

The movement toward ambulatory quality improvement was further supported by the passage of the Patient Protection and Affordable Care Act (ACA) of 2010, which included multiple provisions aiming to improve quality while lowering costs and expanding access. The ACA included requirements for quality measurement, coupled with cost controls, to stimulate more efficient models of care that sought to prevent the overuse, underuse, and inappropriate use of healthcare—a focus regarded as essential for both improving quality and lowering cost (Blumenthal, Abrams, and Nuzum 2015).

Although quality programs in the ACA primarily focused on hospitals, subsequent legislation and regulatory actions expanded quality and value programs to additional venues (Landers et al. 2016). The ACA also provided significant indirect support for the PCMH model, and it created new entities, such as the Patient-Centered Outcomes Research Institute (PCORI), the Hospital Value-Based Purchasing (VBP) Program, and the CMS Innovation Center, that expanded the use of incentives and penalties in connection with inpatient (primarily focused on reducing readmissions) and ambulatory quality measures (CMS 2017a, 2018b; PCORI 2017).

The Hospital VBP Program uses a broad set of performance-based payment strategies to link financial incentives to provider performance on a set of defined measures. It aims to financially reward care providers for delivering appropriate, high-quality care at a lower cost, in an effort to drive quality improvement and to slow the growth in healthcare spending (CMS 2018b). Reports suggest that the Hospital VBP Program has had mixed effectiveness in the care of patients with certain chronic conditions, such as diabetes and hypertension (Chee et al. 2016), and some people have voiced concern that the program might have the unwanted effect of disincentivizing care for these complex patients if it has negative financial repercussions (Ryan and Blustein 2012). Some are also concerned that practices and healthcare organizations might focus their attention on the diseases that are measured, to the exclusion of other important aspects of healthcare. Nonetheless, despite its possible flaws, the Hospital VBP Program's emphasis on providing top quality at a lower price has had a meaningful influence across all care settings, and it is widely viewed as critical to the financial future of healthcare (Keehan et al. 2011).

Accountable Care Organizations

While the Hospital VBP Program brought attention to hospital-based quality and cost, analogous efforts in outpatient sites prompted a move toward accountable care organizations (ACOs). CMS (2018a) defines ACOs as "groups of doctors, hospitals, and other healthcare providers, who come together voluntarily to give coordinated high-quality care to their Medicare patients." The ACO model aims to improve quality and lower costs by guiding healthcare providers and hospitals toward better-coordinated, higher-quality, and patient-centered care for Medicare patients and to replace the often fragmented care received under the traditional fee-for-service system (Marjoua and Bozic 2012).

The ACO model includes an embedded incentive payment in the form of revenue sharing, which represents part of the savings that can be achieved. ACOs require providers to share in the financial risk of the plan, rather than place the financial risk on insurers, as is done under a traditional managed care model. However, savings must also be accompanied by satisfactory performance on quality benchmarks that span various process and outcome measures over multiple domains, including patient experience of care, care coordination, patient safety, preventive health, and health of at-risk populations (Marjoua and Bozic 2012). A list of measures used in ACO performance standards is shown in exhibit 14.1.

Because ambulatory quality is integral to achieving financial savings in an ACO, practices were propelled to become PCMH-recognized, to refine workflows, to integrate EHRs, and to begin viewing their patients as a population that should be proactively managed (Davis, Abrams, and Stremikis 2011). Private insurers took note as well, and they began implementing programs to

EXHIBIT 14.1 Measures for Use in Establishing Quality Performance Standards That ACOs Must Meet for Shared Savings (2017)

Measure	Method of Measurement
Risk-Standardized, All-Condition Readmission	Claims
Skilled Nursing Facility 30-Day All-Cause Readmission Measures	Claims
All-Cause Unplanned Admissions for Patients with Diabetes	Claims
All-Cause Unplanned Admissions for Patients with Heart Failure	Claims
All-Cause Unplanned Admissions for Patients with Multiple Chronic Conditions	Claims
Acute Composite (AHRQ Prevention Quality Indicator [PQI] #91)	Claims
Medication Reconciliation Post-Discharge	Web interface
Falls: Screening for Future Fall Risk	Web interface
Use of Imaging Studies for Low Back Pain	Claims
Preventive Care and Screening: Influenza Immunization	Web interface
Pneumonia Vaccination Status for Older Adults	Web interface
Preventive Care and Screening: Body Mass Index Screening and Follow-Up	Web interface
Preventive Care and Screening: Tobacco Use: Screening and Cessation Intervention	Web interface
Preventive Care and Screening: Screening for Clinical Depression and Follow-Up Plan	Web interface
Colorectal Cancer Screening	Web interface
Breast Cancer Screening	Web interface
Statin Therapy for the Prevention and Treatment of Cardiovascular Disease	Web interface
Depression Remission at 12 Months	Web interface
Diabetes: Hemoglobin A1c Poor Control	Web interface
Diabetes: Eye Exam	Web interface
Controlling High Blood Pressure	Web interface
Ischemic Vascular Disease: Use of Aspirin or Another Antithrombotic	Web interface

Note: The measures listed are in addition to survey measures and EHR certification.

Source: Data from CMS (2017b).

link quality and payment to create more efficient systems of care. These "pay-for-performance" programs would reward providers who met certain quality thresholds, often chosen according to what Medicare was reimbursing for high performance in its Advantage plans (Rosenthal and Dudley 2007). Medicare Advantage plans, which may involve versions of HMOs in the place of traditional fee-for-service Medicare, now serve a third of all Medicare beneficiaries (L&M Policy Research 2016).

Medicare Advantage measures quality and performance using a five-star rating scale. Since 2012, plans that achieve four stars or more have been eligible for additional funds from CMS, and these funds can be invested in additional patient benefits to attract more members and to differentiate the plans from lower-quality plans (L&M Policy Research 2016). Many private insurance plans have copied these strategies and introduced their own ambulatory quality programs, usually focused on payment for reporting results, as well as meeting specific criteria for measures such as patient medication adherence and cost effectiveness.

MACRA and the Shift from Measuring Process to Measuring Outcomes

Historically, the majority of quality measures developed for the ambulatory setting have focused on the completion of processes to care for patients with chronic illnesses, such as diabetes and coronary disease, and to help prevent and detect diseases such as breast cancer and colon cancer. These measures were easy to track and quantify even before the use of well-functioning EHRs, which now can be designed to improve office workflows and drive clinicians and staff to click the appropriate box and order the necessary test, vaccine, or study.

However, although these processes are important, the ultimate goal is to define and measure the health *outcomes* that are affected by these processes. Health outcomes are complicated by nature, and few true measures of health outcomes have yet to be adopted. Some examples may include measuring glycosylated hemoglobin levels in patients with diabetes and gauging the effectiveness of blood pressure control. However, even these examples are not true measures of a disease outcome. To truly measure the end effect of care would require measurement for the prevention of renal disease, a reduction in the rate of cardiac events, or a decrease in the incidence of malignancy. Although such measurement may be possible on a population level, it is extremely difficult at the level of the individual medical office, much less at the level of the individual provider.

The rising costs of healthcare—and the urgent need to control them—have driven a shift away from measures of process and toward more measurements of true disease outcomes, utilization outcomes, and total cost of care. The Medicare Access and CHIP Reauthorization Act of 2015 (MACRA) went into effect in 2017, significantly altering the way physicians are paid by Medicare. MACRA created the Quality Payment Program (QPP), which included two pathways for physician reimbursement: the new Merit-Based Incentive Payment System (MIPS) and Advanced Payment Models (APMs) (CMS 2018c, 2018d). For physicians in MIPS, payment is determined using four domains: cost, clinical practice improvement, advancing care information, and quality (McWilliams 2017). Although the inclusion of quality is laudable, that domain focuses primarily on the achievement of process measures, and the proportion it contributes to the overall MIPS score is set to decrease over the years. In addition, because these programs are built on historical volume-based architecture, they only offer healthcare providers a chance to earn money for quality retroactively through, most commonly, shared savings. As a result, even under the new QPP architecture, US healthcare is still not pursuing truly population-based payment, and thus progress toward true payment for quality is hindered (Landers et al. 2016).

The true value may be that MIPS establishes almost 300 quality measures that will be fine-tuned over time, and that it requires subspecialists to participate in formal clinical practice improvement and submit quality results. Although the most visits occur in primary care, the highest costs arise from specialty (nonprimary care) visits and referrals (McWilliams 2017). Historically, specialty practices have not often been included in ambulatory quality improvement or pay-for-performance efforts to a significant extent, and they continue to derive most of their income from patient visits, procedures, and studies. Therefore, increasing the involvement of specialist providers in quality improvement is a welcome development, with the potential to have a significant impact on quality and cost.

Ambulatory Safety

Evolution of the Patient Safety Movement

In addition to spearheading the drive for quality improvement, the landmark IOM report *To Err Is Human* also brought patient safety to the forefront of healthcare issues, setting a national agenda for reducing medical errors (Kohn, Corrigan, and Donaldson 2000). Shortly after the report's release, the federal government passed the Healthcare Quality and Safety Act, reauthorizing AHRQ and charging it with the responsibility to develop programs to identify causes of medical errors, to evaluate strategies for reducing errors in healthcare delivery, and to disseminate effective strategies throughout the industry (Congress.gov 2017). The years since that landmark IOM report have seen great strides in improving the safety of the American healthcare system.

Hospitals across the United States have designed and implemented programs to identify and address causes of patient safety problems. They have adopted specific approaches such as checklist interventions, antibiotic stewardship programs, and medication reconciliation programs, as well as broader approaches, such as programs to improve patient–provider communication and team-based care. At the same time, policy changes related to reimbursement for hospital-acquired conditions have shifted incentives, increasingly holding hospitals accountable for certain adverse safety events. The implementation of these programs and policies nationally has resulted in significant reductions in common hospital-acquired conditions such as central line–associated bloodstream infections, surgical site infections, hospital-onset *Clostridium difficile* infections, and hospital-onset Methicillin-resistant *Staphylococcus aureus* (MRSA) bacteremia (Centers for Disease Control and Prevention 2016). The benefits that patients experience through improved safety are coupled with benefits to the healthcare system, with billions of dollars in healthcare costs believed to have been saved (AHRQ 2014).

Challenges to Delivery of Safe Care in the Ambulatory Setting

Although much progress has been made in the inpatient hospital setting, systematic programs to improve safety in the ambulatory setting have only been developed more recently. Addressing the safety of healthcare delivery in the ambulatory setting presents myriad challenges. Ambulatory care is often fragmented, with patients receiving care from multiple providers and health systems. Patients may experience long waiting periods, with a number of transitions between healthcare settings. Patient engagement is also a challenge, as patients in the ambulatory setting are held responsible for making decisions about when and where to seek care, managing medications, and performing daily health-related tasks, often without immediate assistance from members of the healthcare team. Furthermore, although numerous evidence-based measures have been developed for the safety of hospital-based care, fewer measures are available to evaluate ambulatory safety. Similarly, fewer evidence-based programs are available for providers and health systems to adopt to improve patient safety in the ambulatory setting.

The relative lack of measures and evidence-based programs for addressing ambulatory patient safety should not be interpreted to mean that ambulatory settings have fewer patient safety problems. To the contrary, a variety of studies have underscored the frequency of medical errors that occur in the ambulatory setting (Sarkar 2016; Panesar et al. 2015).

In 2015, AHRQ sought to address this problem by establishing a task force to provide a comprehensive look at patient safety in the ambulatory setting (Shekelle et al. 2016). The resulting report focused on identifying problems relevant to ambulatory-based care and developing strategies to improve safety. The report identified five concrete patient safety areas that would need to be systematically targeted to meet ambulatory safety goals: (1) medication safety, (2) transitions of care, (3) test tracking, (4) referral tracking, and (5) diagnosis.

Medication safety concerns are analogous to many safety issues in the hospital setting, including errors in prescribing, dispensing, and monitoring medications, as well as failure to note medication interactions. Other medication safety problems are more relevant to the ambulatory setting—for instance, failure to discontinue medications or to identify and address medication nonadherence.

Transitions of care—for instance, during discharge from the hospital or after an emergency department visit—carry a high risk for adverse patient safety events (Forster et al. 2004, 2007; Moore et al. 2003). The risk of adverse drug events is especially high during these transitions, especially for older adults (Kanaan et al. 2013). Changes in medication are common during hospitalizations, including discontinuation of prior medications, initiation of new medications, and dose adjustments. Poor communication between inpatient and outpatient providers is common during transitions, and it has significant implications for safety (Kripalani et al. 2007).

Tracking tests that have been ordered and following up on patient referrals to specialists are essential for reducing errors in healthcare delivery. The tracking of pending test results is especially important during transitions of care. Research suggests that more than 40 percent of patients have pending test results at the time of hospital discharge (Roy et al. 2005). Errors at any step during the testing, reporting, interpretation, and communication processes can lead to errors in the ambulatory setting (Hickner et al. 2008). Ensuring that patients are aware of meaningful test results, both normal and abnormal, is important for the safe provision of care, as is the tracking of test results across the system—including tests that have been ordered but not completed.

Referrals throughout the ambulatory care system also must be tracked. Studies of patient referrals from primary care providers to specialists have revealed poor integration, breakdowns in communication, and process inefficiencies (Mehrotra, Forrest, and Lin 2011). Specialty providers are not always aware of the reasons for the referral, primary care providers are not always aware of specialists' treatment recommendations, and patients are often burdened with transferring information between providers. Shared EHRs can help improve this communication, but they need to be coupled with systematic approaches to referral tracking and communication strategies among providers on a care team.

Finally, diagnostic error has garnered much attention as an area of focus for patient safety efforts. In a 2015 report titled *Improving Diagnosis in Health Care*, the National Academy of Medicine defined *diagnostic error* as either the "failure to (a) establish an accurate and timely explanation of the patient's health problem(s) or (b) communicate that explanation to the patient" (National Academies of Sciences, Engineering, and Medicine 2015, 4). Although diagnostic error rates are difficult to measure, such errors are common. They are believed to affect at least 5 percent of US adults in the outpatient setting, or

12 million adults annually (Singh, Meyer, and Thomas 2014). The figures are even higher in the inpatient setting (Graber 2013). Accurate and timely communication of diagnosis is central to the provision of safe care across all healthcare settings.

Strategies for Safe Care

Although patient safety in the ambulatory setting has challenges distinct from those in the inpatient setting (Wachter 2006), many strategies to improve safety are common to both. Key strategies include establishing and maintaining channels of communication, effectively using health information technology (IT), providing team-based care, fostering patient and family engagement, and developing organizational approaches and a culture of safety (Shekelle et al. 2016). These strategies are essential for organizing and delivering safe, high-quality care in the ambulatory setting.

Patient-centered medical homes and other patient-centered population health models of care can facilitate improved patient safety by leveraging teamwork, information management, population measurement, and patient empowerment (Singh and Graber 2010). These strategies must not be limited to primary care providers; they should engage specialists as well. Patient-centered specialty practices and medical neighborhood models can facilitate the establishment of referral agreements between primary care providers and specialists (Ward et al. 2017). Coupled with effective health IT utilization, such agreements can improve referral tracking and communication between specialists and primary care physicians (Akbari et al. 2008). Health IT measures are also essential for maximizing the safety of test tracking—although, even with advanced EHRs, systems are still needed to ensure that critical results are addressed in a timely manner (Singh et al. 2009).

Future Challenges and Keys to Success

The Role of Primary Care and Subspecialty Providers

Primary care is considered by many to be the foundation for any successful population health strategy, because primary care physicians—including family physicians, general internists, and pediatricians—are the medical providers who most commonly oversee all aspects of their patients' care. They are the main providers for patients with such chronic diseases as coronary artery disease, diabetes, and emphysema, and they are usually the healthcare professionals held responsible for ordering the majority of preventive cancer screenings. They are also the providers most often called upon to manage the numerous ambulatory quality metrics. Primary care physicians have long been central to programs such as PCMHs and the Comprehensive Primary Care Plus (CPC+) model (White 2015). Demand for primary care physicians is likely to increase in the coming years as populations age and grow in size (Health Resources and Services Administration 2013).

Given the ever-increasing demands to deliver higher-quality care at a lower cost across all healthcare settings, a key issue involves incorporating the Institute for Healthcare Improvement's Triple Aim—better experience of care, improved health of populations, and reduced costs (Berwick, Nolan, and Whittington 2008)—in subspecialty offices. MIPS and initiatives such as NCQA's PCSP recognition program have initiated this transformation, but more work remains to be done. A greater emphasis will be placed on educating providers and implementing programs in offices that historically have not been heavily involved in formal ambulatory quality and safety programs (Ward et al. 2017).

Impact of Compensation and Aligning Incentives

Regardless of the practice location, quality and safety metrics should align both with the best clinical care recommendations and with the incentives of medical providers. Incentives for providers may be financial in nature, or they may involve the desire for the most efficient processes for completing the required care, or improved job satisfaction (Bodenheimer and Sinski 2014).

Well-aligned quality measures will promote optimal performance and boost clinicians' motivation by rewarding them for managing patients appropriately. Conversely, poorly aligned measures often add unnecessary work and can even have a negative impact on care by drawing attention away from more important duties (Cassell and Jain 2012; Young, Roberts, and Holden 2014). Furthermore, poor alignment can contribute to physician burnout and cause providers to lose confidence in the overall quality improvement effort (Greenhalgh, Howick, and Maskrey 2014). As healthcare shifts from volume- to value-driven payment approaches, the financial incentives for providers must include appropriate components that reward the delivery of high-quality care.

Number and Standardization of Measures

As the measurement of quality in healthcare has grown and evolved, concerns have arisen about the measures' complexity and the administrative burden they place on providers. For example, the NQF tracks 634 measures through its Quality Positioning System (NQF 2017b). The fact that so many metrics exist—and that a significant number of them must be reported on a regular basis—can be overwhelming. Reporting on such a large number of required measures risks impeding the ability of providers to focus on the metrics that have been proved to be the most important.

Researchers in 2012 estimated that quality measurements and analysis cost healthcare providers $190 billion annually, and that figure is likely to have increased (Meyer et al. 2012). The cost is especially high for organizations that participate in multiple quality initiatives (Blumenthal, Malphrus, and McGinnis 2015). At one such organization, an analysis documented the need to report more than 1,600 quality measures to 49 different sources, at a cost of more than $2 million (Murray et al. 2017).

Additional complexities may result from differences in the measures used from one insurance plan to another. For example, one insurer might choose to rate providers' care of patients with diabetes based on their ability to bring the patients to a glycated hemoglobin (HbA1c) level of less than 9 percent; another might use a threshold of 8 percent. Still another might choose a composite score where HbA1c is only one of multiple metrics used, combined with diabetic eye and kidney care.

This lack of uniformity creates difficulty for provider organizations looking to gather accurate data and perform patient outreach to close gaps in care. It also risks turning providers against the quality improvement movement, if they feel the bar is being set impossibly high or the requirements are too complex for them to understand. To maximize the effectiveness and efficiency of quality improvement programs, all (or, at least, most) insurers must decide upon and utilize a standard set of baseline metrics.

Transparency of Data to Other Providers and the Public

Today, many hospital quality and safety measures are publicly reported, and consumers often compare institutions with one another based on these measures. Experts expect that similar reporting and comparisons with ambulatory measures will not be far behind (Lamb et al. 2013).

This development will require standardized data, but some health plans already have the ability to begin this process. We can easily envision, for instance, a health plan sharing information not only on the cost of care provided by one office compared to another but also on the offices' safety or quality scores. CMS has already reported on PQRS participation, and it might publicly release future MIPS data in a fashion that supports comparisons between medical providers. Through these efforts, pay-for-performance programs become less important than the fact that patients will be able to decide whether to begin a relationship with a provider based on its performance on quality and safety scores.

Conclusion

The growing emphasis on ambulatory quality and safety has had a significant impact on practice operations, the daily workflows of medical providers, and the financial viability of healthcare organizations in the United States. Spurred by such initiatives as the PCMH program and the Value-Based Purchasing Program, ACOs, providers, and health systems are becoming accustomed to measuring quality and safety performance, reporting data, and being reimbursed for the quality of patient care.

The momentum of national strategies to improve healthcare quality has been sustained by public and private funding and by the development of policies that support measurement, public reporting, and accountability. Innovation and collaboration will continue to be a priority for quality improvement efforts, as new care-delivery and population-based models are explored to support integration across healthcare sectors. A key challenge will be to carefully choose quality measures while also limiting redundancies and inefficiencies in the various measures employed across the healthcare landscape. Leaders in quality improvement will also need to continually evaluate the effectiveness of quality programs, incorporate new evidence from scientific research, and reach out to providers across all specialties and healthcare settings.

Case Study: A Private Practice in the Pennsylvania Chronic Care Initiative

Dr. Johnson had been a family medicine physician in Pennsylvania for ten years. He had one physician partner and an office staff of three people: his wife, who functioned as an office manager; a front desk clerk, who greeted visitors, checked patients in and out, and answered phones; and a medical assistant, who assisted with rooming patients, performing electrocardiograms, and drawing blood. The office was under increasing pressure to see more patients and to have shorter appointment times, and Dr. Johnson was concerned about his ability to practice medicine the way he wanted.

In 2008, Dr. Johnson was contacted about a program called the Pennsylvania Chronic Care Initiative (CCI), which was slated to begin the following year. The CCI was an NCQA-accredited program that partnered with his primary professional organization (the Pennsylvania Academy of Family Physicians) and was funded through the predominant local insurance companies, both private and public (Medicare and Medicaid). The CCI sought to create a collaborative network to assist practices in becoming true PCMHs, and it would pay practices monthly for the patients they were caring for on a per-member-per-month basis (Patient Centered Primary Care Collaborative 2015). Excited that this program might alleviate some of his financial burden while also helping him take better care of patients, Dr. Johnson decided to investigate. He learned that many other practices in the area were joining the program, so he decided to do so as well.

Dr. Johnson's local insurers had recently begun offering financial incentives for meeting certain quality metrics, as well as for becoming recognized as a PCMH. He had researched the PCMH concept and thought it

(continued)

sounded like a good idea. However, he was unable to meet the criteria for PCMH recognition without first having funds for additional staff to track his population of patients and to do the necessary outreach to them, along with other required components. He hoped that the CCI would quickly provide him the funds to help him meet the criteria and gain recognition.

Dr. Johnson was accepted into the CCI and quickly saw some benefits for his practice. First, he met with a practice facilitator who helped him develop workflows to meet PCMH criteria and to address the issues of patients who experienced gaps in some aspect of care (e.g., they were due for a mammogram). The facilitator also worked with him to better utilize the EHR system he had purchased a couple years earlier but had not used for anything beyond simple office documentation. Next, Dr. Johnson joined a regional learning collaborative with other practices similar to his own. The collaborative helped provide him and his staff with the education and tools necessary to further redesign his practice. Dr. Johnson was required to submit monthly reports on his performance, and he began to receive additional payments from the insurers.

Dr. Johnson quickly realized how much his office needed to improve to meet the demands of a modern medical practice. In addition to managing the immediate medical needs of his patients, he also had to make sure that the numerous quality metrics (e.g., appropriate cancer screenings, diabetes care metrics) were met. His staff had to track the measures and identify patients who were missing a quality metric—even if those patients had not been seen in the office for up to two years. Significant time had to be devoted to accomplishing these tasks, in addition to writing letters and making phone calls.

Thankfully, Dr. Johnson's performance after the first year of the program was very good, and his rate of meeting many quality metrics had improved significantly. For example, prior to joining the CCI, Dr. Johnson was not regularly tracking his rate of checking the HbA1c levels in patients with diabetes. The practice coaches calculated that he had been checking the levels in 68 percent of patients at some point in the previous year. By both identifying patients when they came to the office and performing outreach to those who did not, his office raised that rate to 90 percent.

Dr. Johnson saw similar improvements in most of the other metrics, with the exception of colon cancer screening. His rate of appropriate screening had improved from 52 percent to 58 percent, but the national average was 70 percent; therefore, he was not satisfied. With the help of his staff and the regional collaborative's suggestions, he sought to evaluate why his performance had not improved as much as he had hoped. Using the

Plan-Do-Study-Act method, the office staff began making changes to their workflows, seeing what effect those changes had, and making the necessary adjustments to improve performance. Their primary discoveries were (1) that patients needed more information to convince them to undergo a colonoscopy and (2) that the gastroenterologist to whom the practice was referring patients was doing a poor job of contacting those patients who were referred for screening. Subsequently, Dr. Johnson improved his explanation to patients of why they needed a colonoscopy and provided supporting written materials. He also began referring patients to a different gastroenterologist who was better able to handle the volume of referrals from his office. After six months, his colon cancer screening rate rose to 74 percent, which qualified him for additional payments from several insurance companies at the end of the year.

Case Study: Comprehensive Primary Care Plus

In 2017, a suburban primary care practice consisting of four physicians and three nurse practitioners applied for and was accepted into a new CMS Innovation Center program called Comprehensive Primary Care Plus, or CPC+ (CMS 2017d). The program was intended as an expansion of the medical home model, which aimed to strengthen primary care through regionally based public/private payer payment reform and care delivery transformation.

The predecessor of CPC+, the CPC initiative, did not achieve financial savings or improvement on quality measures but did demonstrate ways that aligning financial incentives, quality improvement, and data feedback could support practice transformation (CMS 2017c; Dale et al. 2016; Anglin et al. 2017). Building on this knowledge, CPC+ was designed to provide significant funding to practices to make investments, improve quality of care, and reduce the number of unnecessary services their patients receive. As in the previous CPC initiative (and like CCI in the previous case study), CMS provided member practices with a robust learning system, as well as actionable data feedback to guide their decision making. In addition, CPC+ is considered an "advanced" APM for MACRA, which allowed for bonus payments to providers in future years (CMS 2017d). Based on these potential benefits, the providers in the primary care practice decided to join the program.

At the start of the CPC+ program, the practice was notified that it had 1,000 Medicare patients who were attributed (linked) to the practice for the purposes of the program. This attribution made the practice eligible

(continued)

to receive more than $300,000 that year, to be specifically used to hire additional personnel to support the program. After extensive discussion, the practice decided to hire a clinical social worker to assist with behavioral health; a nurse to provide care coordination to patients with complex medical needs; and two additional medical assistants to help close quality gaps and to contact patients soon after visits to hospitals and emergency departments.

The CPC+ program had significant administrative reporting requirements, and satisfying the required quality metrics took substantial effort. At the end of the year, the practice had to submit to CMS the results of nine metrics that they had chosen at the start of the year. Because two of the metrics chosen had never been followed by the practice, and because the providers were unsure whether their EHR system would be able to record measures accurately, they chose to implement an additional two metrics just in case they had problems meeting all the requirements.

The practice hired additional staff and went about implementing the many aspects required by the CPC+ program, including additional care management, tracking and contacting patients after hospital and emergency department visits, and arranging meetings in which patients and practice representatives discuss ways to improve the practice experience. The practice also instituted weekly care team meetings in which physicians and other staff (clinical and nonclinical) would discuss complex patients and review data on hospital readmission rates and quality metrics. Some staff initially viewed these meetings as distractions that interfered with time that could be used to see patients. However, the practice soon realized that, through use of the Plan-Do-Study-Act methodology, results on several of their quality measures had begun to improve. Eventually, staff members came to view the meetings as invaluable opportunities to gather as a group to overcome barriers to improvement (IHI 2017).

Case Study: A New Pay-for-Performance Contract

An eight-member primary care medical practice signed a new contract with an insurance company. The previous contract had paid the practice an average of $90 for each office visit, and the practice had the opportunity to earn an extra $10 per patient, on average, if certain quality measures were met. Over the previous several years under that contract, they had been recognized as a level-3 PCMH, which had earned them an additional $3 per patient.

The practice used the money to hire a nurse and to close quality care gaps. The members of the practice had met all of the quality measures and had successfully maximized their earnings.

Under the new contract, the members agreed to accept a lower average payment of $80 per office visit but hoped to offset that drop by maximizing the new quality payment program, which could earn them an extra $30 per patient. Unfortunately, the insurance company did not renew the extra payments for being a PCMH, stating that such status was now a basic expectation for all practices in the network. Nonetheless, the new contract gave the practice an opportunity to earn more money overall if it was successful in meeting its quality objectives. The members estimated that the practice would earn less money over the next year, because of the drop in payments per visit, but could earn more money when the quality results were tallied at the end of the year, if the practice performed well.

To maximize their chances of success, the practice worked with its EHR vendor to pull data reports from the system, helping to monitor the practice's performance on quality metrics and to identify specific patients who had a gap in care (e.g., patients who needed to have a test completed). A specially trained medical assistant would then use the reports to call patients, briefly explain to them what was needed, and arrange for the test or study to be completed. A provider would write the order, and the medical assistant would make sure all necessary paperwork was completed.

The practice developed a workflow in the EHR that would flag patients with a gap in care so that the appropriate action could be initiated immediately by the front desk or medical assistant and quickly approved by the provider when the patients arrived for office visits. Under this approach, office staff were asked to work "at the top of their license" and felt that they were an integral part of the healthcare team. The approach also allowed providers to focus more on making the complex medical decisions they were trained to make.

A practice report card was developed to track performance and support communication among the staff and providers. The report card was populated with data pulled from the EHR for each metric that was being tracked, and the data were directly linked to the goals stated in the insurance company contract. The report card was updated on a regular basis and shared at each monthly practice meeting, when everyone gathered to discuss current issues. Any metric that was not meeting the performance goal was discussed in detail, and action plans for improvement were developed. The staff then used Plan-Do-Study-Act cycles to fix any problems, with a follow-up report at the next monthly meeting.

Case Study: Referral Follow-Up and Ambulatory Safety

A 57-year-old man, Mr. Young, had experienced three months of burning chest pain after eating and intermittent diffuse abdominal discomfort. His primary care physician prescribed a proton-pump inhibitor for suspected gastroesophageal reflux and ordered a panel of lab tests, including a routine screening for hepatitis C. The physician also noted that Mr. Young had never received a colon cancer screening, so she gave him a referral to a gastroenterologist. The physician included the referral with Mr. Young's visit summary paperwork, but she forgot to explain the reason for the referral. He left the office without talking to any of the other staff members on the team.

Mr. Young took omeprazole as prescribed, and his symptoms improved significantly. Feeling much better, he decided to postpone getting the blood tests done. Mr. Young also misunderstood the reason for the gastroenterology referral, thinking he had been referred to address his now-resolved abdominal symptoms; thus, he felt no urgency to schedule the appointment.

Although this case is fictional, the scenario is typical of many interactions in the ambulatory setting. If the eventual tests revealed that Mr. Young was positive for hepatitis C or if he had abnormal findings on his colonoscopy, he would be at risk for delayed diagnosis. Thus, systematic strategies for test tracking and referral tracking should be implemented to alert the primary care physician if actions ordered for a patient have not been completed in a timely manner. Furthermore, team-based care strategies can be employed both at the time of the visit (e.g., having a medical assistant review the visit summary at check-out) and at a later date (e.g., having a team member use population health approaches to identify patients due for test completion or routine screening).

Study Questions

1. How has passage of the Affordable Care Act affected the emphasis on delivering high-quality care to patients?
2. Construct a possible future timeline for quality improvement activities and legislative initiatives. As healthcare funding moves increasingly to a focus on high-value care, how might measurement and reporting of quality and safety processes and outcomes change? How will these changes affect the way that care is financed by payers and delivered by providers?

3. Discuss the impact that federal quality and safety improvement initiatives will have on healthcare delivery in the state in which you reside. What federal legislative initiatives are controversial in your state or have a high degree of support? Why?
4. Discuss how the mandate to submit quality and safety data to insurance payers might affect a physician office. What would be the positive impact on the office and on the patients it serves? What would be the potential negative impact?

References

Agency for Healthcare Research and Quality (AHRQ). 2014. "Efforts to Improve Patient Safety Result in 1.3 Million Fewer Patient Harms." Published December. www.ahrq.gov/professionals/quality-patient-safety/pfp/interimhacrate2013.html.

Akbari, A., A. Mayhew, M. Al-Alawi, J. Grimshaw, R. Winkens, E. Glidewell, C. Pritchard, R. Thomas, and C. Fraser. 2008. "Interventions to Improve Outpatient Referrals from Primary Care to Secondary Care." *Cochrane Database of Systematic Reviews*. Published October. www.cochranelibrary.com/cdsr/doi/10.1002/14651858.CD005471.pub2/abstract.

American College of Physicians (ACP). 2009. "Controlling Health Care Costs While Promoting the Best Possible Health Outcomes." Accessed November 26. www.acponline.org/system/files/documents/advocacy/current_policy_papers/assets/controlling_healthcare_costs.pdf.

Anglin, G., H. A. Tu, K. Liao, L. Sessums, and E. F. Taylor. 2017. "Strengthening Multipayer Collaboration: Lessons from the Comprehensive Primary Care Initiative." *Milbank Quarterly* 95 (3): 602–33.

Berwick, D. M., T. W. Nolan, and J. Whittington. 2008. "The Triple Aim: Care, Health, and Cost." *Health Affairs* 27 (3): 759–69.

Blumenthal, D., M. Abrams, and R. Nuzum. 2015. "The Affordable Care Act at 5 Years." *New England Journal of Medicine* 372 (25): 2451–58.

Blumenthal, D., E. Malphrus, and J. M. McGinnis (eds.). 2015. *Vital Signs: Core Metrics for Health and Health Care Progress.* Washington, DC: National Academies Press.

Bodenheimer, T., and C. Sinsky. 2014. "From Triple to Quadruple Aim: Care of the Patient Requires Care of the Provider." *Annals of Family Medicine* 12 (6): 573–76.

Cassel, C. K., and S. H. Jain. 2012. "Assessing Individual Physician Performance: Does Measurement Suppress Motivation?" *JAMA* 307 (24): 2595–96.

Centers for Disease Control and Prevention (CDC). 2016. "National and State Healthcare Associated Infections Progress Report." Accessed December 10, 2017. www.cdc.gov/HAI/pdfs/progress-report/hai-progress-report.pdf.

Centers for Medicare & Medicaid Services (CMS). 2018a. "Accountable Care Organizations (ACOs)." Updated May 3. www.cms.gov/Medicare/Medicare-Fee-for-Service-Payment/ACO/.

———. 2018b. "The Hospital Value-Based Purchasing (VBP) Program." Updated August 2. www.cms.gov/Medicare/Quality-Initiatives-Patient-Assessment-Instruments/Value-Based-Programs/HVBP/Hospital-Value-Based-Purchasing.html.

———. 2018c. "MACRA: What's MACRA?" Updated September 21. www.cms.gov/Medicare/Quality-Initiatives-Patient-Assessment-Instruments/Value-Based-Programs/MACRA-MIPS-and-APMs/MACRA-MIPS-and-APMs.html.

———. 2018d. "Quality Payment Program." Updated November 5. www.cms.gov/Medicare/Quality-Payment-Program/Quality-Payment-Program.html.

———. 2017a. "About the CMS Innovation Center." Updated June 23. https://innovation.cms.gov/About.

———. 2017b. "Accountable Care Organization 2017 Program Quality Measure Narrative Specifications." Published January 5. www.cms.gov/Medicare/Medicare-Fee-for-Service-Payment/sharedsavingsprogram/Downloads/2017-Reporting-Year-Narrative-Specifications.pdf.

———. 2017c. "Comprehensive Primary Care Initiative." Updated October 24. https://innovation.cms.gov/initiatives/comprehensive-primary-care-initiative/.

———. 2017d. "Comprehensive Primary Care Plus." Accessed December 6. https://innovation.cms.gov/initiatives/comprehensive-primary-care-plus.

———. 2017e. "Physician Quality Reporting System." Updated October 11. www.cms.gov/Medicare/Quality-Initiatives-Patient-Assessment-Instruments/PQRS/index.html.

———. 2015. "2015 Physician Quality Reporting System (PQRS): Understanding 2017 Medicare Quality Program Payment Adjustments." Updated October 7. www.cms.gov/Medicare/Quality-Initiatives-Patient-Assessment-Instruments/PQRS/Downloads/Understanding2017MedicarePayAdjs.pdf.

Chee, T. T., A. M. Ryan, J. H. Wasfy, and W. B. Borden. 2016. "Current State of Value-Based Purchasing Programs." *Circulation* 133 (22): 2197–205.

Congress.gov. 2017. "S.580—Healthcare Research and Quality Act of 1999." Accessed December 10. www.congress.gov/bill/106th-congress/senate-bill/580.

Dale, S. B., A. Ghosh, D. N. Peikes, T. J. Day, F. B. Yoon, E. F. Taylor, K. Swankoski, A. S. O'Malley, P. H. Conway, R. Rajkumar, M. J. Press, L. Sessums, and R. Brown. 2016. "Two-Year Costs and Quality in the Comprehensive Primary Care Initiative." *New England Journal of Medicine* 374: 2345–56.

Davis, K., M. Abrams, and K. Stremikis. 2011. "How the Affordable Care Act Will Strengthen the Nation's Primary Care Foundation." *Journal of General Internal Medicine* 26 (10): 1201–3.

Donabedian, A. 1966. "Evaluating the Quality of Medical Care." *Milbank Quarterly* 83 (4): 691–729.

Forster, A. J., H. D. Clark, A. Menard, N. Dupuis, R. Chernish, N. Chandok, A. Khan, and C. van Walraven. 2004. "Adverse Events Among Medical Patients After Discharge from Hospital." *CMAJ: Canadian Medical Association Journal* 170 (3): 345–49.

Forster, A. J., N. G. W. Rose, C. van Walraven, and I. Stiell. 2007. "Adverse Events Following an Emergency Department Visit." *Quality & Safety in Health Care* 16 (1): 17–22.

Friedberg, M. W., M. B. Rosenthal, and R. W. Werner. 2015. "Effects of a Medical Home and Shared Savings Intervention on Quality and Utilization of Care." *JAMA Internal Medicine* 175 (8): 1362–68.

Friedberg, M. W., E. C. Schneider, M. B. Rosenthal, K. G. Volpp, and R. M. Werner. 2014. "Association Between Participation in a Multipayer Medical Home Intervention and Changes in Quality, Utilization, and Costs of Care." *JAMA* 311 (8): 815–25.

Future of Family Medicine Project Leadership Committee. 2004. "The Future of Family Medicine: A Collaborative Project of the Family Medicine Community." *Annals of Family Medicine* 2 (Suppl. 1): s3–s32.

Graber, M. L. 2013. "The Incidence of Diagnostic Error in Medicine." *BMJ Quality & Safety* 22 (Suppl. 2): ii21–ii27.

Greenhalgh, T., J. Howick, and N. Maskrey. 2014. "Evidence-Based Medicine: A Movement in Crisis?" *BMJ* 348: g3725.

Health Resources and Services Administration (HRSA). 2013. "Projecting the Supply and Demand for Primary Care Practitioners Through 2020." Published November. https://bhw.hrsa.gov/health-workforce-analysis/primary-care-2020#.

Hickner, J., D. G. Graham, N. C. Elder, E. Brandt, C. B. Emsermann, S. Dovey, and R. Phillips. 2008. "Testing Process Errors and Their Harms and Consequences Reported from Family Medicine Practices: A Study of the American Academy of Family Physicians National Research Network." *Quality & Safety in Health Care* 17 (3): 194–200.

Hospital Consumer Assessment of Healthcare Providers and Systems (HCAHPS). 2017. "HCAHPS Fact Sheet (CAHPS Hospital Survey)." Published November 2. www.hcahpsonline.org/Files/HCAHPS_Fact_Sheet_November_2017.pdf.

Institute for Healthcare Improvement (IHI). 2017. "Plan-Do-Study-Act (PDSA) Worksheet." Accessed December 10. www.ihi.org/resources/Pages/Tools/PlanDoStudyActWorksheet.aspx.

Institute of Medicine (IOM). 2001. *Crossing the Quality Chasm: A New Health System for the 21st Century.* Washington, DC: National Academies Press.

Jackson, G. L., B. J. Powers, R. Chatterjee, J. P. Bettger, A. R. Kemper, V. Hasselblad, R. J. Dolor, R. J. Irvine, B. L. Heidenfelder, A. S. Kendrick, R. Gray, and J. W. Williams Jr. 2013. "The Patient-Centered Medical Home: A Systematic Review." *Annals of Internal Medicine* 158 (3): 169–78.

Kanaan, A. O., J. L. Donovan, N. P. Duchin, T. S. Field, J. Tjia, S. L. Cutrona, S. J. Gagne, L. Garber, P. Preusse, L. R. Harrold, and J. H. Gurwitz. 2013. "Adverse Drug Events After Hospital Discharge in Older Adults: Types, Severity, and Involvement of Beers Criteria Medications." *Journal of the American Geriatrics Society* 61 (11): 1894–99.

Keehan, S. P., A. M. Sisko, C. J. Truffer, J. A. Poisal, G. A. Cuckler, A. J. Madison, J. M. Lizonitz, and S. D. Smith. 2011. "National Health Spending Projections Through 2020: Economic Recovery and Reform Drive Faster Spending Growth." *Health Affairs* 30 (8): 1594–605.

Kohn, L. T., J. M. Corrigan, and M. S. Donaldson (eds.). 2000. *To Err Is Human: Building a Safer Health System*. Washington, DC: National Academies Press.

Kripalani, S., F. LeFevre, C. O. Phillips, M. V. Williams, P. Basaviah, and D. W. Baker. 2007. "Deficits in Communication and Information Transfer Between Hospital-Based and Primary Care Physicians: Implications for Patient Safety and Continuity of Care." *JAMA* 297 (8): 831–41.

Lamb, G. C., M. A. Smith, W. B. Weeks, and C. Queram. 2013. "Publicly Reported Quality-of-Care Measures Influenced Wisconsin Physician Groups to Improve Performance." *Health Affairs (Project Hope)* 32 (3): 536–43.

Landers, S., E. Madigan, B. Leff, R. J. Rosati, B. A. McCann, R. Hornbake, R. MacMillan, K. Jones, K. Bowles, D. Dowding, T. Lee, T. Moorhead, S. Rodriguez, and E. Breese. 2016. "The Future of Home Health Care: A Strategic Framework for Optimizing Value." *Home Health Care Management & Practice* 28 (4): 262–78.

L&M Policy Research. 2016. *Evaluation of the Medicare Quality Bonus Payment Demonstration*. Published February. www.lmpolicyresearch.com/documents/MA-QBP-Demonstration-Final%20Report.pdf.

Marjoua, Y., and K. J. Bozic. 2012. "Brief History of Quality Movement in US Healthcare." *Current Reviews in Musculoskeletal Medicine* 5 (4): 265–73.

Markovich, M. 2003. "The Rise of HMOs." RAND Corporation. Accessed December 2, 2017. www.rand.org/pubs/rgs_dissertations/RGSD172.html.

Marquis, S. M., J. A. Rogowski, and J. J. Escarce. 2004. "The Managed Care Backlash: Did Consumers Vote with Their Feet?" *Inquiry* 41 (4): 376–90.

McWilliams, M. J. 2017. "MACRA: Big Fix or Big Problem?" *Annals of Internal Medicine* 167 (2): 122–25.

Medicare Payment Advisory Commission (MedPAC). 2017. "Ambulatory Care Settings." Accessed November 29. www.medpac.gov/-research-areas-/ambulatory-care-settings.

Mehrotra, A., C. B. Forrest, and C. Y. Lin. 2011. "Dropping the Baton: Specialty Referrals in the United States." *Milbank Quarterly* 89 (1): 39–68.

Meyer, G. S., E. C. Nelson, D. B. Pryor, B. James, S. J. Swensen, G. S. Kaplan, J. I. Weissberg, M. Bisognano, G. R. Yates, and G. C. Hunt. 2012. "More Quality Measures Versus Measuring What Matters: A Call for Balance and Parsimony." *BMJ Quality & Safety* 21 (11): 964–68.

Moore, C., J. Wisnivesky, S. Williams, and T. McGinn. 2003. "Medical Errors Related to Discontinuity of Care from an Inpatient to an Outpatient Setting." *Journal of General Internal Medicine* 18 (8): 646–51.

Murray, K. R., B. Hilligoss, J. L. Hefner, A. Scheck McAlearney, A. VanBuren, T. R. Huerta, and S. Moffatt-Bruce. 2017. "The Quality Reporting Reality at a Large Academic Medical Center: Reporting 1600 Unique Measures to 49 Different Sources." *International Journal of Academic Medicine* 3 (1): 10–15.

National Academies of Sciences, Engineering, and Medicine. 2018. "Our Study Process." Accessed November 26. http://nationalacademies.org/studyprocess/index.html.

———. 2015. *Improving Diagnosis in Health Care*. Washington, DC: National Academies Press.

National Committee for Quality Assurance (NCQA). 2018. "Patient-Centered Medical Home Recognition." Accessed November 26. www.ncqa.org/programs/health-care-providers-practices/patient-centered-medical-home-pcmh/.

———. 2017. *Latest Evidence: Benefits of NCQA Patient-Centered Medical Home Recognition*. Published October. www.ncqa.org/wp-content/uploads/2018/08/20171017_PCMH_Evidence_Report.pdf.

National Quality Forum (NQF). 2017a. "About NQF." Accessed December 8. www.qualityforum.org/About_NQF/Mission_and_Vision.aspx.

———. 2017b. "Field Guide to NQF Resources." Accessed December 10. www.qualityforum.org/Field_Guide/List_of_Measures.aspx.

Panesar, S. S., D. deSilva, A. Carson-Stevens, K. M. Cresswell, S. Angostora Salvilla, S. P. Slight, S. Javad, G. Netuveli, I. Larizgoitia, L. J. Donaldson, D. W. Bates, and A. Sheikh. 2015. "How Safe Is Primary Care? A Systematic Review." *BMJ Quality & Safety* 25 (7): 544–53.

Patient-Centered Outcomes Research Institute (PCORI). 2017. "About Us." Accessed December 8. www.pcori.org/about-us.

Patient Centered Primary Care Collaborative (PCPCC). 2015. "Pennsylvania Chronic Care Initiative (CCI)." Updated September. www.pcpcc.org/initiative/pennsylvania-chronic-care-initiative-cci.

Robert Graham Center. 2007. "The Patient Centered Medical Home: History, Seven Core Features, Evidence and Transformational Change." Published November. www.aafp.org/dam/AAFP/documents/about_us/initiatives/PCMH.pdf.

Rosenthal, M. B., and A. Dudley. 2007. "Pay-for-Performance: Will the Latest Payment Trend Improve Care?" *JAMA* 297 (7): 740–44.

Rosenthal, M. B., R. Fernandopulle, H. S. R. Song, and B. Landon. 2004. "Paying for Quality: Providers' Incentives for Quality Improvement: An Assessment of Recent Efforts to Align Providers' Incentives with the Quality Improvement Agenda." *Health Affairs* 23 (2): 127–41.

Roy, C. L., E. G. Poon, A. S. Karson, Z. Ladak-Merchant, R. E. Johnson, S. M. Maviglia, and T. K. Gandhi. 2005. "Patient Safety Concerns Arising from Test

Results That Return After Hospital Discharge." *Annals of Internal Medicine* 143 (2): 121–28.

Ryan, A., and J. Blustein. 2012. "Making the Best of Hospital Pay for Performance." *New England Journal of Medicine* 366: 1557–59.

Sarkar, U. 2016. "Tip of the Iceberg: Patient Safety Incidents in Primary Care." *BMJ Quality & Safety* 25 (7): 477–79.

Sennett, C. 1998. "An Introduction to the National Committee for Quality Assurance." *Pediatric Annals* 27 (4): 210–14.

Shekelle, P. G., U. Sharkar, K. Shojania, R. M. Wachter, K. McDonald, A. Motala, P. Smith, L. Zipperer, and R. Shanman. 2016. "Patient Safety in Ambulatory Settings." Technical Brief No. 27. Rockville, MD: Agency for Healthcare Research and Quality.

Singh, H., and M. L. Graber. 2010. "Reducing Diagnostic Error Through Medical Home–Based Primary Care Reform." *JAMA* 304 (4): 463–64.

Singh, H., A. N. D. Meyer, and E. J. Thomas. 2014. "The Frequency of Diagnostic Errors in Outpatient Care: Estimations from Three Large Observational Studies Involving US Adult Populations." *BMJ Quality & Safety* 23 (9): 727–31.

Singh, H., E. J. Thomas, S. Mani, D. Sittig, H. Arora, D. Espadas, M. M. Khan, and L. A. Petersen. 2009. "Timely Follow-Up of Abnormal Diagnostic Imaging Test Results in an Outpatient Setting: Are Electronic Medical Records Achieving Their Potential?" *Archives of Internal Medicine* 169 (17): 1578–86.

Steinwachs, D. M., and R. G. Hughes. 2008. "Health Services Research: Scope and Significance." In *Patient Safety and Quality: An Evidence-Based Handbook for Nurses*, edited by R. G. Hughes, 8–43. Rockville, MD: Agency for Healthcare Research and Quality.

Wachter, R. M. 2006. "Is Ambulatory Patient Safety Just Like Hospital Safety, Only Without the 'Stat'?" *Annals of Internal Medicine* 145 (7): 547.

Ward, L. D., R. E. Powell, M. L. Scharf, A. Chapman, and M. Kavuru. 2017. "Patient-Centered Specialty Practice: Defining the Role of Specialists in Value-Based Health Care." *Chest* 151 (4): 930–35.

White, F. 2015. "Primary Health Care and Public Health: Foundations of Universal Health Systems." *Medical Principles and Practice* 24 (2): 103–16.

Young, R. A., R. G. Roberts, and R. J. Holden. 2014. "The Challenges of Measuring, Improving, and Reporting Quality in Primary Care." *Annals of Family Medicine* 15 (2): 175–82.

CHAPTER

15

THE ROLE OF THE NATIONAL COMMITTEE FOR QUALITY ASSURANCE

Michael S. Barr and Frank Micciche

Healthcare Quality: A Novel Concept

This may seem odd to today's students of healthcare policy, but there was a time, in the not-too-distant past, when the idea of concretely measuring healthcare quality was considered aspirational at best. During the 1980s, American businesses and their international counterparts were focused on continuous quality improvement and the Lean-ing of everything from supply chains to manufacturing processes. However, no established, standardized method existed for evaluating the healthcare that these same companies, as well as individuals and governments, were paying for. As healthcare spending rose from about 7 percent of the nation's gross domestic product in 1970 to more than 12 percent in 1990 (Kaiser Family Foundation [KFF] 2011), the need to address this deficiency became increasingly urgent.

Healthcare cost concerns dovetailed with the increasing popularity of various managed care mechanisms, most notably the health maintenance organization (HMO). These prepaid arrangements stood in contrast to the prevailing indemnity insurance model, in which patients paid for healthcare services and were subsequently repaid for some or all of the cost of the services by their insurer. Although indemnity plans represented 95 percent of all employer-sponsored enrollments as recently as 1978, they cover fewer than 1 percent of individuals with job-based health insurance today (KFF 2017).

Indeed, the cost-management capabilities of HMOs and similar products would prove irresistible to employers and other healthcare payers facing steep annual increases in the benefits they were providing. Between 1985 and 1990, enrollment in HMOs more than doubled, to a total of 39 million individuals (Wholey et al. 1997). Still, many purchasers were frustrated by the inability to measure and drive improvement in patient safety and overall healthcare quality among HMOs. As employers and plans sought a credible third-party entity to set healthcare quality standards and measure performance against those standards, they turned to the National Committee for Quality Assurance (NCQA).

Development of the National Committee for Quality Assurance

The National Committee for Quality Assurance (NCQA) had originally been founded in 1979 by representatives of leading HMOs and independent practice associations (IPAs). The groups established a voluntary review system to identify and address problems found within an HMO and to drive internal improvement activities (McPartland 2012). The system did not include a third-party audit of the data used to perform the review or the publication of findings. It was enough, though, to head off the imposition of a more rigorous regimen of federal oversight by the United States Department of Health and Human Services' Office for Health Maintenance Organizations—avoiding such oversight had been a key inspiration behind NCQA's original founding (Iglehart 1996).

In its early years, the opaque nature of NCQA's activities, as well as its ties to the industry it was charged with reviewing, belied any claims to objectivity. By the late 1980s, however, NCQA's board was reconstituted to include representation of payers, consumers, and other healthcare stakeholders, and funding from the Robert Wood Johnson Foundation (RWJF) was secured to study whether NCQA might be reconstituted as an independent, third-party reviewer of managed care performance. With strong support from the purchaser community and with start-up funds from managed care entities used to match a second RWJF grant, NCQA was officially established as an independent, nonprofit organization in April of 1990. Margaret E. "Peggy" O'Kane served as its founding president.

Defining and Measuring Quality

NCQA's rebirth occurred at a time when the debate over what "quality healthcare" entailed was front and center. A seminal report by the Institute of Medicine (IOM)—now the National Academy of Medicine (NAM)—defined *quality* as "the degree to which health services for individuals and populations increase the likelihood of desired outcomes and are consistent with current professional knowledge" (IOM 1990, 4).

The desire to capture how well managed care plans were implementing the latest evidence-based practices for providing high-quality care gave rise to the development of a group of measures now known as the Healthcare Effectiveness Data and Information Set (HEDIS). The idea of developing a single set of standardized measures for healthcare quality had originated in the late 1980s through the collaboration of forward-thinking employers, health plans, and quality experts. Given NCQA's emerging role in assessing healthcare quality, the measure set was officially entrusted to the organization in 1992. HEDIS 2.0, the first public set of HEDIS measures, was released in 1993.

With the HEDIS process established, independent standards for HEDIS collection and reporting procedures and the data they yielded became necessary to verify compliance with HEDIS specifications. In 1995, NCQA convened the HEDIS Audit Committee to develop such standards. The committee established a methodology for verifying the integrity of HEDIS collection and calculation processes—the NCQA HEDIS Compliance Audit. The audit consists of two parts: an overall information systems capabilities assessment (IS standards) and an evaluation of a plan's ability to comply with HEDIS specifications (HD standards).

Many health plans are required to report HEDIS data to employers and government purchasers as a condition of doing business with those entities. Nearly all of the 40 states that used managed care plans to deliver Medicaid benefits in 2017 required those plans to report audited HEDIS data to the state and/or NCQA. HEDIS results are available to the public via NCQA's Quality Compass database, an interactive, web-based comparison tool that allows users to view plan results and benchmark information. The results are also used to develop report cards on health plan performance issued each year by states, other organizations, and NCQA itself.

Since its beginning, HEDIS has transformed in response to changes in medical evidence and best practices. NCQA's Committee on Performance Measurement (CPM) was established in 1995 to oversee the evolution of the measurement set, with representation from purchasers, consumers, health plans, healthcare providers, and policymakers. Multiple Measurement Advisory Panels (MAPs) provide the clinical and technical knowledge required to develop and steward HEDIS measures. Additional expert panels and the Technical Measurement Advisory Panel (TMAP) identify methodological issues and provide feedback on new and existing measures.

Through this process, the list of HEDIS measures grew from a few dozen in the original version to 97 measures in HEDIS 2018. The measures encompass the following domains of care:

- Effectiveness of care
- Access/availability of care
- Experience of care
- Utilization and risk-adjusted utilization
- Health plan descriptive information
- Measures collected using electronic clinical data systems

The curation of HEDIS also involves the retirement of measures that have "done their job" in driving compliance and therefore no longer allow for meaningful performance differentiation between plans. Perhaps the best-known example of such an issue involves the use of beta blockers in patients who have had an acute myocardial infarction. The National Heart, Lung, and Blood Institute had documented in 1982 that beta-blocker treatment could dramatically decrease mortality for such patients, and its findings were reinforced in subsequent studies. Still, as of 1996—the year NCQA updated HEDIS to include a measure tracking adherence to this protocol—only 62 percent of recommended patients were found to have been prescribed a beta-blocker within a week of discharge. Within a decade, the mean was well over 90 percent. The measure was retired in 2007 (Lee 2007).

Health Plan Accreditation

NCQA conducted its first health plan accreditation (HPA, or HP accrediation) survey in 1991. Within six years, nearly a quarter of all large employers (i.e., employers with 5,000 or more workers) offering HMOs to their employees indicated that NCQA accreditation was "very important" in their selection of which plans to offer, with 17 percent of these "jumbo" employers requiring such accreditation. By 1997, three-quarters of all Americans with HMO coverage were in plans accredited by NCQA (Gabel, Hunt, and Hurst 1998). Adapting to the growing range of managed care models in the market, NCQA awarded HP accreditation to a preferred provider organization (PPO) for the first time in 2001. Exclusive provider organizations (EPOs) and point-of-service (POS) plans have since been made eligible for accreditation as well. As of 2017, nearly 182 million people—or 75 percent of all insured Americans—were covered through plans accredited by NCQA.

State and federal officials have also adopted accreditation requirements, in recognition of the growing role that managed care organizations (MCOs) play in providing government-funded health coverage. As of 2017, 25 states required that MCOs bidding to participate in the Medicaid program be accredited by NCQA, with another five imposing a broad mandate for accreditation by any nationally recognized accreditor (including NCQA). Federally, all plans offered through the Affordable Care Act marketplaces must be accredited (roughly 85 percent had NCQA accreditation in 2017), and managed care plans participating in the Medicare Advantage program may be deemed to be in compliance with federal regulations in five areas where accreditation standards and program rules overlap.

A health plan's overall accreditation status is calculated based on its performance in three areas: clinical performance, member satisfaction, and compliance with standards and guidelines. Clinical performance is assessed based on the plan's HEDIS scores relative to national and regional benchmarks. Assessment of member satisfaction centers on the plan's scores on the Consumer Assessment of Health Providers and Systems (CAHPS) survey—a tool maintained by the Agency for Healthcare Research and Quality (AHRQ). Compliance with standards and guidelines—which makes up half of the plan's overall accreditation score—is determined through a review of the plan with regard to the structures and processes contained in NCQA's published *Standards and Guidelines for the Accreditation of Health Plans*.

Accreditation standards and guidelines are established and revisited periodically by the NCQA Standards Committee. Categories include the following (NCQA 2018a):

- Quality Management and Improvement (QI)
- Population Health Management (PHM)
- Network Management (NET)
- Utilization Management (UM)
- Credentialing and Recredentialing (CR)
- Members' Rights and Responsibilities (RR)
- Member Connections (MEM)
- Medicaid Benefits and Services (MED)

Because most organizations offer several product lines (e.g., commercial, marketplace, Medicare, Medicaid), NCQA determines accreditation status by product line for HMO, POS, PPO, and EPO products. Each product line reviewed by NCQA earns an accreditation status level. Levels include *excellent*, *commendable*, *accredited*, *provisional*, *interim*, and *denied*.

Results are reported to the public via the NCQA Health Plan Report Card, using consumer-friendly language for easy comparison of plans. Beyond the plan's accreditation status, the report card provides star ratings in the following areas:

- Access and service—how well a health plan provides its members with access to needed care and good customer service
- Qualified providers—how a health plan ensures that each provider is licensed and appropriately trained to practice and that members are satisfied with their doctors
- Staying healthy—how health plan activities help people maintain good health and avoid illness
- Getting better—how health plan activities help people recover from illness
- Living with illness—how health plan activities help people manage chronic illness

NCQA Adds Practice-Level Focus

For much of its first 10 to 15 years, NCQA focused on improving and expanding health plan accreditation. Beginning around 1999, NCQA started to turn its attention toward the quality of care provided by medical practices. It developed a series of recognition programs that initially targeted specific, highly prevalent, and costly conditions (in terms of human health and health system expense) such as diabetes (the Diabetes Recognition Program, started in 1999), heart disease, and cerebrovascular disease (the Heart/Stroke Recognition Program, started in 2003). In 2002, in anticipation of new health information technology (HIT, or health IT) implementation in medical offices, NCQA developed a program called Physician Practice Connections (PPC) to promote the appropriate use of technology.

Around 2006, escalating healthcare costs, research about the value of primary care, and concerns about its viability in the United States resulted in a major shift in priorities for medical professional societies and health policy experts. These forces led, in part, to the introduction of the patient-centered medical home (PCMH) concept—currently the fastest growing primary care model in the United States. More than 20 medical professional societies, including the American Medical Association, have endorsed the PCMH care model (American College of Physicians 2017).

History of the Patient-Centered Medical Home

Descriptions of the medical home model were first published in the 1960s by the American Academy of Pediatrics (AAP) and Dr. Calvin Sia (AAP 2004; Patient-Centered Primary Care Collaborative 2017a). The central idea was to organize pediatric practices around the needs of children with chronic diseases and disabling conditions. Subsequently, AAP expanded the role of medical homes to include the provision of the same high-quality care for all children. Over the ensuing years, AAP promoted the model through its membership chapters and advocacy efforts, with support from the federal Maternal Child Health Bureau (MCHB).

A parallel effort focusing on patients with chronic conditions started in the mid-1990s. Led by Dr. Ed Wagner, the MacColl Center for Health Care Innovation at the Group Health Research Institute developed the Chronic Care Model (CCM) to guide the development of well-organized care for people with chronic conditions (Improving Chronic Illness Care 2017). Elements of the model include health system organization and culture, delivery system design, decision support, clinical information systems, self-management support, and inclusion of the community. The idealized output of the CCM is improved outcomes through the engagement of an informed, active patient by a prepared, proactive team.

The pediatric medical home and the CCM were eventually adapted by the American College of Physicians (ACP) into a new approach, labeled the "advanced medical home." The concept was detailed in a 2006 position paper and released with an ACP report titled "The Impending Collapse of Primary Care Medicine and Its Implications for the State of the Nation's Health Care" (Barr and Ginsburg 2006; ACP 2006). The first two sentences of the report set the stage for the recommendations (ACP 2006): "Primary care, the backbone of the nation's healthcare system, is at grave risk of collapse due to a dysfunctional financing and delivery system. Immediate and comprehensive reforms are required to replace systems that undermine and undervalue the relationship between patients and their personal physicians."

The authors pushed for tests of the advanced medical home in the first recommendation of the report (ACP 2006):

> First, we are calling on policymakers to implement and evaluate a new way of financing and delivering primary care called the *advanced medical home*. The advanced medical home is a physician practice that provides comprehensive, preventive and coordinated care centered on their patients' needs, using health information technology and other process innovations to assure high quality, accessible and efficient care. Practices would be certified as advanced medical homes, and certified practices would be eligible for new models of reimbursement to provide financing commensurate with the value they offer. These practices would also be accountable for results based on quality, efficiency and patient satisfaction measures. The advanced medical home would be particularly beneficial to patients with multiple chronic diseases—a population of patients that is growing rapidly and that consumes a disproportionate share of healthcare resources.

The ACP's recommendations were accompanied by similar calls from the American Academy of Family Physicians (AAFP) in its "Future of Family Medicine" report (Kahn 2004) and by ongoing promotion of the medical home concept by AAP. In 2006, the ACP, AAFP, and AAP assembled in a series of meetings, with strong encouragement from two executives at IBM, Martin Sepulveda and Paul Grundy. As physicians responsible for the health of IBM employees worldwide, Sepulveda and Grundy were passionate about primary care and concerned about the challenges described by the three professional societies and other health policy experts. They challenged the professional societies to develop a unified model for primary care—one that could be described in no more than two pages—and promised to convene the largest employers in the country to listen to the final concept.

The Joint Principles of the Patient-Centered Medical Home

The ACP and AAFP took the challenge and drafted a set of principles based on their respective position papers. The initial draft of the principles became part of the ongoing advocacy efforts of the ACP and AAFP prior to public release. The collaborative effort resulted in the first call for a Medicare medical home demonstration project in the Tax Relief and Health Care Act of 2006.

AAP and the American Osteopathic Association (AOA) soon joined the effort, and in March 2007 the four organizations collectively released the

"Joint Principles of the Patient-Centered Medical Home" (ACP 2007). The collection of seven principles focused on personal physicians, physician-directed medical practice, whole-person orientation, care coordination/integration, quality and safety, enhanced access, and payment, and together they reflected the organizations' definition of excellent primary care: Every person should have a primary care physician who leads a well-organized team that addresses all the needs of the individual either directly or through coordination with other healthcare professionals while delivering high-quality, safe, accessible care. The seventh principle—that payment for services should support the necessary infrastructure and deviate from the traditional volume-based, fee-for-service (FFS) model—indirectly led to the involvement of NCQA and other accrediting entities.

NCQA Launches the First PCMH Recognition Program

Representatives from the medical societies soon turned to NCQA for help. NCQA's PPC program had been in place for approximately four years, and despite its heavy emphasis on technology implementation, the program aligned reasonably well with the core tenets of the PCMH. Over a series of meetings in 2007, NCQA agreed to modify the PPC program to better reflect the Joint Principles. In 2008, NCQA launched the first US recognition program for the PCMH, called the Physician Practice Connections—Patient-Centered Medical Home (PPC-PCMH).

Initial uptake by practices was relatively slow. However, in parallel to the discussions with NCQA, the medical societies had initiated conversations with several insurance plans around the country to encourage PCMH pilots in tandem with new financial incentives. One of the earliest pilots was implemented by UnitedHealthcare and IBM in Arizona (Merrill 2009), and the number of projects increased significantly in the years that followed (Bitton, Martin, and Landon 2010). As of November 2017, roughly 65,000 clinicians were working in more than 13,000 NCQA-recognized medical homes in the United States (PCPCC 2017b).

Other organizations—including The Joint Commission, URAC, and the Accreditation Association for Ambulatory Health Care—have also developed medical home accreditation and certification programs, as have several health plans, including Blue Cross Blue Shield of Michigan.

Since its inception, the NCQA PCMH program has evolved in response to feedback from key stakeholders and research literature. Major updates to the PCMH standards occurred in 2011, 2014, and 2017. The 2017 revisions were accompanied by major changes to the process for attaining recognition. In addition, the previous three-year cycle for renewal of recognition was modified so that practices get initial recognition and then provide a limited set of data and reports annually to sustain their recognition status (NCQA 2017b).

The research literature about the success of the PCMH probably raises more questions than it answers. Many peer-reviewed studies demonstrate at least some benefit to quality of care, but improvements are often small and not seen across all metrics assessed (Jabbarpour et al. 2017). Similarly, patient experience results are mixed. Both proponents and critics of the model generally agree that evaluation of the PCMH concept is challenging and complex, given the various implementation approaches, incentives, metrics, and compromises in study design (AHRQ 2011, 2013a, 2013b). However, several health systems, insurance plans, and networks have published or presented encouraging results and continue to promote and expand their use of the program. The PCPCC compiles evidence from a variety of sources every year (PCPCC 2017c).

Expansion of the PCMH Concept to Specialties and Additional Sites of Care

Following the launch of the NCQA PPC-PCMH in 2008, the ACP's Council of Subspecialty Societies began to contemplate the involvement of specialists and subspecialists. In 2010, the ACP published a policy paper titled "The Patient-Centered Medical Home Neighbor: The Interface of the Patient-Centered Medical Home with Specialty/Subspecialty Practices" (Kirschner and Greenlee 2010). According to the authors, a specialty/subspecialty practice adhering to the model would engage in the following behaviors:

- Ensure effective communication, coordination, and integration with PCMH practices in a bidirectional manner to provide high-quality and efficient care
- Ensure appropriate and timely consultations and referrals that complement the aims of the PCMH practice
- Ensure the efficient, appropriate, and effective flow of necessary patient and care information
- Effectively guide determination of responsibility in co-management situations
- Support patient-centered care, enhanced care access, and high levels of care quality and safety
- Support the PCMH practice as the provider of whole-person primary care to the patient and as having overall responsibility for ensuring the coordination and integration of the care provided by all involved physicians and other healthcare professionals.

On the basis of this policy paper, and with input from ACP and other societies, NCQA developed and launched the Patient-Centered Specialty Practice Program (PCSP) in 2013. NCQA's vision for the program was that "specialty practices committed to access, communication and care coordination [could] earn accolades as the 'neighbors' that surround and inform the medical homes and colleagues in primary care" (PCPCC 2014).

This concept of the medical home "neighborhood" was extended even further through NCQA's Patient-Centered Connected Care (in 2015) and Oncology Medical Home (in 2017) programs. NCQA (2018b) has stated that these programs "empower employers, health plans, patients and consumers to make informed healthcare decisions based on quality. Participation in a NCQA Recognition Program demonstrates that the practice or clinician values quality healthcare delivery and the latest clinical protocols to ensure that patients receive the best care at the right time." The scope of NCQA recognition programs and patient-centered care is illustrated in exhibit 15.1.

In the absence of any significant financial incentives, the PCSP program has not experienced the same pace of growth as the PCMH program. However, several health systems and certain specialty practices have leveraged the program to differentiate themselves from nonrecognized practices and to prepare their offices for value-based payment models. In 2014, the Thomas Jefferson University (now Jefferson) practices in oncology and pulmonary medicine achieved level-3 recognition in the PCSP program (Thomas Jefferson University 2014).

EXHIBIT 15.1 NCQA Recognition Programs and Patient-Centered Care

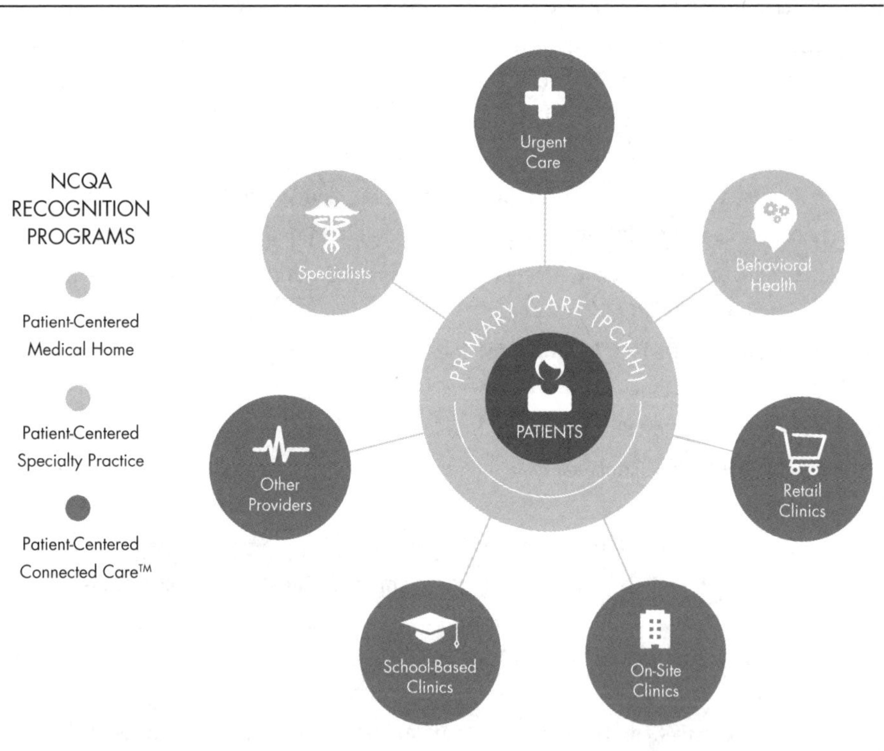

Source: Content reproduced with the permission of the National Committee for Quality Assurance (NCQA). NCQA disclaims all liability for the use and interpretation of the content.

Dr. Lawrence Ward and colleagues (2017, 935) from Jefferson offered their perspective on the PCSP program, concluding with the following statement:

> The US health-care system is under scrutiny from the public, regulators, and payers, and innovative models are needed to deliver timely, high-quality care, using appropriate resources. The PCSP model, like its predecessor, PCMH, offers a path for specialty practices to coordinate care, improve access and communication, and reduce duplicate testing. As health reform efforts to improve quality and experience of care move forward, pulmonary and other specialists have an opportunity to shape the vision of patient-centered care through adoption of the PCSP model of care.

The PCSP program has not yet been studied to any significant extent, given the limited uptake of the program, but its importance has been recognized. Writing in the *New England Journal of Medicine*, Huang and Rosenthal (2014, 1378–79) state that "active engagement of most specialties in a more patient- and population-centered model of care is necessary, however, and will require payers and systems to ensure that the status quo is no longer a feasible option, while providing support and a compelling clinical rationale for change." Most of the current literature about the PCSP program is qualitative rather than quantitative, with examples focusing on gastroenterology (Meier, Shah, and Talwalkar 2016), radiology (Greene et al. 2017), and oncology (Tirodkar et al. 2015).

In the coming years, NCQA expects participation in the PCSP program to grow, in part because of the Medicare Access and CHIP Reauthorization Act of 2015 (MACRA). MACRA, which is discussed in greater detail later in the chapter, credits recognized PCMH and PCSP practices with 100 percent of the points available—or 15 percent of the total—in the "Improvement Activities" category of the Merit-Based Incentive Payment System (MIPS). In addition, as value-based payment models and risk-sharing formulas drive changes in reimbursement, accountable care organizations (ACOs) and clinically integrated networks (CINs) will look for models of transformation to enhance their readiness to succeed. The PCMH and PCSP programs could support such efforts.

The Future of NCQA Recognition Programs

With the launch of the 2017 PCMH program, NCQA signaled a major shift in the way its recognition programs will operate. The process by which practices attain and sustain recognition was changed significantly based on a review of the literature, stakeholder and technical expert input, and analysis of data from prior versions. The major differences in the standards are the following:

- Reduction from 167 factors to 100 criteria
- Introduction of core and elective criteria instead of "must-pass" elements
- Scoring based on achievement of all 40 core criteria and 25 elective credits from a set of 60 elective options (some electives are worth two credits)
- Elimination of the three levels; practices instead achieve recognition on the basis of satisfying the 40 core and 25 elective credits
- Transition from a three-year recognition cycle to initial recognition (for practices new to PCMH) and annual reporting

The six concepts, or overarching themes, of the 2017 PCMH program are shown in exhibit 15.2 (NCQA 2017b).

2009–2017: A New Era of Health Reform

Although the first decade of the 2000s saw important progress for the quality movement—most notably an increased focus on setting standards and measuring performance at the primary care level—it represented the calm before the storm that was to come in US healthcare policy. Republicans had held

EXHIBIT 15.2 Concepts in the 2017 NCQA Patient-Centered Medical Home Program

2017 Standards

Concepts

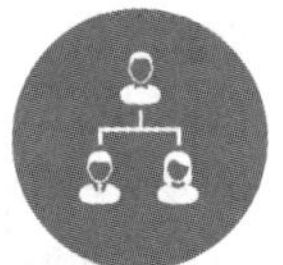

Team-Based Care and Practice Organization

Knowing and Managing Your Patients

Patient-Centered Access and Continuity

Care Management and Support

Care Coordination and Care Transitions

Performance Measurement & Quality Improvement

Source: Content reproduced with the permission of the National Committee for Quality Assurance (NCQA). NCQA disclaims all liability for the use and interpretation of the content.

the White House and a majority in Congress for much of that decade, during which time they displayed little interest in challenging the status quo in the commercial insurance markets or making a significant dent in the size of the uninsured population. The party instead seemed content to take limited steps to promote certain favorite proposals, such as the use of health savings accounts, while leaving their largest mark on the Medicare program, to which they added a prescription drug benefit in 2003.

For most of the decade, the overall uninsured rate hovered just above 16 percent, although Medicaid enrollment rose from 39 million to 54 million between 2001 and 2009 (KFF 2014). Several factors drove the increase, including the "post-bubble" recession of the early 2000s and an interest among the states in extending coverage beyond statutorily mandated Medicaid populations via Section 1115 waivers. Between these expansion activities and innovative coverage reforms, such as those implemented in Massachusetts by then-Governor Mitt Romney (which were largely funded through a repurposing of Medicaid dollars), a clear devolution of healthcare policymaking authority to the states was underway prior to 2009.

The Health Information Technology for Economic and Clinical Health Act

The 2008 election of Democrat Barack Obama to presidency reversed the complacency in health policy and spurred NCQA's next sustained period of growth. In February 2009, in response to a crippling meltdown on Wall Street and the Great Recession that followed, Obama proposed and the Democratic majority in Congress passed a nearly $800 billion economic stimulus bill, the American Recovery and Reinvestment Act (ARRA). Title XII of the law was known as the Health Information Technology for Economic and Clinical Health (HITECH) Act and included the Electronic Health Records (EHR) Incentive Program (also known as Meaningful Use). By September of 2017, more than 530,000 Medicare and/or Medicaid providers and nearly 5,000 hospitals had received incentive payments for the adoption and meaningful use of EHRs through the program, at a cost to the federal government of $37.7 billion (CMS 2017c).

The growth in EHR adoption spurred by the HITECH Act was an important step forward for quality measurement, given the potential for EHR systems to revolutionize data reporting. By 2016, four out of five US physicians and almost all hospitals possessed EHRs certified to meet the standards set by the Office of the National Coordinator of Health Information Technology (ONC). For comparison, just 17 percent of physicians and 9 percent of hospitals used "basic" EHRs in the year prior to ARRA's passage (ONC 2016).

Although widespread adoption of EHR technology is a precursor to realizing maximum gains from quality measurement and value-based care, it is not sufficient in and of itself. Large numbers of providers and health systems that use EHRs are incapable of easily sharing data with the various payers (e.g., health plans, ACOs, government agencies) that could use the data to drive pay-for-performance initiatives. Also, the burden of inputting the data remains a concern for doctors and policymakers. Indeed, many of NCQA's most ambitious agenda items hinge on a level of HIT sophistication and data-sharing fluidity that simply does not exist at the time of this writing.

The Affordable Care Act

If the HITECH Act was the appetizer of this new era of health policy reform, the Patient Protection and Affordable Care Act (ACA), also known as "Obamacare," was undoubtedly the main course. Passed by Democrats in March of 2010 by a razor-thin, party-line vote, the ACA included a broad expansion of Medicaid eligibility to include all individuals up to 138 percent of the federal poverty level (FPL). The law also established health insurance exchanges (officially known as "marketplaces") to parallel the individual insurance market, through which people earning as much as 400 percent of the FPL could receive subsidies to cover the cost of their coverage, on a sliding scale. It also federalized the health insurance market in unprecedented fashion, establishing national minimum standards for coverage and abolishing the ability for insurers to deny coverage based on preexisting medical conditions, among other reforms.

By 2017, 16 million more Americans had coverage through Medicaid and the Children's Health Insurance Program (CHIP) than did immediately before the provisions went into effect in 2014. In addition, 12 million people were enrolled in an ACA marketplace plan, and the overall uninsured rate had fallen to just over 10 percent (CMS 2017b, 2017d). These developments increased the demand for NCQA's accreditation services, given that many of the newly insured were receiving coverage through private health plans. Plans offered via the federal government website www.healthcare.gov or a state-based exchange were required to be accredited—with NCQA accrediting more than four out of five of these plans. Moreover, an increasing amount of Medicaid coverage—particularly for the ACA expansion population—was offered through managed care plans with which states contracted to provide services, and the majority of these plans were also accredited by NCQA.

Center for Medicare & Medicaid Innovation

Perhaps the ACA's greatest impact on NCQA, and the nation, involved the provisions in the law that funded sweeping delivery system reforms designed to focus payment on value rather than the volume of services. Most of the reforms originated in the Center for Medicare & Medicaid Innovation (CMMI), which is tasked with testing innovative healthcare payment and service delivery models with the potential to improve the quality of care and reduce Medicare,

Medicaid, and CHIP expenditures. CMMI was granted a cumulative $10 billion for fiscal years 2011 through 2019 to pursue these goals. CMMI initiatives have included a series of ACO experiments, several efforts to incentivize value-based care, and the State Innovation Model (SIM) grants program. The latter has provided states with more than $1 billion to design and implement cross-cutting reforms involving multiple healthcare payers in addition to Medicaid and Medicare. NCQA has partnered with several states to help implement SIM grants and to measure the quality of care under the revised delivery systems being tested.

More broadly, the ACA's focus on moving healthcare toward achieving the Institute for Healthcare Improvement's Triple Aim—improving the patient experience of care, improving the health of populations, and reducing the per capita cost of healthcare (Berwick, Nolan, and Whittington 2008)—has put quality measurement at the forefront of the quickly evolving landscape. Measure development and attention to quality have surged under the law, as organizations seek to balance the cost-saving potential of various initiatives with concerns that the care provided continue to meet the latest quality standards.

By applying its expertise in the field of quality measurement to the rapid increase in demand for such capabilities in the transition to value-based care, NCQA more than doubled its contracting revenue, primarily from federal government work. Coupled with the growth in the nascent PCMH recognition program and a steady stream of health plan accreditation customers, these events raised NCQA's overall revenue to nearly $65 million by 2016, from $27 million in 2006.

The Medicare Access and CHIP Reauthorization Act of 2015

At the time of this writing, the future of the ACA remains in flux, at least in part because of the partisan nature of its passage. Democrats and Republicans have thus far been unable to reach the compromises necessary to amend the law in a way that will make it more workable. The Democrats have mainly sought to bolster funding for healthcare subsidies, whereas the Republicans have attempted to dismantle the federal mandates on insurers or repeal the law outright. Amid the standoff, MACRA—which passed in 2015 with strong Republican and Democratic support in both chambers of Congress—stands as strong evidence that health policy can in fact be made across party lines.

MACRA encourages the shift toward more coordinated delivery systems by disrupting the way providers participating in FFS Medicare are paid, tacking bonuses onto the FFS payments of high-performing practices and imposing penalties on their lower-performing counterparts. Practices participating at a significant level in value-based alternative payment models (APMs) can avoid the risk of penalties and earn an automatic 5 percent bonus. As a nod to the importance of coordinated care in increasing quality and value, MACRA provides an automatic credit for 15 percent of a practice's overall score on the non-APM track if it is a recognized PCMH.

Under both Obama and President Donald Trump, the government refrained from pushing too hard on providers to meet MACRA's quality reporting requirements. Program regulations for 2017 (the reporting year on which 2019 penalties and bonuses will be based) and 2018 set an extremely low bar for reporting and exempted tens of thousands of low-volume providers from any reporting at all. Still, MACRA promises to be another important catalyst in the transition to value-based care.

The Future of Policy and the Politics of Healthcare Quality

Several policy and political factors will dictate how the future of quality measurement—and of NCQA—unfolds. Central to the question is the role that governments at every level will play in providing and regulating care. Will free-market sentiments among Republicans lead to a diminished role for evidence-based standards and minimum quality expectations? Will the push by Democrats for a single-payer system bring about the eventual demise of the commercial health insurance market? Or will the drive for high-quality, lower-cost care based on reforms that incentivize coordination, communication, and the measurement of outcomes remain a beacon of bipartisanship amid otherwise paralyzed policymakers? And how will public policy evolve in response to the challenge of balancing consumer privacy with the free flow of clinical data that is essential to meaningful improvement? Predicting exactly how these and other questions will play out is difficult, if not impossible.

Quality Measurement: Assessing Healthcare Performance Across the United States

Throughout this period of healthcare reform, the effort to measure quality and cost and to assign accountability has been questioned by a variety of stakeholders and experts. CMS continues to include a large set of measures from which clinicians can choose to report for programs such as the Physicians Quality Reporting System (PQRS), the EHR Incentive Program, and now MACRA (which replaces PQRS and the Incentive Program). However, other groups have called for a more parsimonious set of measures. In 2015, the IOM released "Vital Signs: Core Metrics for Health and Health Care Progress," which listed a core measure set with related priority measures. The report called for the implementation of standardized measures to "reduce the burden of unnecessary measurement but also align the incentives and actions of multiple organizations and multiple levels . . . to yield better health at lower costs for all Americans" (IOM 2015).

The IOM effort was not the first attempt to develop a core set of measures, and it probably will not be the last. In 2004, the AAFP, ACP, America's Health Insurance Plans (AHIP), and AHRQ created the Ambulatory Care Quality Alliance (AQA), which aimed to develop "a starter set of measures for ambulatory care that stakeholders can use in January 2006 contracts" (AHRQ 2005; White 2007). AQA used a consensus-based process to identify a set of 26 measures for primary care that became part of the measure set used in the Physician Voluntary Reporting Program (a precursor to the PQRS) in 2006 (Quality & Patient Safety 2017). Around that same time, a number of other alliances were supported through public–private collaboration with CMS, including the Hospital Quality Alliance, Pharmacy Quality Alliance, Kidney Care Quality Alliance, Cancer Care Quality Alliance, Nursing Home Quality Initiative, and Quality Alliance Steering Committee (CMS 2006).

In 2011, AHRQ established what is now referred to as the National Quality Strategy (NQS) through a "transparent and collaborative process with input from a range of stakeholders" (AHRQ 2017). The NQS aims to improve care by advancing three aims (consistent with the Triple Aim), six priorities, and nine levers, which are applied as follows (AHRQ 2017):

- Adopt the three aims to provide better, more affordable care for the individual and the community.
- Focus on the six priorities to guide efforts to improve health and health care quality.
- Use one or more of the nine levers to identify core business functions, resources, and/or actions that may serve as means for achieving improved health and health care quality.

CMS created the Health Care Payment Learning and Action Network (HCPLAN, or LAN) in 2015 to help move payment for healthcare services in the United States from fee-for-service models to alternative payment models based on quality and value (CMS 2018). A stated aim was to have 50 percent of healthcare payments made through alternative payment models by 2018. HCPLAN is organized into several work groups to address payment models, attribution, data sharing, and performance measurement. The Population-Based Payment Work Group, rather than identifying specific measures for performance-based payment, created a set of principles and recommendations to guide the selection of measures appropriate for use in population-based payment models. A key recommendation was to address overall system performance, not the processes used to produce the performance. The work group characterized system-level outcomes, such as total cost of care, as "big dot" measures. Process or intermediate outcome measures were regarded as "atomistic performance measures" or "little dot" measures (HCPLAN 2016).

Efforts to define core sets of measures continue, a notable example being the Core Quality Measure Collaborative led by AHIP, CMS, and the National Quality Forum (NQF), with participation from physician organizations, employers, consumers, and measure developers (CMS 2017a). The collaborative produced eight sets of measures in 2016:

- Accountable care organizations, patient-centered medical homes, and primary care
- Cardiology
- Gastroenterology
- HIV and hepatitis C
- Medical oncology
- Obstetrics and gynecology
- Orthopedics
- Pediatrics

During an address at the HCPLAN summit in October 2017, CMS administrator Seema Verma stated that "one of our top priorities is to ease regulatory burden that is destroying the doctor–patient relationship. We want doctors to be able to deliver the best quality care to their patients" (CMS 2017e).

Dealing with the Measurement Burden

All of these worthy efforts to define core measure sets have struggled—and will likely continue to struggle—with three underlying issues: (1) the misalignment of measures across the health system; (2) challenges of data collection and reporting; and (3) questions about the accuracy and validity of quality reports. If these issues were to be appropriately addressed, the focus on reducing the number of measures could conceivably shift to a focus on the selection and/or development of more measures to address known gaps in care.

One of the main causes of the excessive reporting burden associated with quality measures is that the specifications developed by the measure stewards for federal programs (i.e., numerator/denominator inclusion and exclusion criteria) are not always adopted "as is" by commercial health plans, state Medicaid agencies, and Medicare Advantage plans. In addition, measures designed for national reporting and benchmarking are not always useful in the day-to-day assessment of quality at the level of the delivery system or for population health activities needed for the operation of ACOs and CINs. Under risk-based contracts, these entities are often more interested in patient- and population-specific measure results provided at the point of care to reduce costs than measures that do not provide timely information or a sufficient level of detail upon which clinicians can act.

For example, health plan measures often require a long look-back period and rely on beneficiary enrollment for attribution, and clinician-level measures typically need for an encounter to occur to be counted. Therefore, ACOs and CINs often add unique measures or modify national measures to suit their purposes. In addition, ACOs and CINs can be subjected to different attribution models (e.g., prospective or performance year) than are typically used for national measures (National Quality Forum 2016; Lewis et al. 2013). Similarly, health plans and state Medicaid agencies sometimes adjust measure specifications to suit their programs' needs.

Another key issue is that clinicians and their teams, even if they had a defined set of core measures, would remain highly dissatisfied with the usability and efficiency of most EHR systems. A survey of 142 family medicine physicians using a single EHR system found that the physicians spend 5.9 hours of an 11.4-hour workday on the EHR, with 44 percent of that time spent doing clerical and administrative tasks that, in theory, could have been done by other members of the practice team if facilitated by the system (Arndt et al. 2017).

Current clinician-level measures are heavily process related and often require clinicians and their teams to document specific activities solely for the purpose of satisfying measure needs. Combined with the variation in measure specifications, the task becomes frustrating and often detracts from time spent caring for patients (Dunlap et al. 2016). It is also very costly: A 2016 report estimated that US physician practices in four specialties (cardiology, orthopedics, primary care, and multispecialty practices that include primary care) spend 785 hours per physician and more than $15.4 billion annually to report quality measures (Casalino et al. 2016).

Measure developers, EHR designers, and policymakers should not forget the most important purpose of EHR-generated documentation, as described in an ACP policy paper (Kuhn et al. 2015, 301):

> The primary goal of EHR-generated documentation should be concise, history-rich notes that reflect the information gathered and are used to develop an impression, a diagnostic and/or treatment plan, and recommended follow-up. Technology should facilitate attainment of these goals in the most efficient manner possible without losing the humanistic elements of the record that support ongoing relationships between patients and their physicians.

Getting to Meaningful Measures

Given the dynamic healthcare environment and the associated stress already pervasive within the field, NCQA is approaching measure alignment, development, and use with the aim of reducing the burden associated with quality measurement as well as the work associated with measure updates and accuracy.

A key strategy is to align measures throughout the healthcare system using industry-standard specifications as building blocks and to use the same clinical concepts and the relevant codes and value sets. Built using a modular approach, such measures would allow the application of different attribution models suited to purpose for the same clinical measures (e.g., beneficiaries for health plans, prospective or performance year for ACOs).

Many practices, health systems, and health plans already use data analytics companies to support their analytic and reporting needs. Others participate in health information exchanges. Still others have invested heavily in the technical infrastructure to carry out their own measurement and reporting activities. In each case, the use of clinical and claims data collected and reused for multiple measurement needs would significantly reduce the burden associated with measure collection and reporting—and eventually lower the cost of collecting and reporting measures (Schuster, Onorato, and Meltzer 2017).

To truly get to meaningful measures, the art and science of measurement have to move beyond snapshot/threshold types of assessments. Given that the goal should be to get to "big dot" measures as defined by HCPLAN, new types of process measures may be more relevant than the current set. The use of technical standards, such as the Health Level Seven (HL7) standard for trial-use Clinical Quality Language (CQL), and updates to data models, such as the Quality Data Model (QDM), will open the door to measuring changes over time and will allow sharing of logic with decision support (eCQI Resource Center 2018). In 2017, CMS announced the transition of its electronic clinical quality measures (eCQMs) to CQL for the calendar year 2019 reporting/performance periods (eCQI Resource Center 2017).

A final issue involves the accuracy and validity of measure calculations. As public and private payers begin to compensate clinicians and hospitals based on their quality performance, they need to have confidence that the reported results accurately reflect performance. To date, the ONC Health IT Certification Program's testing of EHR systems for accuracy of measure reporting has been limited to use of the Project Cypress (ONC 2018; Cypress 2018). Recognizing the importance of testing, ONC is taking steps to diversify. In June 2017, it approved NCQA's eCQM testing method as an alternative to the existing method (NCQA 2017a; Posnack 2017). Both Project Cypress and NCQA's eMeasure Certification program use synthetic EHR data to test the ability of health IT systems to accurately calculate measure results. The programs differ in the scope of their test decks and processes, but the aim is the same—to ensure that comparisons of quality and payment are based on valid, reliable information.

Conclusion

Since its founding in 1990, NCQA, under Margaret E. O'Kane's leadership, has pursued its vision of transforming healthcare quality through measurement, transparency, and accountability. Starting with the assessment of health plan quality through HEDIS, NCQA expanded to clinicians, practices, and networks. NCQA is now in the midst of updating its programs and its approach to quality measurement and accountability. The complexities of healthcare and the associated politics make the present day an exciting and uncertain time for everyone dedicated to improving the health of individuals and populations.

Study Questions

1. Why did employers and health plans agree to an external third-party evaluation program?
2. What role can or should accreditation and quality measurement/reporting play in the future, as the public availability of performance data increases and payment is linked to performance (or value)?
3. What policy drivers could states and the federal government use to bring quality up and cost down? Are the current efforts effective?
4. Does the current quality measurement approach lead to better quality and lower cost? Whether your answer is yes or no, how could the approach to measurement improve?
5. As CMS and states push to introduce value-based payment models, what mechanisms would you employ to ensure the accuracy and validity of measurement data? Would you adjust reported performance rates and/or payment to account for population differences?

References

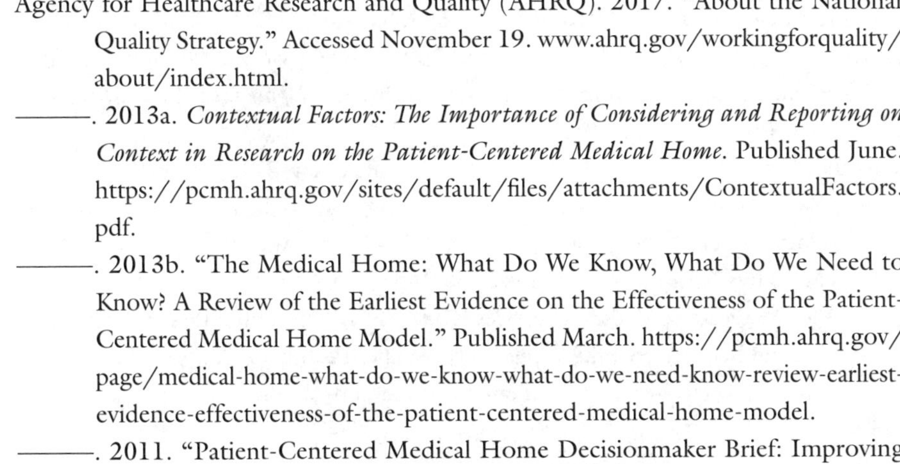

Agency for Healthcare Research and Quality (AHRQ). 2017. "About the National Quality Strategy." Accessed November 19. www.ahrq.gov/workingforquality/about/index.html.

———. 2013a. *Contextual Factors: The Importance of Considering and Reporting on Context in Research on the Patient-Centered Medical Home.* Published June. https://pcmh.ahrq.gov/sites/default/files/attachments/ContextualFactors.pdf.

———. 2013b. "The Medical Home: What Do We Know, What Do We Need to Know? A Review of the Earliest Evidence on the Effectiveness of the Patient-Centered Medical Home Model." Published March. https://pcmh.ahrq.gov/page/medical-home-what-do-we-know-what-do-we-need-know-review-earliest-evidence-effectiveness-of-the-patient-centered-medical-home-model.

———. 2011. "Patient-Centered Medical Home Decisionmaker Brief: Improving Evaluations of the Medical Home." Published September. https://pcmh.ahrq.

gov/page/patient-centered-medical-home-decisionmaker-brief-improving-evaluations-medical-home.

———. 2005. "The Ambulatory Care Quality Alliance: Improving Clinical Quality and Consumer Decisionmaking." Published May. https://archive.ahrq.gov/professionals/quality-patient-safety/quality-resources/tools/ambulatory-care/background.html.

American Academy of Pediatrics (AAP). 2004. "The Medical Home." *Pediatrics* 113 (4): 1545–47.

American College of Physicians (ACP). 2017. "Who Supports the PCMH Care Model?" Accessed November 17. www.acponline.org/practice-resources/business-resources/payment/models/pcmh/understanding/who-supports-the-pcmh-care-model.

———. 2007. "Joint Principles of the Patient-Centered Medical Home." Published March. www.acponline.org/system/files/documents/running_practice/delivery_and_payment_models/pcmh/demonstrations/jointprinc_05_17.pdf.

———. 2006. "The Impending Collapse of Primary Care Medicine and Its Implications for the State of the Nation's Health Care: A Report from the American College of Physicians." Published January 30. www.acponline.org/acp_policy/policies/impending_collapse_of_primary_care_medicine_and_its_implications_for_the_state_of_the_nation's_health_care_2006.pdf.

Arndt, B. G., J. W. Beasley, M. D. Watkinson, J. L. Temte, W.-J. Tuan, C. A. Sinsky, and V. J. Gilchrist. 2017. "Tethered to the EHR: Primary Care Physician Workload Assessment Using EHR Event Log Data and Time-Motion Observations." *Annals of Family Medicine* 15 (5): 419–26.

Barr, M. S., and J. Ginsburg. 2006. *The Advanced Medical Home: A Patient-Centered, Physician-Guided Model of Health Care*. American College of Physicians. Accessed November 17, 2017. www.acponline.org/acp_policy/policies/adv_medicalhome_patient_centered_model_healthcare_2006.pdf.

Berwick, D. M., T. W. Nolan, and J. Whittington. 2008. "The Triple Aim: Care, Health and Cost." *Health Affairs* 27 (3): 759–69.

Bitton, A., C. Martin, and B. E. Landon. 2010. "A Nationwide Survey of Patient Centered Medical Home Demonstration Projects." *Journal of General Internal Medicine* 25 (6): 584–92.

Casalino, L. P., D. Gans, R. Weber, M. Cea, A. Tuchovsky, T. F. Bishop, Y. Miranda, B. A. Frankel, K. B. Ziehler, M. M. Wong, and T. B. Evenson. 2016. "US Physician Practices Spend More than $15.4 Billion Annually to Report Quality Measures." *Health Affairs* 35 (3): 401–6.

Centers for Medicare & Medicaid Services (CMS). 2018. "Health Care Payment Learning and Action Network." Updated November 14. https://innovation.cms.gov/initiatives/Health-Care-Payment-Learning-and-Action-Network/.

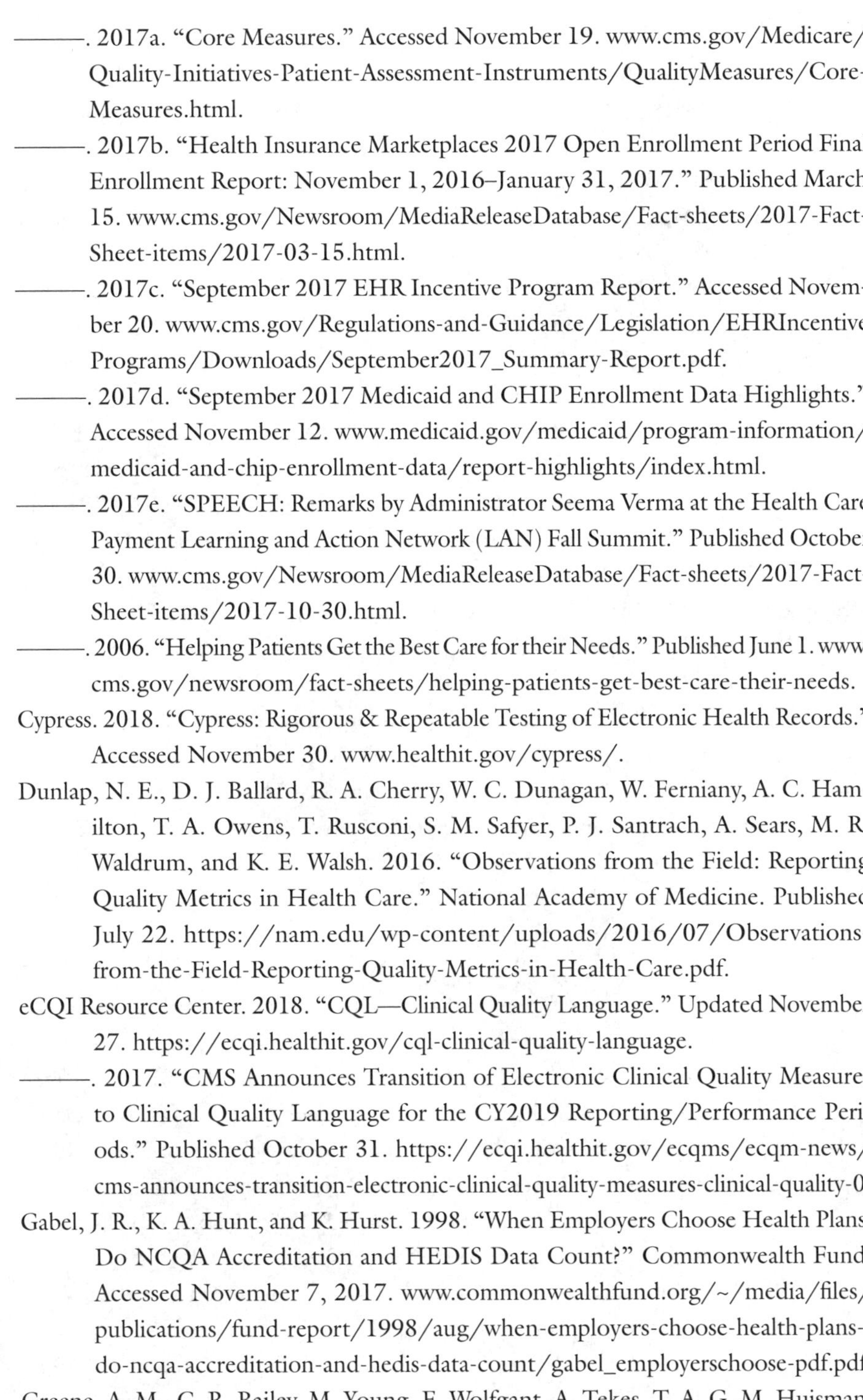

———. 2017a. "Core Measures." Accessed November 19. www.cms.gov/Medicare/Quality-Initiatives-Patient-Assessment-Instruments/QualityMeasures/Core-Measures.html.

———. 2017b. "Health Insurance Marketplaces 2017 Open Enrollment Period Final Enrollment Report: November 1, 2016–January 31, 2017." Published March 15. www.cms.gov/Newsroom/MediaReleaseDatabase/Fact-sheets/2017-Fact-Sheet-items/2017-03-15.html.

———. 2017c. "September 2017 EHR Incentive Program Report." Accessed November 20. www.cms.gov/Regulations-and-Guidance/Legislation/EHRIncentivePrograms/Downloads/September2017_Summary-Report.pdf.

———. 2017d. "September 2017 Medicaid and CHIP Enrollment Data Highlights." Accessed November 12. www.medicaid.gov/medicaid/program-information/medicaid-and-chip-enrollment-data/report-highlights/index.html.

———. 2017e. "SPEECH: Remarks by Administrator Seema Verma at the Health Care Payment Learning and Action Network (LAN) Fall Summit." Published October 30. www.cms.gov/Newsroom/MediaReleaseDatabase/Fact-sheets/2017-Fact-Sheet-items/2017-10-30.html.

———. 2006. "Helping Patients Get the Best Care for their Needs." Published June 1. www.cms.gov/newsroom/fact-sheets/helping-patients-get-best-care-their-needs.

Cypress. 2018. "Cypress: Rigorous & Repeatable Testing of Electronic Health Records." Accessed November 30. www.healthit.gov/cypress/.

Dunlap, N. E., D. J. Ballard, R. A. Cherry, W. C. Dunagan, W. Ferniany, A. C. Hamilton, T. A. Owens, T. Rusconi, S. M. Safyer, P. J. Santrach, A. Sears, M. R. Waldrum, and K. E. Walsh. 2016. "Observations from the Field: Reporting Quality Metrics in Health Care." National Academy of Medicine. Published July 22. https://nam.edu/wp-content/uploads/2016/07/Observations-from-the-Field-Reporting-Quality-Metrics-in-Health-Care.pdf.

eCQI Resource Center. 2018. "CQL—Clinical Quality Language." Updated November 27. https://ecqi.healthit.gov/cql-clinical-quality-language.

———. 2017. "CMS Announces Transition of Electronic Clinical Quality Measures to Clinical Quality Language for the CY2019 Reporting/Performance Periods." Published October 31. https://ecqi.healthit.gov/ecqms/ecqm-news/cms-announces-transition-electronic-clinical-quality-measures-clinical-quality-0.

Gabel, J. R., K. A. Hunt, and K. Hurst. 1998. "When Employers Choose Health Plans: Do NCQA Accreditation and HEDIS Data Count?" Commonwealth Fund. Accessed November 7, 2017. www.commonwealthfund.org/~/media/files/publications/fund-report/1998/aug/when-employers-choose-health-plans--do-ncqa-accreditation-and-hedis-data-count/gabel_employerschoose-pdf.pdf.

Greene, A. M., C. R. Bailey, M. Young, E. Wolfgant, A. Tekes, T. A. G. M. Huisman, and D. J. Durand. 2017. "Applying the National Committee for Quality Assurance Patient-Centered Specialty Practice Framework to Radiology." *Journal of the American College of Radiology* 14 (9): 1173–76.

Health Care Payment Learning and Action Network (HCPLAN). 2016. *Accelerating and Aligning Population-Based Payment Models: Performance Measurement.* Accessed November 19, 2017. http://hcp-lan.org/workproducts/pm-whitepaper-final.pdf.

Huang, X., and M. B. Rosenthal. 2014. "Transforming Specialty Practice—The Patient-Centered Medical Home Neighborhood." *New England Journal of Medicine* 370 (15): 1376–79.

Iglehart, J. K. 1996. "The National Committee for Quality Assurance." *New England Journal of Medicine* 335 (13): 995–99.

Improving Chronic Illness Care. 2017. "The Chronic Care Model." Accessed November 17. www.improvingchroniccare.org/index.php?p=The_Chronic_Care_Model&s=2.

Institute of Medicine (IOM). 2015. "Report Brief: Vital Signs: Core Metrics for Health and Health Care Progress." Published April. www.nationalacademies.org/hmd/~/media/Files/Report%20Files/2015/Vital_Signs/VitalSigns_RB.pdf.

———. 1990. *Medicare: A Strategy for Quality Assurance.* Washington, DC: National Academies Press.

Jabbarpour, Y., E. DeMarchis, A. Bazemore, and P. Grundy. 2017. *The Impact of Primary Care Practice Transformation on Cost, Quality, and Utilization. A Systematic Review of Research Published in 2016.* Patient-Centered Primary Care Collaborative. Published July. www.pcpcc.org/sites/default/files/resources/pcmh_evidence_report_08-1-17%20FINAL.pdf.

Kahn, N. B. 2004. "The Future of Family Medicine: A Collaborative Project of the Family Medicine Community." *Annals of Family Medicine* 2 (Suppl. 1): S3–S32.

Kaiser Family Foundation (KFF). 2017. "2017 Employer Health Benefits Survey." Published September 19. www.kff.org/health-costs/report/2017-employer-health-benefits-survey.

———. 2014. "Medicaid Enrollment: An Overview of the CMS April 2014 Update." Published June 10. www.kff.org/medicaid/fact-sheet/medicaid-enrollment-an-overview-of-the-cms-april-2014-update/.

———. 2011. "Snapshots: Health Care Spending in the United States & Selected OECD Countries." Published April 12. www.kff.org/health-costs/issue-brief/snapshots-health-care-spending-in-the-united-states-selected-oecd-countries.

Kirschner, N., and C. M. Greenlee. 2010. "The Patient-Centered Medical Home Neighbor: The Interface of the Patient-Centered Medical Home with Specialty/Subspecialty Practices." American College of Physicians. Accessed November 19, 2017. www.acponline.org/system/files/documents/advocacy/current_policy_papers/assets/pcmh_neighbors.pdf.

Kuhn, T., P. Basch, M. Barr, and T. Yackel. 2015. "Clinical Documentation in the 21st Century: Executive Summary of a Policy Position Paper From the American College of Physicians." *Annals of Internal Medicine* 162 (4): 301–3.

Lee, T. H. 2007. "Eulogy for a Quality Measure." *New England Journal of Medicine* 357: 1175–77.

Lewis, V. A., A. B. McClurg, J. Smith, E. S. Fisher, and J. P. W. Bynum. 2013. "Attributing Patients to Accountable Care Organizations: Performance Year Approach Aligns Stakeholders' Interests." *Health Affairs* 32 (3): 587–95.

McPartland, G. 2012. "Birth of the National Committee for Quality Assurance." Kaiser Permanente. Published March 21. http://kaiserpermanentehistory.org/latest/birth-of-the-national-committee-for-quality-assurance/.

Meier, S. K., N. D. Shah, and J. A. Talwalkar. 2016. "Adapting the Patient-Centered Specialty Practice Model for Populations with Cirrhosis." *Clinical Gastroenterology and Hepatology* 14 (4): 492–96.

Merrill, M. 2009. "IBM, UnitedHealthcare Collaborate on Medical Home Initiative for Ariz. Docs." Published February 9. www.healthcareitnews.com/news/ibm-unitedhealthcare-collaborate-medical-home-initiative-ariz-docs.

National Committee for Quality Assurance (NCQA). 2018a. "Health Plan Accreditation (HPA)." Accessed November 29. www.ncqa.org/programs/health-plans/health-plan-accreditation-hpa/.

———. 2018b. "Recognition." Accessed November 29. http://store.ncqa.org/index.php/recognition.html.

———. 2017a. "eMeasure Certification." Accessed November 19. www.ncqa.org/hedis-quality-measurement/data-reporting-services/emeasure-certification.

———. 2017b. "The PCMH Recognition Process." Accessed November 19. www.ncqa.org/programs/recognition/practices/patient-centered-medical-home-pcmh/getting-recognized/get-started/process-becoming-a-pcmh.

National Quality Forum (NQF). 2016. "Attribution: Principles and Approaches. Final Report. December 2016." Published December. www.qualityforum.org/Publications/2016/12/Attribution_-_Principles_and_Approaches.aspx.

Office of the National Coordinator for Health Information Technology (ONC). 2018. "About the ONC Health IT Certification Program." Reviewed September 21. www.healthit.gov/policy-researchers-implementers/about-onc-health-it-certification-program.

———. 2016. "2016 Report to Congress on Health IT Progress: Examining the HITECH Era and the Future of Health IT." Published November. https://dashboard.healthit.gov/report-to-congress/2016-report-congress-examining-hitech-era-future-health-information-technology.php#critical-actions.

Patient-Centered Primary Care Collaborative (PCPCC). 2017a. "Calvin Sia, MD." Accessed November 17. www.pcpcc.org/profile/calvin-sia.

———. 2017b. "Primary Care Innovations and PCMH Programs by Title." Accessed November 19. www.pcpcc.org/initiatives/list.

———. 2017c. "Snapshot of the Evidence." Accessed November 19. www.pcpcc.org/results-evidence.

———. 2014. "Introduction to NCQA's Patient-Centered Specialty Practice Recognition." Accessed November 29, 2018. www.pcpcc.org/event/2014/06/introduction-ncqa%E2%80%99s-patient-centered-specialty-practice-recognition.

Posnack, S. 2017. "A First Step to Diversify the Certification Program's Testing Portfolio." *Health IT Buzz.* Published June 22. www.healthit.gov/buzz-blog/healthit-certification/step-diversify-certification-programs-testing-portfolio/.

Quality & Patient Safety. 2017. "Performance Measures: Ambulatory Care Quality Alliance (AQA)." Accessed November 19. http://qups.org/perf_measure.php?c=18#clinmeasures.

Schuster, M. A., S. E. Onorato, and D. O. Meltzer. 2017. "Measuring the Cost of Quality Measurement. A Missing Link in Quality Strategy." *Journal of the American Medical Association* 318 (13): 1219–20.

Thomas Jefferson University. 2014. "Thomas Jefferson University Earns National Recognition for Quality Care." Published May 1. www.jefferson.edu/university/news/2014/05/01/thomas-jefferson-university-earns-national-recognition-for-quali.html.

Tirodkar, M. A., N. Acciavatti, L. M. Roth, E. Stovall, S. F. Nasso, J. Sprandio, S. Tofani, M. Lowry, M. W. Friedberg, A. Smith-McLallen, J. Chanin, and S. H. Scholle. 2015. "Lessons from Early Implementation of a Patient-Centered Care Model in Oncology." *Journal of Oncology Practice* 11 (6): 456–61.

Ward, L., R. E. Powell, M. L. Scharf, A. Chapman, and M. Kavuru. 2017. "Patient-Centered Specialty Practice: Defining the Role of Specialists in Value-Based Health Care." *Chest* 151 (4): 930–35.

White, J. 2007. "The AQA Alliance." National Committee for Vital and Health Statistics. Published July 19. www.ncvhs.hhs.gov/wp-content/uploads/2014/08/070719p1.pdf.

Wholey, D. R., J. B. Christianson, J. Engberg, and C. Bryce. 1997. "HMO Market Structure and Performance: 1985–1995." *Health Affairs* 16 (6): 77.

CHAPTER

16

VALUE-BASED INSURANCE DESIGN

A. Mark Fendrick, Susan Lynne Oesterle,
Marianthi N. Hatzigeorgiou, and Margaret F. Shope

Introduction

The current level of healthcare spending in the United States, experts widely agree, does not deliver sufficient value in terms of individual or population health. This finding was strongly reinforced by a Commonwealth Fund study that compared the United States with ten other industrialized nations. The study found that the United States spent 16.4 percent of its gross domestic product (GDP) on healthcare in 2014, about 50 percent more than Switzerland, the next highest nation. At the same time, the United States ranked eleventh—last—in overall health system performance, with rankings of fifth in care process, and eleventh in access, administrative efficiency, equity, and healthcare outcomes (Schneider et al. 2017).

The high level and rapid rise of medical expenditures create tremendous pressures for public and private purchasers, who seek to reduce the rate of spending growth. Simultaneously, the quality gaps and underutilization of high-value clinical services across the entire spectrum of clinical care necessitate incremental payments. Given the well-documented shortcomings of individual and population health metrics and the trillions of dollars invested in American healthcare annually, policy deliberations should turn from *how much* we spend to *how well* we spend our healthcare dollars.

The transition from a volume-driven healthcare system to a value-based system requires changes in both how purchasers pay for healthcare and how consumers are engaged and motivated to seek care. Most efforts to control costs or improve quality of care have concentrated on provider-facing, "supply-side" initiatives. These efforts have addressed the infrastructure, processes, and financing of care delivery (e.g., accountable care, medical homes). Far less attention has been devoted to "demand-side" programs that directly engage consumers (e.g., price transparency). This chapter focuses on value-based insurance design (V-BID), a consumer-facing tool that, when combined with quality-driven payment programs, has the potential to improve patient-centered outcomes and contain costs.

Key Concepts in the Shift from Volume to Value

Consumer Cost Sharing

One commonly used strategy for slowing the growth of healthcare spending is to increase consumer cost sharing, making insured individuals pay more for their healthcare (e.g., through deductibles, copayments, coinsurance). The Kaiser Family Foundation (KFF) and the Health Research and Educational Trust (HRET) reported cumulative increases of 224 percent in family premiums and 270 percent in worker contributions to those premiums between 1999 and 2017, compared with a 64 percent rise in workers' earnings (Claxton et al. 2017). At the same time, a marked change occurred in the types of consumer cost sharing being used, as shown in exhibit 16.1. The use of deductibles increased dramatically, while the use of coinsurance saw a moderate increase and the use of copayments declined.

People enrolled in plans with a deductible are required to pay the full cost of most medical care until the deductible is met; only after that point will the insurance cover the costs of care. The 2016 National Health Interview Survey, by the US National Center for Health Statistics, revealed that 40 percent of people younger than 65 years with private health insurance were enrolled in high-deductible health plans (HDHPs)—a sharp increase from the 25 percent who were enrolled in HDHPs in 2010 (Cohen and Zammitti 2017). Additionally, a KFF (2016) survey found that the average health plan deductible increased

EXHIBIT 16.1
Distribution of Cost-Sharing Payments by Type (2004–2014)

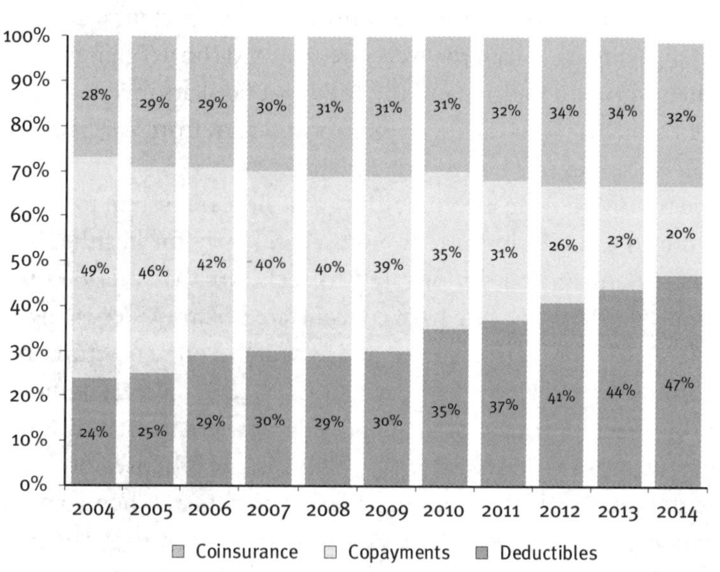

Source: Data from Claxton, Levitt, and Long (2016).

from $818 in 2006 to $2,069 in 2015. Other research indicates that 22 percent of covered workers face deductibles of $2,000 or more for single coverage, and 11 percent face deductibles of $3,000 or more (Claxton et al. 2017).

HDHP enrollees, though insured, often struggle to afford their medical care. According to a 2017 KFF survey, 46 percent of HDHP enrollees report difficulty paying deductibles. Approximately one-third of members with chronic conditions report delaying or avoiding care due to the high cost, and nearly half of HDHP enrollees with a family member with a chronic condition report problems paying medical bills or other bills because of healthcare costs (Claxton et al. 2017). Consequently, racial/ethnic minorities, lower-income individuals, and people in fair or poor health are more negatively affected than other groups by increasing out-of-pocket costs.

Most health insurers—including Medicare—implement consumer cost-sharing in a "one-size-fits-all" manner, such that beneficiaries are expected to pay the same out-of-pocket amount for every service within a particular category of care (e.g., office visits, diagnostic tests, formulary tiers of prescription drugs). Thus, in nearly every instance, consumer cost sharing is based on the type and price of service provided, not the clinical value.

The theoretical motivation for cost sharing is to simultaneously increase consumer engagement and to reduce the use of low-value, unnecessary services. However, a robust evidence base has demonstrated that increases in consumer cost sharing on all services, regardless of their clinical value, lead to decreases in the use of both nonessential and essential care. For example, when consumers are asked to pay more for high-value cancer screenings, clinician visits, and potentially lifesaving drugs, they use significantly fewer of these services. When cost sharing was increased for office visits in Medicare Advantage plans, patients visited their physicians less often. Consequently, individuals with increased cost sharing for office visits were also hospitalized more frequently, and their total costs outpaced those of patients whose out-of-pocket costs did not rise (Trivedi, Moloo, and Mor 2010).

Clinical Nuance

Given the shortcomings of "blunt" cost-sharing approaches, we need a smarter approach that encourages consumers to use more high-value services and providers while discouraging the use of low-value ones. To achieve these desired behaviors, insurance benefits and payment models must be redesigned with the basic tenets of *clinical nuance* in mind. These tenets recognize that the clinical benefit derived from a specific service depends on the consumer using the service, the provider of the service, and the place in which the service is delivered. A key takeaway is that the same clinical service that strongly benefits one person might not benefit another person and can, in some instances, even harm yet another (e.g., antibiotic use for bacterial infections and viral infections).

Two common clinical examples demonstrate how a clinically nuanced cost-sharing approach can improve the outcomes and efficiency of healthcare: (1) colorectal screening and (2) eye examinations. Screening for colorectal cancer (CRC) is an important, potentially lifesaving service that is provided with no cost sharing under the preventive health provisions of the Affordable Care Act. The US Preventive Services Taskforce recommends CRC screening only for adults of average risk between the ages of 50 and 75; it states that screening beyond the age of 85 is generally harmful.

This recommendation demonstrates the crucial principle of clinical nuance: The value of the service depends on the needs of the consumers receiving it. In this case, average-risk individuals benefit from the CRC screening and therefore should forego cost sharing. In contrast, patients outside the recommended age range should not be eligible to forego cost sharing unless they have a family history of colorectal cancer (for those under 50) or have had precancerous polyps on prior screenings (for those over 75). This nuanced approach ensures that patient cost sharing is eliminated or substantially reduced when the service is clinically necessary, thereby encouraging usage, while allowing health plans to impose higher cost sharing for services that lack strong clinical evidence to support their use.

The second example of using clinical nuance to make health plans more efficient involves eye examinations for people with diabetes. Current evidence-based quality metrics call for individuals with diabetes to undergo routine eye examinations. Hence, in a nuanced design, cost sharing for eye examinations would be substantially lower for people with diabetes than for those without.

Clinical evidence and specialty guidelines frequently indicate treatment recommendations for specific diagnoses (e.g., asthma, cardiovascular disease, depression), but most benefit designs do not tailor consumer cost sharing in a similar manner. Although cost sharing without clinical nuance may, in the short term, reduce medical expenditures through reduced utilization, it may also lead to lower rates of adherence to evidence-based recommendations—especially by specific patient groups most likely to benefit—thus leading to inferior health outcomes and, in the long term, higher overall costs.

The use of high cost-sharing levels on high-value services in targeted populations demonstrates the aphorism "penny wise and pound foolish" as applied to healthcare. Conversely, when cost sharing is set too low—as in certain Medicare supplemental insurance plans—people who do not have an appropriate clinical need may overuse services that are low in value or even potentially harmful, resulting in wasteful spending.

Implementing Clinical Nuance in Value-Based Insurance Design

During the first decade of the 2000s, private-sector payers began implementing V-BID to encourage consumers to take better advantage of high-value services and actively participate in decision making about treatments that are often subject to misuse. The basic V-BID premise calls for a clinically nuanced benefit structure that reduces consumer cost sharing for evidence-based services and high-performing providers.

Research on the clinical and economic impact of V-BID programs that lower cost sharing for targeted services has consistently demonstrated improved medication adherence with no net increases in aggregate expenditures when compared with plans without such clinically nuanced cost sharing. A number of studies have found that such programs increased adherence to prescriptions and services for management of chronic illnesses by several percentage points (Choudhry, Rosenthal, and Milstein 2010; Chernew et al. 2008; Farley et al. 2012; Maciejewski et al. 2014; Gibson et al. 2011; Hirth et al. 2016).

Most initial V-BID programs, including those implemented by early adopter Pitney Bowes, focused on prescription drugs. However, more recent implementations, such as Connecticut's state employee Health Enhancement Plan, have improved access to clinical services across the entire spectrum of clinical care (e.g., visits, diagnostic tests, treatments). According to a PricewaterhouseCoopers (2017) survey of US employers across various industries, 9 percent of employers were using V-BID in their benefit plans in 2017, and 36 percent were considering it for the future. The strong private-sector support for V-BID has created momentum to spur its uptake in public programs.

Putting Innovation into Action

The Affordable Care Act

The passage of the Patient Protection and Affordable Care Act (ACA) of 2010 (H.R. 3590) solidified the role of V-BID in national healthcare reform. Section 2713 of the ACA, titled "Coverage of Preventive Health Care Services," requires that issuers offering group or individual health insurance plans provide coverage for specified preventive services without a beneficiary copayment or a contribution toward a deductible (Congress.gov 2018b). These services include (1) those services receiving an "A" or "B" rating from the US Preventive Services Taskforce; (2) immunizations recommended by the Advisory Committee on Immunization Practices; and (3) preventive care and screenings supported by the Health Resources and Services Administration. The final subsection of the law specifically allows the secretary of health and human services to develop guidelines for value-based insurance designs. Since the ACA's passing, more than 137 million Americans have received expanded coverage of preventive services, and more than 76 million have accessed them without any level of cost sharing (Kaiser Family Foundation 2015).

In 2016, a KFF survey reported that the elimination of out-of-pocket costs for many preventive services was the second most popular ACA provision, after the provision allowing young adults to stay on their parents' insurance until age 26 (Kirzinger, Sugarman, and Brodie 2016). The widespread popularity of the measure was indicative of the growing bipartisan support for V-BID.

Medicare Advantage

Policymakers have begun exploring consumer-facing strategies and complementary provider-facing payment reforms as a means to contain Medicare spending increases while improving quality of care (Chernew, Fendrick, and Spangler 2013; Chernew and Fendrick 2016). Given the success of V-BID principles in the private sector and the special needs of the high-risk population of beneficiaries covered by Medicare, V-BID strategies have become a particularly attractive option for the Medicare Advantage (MA) program.

With the goal of improving health outcomes and reducing spending, the incorporation of V-BID principles into MA plans has garnered support from multiple stakeholder groups across both major political parties. The Seniors' Medication Copayment Reduction Act of 2009 (S. 1040); the Better Care, Lower Cost Act of 2014 (S. 1932); and the Strengthening Medicare Advantage Through Innovation and Transparency for Seniors Act of 2015 (H.R. 2570) have all proposed incorporating V-BID principles into Medicare and MA (Center for Value-Based Insurance Design 2015, 2017c). In its 2012 report to Congress, the Medicare Payment Advisory Commission (MEDPAC) proposed allowing greater flexibility in the provision of supplemental services in MA benefit design and recommended that the secretary of health and human services be given the authority to alter or eliminate cost sharing based on the evidence of the value of the service (Bipartisan Policy Center 2017; MEDPAC 2013).

In 2016, an actuarial analysis of the fiscal implications of condition-specific MA V-BID programs from the patient, plan, and societal perspectives was undertaken for diabetes mellitus (DM), chronic obstructive pulmonary disease (COPD), and congestive heart failure (CHF) (see exhibit 16.2). The actuarial model estimated that, after one year, V-BID programs reduced consumer out-of-pocket costs in all three conditions. Plan costs increased slightly for DM and COPD, but the plan realized cost savings for CHF. From a societal perspective, the DM program was close to cost neutral, while the COPD and CHF programs led to net societal savings one year after implementation (Fendrick et al. 2016).

Medicare Advantage V-BID Model Test

In September 2015, the Center for Medicare & Medicaid Innovation (CMMI) announced the Medicare Advantage Value-Based Insurance Design Model Test, which began at the beginning of the 2017 contract year (Fendrick et al. 2016; Centers for Medicare & Medicaid Services [CMS] 2016). CMMI specified nine clinical conditions for which plans can test V-BID with clinically nuanced changes in benefits that

EXHIBIT 16.2 Actuarial Analysis of Medicare Advantage Value-Based Insurance Design Programs, by Condition and Stakeholder

Projected Financial Impact of MA V-BID Program, Year 1

Cost Paid per Month ($)	Diabetes Mellitus	COPD	CHF
Member Cost Share	↓ $21.64	↓ $17.63	↓ $12.73
Plan Paid Amount	↑ $24.56	↑ $14.36	↓ $.56
Total Societal Costs	↑ $2.94	↓ $3.27	↓ $13.29

Note: MA = Medicare Advantage; V-BID = value-based insurance design; COPD = chronic obstructive pulmonary disease; CHF = congestive heart failure.

Source: Adapted from Fendrick et al. (2016).

- reduce cost sharing for high-value services,
- reduce cost sharing for high-value providers,
- reduce cost sharing for participants in disease management or related programs, and
- support coverage of additional supplemental benefits.

CMMI specifies that changes in benefit design through this model can only encourage use of high-value care or services for the targeted enrollees within the designated clinical conditions. In other words, members of the V-BID model plans can never be subject to higher cost sharing than other beneficiaries. Nine MA plans in three states started the program in January 2017 (see exhibit 16.3).

For 2018, CMS announced the expansion of the model to ten states and the addition of two more clinical conditions: dementia and rheumatoid arthritis. For 2019, the MA V-BID demonstration expanded further to include MA plans in 15 additional states, as well as special needs plans (see exhibit 16.4) (CMS 2016).

Bipartisan congressional interest to include all 50 states in the MA V-BID demonstration continues. The Bipartisan Budget Act of 2018, signed by President Donald Trump, provides funding for the Creating High-Quality Results and Outcomes Necessary to Improve Chronic (CHRONIC) Care Act of

EXHIBIT 16.3 Medicare Advantage Value-Based Insurance Design Model Test Plans and Conditions, Year 1

Medicare Advantage Organization	Conditions
BCBS of Massachusetts	Hypertension
Fallon Community Health Plan, MA	Diabetes
Tufts Associated Health Plan, MA	COPD and/or CHF
Geisinger Health Plan, PA	COPD
Aetna, PA	CHF
Independence Blue Cross, PA	Diabetes and CHF
Highmark, PA	Diabetes and/or COPD
UPMC Health Plan, PA	CHF and COPD or CHF and diabetes
Indiana University Health Plan	CHF

EXHIBIT 16.4 States Eligible for Medicare Advantage Value-Based Insurance Design Model Test, Year 2

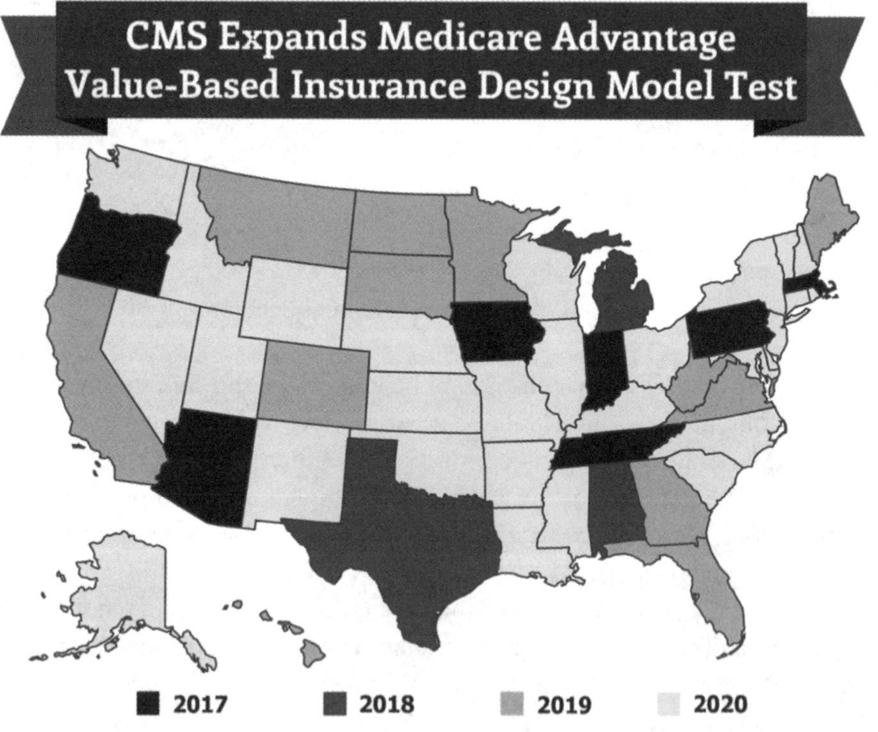

Source: CMS (2016).

2017 (S. 870), which was unanimously passed by the Senate. The CHRONIC Care Act specifically calls for the expansion of the MA V-BID demonstration to all 50 states by 2020. Mirroring the Senate version of the legislation, the V-BID for Better Care Act of 2017 (H.R. 1995)—sponsored in the House by Diane Black (R-TN), along with cosponsors Earl Blumenauer (D-OR), Cathy McMorris Rodgers (R-WA), and Debbie Dingell (D-MI)—also seeks to provide national testing of the MA V-BID model across all 50 states.

Beyond the model, a CMS proposed rule recommends greater flexibility around the MA uniformity requirement that originally deterred MA plans from offering clinically nuanced benefits. This change would allow for the implementation of V-BID principles throughout the MA program.

V-BID principles can be used to create MA plan designs that are better aligned with value. Encouraging the use of high-value services and providers while discouraging the use of those with low value will decrease cost-related nonadherence, reduce healthcare disparities, and improve the efficiency of healthcare spending without compromising quality. The use of clinical nuance to establish out-of-pocket costs for Medicare beneficiaries would have significant positive impacts, providing consumers with better access to quality services, resulting in a healthier population, and containing the growth of healthcare expenditures (Fendrick et al. 2016).

Changes to High-Deductible Health Plans

High-deductible health plans (HDHPs) differ from traditional plans in that they have lower premiums and higher deductibles. HDHPs coupled with tax-free health savings accounts (HSAs)—together known as HSA-HDHPs—are among the fastest-growing plan types in the United States.

For an HDHP to be HSA-eligible, it must meet Internal Revenue Service (IRS) guidelines for minimum individual and family deductibles. For 2017, the minimum deductible was $1,300 for an individual and $2,600 for a family (IRS 2016). Deposits into HSAs are made with pre-tax dollars, savings grow tax-free, and eligible withdrawals incur no tax liability; hence, they are said to have a "triple tax advantage." To open an HSA, the account holder must be enrolled in an IRS-qualified HDHP.

The appeal of a tax-advantaged savings account coupled with low annual HDHP premiums has propelled HSA-HDHP enrollment from 3.2 million in 2006 to 21.8 million in 2017 (America's Health Insurance Plans 2018). Unfortunately, yearly out-of-pocket maximums—the maximum amount that individuals and families must pay out-of-pocket before the insurance plan covers the remainder of expenses—are rapidly increasing as well. In 2006, the out-of-pocket maximums were $5,000 for individuals and $10,000 for families; these numbers rose to $6,550 and $13,100 by 2017 (IRS 2016). With rising out-of-pocket costs, patients often delay seeking essential medical care to avoid heavy financial burdens.

The IRS determines the coverage limits of HSA-HDHPs because of their tax implications. Under current IRS guidance, select preventive care services (e.g., screenings, vaccinations) must be fully covered prior to meeting the plan deductible. This collection of services is commonly referred to as the "safe harbor." Services used to treat any "existing illness, injury, or condition," however, are currently excluded from the safe harbor (IRS 2004). Thus, the portion of the 133 million Americans enrolled in HSA-HDHPs diagnosed with chronic conditions such as diabetes, HIV, or depression must pay the entire cost of their clinician visits, tests, and prescriptions until they reach their plan's deductible. This lack of pre-deductible coverage for services and medications essential for managing chronic conditions markedly deters those who may be interested from opening an HSA.

Broad stakeholder and bipartisan political support exist to amend the IRS code to expand the safe harbor, allowing HSA-HDHPs the option to cover certain high-value clinical services and medications for treating chronic medical conditions prior to meeting the plan deductible. Such a change would lead to a new generation of HDHPs known as "high-value health plans" (HVHPs) (Center for Value-Based Insurance Design 2017b). HVHPs would better meet the clinical and financial needs of millions of Americans, premiums would be lower than most existing commercial health plans, and coverage would be more generous than existing HSA-HDHPs.

Potential Impact of High-Value Health Plans

An extreme scenario involving a hypothetical HVHP that provides first-dollar, pre-deductible coverage for selected, well-established health plan quality metrics was created to estimate HVHP plan premiums and HVHPs' potential uptake in the individual and employer markets. The selected quality metrics included diagnostic tests (e.g., hemoglobin A1c test for diabetes), durable medical equipment (e.g., peak flow meter for asthma), and chronic disease medications (e.g., medications for patients with major depression).

Compared to an existing baseline HSA-HDHP (actuarial value of 71.7 percent), coverage of targeted services pre-deductible led to an estimated 5.63 percent increase in premiums, when no offsets are included for other clinical services that might be prevented (e.g., emergency room visits, hospitalizations). When the analysis included the Congressional Budget Office's (CBO's) offset estimate—one-fifth of 1 percent decrease in spending for every 1 percent increase in expenditures on targeted services—the HVHP resulted in a slightly lower premium increase of 5.08 percent. The actuarial value of the HVHP increased by less than 3 percent, to 74.18 percent when assuming no offset and to 74.20 percent when the CBO offset estimate was included. If cost sharing were applied to the pre-deductible services, the impact on premiums and actuarial value would be less (Center for Value-Based Insurance Design 2017b).

The Adjusted Risk Choice & Outcomes Legislative Assessment (ARCOLA) simulation model was used to forecast the demand for the hypothetical HVHP among currently available plan choices in the individual and employer insurance market. Holding a plan's generosity constant, an increase in premium would decrease the demand for that particular type of plan. Similarly, an increase in the generosity of a plan (i.e., higher actuarial value) would increase demand. The model accounts for the fact that, compared to the HVHP, some existing plan choices—such as preferred provider organizations (PPOs) and health maintenance organizations (HMOs)—have higher premiums and are more generous, whereas other options have lower premiums and provide less generous coverage (e.g., current HDHPs). Thus, if an HVHP were an alternative plan choice, some consumers could "buy down" from more expensive PPO and HMO plans, while others enrolled in less generous HDHPs could "buy up" and substitute an HVHP with more generous coverage.

The ARCOLA model estimated that the introduction of the hypothetical HVHP would be in high demand in the individual and employer market (see exhibit 16.5). HSA-HDHPs have experienced considerable growth in the employer sector, as PPO enrollment declines (Center for Value-Based Insurance Design 2017b).

Removing Regulatory Barriers to Expand HSA-HDHP Options and Increase Uptake

Out-of-pocket payments—such as those required by HDHPs—are a helpful tool in establishing a consumer-centric system by better engaging patients in their healthcare decision-making. However, existing IRS regulations that

EXHIBIT 16.5 Projected High-Value Health Plan Uptake in the Employer Market

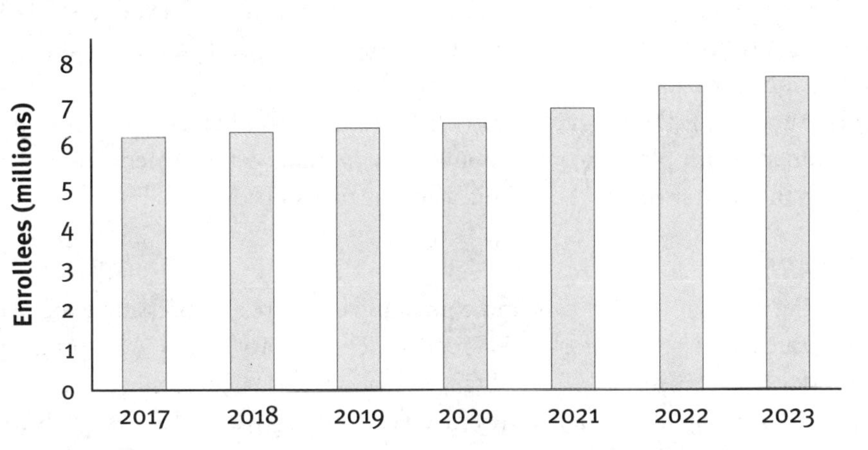

Source: Adapted from Center for Value-Based Insurance Design (2017b).

limit what services can be covered in HSA-HDHPs before meeting the plan deductible substantially restrain the breadth of plan options and thus stifle consumers' ability to benefit from the financial advantages of a tax-free HSA.

Preferably, insurers would have the flexibility to offer plans that provide pre-deductible coverage of high-value services across the entire spectrum of clinical care. HVHPs would allow Americans with chronic conditions to better afford the care they need while maintaining the original intent and spirit of consumer-directed health plans.

Expansion of the IRS safe harbor enjoys bipartisan, bicameral support from congressional leaders. In 2016, representatives Diane Black (R-TN) and Earl Blumenauer (D-OR) introduced the Access to Better Care Act (H.R. 5652), and senators Thomas R. Carper (D-DE) and John Thune (R-SD) sent a letter to the Secretary of the Treasury urging the modernization of the preventive care safe harbor to ensure that patients "have full access to adequate preventive care and chronic care management services"(Thune and Carper 2016). In 2017, a draft executive order included a provision directing the IRS commissioner to expand the preventive care safe harbor under section 223(c)(2)(C) of the Internal Revenue Code to include services and benefits, including medications, related to the management of chronic diseases (Center for Value-Based Insurance Design 2017a). In February 2018, the bipartisan Chronic Disease Management Act of 2018 (S. 2410, H.R. 4978) was introduced to amend the IRS safe harbor and "permit high-deductible health plans to provide chronic disease prevention services to plan enrollees prior to satisfying their plan deductible" (Center for Value-Based Insurance Design 2018).

Rising healthcare spending has created serious fiscal challenges and demonstrated the need for novel benefit designs that better engage consumers in their healthcare decisions. HSA-HDHPs that cover essential chronic disease services have the potential to mitigate cost-related nonadherence, enhance patient-centered outcomes, allow for premiums lower than those of most PPOs and HMOs, and substantially reduce aggregate US healthcare expenditures. The voluntary expansion of the IRS safe harbor would enhance the clinical effectiveness of HDHPs and increase the attractiveness of HSAs. By expanding consumer health plan choice, it could provide millions of Americans a plan option that better meets their clinical and financial needs.

TRICARE

Ensuring access to quality care and containing costs are also pressing issues for healthcare administrators for the US military. The military's TRICARE program provides health insurance for military personnel and their families—totaling more than 9 million beneficiaries in 2017 (TRICARE 2017). As in other sectors, a shift in TRICARE from a volume-driven system to a value-based system requires a change in how healthcare is paid for and how consumers are engaged and motivated to seek care. Less attention, however, has been focused on how we can alter consumer behavior as a policy lever to bring about a more efficient delivery system.

As TRICARE members have been asked to pay more for their medical care, a growing body of evidence has demonstrated that increases in consumer cost sharing lead to decreases in the use of both nonessential and essential care. Because analysis of TRICARE usage shows evidence of both underuse of high-value services and overuse of low-value services, "smarter" cost sharing is a potential solution. Such an approach would encourage TRICARE members to use more of the services that make them healthier and discourage the use of services that do not.

In 2016, the US Senate Committee on Armed Services began exploring the role of V-BID in defense healthcare reform, and the National Defense Authorization Act (NDAA) of 2017 (S. 2943) called for a pilot program incorporating V-BID into the TRICARE program no later than January 1, 2018. Specifically, the reforms would reduce copayments for high-value medications and services and the use of high-value providers for targeted populations, while evaluating how reducing or eliminating cost sharing for specified high-value medications and services affects adherence to medication regimens, quality measures, health outcomes, and beneficiary experience. The NDAA states that, by "reducing copayments . . . for targeted populations of covered beneficiaries in the receipt of high-value medications and services and the use of high-value providers," the pilot could improve health outcomes and enhance the experience of care for US Armed Forces military personnel, military retirees, and their dependents (Congress.gov 2018c).

The National Defense Authorization Act for Fiscal Year 2018 (H.R. 2810) includes the incorporation of V-BID principles within section 702, which calls for "modifications of cost-sharing requirements for the TRICARE Pharmacy Benefits Program and treatment of certain pharmaceutical agents" (Congress.gov 2018a).

To achieve better care and lower costs for the military healthcare system, value-driven consumer incentives—through benefit design reforms promoting smart decisions and enhanced responsibility—must align with payment reform initiatives. Permitting clinically nuanced cost sharing will give TRICARE plans a valuable tool to better encourage members to receive high-value services.

State Health Reform

V-BID principles have also been incorporated into a variety of state health reform initiatives, including exchanges, Medicaid, and state employee health plans.

Medicaid policy includes substantial constraints on cost sharing. Given that the program serves people with low income, even relatively nominal cost-sharing amounts could represent barriers to care for the beneficiary. CMS regulations finalized in 2013 allow states to implement certain forms of V-BID-based flexibility within the cost sharing bounds. For example, states may incorporate clinical nuance by targeting cost-sharing variations, such as exempting patients from the nominal cost sharing included in a plan for those with certain clinical conditions, as well as for preferred drugs (CMS 2013).

For example, Michigan's Medicaid expansion under the ACA—a plan known as Healthy Michigan—was implemented under a CMS waiver that includes a V-BID component. Michigan's plan includes the potential for premiums and cost sharing of up to 7 percent of income for people with income above 100 percent of the federal poverty level, but it eliminates copays to promote access to services that prevent the progress and complications of chronic disease. Healthy Michigan also allows other cost-sharing reductions for enrollees who participate in healthy behaviors defined by the state (Udow-Phillips et al. 2015).

With more than 22 million state employees (almost 15 percent of the US workforce) receiving care through a public employee health plan, a major opportunity exists for state employers—who spend more than $31 billion annually—to incorporate clinically nuanced designs to improve employee health and spend more efficiently (US Bureau of Labor Statistics 2018; Pew Charitable Trusts 2014).

Applied Example: The Connecticut Health Enhancement Program

In 2011, Connecticut implemented the Connecticut Health Enhancement Program (HEP) for state employees. This voluntary program followed the principles of V-BID by lowering patient costs for certain high-value primary care and chronic disease preventive services, coupled with requirements that enrollees receive these services. HEP reduced cost sharing for evidence-based preventive services, provided $100-per-month discounts on premiums, and eliminated the deductible (Center for Value-Based Insurance Design 2017d).

The plan encouraged better management of conditions and alignment of provider and consumer incentives by offering free physicals, two free dental cleanings per year, and appropriate diagnostic tests, hoping to emphasize appropriate and well-managed care. Employees with at least one specified chronic condition (asthma, COPD, diabetes, heart disease, hypertension, or hyperlipidemia) were eligible to participate in disease management programs and offered chronic care appointments with $0 copay. A $35 copayment was added to the plan for emergency room visits but applied only when "reasonable medical alternatives" were available, thereby deterring patients from using emergency departments to treat care that could have been provided in urgent care or primary care physician facilities. A novel feature of HEP was a requirement that members receive certain services, including preventive care office visits and age-appropriate screenings, to remain enrolled. Nonparticipants in the program, including those removed for noncompliance with its requirements, were assessed a premium surcharge (Hirth et al. 2016).

The program was intended to curb cost growth and to improve health through adherence to evidence-based preventive care. To evaluate its efficacy in doing so, changes in service use and spending after implementation of the program were compared to trends among employees of six other states. Enrollment in the first year exceeded 98 percent, and 98 percent of enrollees remained compliant. The use of the targeted services and adherence to medications increased over the two-year study period. Preventive office visits increased by 13.5 percentage points in year one and 4.8 percentage points in year two. The number of ER visits without an accompanying admission decreased by 10 visits per 1,000 enrollees in year one and 25 visits per 1,000 enrollees in year two—a reduction of about 10 percent relative to the comparison states (Hirth et al. 2016). The program's impact on costs was inconclusive and requires a longer follow-up period.

The Future of V-BID

Identifying and Reducing Low-Value Care

As stated at the start of the chapter, the United States spends more on healthcare per capita than any other country, yet it does not achieve better outcomes. A substantial share of this spending is devoted to services that carry no additional health benefit and, in some instances, expose patients to serious risk of harm. A 2016 *Health Affairs* article estimated that low-value care accounted for more than $765 billion in wasteful expenditures in 2013 (Beaudin-Seiler et al. 2016). Separate research has estimated that between 23 and 37 percent of Medicare beneficiaries receive at least one low-value service per year, and many believe that these estimates, even those at the higher end, are too conservative (VBID Health 2017).

Beyond the heavy price that public and private purchasers pay, use of low-value care can be harmful for patients. Risks include the following:

- Low-value care can expose patients to iatrogenic harm. For example, inappropriate computed tomography (CT) studies raise the lifetime risk of cancer without commensurate benefit, screening for colorectal cancer can raise the risk of perforation without reducing mortality, and inappropriate use of antibiotics can raise the risk of serious infection (VBID Health 2017).
- Low-value care can impose high out-of-pocket costs. In an era of high-deductible plans, analyses have found that between 17 and 33 percent of spending on low-value care is paid by patients, leading to hundreds of thousands in financial exposure (Chua et al. 2016).
- Low-value care can lead to lost time, lost productivity, and "botheredness" (VBID Health 2017).

As states, plans, and employers work toward creating better systems that discourage spending on unnecessary services and promote the use of high-value services, one of the greatest challenges will be addressing, identifying, and measuring low-value care. Progress has been fragmented and slow, primarily because of complexities in defining low-value care services, discrepancies in how to incorporate patient preferences and satisfaction with the concept of low-value care, and lack of consensus on how pricing information should be incorporated.

In response to growing concerns surrounding low-value care, the Choosing Wisely campaign, an initiative launched by the American Board of Internal Medicine (ABIM) Foundation in partnership with more than 70 professional societies, has identified about 500 commonly overused services across the spectrum of medical care (Reid, Rabideau, and Sood 2016). Generally, a particular type of service is not going to be high-value or low-value in every instance. Rather, a service that benefits one person often may harm another. Thus, clinical nuance comes into play.

Although the Choosing Wisely campaign has brought greater attention to the issue of low-value care, broad dissemination of its recommendations has had only a modest impact on the receipt of targeted services (Schwartz et al. 2014, 2015). Several additional approaches (shown in exhibit 16.6) merit the attention of payers and purchasers seeking to cut down on commonly overused services while respecting the need for clinical nuance. The most effective initiatives in this area will likely couple interventions to change provider behavior with carefully designed incentives for consumers.

EXHIBIT 16.6
Provider- and Patient-Facing Methods of Reducing Low-Value Care

Provider-Facing	Patient-Facing
Coverage policies—No reimbursement for services that are clearly inappropriate based on administrative data. **Payment rates**—Consider the risk of overuse across services in negotiating or setting allowed amounts. **Provider profiling information**—Provide reports benchmarking the practice patterns of a clinician or practice against those of peers. **Payment models**—Accelerate adoption of new approaches to reimbursement that reduce financial incentives for overuse.	**Network design**—Steer patients to providers and plans that minimize use of inappropriate medical services. **Utilization management**—While minimizing administrative burden, selectively consider prior authorization programs. **Value-based insurance designs**—Align patients' out-of-pocket cost-sharing with the value of the underlying service. For commonly overused services, selectively allow cost sharing to serve as a "speed bump."

Source: Adapted from VBID Health (2017).

Promising examples of each of these strategies can be seen in the field today. By learning from existing work and pioneering new approaches, payers and purchasers can better protect patients from the physical, financial, and time-related harms of overuse; support allied efforts in the provider community; and free limited healthcare resources for more productive uses.

The Role of V-BID in Low-Value Care

Most V-BID interventions have focused on reducing cost sharing for high-value services in an effort to encourage access and patient adherence to recommended clinical protocols, especially for chronic conditions. V-BID interventions can also improve healthcare quality and efficiency through the reverse approach, by increasing cost sharing for low-value services, thereby ensuring more effective care and achieving net cost savings. However, defining what is meant by "low-value services" and implementing programs to restrict those services' use can be challenging.

A number of writers have explored the complexities in identifying and eliminating low-value services, particularly given the V-BID core principle of "clinical nuance":

- Fendrick, Smith, and Chernew (2017) identify options for addressing lower-value services, including untargeted increases in cost sharing for all services not designated as high-value and service-specific increases in cost sharing with particular attention to the value of a service compared with alternative modes of treatment.
- Robinson (2010) notes that coinsurance (rather than copayments) generally tends to affect higher-cost services, and he reviews various types of high-cost services for which V-BID principles can be applied. Examples may include self- and office-administered specialty drugs, implantable devices, advanced imaging, and high-cost surgical procedures.
- Neumann and colleagues (2010) set explicit criteria for defining low-value services based on studies of cost-effectiveness compared with alternatives, and they provide a list of potential low-value services, including several cancer drugs. They also note the challenges in moving forward, including the need for a clear process and approach for identifying low-value services and the subgroups of people for whom the services are low-value, as well as the challenge of extending the process beyond prescription drugs.

The identification, measurement, and removal of low-value care must be part of a strategy to move to a high-performing healthcare delivery system. Key stakeholders—including a large number of medical professional societies—agree that discouraging consumers from using specific low-value services must be an essential element of this strategy. The removal of wasteful spending is challenging, but the immediate and substantial savings that result can provide payers "headroom" to buy more high-value services.

Precision Medicine

Precision medicine—the integration of molecular science into the clinical care of individual patients—has spurred efforts to develop targeted preventive strategies and disease-specific therapies. This personalized approach to clinical medicine has vast potential to improve quality of care, enhance the patient experience, and allow more efficient healthcare expenditures. V-BID principles can be applied to create "precision benefit designs" that encourage the appropriate usage of high-value, targeted clinical services and therapies.

The common recommendation that patients *initially* be prescribed a lower-cost treatment is a reasonable population health strategy, given that a first-line therapy will often be effective and will be considered high value for the patient and for the payer. The designation of first-line therapies is often based on a tiered formulary design and requires patients to progress through an established sequence of treatment options before being granted coverage for targeted therapies. However, advances in precision medicine may specify the immediate use of more expensive, targeted therapies, nullifying recommendations for use of the standard first-line treatment. Thus, in the increasingly frequent scenario in which a person tests positive for a specific marker, a targeted therapy may be indicated to optimize patient-centered outcomes. Here, the standard first-line therapy is no longer high-value, and a clinically indicated "precision" alternative becomes a higher-value choice.

Generally, current cost-sharing levels are fixed and do not reflect the varying nature of many clinical conditions. Precision medicine, meanwhile, is founded on the V-BID principle that the health benefits provided by a particular service depend on the specific clinical circumstances around its use. The use of targeted and sequential therapies in a growing number of clinical circumstances supports the elimination of the archaic prescription drug cost-sharing model, which does not share this fundamental premise. The V-BID-based precision medicine approach would involve setting the level of consumer cost sharing based on the clinical value—not solely the price—of a therapy when used in a specific circumstance. The implementation of such a cost-sharing model enhances access to effective, clinically appropriate therapies; improves patient outcomes; aligns with quality-driven provider initiatives; and promotes efficient expenditures for the payer.

As evidence supporting the promise of precision medicine accumulates, several systemwide obstacles remain that hinder its implementation in clinical practice. Challenges may include minimizing administrative complexities, establishing incentives that engage patients, integrating provider- and patient-focused initiatives, and recognizing that "the perfect must not be the enemy of the good" in the financing and delivery of targeted care. If the full potential of precision medicine is to be realized, system-based reforms must encourage—not deter—its adoption by clinicians and consumers.

Conclusion

The ultimate test of health reform will be whether it expands coverage in a way that improves health and addresses rapidly rising costs. To generate public support, efforts to bend the healthcare cost curve must be linked with a focus on patient-centered, high-quality care. By basing consumer cost sharing on the clinical value—not the price—of services, payers can actively engage consumers in seeking high-value care and foster more regular conversations with providers about low-value services. Moreover, as provider-facing initiatives are implemented, these supply-side programs must be closely aligned with approaches to assist consumers. The potential impact of such carefully aligned approaches to contain costs and improve quality will be far greater than what any single strategy can achieve on its own.

Study Questions

1. Under what circumstances might increasing out-of-pocket costs for consumers increase the value and efficiency of healthcare provided? Under what circumstances might doing so have an undesirable effect?
2. What is clinical nuance? What role does it play in value-based insurance design?
3. What are some of the obstacles that stand in the way of the next generation of high-value health plans?
4. What are the main risks associated with low-value care?

Case Study: Implementation of Connecticut's Health Enhancement Plan

Mr. Arnold is a bridge safety supervisor for the state of Connecticut. He has worked in many regions throughout the state and relies on state insurance plans for coverage. Within the past few years, he sustained an injury on the job and, while at the hospital, was diagnosed with COPD, after many years

(continued)

of smoking. He has begun paying closer attention to his health, but he still requires multiple medications and physician visits throughout the year.

The year is 2010, and Mr. Arnold has heard that, starting next year, Connecticut will implement the Health Enhancement Plan for its state employees. The program follows V-BID principles by lowering patient costs for certain high-value primary and chronic disease preventive services and coupling services with enrollment requirements.

As Mr. Arnold reads the informational booklets provided by the state, he discovers that HEP is unlike previous plans he has known in that it requires members to receive certain services, including preventive care office visits and age-appropriate screenings, to remain enrolled in the plan. The plan encourages better management of chronic conditions and aligns with existing incentives by offering services in the form of free physicals, two free dental cleanings per year, and appropriate diagnostic tests. Members who choose not to participate in the services are unenrolled from the program and assessed a premium surcharge of $100.

Employees with at least one of the specified chronic conditions (asthma, COPD, diabetes, heart disease, hypertension, or hyperlipidemia) are eligible to participate in disease-management programs and offered chronic care appointments with $0 copay. To deter enrollees from using emergency departments for care that could have been provided in less expensive urgent care or primary care facilities, HEP features a $35 copayment for emergency room visits, but the copay is applied only when "reasonable medical alternatives" are available.

Mr. Arnold is asked by his supervisor, Mr. Joseph, to train new employees on the basics of the new HEP plan. Mr. Joseph, a healthy individual with no chronic conditions, is worried that these plans will create confusion for his employees and increase his own healthcare costs.

Case Study Discussion Questions

1. What should Mr. Arnold consider the key takeaways in the HEP plan when training new employees? Is Mr. Joseph correct that the plan will increase his costs? Additionally, what should Mr. Arnold tell Harry, a diabetic employee who is starting at his department?
2. In drafting your response, think about the population and health of state employees. Do these factors affect HEP plan profitability? Why or why not?

References

America's Health Insurance Plans. 2018. "Health Savings Accounts: Providing High-Quality Coverage to 21.8 Million People." Published April 12. www.ahip.org/health-savings-accounts-infographic/.

Beaudin-Seiler, B., M. Ciarametaro, R. W. Dubois, J. Lee, and A. M. Fendrick. 2016. "Reducing Low-Value Care." *Health Affairs*. Published September 20. www.healthaffairs.org/do/10.1377/hblog20160920.056666/full/.

Bipartisan Policy Center. 2017. *Challenges and Opportunities in Caring for High-Need, High-Cost Medicare Patients: BPC Preliminary Findings and Policy Options*. Published February. https://cdn.bipartisanpolicy.org/wp-content/uploads/2017/02/BPC-Health-High-Need-High-Cost-Medicare-Patients.pdf.

Center for Value-Based Insurance Design. 2018. "Chronic Disease Management Act of 2018 Introduced in Congress." Published February 6. http://vbidcenter.org/chronic-disease-mngmt-act-2018/.

———. 2017a. "Draft Executive Order Enables Innovation in HSA-HDHPs." Published August 1. http://vbidcenter.org/draft-executive-order-enables-innovation-in-hsa-hdhps/.

———. 2017b. "The Next Generation Health Savings Account: The 'High-Value Health Plan'." Accessed December 1. http://vbidcenter.org/wp-content/uploads/2016/12/HSA-HDHP-Summary-UPDATED-8.8.17-Final.pdf.

———. 2017c. "V-BID Concepts Included in New Medicare Legislation to Improve Care and Lower Costs." Published January 15. http://vbidcenter.org/v-bid-concepts-included-in-new-medicare-legislation-to-improve-care-and-lower-costs/.

———. 2017d. "V-BID in Action: A Profile of Connecticut's Health Enhancement Program." Published February 21. http://vbidcenter.org/v-bid-in-action-a-profile-of-connecticuts-health-enhancement-program-2/.

———. 2015. "News Update: V-BID Medicare Advantage Bill Passes House of Representatives." Published June 18. http://vbidcenter.org/news-update-v-bid-medicare-advantage-bill-passes-house-of-representatives/.

Centers for Medicare & Medicaid Services (CMS). 2016. "Medicare Advantage Value-Based Insurance Design Model Test—Advanced Notice of CY 2018 Model Changes." Published August 7. http://vbidcenter.org/wp-content/uploads/2016/08/CMS-Update-V-BID-MA-Demo-8-10-16-includes-MI.pdf.

———. 2013. "Final Rule for Strengthening Medicaid, the Children's Health Insurance Program and the New Health Insurance Marketplace (CMS-2334-F)." Published July. www.cms.gov/newsroom/fact-sheets/final-rule-strengthening-medicaid-childrens-health-insurance-program-and-new-health-insurance.

Chernew, M. E., and A. M. Fendrick. 2016. "Improving Benefit Design to Promote Effective, Efficient, and Affordable Care." *JAMA* 316 (16): 1651–52.

Chernew, M. E., A. M. Fendrick, and K. Spangler. 2013. "Implementing Value-Based Insurance Design in the Medicare Advantage Program." VBID Health. Published May. http://vbidcenter.org/wp-content/uploads/2015/01/ImplementingVBIDintheMedicareAdvantageProgram_May2013.pdf.

Chernew, M. E., M. R. Shah, A. Wegh, S. N. Rosenberg, I. A. Juster, A. B. Rosen, M. C. Sokol, K. Yu-Isenberg, and A. M. Fendrick. 2008. "Impact of Decreasing Copayments on Medication Adherence Within a Disease Management Environment." *Health Affairs* 27 (1): 103–12.

Choudhry, N. K., M. B. Rosenthal, and A. Milstein. 2010. "Assessing the Evidence for Value-Based Insurance Design." *Health Affairs* 29 (11): 1988–94.

Chua, K.-P., A. L. Schwartz, A. Volerman, R. M. Conti, and E. S. Huang. 2016. "Use of Low-Value Pediatric Services Among the Commercially Insured." *Pediatrics*. Published December. http://pediatrics.aappublications.org/content/138/6/e20161809.

Claxton, G., L. Levitt, and M. Long. 2016. "Payments for Cost-Sharing Increasing Rapidly over Time." Peterson-Kaiser Health System Tracker. Published April 12. www.healthsystemtracker.org/brief/payments-for-cost-sharing-increasing-rapidly-over-time/.

Claxton, G., M. Rae, M. Long, A. Damico, G. Foster, and H. Whitmore. 2017. *Employer Health Benefits: 2017 Annual Survey*. Kaiser Family Foundation and Health Research and Educational Trust. Accessed December 3, 2018. www.eesipeo.com/media/24-Report-Employer-Health-Benefits-Annual-Survey-2017.pdf.

Cohen, R. A., and E. P. Zammitti. 2017. "High-Deductible Health Plans and Financial Barriers to Medical Care: Early Release of Estimates from the National Health Interview Survey, 2016." Centers for Disease Control and Prevention. Published June. www.cdc.gov/nchs/data/nhis/earlyrelease/ERHDHP_Access_0617.pdf.

Congress.gov. 2018a. "H.R. 2810—National Defense Authorization Act for Fiscal Year 2018." Accessed December 4. www.congress.gov/bill/115th-congress/house-bill/2810/text.

———. 2018b. "H.R. 3590—Patient Protection and Affordable Care Act." Accessed December 3. www.congress.gov/bill/111th-congress/house-bill/3590.

———. 2018c. "S. 2943—National Defense Authorization Act of Fiscal Year 2017." Accessed November 30. www.congress.gov/bill/114th-congress/senate-bill/2943/text.

Farley, J. F., D. Wansink, J. H. Lindquist, J. C. Parker, and M. L. Maciejewski. 2012. "Medication Adherence Changes Following Value-Based Insurance Design." *American Journal of Managed Care* 18 (5): 265–74.

Fendrick, A. M., S. L. Oesterle, H. M. Lee, P. Padaley, T. Eagle, M. Chernew, P. P. Mueller, J. Adams, J. V. Agostini, and C. Montagano. 2016. "Incorporating Value-Based Insurance Design to Improve Chronic Disease Management in the Medicare Advantage Program." Center for Value-Based Insurance Design. Published August. http://vbidcenter.org/wp-content/uploads/2016/08/MA-White-Paper_final-8-16-16.pdf.

Fendrick, A. M., D. G. Smith, and M. E. Chernew. 2017. "Applying Value-Based Insurance Design to Low-Value Health Services." *Health Affairs*. Published November. www.healthaffairs.org/doi/10.1377/hlthaff.2010.0878.

Gibson, T. B., S. Wang, E. Kelly, C. Brown, C. Turner, F. Frech-Tamas, J. Doyle, and E. Mauceri. 2011. "A Value-Based Insurance Design Program at a Large Company Boosted Medication Adherence for Employees with Chronic Illnesses." *Health Affairs* 30 (1): 109–17.

Hirth, R. A., E. Q. Cliff, T. B. Gibson, M. R. McKellar, and A. M. Fendrick. 2016. "Connecticut's Value-Based Insurance Plan Increased the Use of Targeted Services and Medication Adherence." *Health Affairs* 35 (4): 637–46.

Internal Revenue Service (IRS). 2016. "Tax Forms and Instructions." Accessed December 1, 2017. www.irs.gov/pub/irs-drop/rp-16-28.pdf.

———. 2004. "Notice 2004-23." Accessed December 1, 2017. www.irs.gov/irb/2004-15_IRB#NOT-2004-23.

Kaiser Family Foundation (KFF). 2016. "2016 Employer Health Benefits Survey." Published September 14. www.kff.org/report-section/ehbs-2016-summary-of-findings/.

———. 2015. "Preventive Services Covered by Private Health Plans under the Affordable Care Act." Published August 4. www.kff.org/health-reform/fact-sheet/preventive-services-covered-by-private-health-plans/.

Kirzinger, A., E. Sugarman, and M. Brodie. 2016. "Kaiser Health Tracking Poll: November 2016." Kaiser Family Foundation. Published December 1. www.kff.org/health-costs/poll-finding/kaiser-health-tracking-poll-november-2016/.

Maciejewski, M. L., D. Wansink, J. H. Lindquist, J. C. Parker, and J. F. Farley. 2014. "Value-Based Insurance Design Program in North Carolina Increased Medication Adherence but Was Not Cost Neutral." *Health Affairs* 33 (2): 300–8.

Medicare Payment Advisory Commission (MEDPAC). 2013. *Report to the Congress: Medicare Payment Policy*. Published March. http://medpac.gov/docs/default-source/reports/mar13_entirereport.pdf.

Neumann, P. J., H. R. Auerbach, J. T. Cohen, and D. Greenberg. 2010. "Low-Value Services in Value-Based Insurance Design." *American Journal of Managed Care* 16 (4): 280–86.

Pew Charitable Trusts. 2014. "State Employee Health Plan Spending." Published August 12. www.pewtrusts.org/en/research-and-analysis/reports/2014/08/state-employee-health-plan-spending.

PricewaterhouseCoopers. 2017. *Health and Well-being Touchstone Survey Results*. Published June. www.pwc.com/us/en/hr-management/publications/pdf/pwc-touchstone-2017.pdf.

Reid, R. O., B. Rabideau, and N. Sood. 2016. "Low-Value Health Care Services in a Commercially Insured Population." *JAMA Internal Medicine* 176 (10): 1567–71.

Robinson, J. C. 2010. "Applying Value-Based Insurance Design to High-Cost Health Services." *Health Affairs* 29 (11): 2009–16.

Schneider, E. C., D. O. Sarnak, D. Squires, A. Shah, and M. M. Doty. 2017. "Mirror, Mirror 2017: International Comparison Reflects Flaws and Opportunities for Better U.S. Health Care." Commonwealth Fund. Accessed December 3, 2018. https://interactives.commonwealthfund.org/2017/july/mirror-mirror/.

Schwartz, A. L., M. E. Chernew, B. E. Landon, and J. M. McWilliams. 2015. "Changes in Low-Value Services in Year 1 of the Medicare Pioneer Accountable Care Organization Program." *JAMA Internal Medicine* 175 (11): 1815–25.

Schwartz, A. L., B. E. Landon, A. G. Elshaug, M. E. Chernew, and J. M. McWilliams. 2014. "Measuring Low-Value Care in Medicare." *JAMA Internal Medicine* 174 (7): 1067–76.

Thune, J., and T. R. Carper. 2016. "Letter to the Treasury and IRS on Safe Harbor Expansion." Center for Value-Based Insurance Design. Accessed December 2, 2017. http://vbidcenter.org/wp-content/uploads/2016/03/Letter-to-Treasury-and-IRS-on-Expansion-of-Safe-Harbor.pdf.

TRICARE. 2017. "Number of Beneficiaries." Accessed December 2. www.tricare.mil/About/Facts/BeneNumbers.

Trivedi, A. N., H. Moloo, and V. Mor. 2010. "Increased Ambulatory Care Copayments and Hospitalizations Among the Elderly." *New England Journal of Medicine* 362 (4): 320–28.

Udow-Phillips, M., K. Burns Lausch, E. Shigekawa, R. Hirth, and J. Ayanian. 2015. "The Medicaid Expansion Experience in Michigan." *Health Affairs*. Published August 28. www.healthaffairs.org/do/10.1377/hblog20150828.050226/full/.

US Bureau of Labor Statistics. 2018. "Databases, Tables & Calculators by Subject." Accessed December 14. www.bls.gov/data/.

VBID Health. 2017. "Reducing Use of Low-Value Medical Care." Accessed December 3. www.vbidhealth.com/docs/TF-LVC%20-%20One-Pager.pdf.

CHAPTER

17

VALUE-BASED PURCHASING: THE INCREASING IMPORTANCE OF QUALITY CONSIDERATIONS IN FUNDING THE HEALTHCARE SYSTEM

Neil Goldfarb

Introduction and Definitions

Measurement plays a key role in driving improvements in healthcare quality and safety. In this chapter, we will consider how purchasers are using quality measurement and improvement principles to derive better value from their purchasing decisions.

Value has many definitions in healthcare, but it is generally considered to be the relationship between quality (usually with a focus on outcomes and patient centeredness) and costs (Porter 2010). The US healthcare system has tended to deliver relatively low value, in that it has much room for improvement in quality and safety, despite costs being high. The value of our health benefits spend will increase as efforts to improve quality, lower costs, or do both simultaneously succeed.

Purchasers are the entities that fund the healthcare system. Typically, we think about two categories of purchasers—public and private. The Centers for Medicare & Medicaid Services (CMS) is the largest public purchaser in the United States, funding and administering benefits on behalf of the elderly and disabled (via Medicare) and the poor and medically indigent (via Medicaid, which is also funded and administered by the states). Private purchasers are primarily employers who fund health benefits for workers, their families, and, in some cases, retirees. As of 2017, 49 percent of Americans received health insurance coverage through employer-sponsored insurance, 14 percent were covered through Medicare, and 21 percent were covered through Medicaid (Kaiser Family Foundation [KFF] 2018).

Consumers also fund the healthcare system through premium payments or shares; out-of-pocket payments (e.g., deductibles, copayments, coinsurance associated with employer-sponsored insurance); and direct payments for services, drugs, and supplies. However, because consumers individually have minimal market power, this chapter will focus primarily on federal governmental programs and private employers—the purchasers most likely to pursue value-based purchasing (VBP) strategies. Nonetheless, the chapter will address these purchasers' roles in seeking to educate and empower consumers.

Based on our definitions of *value* and *purchasers*, the phrase *value-based purchasing*, in the broadest sense, refers to any activities by public or private purchasers to achieve greater value for the benefits spend—actions aimed at improving quality of care, lowering costs, or doing both.

Overview of Value-Based Purchasing Strategies

A 2003 literature review and series of stakeholder interviews supported by the Commonwealth Fund identified six VBP strategies (Goldfarb et al. 2003). This categorization has been maintained and periodically updated by the College for Value-Based Purchasing of Health Benefits and now encompasses the following:

1. Collecting information on quality and fostering transparency
2. Taking a value-based insurance design (V-BID) approach to plan design
3. Selectively contracting with higher-value health plans and providers
4. Pursuing payment reform—moving away from fee-for-service to models that promote value
5. Engaging consumers in seeking higher-value care
6. Supporting population health through wellness, disease prevention, and disease management

In this section, we will take a closer look at each of these strategies and examine how they are being implemented by CMS and by large employers and employer coalitions.

Collecting Information on Quality and Fostering Transparency

To move toward higher value, purchasers first need to understand their present situation. What are the diagnoses and conditions most prevalent and most costly in their populations? To what extent are guidelines associated with higher-quality care (e.g., immunization rates, preventive testing rates, diabetes testing rates) being met? What outcomes are being achieved, including clinical outcomes such as diabetes control rates, humanistic outcomes such as well-being and emotional health, and economic outcomes (both direct and indirect costs)? Are there differences in processes and outcomes by demographic group, region, provider group or health system, or other characteristics? Where are the opportunities for greatest improvement? Looking at data to answer these types of questions serves several purposes:

1. It helps to identify the most significant opportunities for improvement in value.
2. It creates a baseline against which the effectiveness of improvement efforts can be assessed.
3. Perhaps most importantly, health plans, providers, and service vendors are more likely to make efforts to assess and improve quality when they know that the purchasers who fund them are watching.

Recognizing the significant variation across healthcare providers, many national and regional purchaser and consumer-driven efforts are promoting transparency of price and quality information—making detailed data publicly available about a provider's performance and the costs of seeing that provider. Creating transparency of quality information presents a number of challenges related to sample size adequacy, measurement and risk-adjustment methodologies, and data availability, and transparency of cost or price information can be equally problematic. According to one systematic review of the transparency literature, "Evidence suggests that publicly releasing performance data stimulates quality improvement activity at the hospital level. The effect of public reporting on effectiveness, safety, and patient-centeredness remains uncertain" (Fung et al. 2008, 111).

Taking a Value-Based Insurance Design Approach to Plan Design

The University of Michigan's Center for Value-Based Insurance Design (2016) offers the following definition:

> Value-Based Insurance Design (V-BID) is a potential solution built on the principle of lowering or removing financial barriers to essential, high-value clinical services. V-BID plans align patients' out-of-pocket costs, such as copayments and deductibles, with the value of services and are designed with the tenets of "clinical nuance" in mind, which recognize that 1) medical services differ in the amount of health produced, and 2) the clinical benefit derived from a specific service depends on the consumer using it, as well as when, where, and by whom the service is provided.

In simpler terms, V-BID involves promoting the use of high-value services and discouraging use of low-value services.

The Asheville Project—a diabetes care improvement initiative implemented by two employers in Asheville, North Carolina, in the late 1990s—is a well-known example of a value-based program incorporating V-BID and a formal evaluation. The project combined a community-based pharmacist counseling intervention with waived out-of-pocket payments for diabetes drugs and supplies for program participants. Short- and long-term (up to five years) outcomes demonstrated that diabetes control had improved and total costs of care had decreased for program participants (Cranor, Bunting, and Christensen 2003).

Selectively Contracting with Higher-Value Health Plans and Providers

When purchasers are able to access quality and cost information, they can use these data to contract with, and/or promote use of, higher-performing health plans and providers. At the health plan level, performance metrics are made available through National Committee for Quality Assurance (NCQA) accreditation and Healthcare Effectiveness Data and Information Set (HEDIS) data. Purchasers can drive performance improvement in specific areas by discussing with currently contracted plans the need for such improvement and expressing their willingness to take their business elsewhere if the plans do not improve. The data also can be used to select which plans will be offered by the purchaser in the future.

The National Alliance of Healthcare Purchaser Coalitions' (2018b) eValue8 tool was created by large employers and regional coalitions to "define, measure and evaluate health plan performance." The employers and coalitions "want evidence that that they are purchasing quality health care and demand administrative excellence and consumer satisfaction at cost-effective prices." According to the National Alliance, purchasers can use eValue8 data to accomplish the following:

- Establish performance goals and measure quality based on leading edge purchaser expectations
- Identify results-oriented disease management programs
- Designate "best-in-class" performers
- Determine health promotion and education opportunities
- Develop targeted strategies for improving the value of your health care investments
- Collaborate with purchasers and health care providers to improve community health quality

In 2018, the National Alliance announced that it was developing "deeper dives" into specific clinical areas, such as oncology care and mental health care, to further foster health plan transparency and drive improvement in these areas.

At the provider level, purchasers also are beginning to selectively contract with systems, hospitals, and groups for specific services, with their decisions based on quality and cost criteria. The contracting may be done by a health plan on behalf of its purchaser clients, or directly by a large employer or coalition of employers. For example, the Alliance (2018), a Wisconsin-based purchaser coalition, has developed a narrow network called QualityPath that includes providers for select conditions and procedures who have been identified based on performance metrics. QualityPath's innovative approach includes the following elements (Alliance 2018):

- Identifying doctors, hospitals and other facilities that meet or exceed national measures for delivering quality care for selected surgeries and tests. For surgeries, measures are based on the performance of a specific doctor working at a specific hospital.
- Asking designated doctors and facilities to adopt processes that are shown to improve care.
- Requiring providers to adopt decision-support tools system-wide to benefit all patients.
- Focusing on non-emergency surgeries and tests that allow patients to "shop" for care.
- Assisting employers in creating health benefit plans that encourage employees and family members to choose high-quality care.
- Exploring new ways to pay for care, such as bundled payments and warranties.

QualityPath is one of many examples across the United States of direct contracting efforts aimed at improving value.

Pursuing Payment Reform

Healthcare system stakeholders in the United States widely agree that one of the main causative factors of excessive utilization, high costs, and sluggish improvement in performance is fee-for-service payment arrangements, in which providers are paid based on the volume of services provided, rather than on the quality or outcomes of services. The National Commission on Physician Payment Reform (2013) called for a phase-out of fee-for-service payment over time because of its "inherent inefficiencies and problematic financial incentives" and urged a transition toward "an approach based on quality and value."

Both public and private purchasers are actively engaged in payment reform initiatives and demonstration projects, and several ways of thinking about models of payment reform have emerged. For example, the Health Care Payment Learning and Action Network (HCP-LAN), a multistakeholder public–private partnership initiative to foster the payment reform movement, issued an Alternative Payment Model (APM) Framework with the following typology (Alternative Payment Model Framework and Progress Tracking Work Group 2016):

- Category 1: Fee-for-service payment with no link to quality and value
- Category 2: Fee-for-service with a link to quality and value
  - Category 2A: Foundational payments for infrastructure and operations (e.g., bonus payments to physicians whose offices use electronic health records and e-prescribing)

  - Category 2B: Pay for reporting (e.g., bonus payments to physician practices that self-assess and report their quality metrics, regardless of whether those metrics indicate good or bad performance)
  - Category 2C: Rewards for performance (e.g., providing additional compensation to practices that demonstrate high-quality performance on process and outcomes measures, such as HbA1c testing and control rates for people with diabetes)
  - Category 2D: Rewards and penalties for performance (e.g., in addition to providing additional payment to high performers on diabetes care measures, withholding some portion of payment from providers who score poorly on these measures)
- Category 3: APMs built on a fee-for-service architecture
  - Category 3A: APMs with upside gain sharing (e.g., systems that measure baseline utilization and cost and provide a financial incentive, such as a share of the savings, if savings are achieved through care management performance improvement efforts)
  - Category 3B: APMs with upside gain sharing and downside risk (similar to the difference between categories 2C and 2D)
- Category 4: Population-based payment
  - Category 4A: Condition-specific population-based payment (e.g., "bundled payments" for maternity care that reimburse the provider group or system one global payment for prenatal, delivery, and postpartum care services, regardless of how many individual services are provided for that spectrum of care; such payments need to appropriately adjust for patient risk, and quality thresholds must be met to qualify for full payment)
  - Category 4B: Comprehensive population-based payment (e.g., accountable care organizations—provider organizations that agree to accept financial risk and to meet quality targets in managing an enrolled population; such organizations may be paid a global payment, such as through demographically- or risk-adjusted capitation, per enrolled individual per time period, regardless of how much or how little service that individual uses)

HCP-LAN brings together a variety of organizations that are engaged in the payment reform movement. For example, Catalyst for Payment Reform (CPR), one active partner, is "an independent, nonprofit organization on a mission to help employers and other health care purchasers get better value for their health care dollar." CPR aims to "empower health care purchasers who want to proactively improve the way the health care market functions" (CPR 2018).

Engaging Consumers in Seeking Higher-Value Care

Patients' demand for services, care-seeking behaviors, lifestyle choices, and adherence to provider recommendations all play a significant role in fostering (or impeding) high-quality care and optimizing (or worsening) health outcomes. A key consideration for purchasers, therefore, is how to engage consumers in behaviors that will drive health and healthcare improvement.

The field of behavioral economics—which combines principles of economics and psychology to better understand consumer behaviors—has attracted significant interest as a way to address consumer engagement, and a growing body of evidence supports this approach. Whereas economics holds as a central tenet the idea that consumers make rational decisions when presented with information, behavioral economics suggests that decisions often seem irrational because consumers prefer to accept the status quo, resulting in inertia, and because "decision fatigue" leads to snap judgments, especially when the amount of information presented to consumers is overwhelming (Rice 2013).

Principles of behavioral economics can be incorporated into tools that present quality and cost information to consumers and help drive consumers to higher-value providers. For example, Judith Hibbard and colleagues (2012) found that, in the absence of being presented with information on quality of care, consumers equate lower cost with lower quality, and many will select higher-cost providers as a result. However, presenting quality information in clearly understood formats with strong signals as to how to interpret information resulted in significant gravitation toward the higher-value providers.

Financial incentives also can be used to drive consumer behavior. Many private purchasers and insurers now offer tiered networks in which providers (systems, hospitals, groups, individual providers) are assigned to different tiers based on cost, quality, or both (value). The financial incentives may take the form of waived or reduced coinsurance rates or copayments to induce selection of providers in the purchaser-preferred tier. (Coinsurance is the percentage of the total allowable charge that the consumer pays out-of-pocket, whereas copayments are flat dollar amounts.)

One specific type of financial incentive is "reference pricing," a way of controlling spending on a specific service by setting a defined contribution to the total cost of that service, with the balance paid by the consumer using the service. Services subjected to reference pricing are typically those with high volume, where price variation exists across multiple suppliers, and where variation in quality of care is believed to be (but not necessarily) minimal (e.g., magnetic resonance imaging [MRI], computed tomography [CT] scans, other imaging procedures). For example, suppose that colonoscopy costs within a region were observed to vary from $500 to $5,000, depending on provider, and that the median colonoscopy cost was $1,200. A purchaser could set the reference price (the amount the purchaser pays) at $1,200, and the consumer who sought a colonoscopy with a provider charging $5,000 (allowable reimbursable amount) would be responsible for the $3,800 balance after the reference price was paid.

For a reference pricing program to be successful, the purchaser needs to make data on costs per provider accessible to consumers. An analysis by the Employee Benefits Research Institute found that "potential aggregate savings could reach $9.5 billion if all employers adopted reference pricing" for such procedures as hip and knee replacement, colonoscopy, MRI of the spine, CT of the head, nuclear stress test of the heart, and echocardiogram (Fronstin and Roebuck 2014).

Supporting Population Health Through Wellness, Disease Prevention, and Disease Management

Generally speaking, a healthier population is going to use fewer—and less intensive and costly—healthcare services, so promoting population health is a major focus of purchaser efforts. *Zero Trends* is a seminal work summarizing Dee Edington's (2009) many years of employer-focused research, with a focus on producing a "zero trend," or no increase in health-related annual costs for a purchaser. Edington identifies five key pillars for achieving such a trend: (1) strong senior leadership, (2) operational leadership, (3) promotion of self-leadership for consumers, (4) rewards for positive behaviors, and (5) measurement of results. Edington (2009) also identifies three key strategies for employers:

- Don't get worse. Focus wellness efforts on preventing further worsening of a less-than-optimal health state, rather than on returning to the optimal health state (e.g., help overweight and obese individuals maintain their present weight, at a minimum).
- Keep healthy employees healthy. Unhealthy individuals are often the focus of wellness initiatives, but employers should also pay attention to keeping the healthy (low-cost) employees healthy; investments in maintaining health can have larger returns than investments in trying to reverse unhealthy states.
- Create a culture of health within the organization.

HealthNEXT is one example of an innovative organization trying to help employers measure and improve their cultures of health. The company's central philosophy is that "what's measured gets improved" (HealthNEXT 2018). A proprietary methodology developed by the organization's leadership helps employers quantify their culture of health; benchmark against other employers; and identify population health practices that, if implemented, could measurably improve the culture score, leading to improved health and lower costs.

The organization's experience in assessing cultures of health across a variety of organizations has identified seven key "pressure points" (HealthNEXT 2018):

- Empowering a dedicated physician executive / clinical support team to assist in program design, implementation and vendor integration
- Developing integrated multi-year strategic roadmaps for improving the wellbeing of the workforce
- Creating awareness, affiliation and accountability within the workforce and covered lives
- Expanding sick care focus to integrated population health management
- Engaging management, employees and their spouses in "high-touch" early detection and prevention programs; while aligning the workplace with "culture of health" environment and cues
- Recruiting and rewarding the most relevant community providers to actively engage and participate in this mission
- Creating centers of excellence that focus attention on complex medical problems that generate high cost claimants

Public Purchaser Value-Based Purchasing: CMS and Medicare

CMS administers the Medicare program, which is the largest single purchaser of healthcare in the United States, covering approximately 13 percent of Americans and representing 15 percent of total federal spending (KFF 2018; Cubanski and Neuman 2018). As a result, CMS has significant purchasing power to influence healthcare quality and value. The traditional Medicare program is slowly moving from a fee-for-service approach to a value-based system. The introduction of the Prospective Payment System, using diagnosis-related groups (DRGs), or case rates, to reimburse hospitals for inpatient services, is one of CMS's earliest and enduring VBP initiatives.

Although we cannot describe the full range of CMS initiatives in a single chapter, this section will present some examples of initiatives focused on inpatient care.

Nonpayment (Never) Events

In 2007, CMS announced that Medicare would cease paying for the additional care associated with "never events"—extreme cases of medical errors that should never occur. By definition, never events are unambiguous (i.e., they can be identified and measured), serious (i.e., they result in death or significant harm), and preventable. Examples include wrong-site surgeries, retention of foreign objects in surgery cases, harm resulting from medication errors or patient falls, and occurrence of stage-3 or stage-4 pressure ulcers. The National Quality Forum maintains a list of never events, which now includes 29 events grouped into seven categories (Patient Safety Network 2018). Many public and private insurers have followed CMS's lead in implementing similar nonpayment policies.

Hospital Readmissions Reduction Program (HRRP)

The Affordable Care Act (ACA) of 2010 established the Hospital Readmissions Reduction Program (HRRP), calling for CMS to reduce payments to inpatient facilities that have excessive rates of readmissions. An excess readmission ratio (ERR) compares a facility's experienced 30-day readmission rate to the expected, risk-adjusted rate for six common diagnoses and procedures: acute myocardial infarction, chronic obstructive pulmonary disease, heart failure, pneumonia, coronary artery bypass graft surgery, and elective primary total hip arthroplasty and/or total knee arthroplasty. Hospital penalties for hospitals with high ERR's range from 1 percent to 3 percent of total Medicare payment (not just payment for the identified diagnoses and procedures).

An analysis of data for the first five years of the HRRP found that "beneficiary readmission rates started to fall in 2012, and have continued to drop since then, suggesting that hospitals and clinicians may have adopted new, system-wide interventions soon after the HRRP was enacted" (Boccuti and Casillas 2017). One finding of concern, however, was that hospitals in underserved areas and teaching hospitals were more likely to experience penalties under the HRRP, highlighting the need for a socioeconomic adjustment methodology to be implemented in the future.

Other CMS VBP Programs

In addition to the programs already mentioned, CMS has operated a Hospital VBP Program and a Hospital-Acquired Condition (HAC) Reduction Program to drive value improvement for Medicare. The Hospital VBP program employs a complex algorithm that scores hospitals on patient experience (via the Hospital Consumer Assessment of Healthcare Providers and Systems, or HCAHPS, survey); clinical process measures; efficiency measures; and outcomes, including mortality, complications, and infections. Up to 1.5 percent of Medicare payment is at risk under this program. The HAC Reduction Program imposes up to a 1 percent penalty for hospitals in the top quartile of HAC rates as measured by CMS and reported on CMS's Hospital Compare database. CMS has been moving to consolidate its VBP initiatives into a single comprehensive measurement, reporting, and payment system for inpatient providers.

MACRA and MIPS

The Medicare Access and CHIP Reauthorization Act of 2015 (MACRA) established a new Quality Payment Program (QPP) for Medicare-participating clinicians. Eligible practices can participate in this VBP program through one of two tracks: Advanced Alternative Payment Models (APMs) and the Merit-Based Incentive Payment System (MIPS). Interested readers are encouraged to stay abreast of program rules, measurement specifications, and incentive levels, as they continue to evolve as of this writing. Information is available via the CMS website at https://qpp.cms.gov/.

Employers as Value-Based Purchasers

Employer-sponsored health insurance covers nearly half of all Americans, and annual premiums for individual and family coverage have continued to increase. In 2017, the cost of individual coverage was estimated at $6,690 per year, and family coverage was $18,764 per year (KFF 2017). As the majority of mid-size and large employers continue to offer health benefits, pursuing a VBP strategy has become increasingly important in the private purchaser market.

Before providing examples of employer-focused VBP initiatives, we should point out that most mid-size and large employers are self-funded rather than fully insured. A fully insured employer buys a complete set of services and transfers risk of high-cost cases or a high-cost year to the insurer; in return for premium payments, the insurer provides the full range of services and bears the risk. By contrast, under self-funding, the insurer manages the provider network, claims processing, and other functions in return for an administrative fee, and the employer bears the risk. (The employer typically will purchase "stop loss insurance," a secondary insurance that mitigates the risk of high-cost individual cases or overall population costs.) This distinction is important, because it gives the self-funded employer more flexibility to implement innovative purchasing approaches, and more incentive to do so.

Another important distinction between public purchasers and employers is that total costs to the employer include not only the direct medical cost (i.e., the cost of delivered care services), but also the indirect cost associated with health-related productivity loss. The two components of indirect cost are absenteeism, or not showing up to work because of a health issue for oneself or a family member, and presenteeism, which involves physically presenting to the workplace but not being able to fully perform because of a health issue. (Presenteeism may also occur when a worker has to check in on or worry about a direct family member with a health condition).

Ill health can threaten the bottom line for an employer if it affects work engagement, employee turnover rates, and occupational safety (e.g., health-related accidents associated with drowsiness). The Total Worker Health movement, promoted by the Centers for Disease Control and Prevention, recognizes these effects and understands their relevance to healthcare system quality and value (National Institute for Occupational Safety and Health 2018).

Examples of Employer-Focused VBP programs

The Leapfrog Group and the Leapfrog Value-Based Purchasing Platform

A group of large employers and other purchasers founded the Leapfrog Group, an organization dedicated to advancing quality and safety in US healthcare, in 2000 (Leapfrog Group 2018b). The group was established in response to a finding in the Institute of Medicine's landmark *To Err Is Human* report that medical errors are responsible for as many as 98,000 deaths in hospitals each year (Kohn, Corrigan, and Donaldson 2000).

In 2001, Leapfrog launched the Leapfrog Hospital Survey, a national voluntary survey of hospitals. The survey project set out to identify and share information about which hospitals meet safety standards in the following key areas that can significantly reduce the risk of error: computerized order entry, the use of intensivists in intensive care units, and referral of patients to other facilities when the hospital has a low volume of select procedures. The Leapfrog Hospital Survey has grown to include many other measures that are believed to significantly influence patient safety, that are relevant to consumers, and that show variation across hospitals. In 2017, more than 1,900 hospitals participated in the voluntary reporting and improvement initiative (Leapfrog Group 2018c).

Recognizing that not all hospitals were willing to complete the survey and have their data published on the Leapfrog website, the Leapfrog Group in 2012 began calculating the Hospital Safety Grade (formerly the Hospital Safety Score) and publishing the grading information online at www.hospitalsafetygrade.org. The Hospital Safety Grade applies a standardized methodology, developed by a national expert panel, to publicly available data on hospital performance (including Leapfrog Hospital Survey data for hospitals that choose to report that information), along with other measures such as infection rates for Medicare beneficiaries, available through CMS. Hospitals are graded on a scale from "A" to "F" and given a summary score that is readily interpretable by consumers (Leapfrog Hospital Safety Grade 2018).

These Leapfrog transparency products are designed to drive improvement by educating consumers and increasing the pressure on providers to adequately invest in improvement. Leapfrog also offers a VBP Program to health plans and encourages employers and coalitions to promote this product with their plans. The Leapfrog Group (2018a) makes clear that "health plans that utilize the Leapfrog VBP Program request that hospitals in their network participate in the annual Leapfrog Hospital Survey." Leapfrog applies a scoring algorithm to hospitals' survey results and gives each facility an overall value score. Plans can use these scores "to rank the hospitals and set benchmarks for financial awards or incentives, such as allocating the highest rewards to hospitals scoring in the top decile" (Leapfrog Group 2018a). Participating hospitals receive a report that details their survey performance and results twice annually.

Bridges to Excellence

In 2003, several large employers—including General Electric, Ford, Procter & Gamble, and UPS—launched the Bridges to Excellence (BTE) program to tie physician payments to the achievement of certain quality criteria. The concept was simple and continues to be implemented by employers and health plans throughout the United States. It asks physicians to demonstrate the quality of care delivered by submitting clinical data to an independent third-party evaluator. Physicians receive a financial reward per patient managed if their quality score exceeds a certain threshold. Like most pay-for-performance programs, BTE is an upside-only program. Physicians are never penalized; they are only rewarded based on the premise that better-quality care will lead to better financial outcomes (BTE 2018).

Purchaser Value Network

The Pacific Business Group on Health (PBGH), a coalition of large employers, established the Purchaser Value Network (PVN) as a "network of and for purchasers that aims to accelerate the adoption of high value healthcare delivery and payment models through policy advocacy, education, and purchaser engagement" (PBGH 2018). The network provides education and tools to public and private purchasers and advocates for policies that will promote value. Toolkits developed by PVN thus far have focused on improving maternity care, evaluating accountable care organizations, and entering into bundled payment arrangements for orthopaedic procedures and oncology care.

The PVN Maternity Care Toolkit illustrates how many of the VBP concepts discussed in this chapter can be pursued by an employer to drive value in maternity-related services, particularly with regard to reducing C-section rates. Recommended actions for employers in this area include the following (PVN 2016):

- Assess the problem by obtaining and analyzing data.
- Identify potential local collaborators and partners (e.g., community organizations and providers who share a commitment to improving maternity care and lowering C-section rates).
- Meet with local providers to express concern about high C-section rates.
- Eliminate financial incentives for inappropriate C-sections in hospital contracts (e.g., reduce or eliminate payment for clearly inappropriate

C-sections, pay the same blended rate for vaginal deliveries and C-sections, create a bundled payment).
- Drive beneficiaries toward higher-value providers.
- Review benefits coverage for high-value services such as midwives, birth assistants, and doulas.

Choosing Wisely

Another initiative, the Choosing Wisely campaign, was developed in 2012 by the American Board of Internal Medicine Foundation. Under the program, physician professional societies identify clinical services offered by their specialties that are overutilized and potentially wasteful (Choosing Wisely 2018). The campaign seeks to promote services that are supported by evidence, free from harm, truly necessary, and not duplicative of tests or procedures already performed. Choosing Wisely maintains educational materials for providers and consumers to foster meaningful conversations and reduce unnecessary care. Consumers, particularly those in high-deductible health plans (who have more "skin in the game," given the size of the deductibles), are encouraged to ask questions about whether certain tests and procedures are truly necessary.

Although Choosing Wisely in itself is not a VBP initiative, purchasers are increasingly exploring applications of the Choosing Wisely lists for such initiatives. Lists of tests and procedures identified by the campaign as potentially wasteful may ultimately lead to purchasers discontinuing coverage, requiring prior authorization, or otherwise implementing value-based strategies to reduce their utilization.

The MedInsight Waste Calculator, a proprietary tool developed by Milliman in partnership with VBID Health, examines purchaser claims data sets to identify opportunities for reducing waste, lowering cost, and improving care, using Choosing Wisely lists and other sources of information (Milliman 2018). Several employers and coalitions working with this tool have reported the identification of significant potential savings through the initial analysis.

For example, a report from the Washington Health Alliance (2018) examined 47 common procedures that are potentially wasteful and found that "more than 45% of the health care services examined were determined to be low value (likely wasteful or wasteful) [and] 36% of spending on the health care services examined went to low value treatment and procedures. This amounts to an estimated $282 million in wasteful spending." Elements of the Washington Health Alliance's "Call for Action" include honest multistakeholder discussions about healthcare value and waste in Washington state, greater clinical leadership in changing the culture, increased emphasis on "choosing wisely" and shared decision making, expedited efforts to transition from paying for volume to paying for value, and increased provider attention (via contracts) to reporting on overuse.

Driving Toward a Value-Based Marketplace

Few employers have sufficient market power to drive change in a meaningful and sustained manner. Large national and global purchasers such as General Electric, Boeing, Walmart, Intel, and Comcast, among others, are on the forefront of value-based purchasing on behalf of their employees, but even these purchasers recognize the value of joining with other employers to create a value-based marketplace.

Purchaser organizations working at the national level to drive change include the National Business Group on Health (2018), which focuses on representing large national employers, and the National Alliance of Healthcare Purchaser Coalitions (2018a), which represents regional business coalitions, with employers of all sizes. Many other organizations are supporting the VBP movement through their work, including the Integrated Benefits Institute (IBI), the Employee Benefits Research Institute, the American Benefits Council, the Wellness Council of America, the Network of Regional Health Initiatives (NRHI), and the Health Enhancement Research Organization (HERO).

Newer players on the VBP scene demonstrate growing interest on the part of large employers to invest in health system improvement. The Health Transformation Alliance (HTA) announced its launch early in 2016 with a mission of "fixing our broken healthcare system" (HTA 2018), and it grew from 20 to more than 40 members in its first two years. The HTA has begun offering its members national group purchasing contracts for pharmacy and other services, and it has developed pilot quality- and value-focused network development demonstrations in several key markets.

Early in 2018, Amazon, JP Morgan Chase, and Berkshire Hathaway made headlines and sent ripples through the healthcare system when they announced a joint venture to transform healthcare and increase value, with a focus on technology (Wingfield, Thomas, and Abelson 2018). What they will do and how they will do it—and whether they, or others, will succeed—are unclear. However, what is certain is that purchasers, both public and private, are increasingly investing in efforts to derive greater value from their spend, and these efforts will almost certainly result in more transparency of quality information, more pressure on plans and providers to improve quality and safety, and more informed and engaged consumers.

Study Questions

1. An employer would like to put in a value-based purchasing program to improve care for diabetes. Using the typology of VBP strategies, what are some of the things an employer could do?

2. What are the main components of the CMS Hospital VBP Program? What are those components' key properties?
3. Employers are increasingly engaging in value-based purchasing activities. From a provider perspective, is this movement a good thing? What are some of the key advantages or disadvantages?

References

Alliance. 2018. "QualityPath Frequently Asked Questions (FAQs)." Accessed December 5. www.the-alliance.org/qualitypath/qualitypath-frequently-asked-questions-faqs.

Alternative Payment Model Framework and Progress Tracking Work Group. 2016. "Alternative Payment Model (APM) Framework: Final White Paper." Health Care Payment Learning and Action Network. Published January 12. https://hcp-lan.org/workproducts/apm-whitepaper.pdf.

Boccuti, C., and G. Casillas. 2017. "Aiming for Fewer Hospital U-Turns: The Medicare Hospital Readmission Reduction Program." Kaiser Family Foundation. Published March 10. www.kff.org/medicare/issue-brief/aiming-for-fewer-hospital-u-turns-the-medicare-hospital-readmission-reduction-program/.

Bridges to Excellence (BTE). 2018. "Bridges to Excellence Mission." Accessed December 5. www.bridgestoexcellence.org/.

Catalyst for Payment Reform (CPR). 2018. "Who We Are." Accessed December 5. www.catalyze.org/about-us/.

Center for Value-Based Insurance Design. 2016. "Value-Based Insurance Design—Why Clinically Nuanced Care Became a Game Changer." Accessed December 5, 2018. http://vbidcenter.org/wp-content/uploads/2016/10/V-BID-1-Pager-updated-2-8-18.pdf.

Choosing Wisely. 2018. "Our Mission." Accessed December 5. www.choosingwisely.org/our-mission/.

Cranor, C. W., B. A. Bunting, and D. B. Christensen. 2003. "The Asheville Project: Long-Term Clinical and Economic Outcomes of a Community Pharmacy Diabetes Care Program." *Journal of the American Pharmaceutical Association* 43 (2): 173–84.

Cubanski, J., and T. Neuman. 2018. "The Facts on Medicare Spending and Financing." Kaiser Family Foundation. Published June 22. www.kff.org/medicare/issue-brief/the-facts-on-medicare-spending-and-financing/.

Edington, D. W. 2009. *Zero Trends: Health as a Serious Economic Strategy.* Ann Arbor, MI: Health Management Research Center.

Fronstin, P., and M. C. Roebuck. 2014. "Reference Pricing for Health Care Services: A New Twist on the Defined Contribution Concept in Employment-Based Health Benefits." Employee Benefits Research Institute. www.shrm.org/ResourcesAndTools/hr-topics/benefits/Documents/EBRI_IB_398_Apr14.RefPrcng.pdf.

Fung, C. H., Y. W. Lim, S. Mattke, C. Damberg, and P. G. Shekelle. 2008. "Systematic Review: The Evidence That Publishing Patient Care Performance Data Improves Quality of Care." *Annals of Internal Medicine* 148 (2): 111–23.

Goldfarb, N. I., V. Maio, C. T. Carter, L. Pizzi, and D. B. Nash. 2003. "How Does Quality Enter into Health Care Purchasing Decisions?" Commonwealth Fund. Published May. https://core.ac.uk/download/pdf/46965160.pdf.

HealthNEXT. 2018. "Our Approach." Accessed December 5. http://healthnext.com/what-we-do/our-approach/.

Health Transformation Alliance (HTA). 2018. "We're the HTA." Accessed December 6. www.htahealth.com/.

Hibbard, J. H., J. Greene, S. Sofaer, K. Firminger, and J. Hirsh. 2012. "An Experiment Shows That a Well-Designed Report on Costs and Quality Can Help Consumers Choose High-Value Health Care." *Health Affairs* 31 (3): 560–68.

Kaiser Family Foundation (KFF). 2018. "Health Insurance Coverage of the Total Population." Accessed December 5. www.kff.org/other/state-indicator/total-population/?currentTimeframe=0&sortModel=%7B%22colId%22:%22Location%22,%22sort%22:%22asc%22%7D.

———. 2017. "2017 Employer Health Benefits Survey." Published September 19. www.kff.org/report-section/ehbs-2017-section-1-cost-of-health-insurance/.

Kohn, L. T., J. M. Corrigan, and M. S. Donaldson (eds.). 2000. *To Err Is Human: Building a Safer Health System*. Washington, DC: National Academies Press.

Leapfrog Group. 2018a. "Leapfrog Value-Based Purchasing Program." Accessed December 5. www.leapfroggroup.org/VBP-Program.

———. 2018b. "Raising the Bar for Safer Healthcare." Accessed December 5. www.leapfroggroup.org/about.

———. 2018c. "Welcome to the 2018 Leapfrog Hospital Survey." Accessed December 5. www.leapfroggroup.org/survey-materials/survey-login-and-materials.

Leapfrog Hospital Safety Grade. 2018. "About the Grade." Updated November 8. www.hospitalsafetygrade.org/your-hospitals-safety-grade/about-the-grade.

Milliman. 2018. "MedInsight Waste Calculator." Accessed December 6. www.milliman.com/Solutions/Products/MedInsight-Waste-Calculator/#.

National Alliance of Healthcare Purchaser Coalitions. 2018a. "About the National Alliance of Healthcare Purchaser Coalitions." Accessed December 6. www.nationalalliancehealth.org/about/new-overview.

———. 2018b. "eValue8." Accessed December 5. www.nationalalliancehealth.org/initiatives/initiatives-market-assessments/evalue8.

National Business Group on Health. 2018. "About the Business Group." Accessed December 6. www.businessgrouphealth.org/.

National Commission on Physician Payment Reform. 2013. *Report of the National Commission on Physician Payment Reform*. Published March. http://physicianpaymentcommission.org/wp-content/uploads/2013/03/physician_payment_report.pdf.

National Institute for Occupational Safety and Health (NIOSH). 2018. "NIOSH Total Worker Health: Webinar Series." Centers for Disease Control and Prevention. Accessed December 5. www.cdc.gov/niosh/twh/default.html.

Pacific Business Group on Health (PBGH). 2018. "The Purchaser Value Network (PVN)." Accessed December 5. www.pbgh.org/pvn.

Patient Safety Network. 2018. "Never Events." Updated August. https://psnet.ahrq.gov/primers/primer/3/never-events.

Porter, M. E. 2010. "What Is Value in Health Care?" *New England Journal of Medicine* 363: 2477–81.

Purchaser Value Network (PVN). 2016. "Maternity Toolkit: Reducing Unnecessary C-Sections." Published April. www.pvnetwork.org/storage/documents/PVN%20Maternity%20Toolkit%20(Online)%20Final.pdf.

Rice, T. 2013. "The Behavioral Economics of Health and Health Care." *Annual Review of Public Health* 34: 431–47.

Washington Health Alliance. 2018. *First, Do No Harm. Calculating Health Care Waste in Washington State.* Published February. http://wahealthalliance.org/alliance-reports-websites/alliance-reports/first-do-no-harm/.

Wingfield, N., K. Thomas, and R. Abelson. 2018. "Amazon, Berkshire Hathaway and JPMorgan Team Up to Disrupt Health Care." Published January 30. www.nytimes.com/2018/01/30/technology/amazon-berkshire-hathaway-jpmorgan-health-care.html.

CHAPTER

18

MEDICATION USE QUALITY

Mel L. Nelson, Matthew K. Pickering, Hannah M. Fish, and Laura Cranston

Introduction

Healthcare spending in the United States now totals $3.5 trillion per year, or $10,739 per person, which is the largest amount per capita in the world (Centers for Medicare & Medicaid Services 2018b). A large portion of healthcare spending is attributable to prescription drug costs. In 2016, an estimated $450 billion was spent on therapeutic drugs. Not surprisingly, drug spending is expected to continue rising, reaching $580 to $610 billion by 2021 (IQVIA Institute for Human Data Science 2017). This expected increase is a result of not only the high rate of prescription drug use (48.9 percent of Americans have used at least one medication in the past 30 days, 23.1 percent use three or more medications, and 11.9 percent use five or more) but also the country's aging population and its corresponding need for polypharmacy (National Center for Health Statistics 2017). With this increased medication use comes the increased potential for medication errors, which can also drive up costs and decrease quality.

According to the Institute of Medicine (IOM)—now the National Academy of Medicine (NAM)—most medication errors and more than a quarter of adverse drug events are preventable (Aspden et al. 2007). The IOM's *Preventing Medication Errors* report followed an earlier call to action in its landmark *To Err Is Human* report (discussed in earlier chapters), which focused on building a safer healthcare system (Kohn, Corrigan, and Donaldson 2000). In the years since that report, the US healthcare system has heightened its emphasis on quality improvement and containment of costs. However, with the high prevalence of medication use, and its associated costs and side effects, an increased focus on the quality of medication use is necessary.

The Shift from Volume to Value in Healthcare

Using the National Quality Strategy as a Road Map

Despite continued efforts to control healthcare spending, costs have continued to escalate over the past several decades. To better address this problem, US healthcare has taken steps to transition from a volume-based, fee-for-service system to a system driven by value. Value considers both quality and cost, with the aim of optimizing the level of care and improving health outcomes while minimizing cost and resource use. This seismic shift in focus for our healthcare system has resulted in the evolution of quality rating systems and quality-based payment programs that use medication-related metrics, forging a fast-paced, ever-evolving environment that is continually redefining how pharmacists, other healthcare practitioners, and patients interact.

The Affordable Care Act (ACA) of 2010 required the secretary of the Department of Health and Human Services (HHS) to establish a National Strategy for Quality Improvement in Health Care—commonly known as the National Quality Strategy (NQS)—to guide our efforts to transform the healthcare system. The initial version of the NQS was submitted to Congress on March 21, 2011, but the strategy is maintained as a "living, breathing" document, updated on a yearly basis by the Agency for Healthcare Research and Quality (AHRQ) on behalf of HHS (AHRQ 2017a). These updates are shared with Congress and made available to the general public. Key elements of the NQS, as of 2017, are shown in exhibit 18.1.

The NQS was developed through a transparent, collaborative process, incorporating input from more than 300 groups, organizations, and individuals representative of all healthcare sectors, as well as the general public. The strategy itself is based on the Institute for Healthcare Improvement's (IHI's) Triple Aim—a framework for optimizing health system performance by simultaneously focusing on the health of a population, the experience of care for individuals within that population, and the per capita cost of providing that care (IHI 2017). The Triple Aim concept was a product of the leadership and vision of IHI president and CEO Donald Berwick. In 2010, President Barack Obama tapped Berwick to serve as the administrator of the Centers for Medicare & Medicaid Services (CMS) (Branigin and Aizenman 2010). During his tenure in this position, Berwick's vision for the Triple Aim began to infiltrate the nation's largest healthcare agency. Today, the Triple Aim concept is widely adopted, supported through the NQS and the IHI's collaborative work with various organizations.

Performance Measurement

Increasingly, measurement has become a major area of focus in US healthcare quality improvement efforts. Various public and private value-based initiatives are requiring healthcare providers (e.g., payers, practitioners) to collect and report on performance measures (Blumenthal, Malphrus, and McGinnis 2015). Measuring the quality of healthcare helps to identify and address gaps in care, inform patients of good versus poor care quality, and promote accountability across settings. Furthermore, healthcare quality measurement aligns with the NQS, as evident through the implementation of measures across various federal

EXHIBIT 18.1
The National Quality Strategy: Three Aims, Six Priorities, Nine Levers

THE THREE BROAD AIMS

The National Quality Strategy (NQS) has incorporated three broad aims that are used to guide and assess local, state, and national efforts to improve health and healthcare quality.

1. Better Care: Improve the overall quality, by making healthcare more patient centered, reliable, accessible, and safe.
2. Healthy People/Healthy Communities: Improve the health of the US population by supporting proven interventions to address behavioral, social, and environmental determinants of health in addition to delivering higher-quality care.
3. Affordable Care: Reduce the cost of quality healthcare for individuals, families, employers, and government.

THE SIX HIGHEST PRIORITIES

To advance the three aims, the NQS focuses on six priorities:

1. Making care safer by reducing harm caused in the delivery of care
2. Ensuring that each person and family is engaged as partners in their care
3. Promoting effective communication and coordination of care
4. Promoting the most effective prevention and treatment practices for the leading causes of mortality, starting with cardiovascular disease
5. Working with communities to promote wide use of best practices to enable healthy living
6. Making quality care more affordable for individuals, families, employers, and governments by developing and spreading new healthcare delivery models

USING THE NINE LEVERS

The nine levers represent core business functions, resources, and/or actions that stakeholders can use to achieve alignment with the NQS.

1. Measurement and Feedback: Provide performance feedback to plans and providers to improve care.
2. Public Reporting: Compare treatment results, costs, and patient experience for consumers.
3. Learning and Technical Assistance: Foster learning environments that offer training, resources, tools, and guidance to help organizations achieve quality improvement goals.
4. Certification, Accreditation, and Regulation: Adopt or adhere to approaches to meet safety and quality standards.
5. Consumer Incentives and Benefit Designs: Help consumers adopt healthy behaviors and make informed decisions.
6. Payment: Reward and incentivize providers to deliver high-quality, patient-centered care.
7. Health Information Technology: Improve communication, transparency, and efficiency for better coordinated health and healthcare.
8. Innovation and Diffusion: Foster innovation in healthcare quality improvement, and facilitate rapid adoption within and across organizations and communities.
9. Workforce Development: Invest in people to prepare the next generation of healthcare professionals and support lifelong learning for providers.

Source: Adapted from AHRQ (2017a).

quality improvement programs (CMS 2018a). Specifically, CMS committed to tying 90 percent of all Medicare fee-for-service payments to quality by 2018, thereby advancing value-based healthcare (Burwell 2015).

When attempting to measure various aspects of healthcare, we need to make sure we have the right tools for the job. A conceptual model from Avedis Donabedian (1988), a physician and health services researcher, provides a framework for assessing health services and evaluating the quality of care. The model calls for approaching the healthcare system in terms of structure, process, and outcomes (see exhibit 18.2).

Structure refers to the organizational culture and the instruments used to provide care. It includes such elements as hospitals, the number of pharmacists on staff, standards and procedures for medication error response and reporting, and so on. *Process*, meanwhile, refers to how the structure is used. Process might be reflected by the number of pharmacy interventions per 100 admissions, or the percentage of adult patients discharged from an inpatient facility (e.g., hospital, skilled nursing facility, rehabilitation facility) whose discharge medication list was reconciled with the current medication list in the outpatient medical record. Finally, *outcomes* are the changes in patient health status attributable to care, and they may be viewed in terms of the prevention of medication errors or the prevention of hospital readmissions due to a medication-related event (e.g., hypoglycemia).

The structure/process/outcomes triad framework is useful for identifying appropriate measures to assess the quality of services provided to a patient or population. Structure measures are not task oriented; rather, they assess provider or organization capacity. They determine whether the people, technologies, and infrastructure are in place to deliver adequate healthcare services. An example

EXHIBIT 18.2 Types of Quality Measures, with Examples for Medication Use Quality

Structure	Process	Outcomes
Inputs • Number of pharmacists on staff • Standards and procedures for medication error response and reporting	**Steps** • Number of pharmacy interventions per 100 admissions • Percentage of medication reconciliation at discharge	**Outputs** • Prevention of medication errors • Prevention of hospital readmissions due to hypoglycemic event
Assesses provider/organization capacity, technologies, and infrastructure to deliver healthcare services	Measures provider application of recommended practices when interacting with patients	Reflects changes (desirable or undesirable) in patient or population health due to healthcare processes

of a structure measure might be the number of qualified staff members who can adequately identify medication errors and provide appropriate medication interventions (i.e., the number of pharmacists, in the example in exhibit 18.2). Process measures determine whether current recommended practices or guidelines are being adequately applied, such as whether a pharmacist reviews a patient's medication list to reconcile discrepancies, identify errors, and make any necessary changes (e.g., performing a medication reconciliation that discovers a drug–drug interaction that led to a hypoglycemic event, and then modifying the medication list accordingly). Lastly, outcomes measures reflect the desirable or undesirable results of the healthcare processes and structures that are in place. For instance, prevention of medication errors or medication-related rehospitalizations, such as those related to hypoglycemia, would indicate that the processes and structure are resulting in desirable outcomes for patients.

Quality measures have been developed by a variety of entities, including but not limited to government agencies, academic institutions, business coalitions, and professional societies. The Pharmacy Quality Alliance (PQA) is a leader in the development of quality measures that target appropriate medication use and safety. Founded in 2006 as a public–private partnership with CMS, PQA is now a nonprofit (501(c)(3)), multistakeholder, consensus-based organization that collaboratively promotes appropriate medication use and develops strategies for measuring and reporting performance information related to medications (PQA 2017a).

Most notably, PQA metrics (e.g., measures focused on patient adherence to certain chronic medications) reside within the CMS Five-Star Quality Rating System for Medicare Part C (Medicare Advantage) and Part D (PQA 2017b). In this program, CMS assigns ratings—on a scale of one to five stars, with five stars being the highest rating—that indicate the quality of Medicare plans. With the passage of the ACA, a new system emerged to compensate plans that had high quality ratings (i.e., four or more stars). Highly rated Medicare Advantage (MA) plans have been receiving quality bonus payments (QBPs) since 2012.

The star ratings and bonus payments have been a key component in the financing of healthcare benefits for MA plan enrollees. In addition, the ratings are posted on the CMS consumer website (www.medicare.gov) to assist beneficiaries in choosing from among the MA and MA-Prescription Drug plans offered in their area. In 2017, 66 percent of MA enrollees were in plans with four or more stars (Kaiser Family Foundation 2017).

The heightened focus on quality measures is not just limited to Medicare. Accountable care organizations (ACOs) are striving to meet quality measures and achieve shared savings, and Medicaid has seen a significant shift to managed care, with an Adult and Pediatric Core Set of Measures in use in many states. The health insurance exchange market also has a quality rating system.

High-Stakes Implications: The Drive to Five

With health plan reimbursement increasingly tied to performance, billions of dollars are now at stake in the form of QBPs. Thus, health plans have had to evolve their business practices to achieve higher performance ratings—focusing on the "drive to five"—and receive larger QBPs (see exhibit 18.3). In addition, Medicare plans that are considered low-performing (i.e., 2.5 stars or lower for three consecutive years) are identified on the CMS consumer website with a Low Performing Icon (LPI) that serves as a warning to consumers (CMS 2016c). CMS (2016a) notifies beneficiaries who are enrolled in low-performing plans and advises them to instead join higher-rated plans. Yet another bonus for five-star health plans is that they can accept new enrollees at any time, whereas other plans must wait for the Medicare open enrollment period.

In an effort to drive higher star ratings and benefit from the associated incentives, health plans are investing significant finances and resources in strategies aimed at performance improvement, with many plans introducing new programs or changing their business structure. One potential approach to drive higher ratings focuses on formulary management (Shrank et al. 2009). Many plans have closely examined lists of high-risk medications (HRMs) and identified alternatives that are less risky. These alternatives are then designated as "preferred" drugs and offered at a lower cost to patients. Health plans have also developed clinical strategies to target specific measures for improvement in their patients (Shrank et al. 2009). Some health plans have begun reaching out to providers who prescribe HRMs to inform them of potentially safer clinical options. Health plans have similarly reached out to providers to promote appropriate treatment of hypertension, targeting diabetic patients who do not have an appropriate hypertensive agent prescribed. Some plans have used third-party vendors to help pharmacists identify and reach out to providers.

EXHIBIT 18.3
The Drive to Five: Strategies to Improve Health Plan Performance

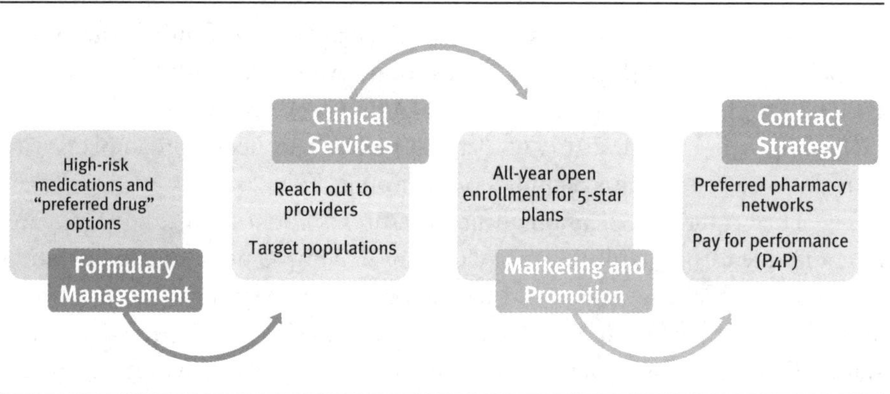

Source: Used with permission from Pharmacy Quality Alliance.

Health plans can also use contract strategy to meet their quality goals, selectively contracting with downstream entities that have the capacity to improve performance. Plans may choose to limit their pharmacy networks to pharmacies that provide the highest performance on relevant metrics to maximize the health plan's overall star rating. This type of arrangement has been achieved through two primary mechanisms thus far: (1) a pay-for-performance network, whereby bonus payments can be awarded to pharmacies themselves for achieving specified star ratings, and (2) a preferred pharmacy network that only includes high-performing pharmacies (Bonner 2016). These strategies have major impacts for pharmacists and pharmacies, as discussed in the next section.

Medication Use Expert: The Pharmacist

Many of the metrics for which health plans are held accountable are related to medication. For example, the 2017 Medicare Part D program included 15 measures across four domains. The measures cover such areas as customer service, member complaints, member experience, and drug safety, and they are each weighted depending on the type (e.g., process, intermediate outcome). The individual measures and weights determine the overall star rating (CMS 2016b). The 2017 metrics are shown in exhibit 18.4. Notice that the medication-related measures are weighted more heavily than the others. Thus, 43 percent of a Part D plan's overall star rating score is dependent on the PQA-developed medication-use metrics, for which pharmacists themselves naturally play a major role. Given the importance of medication-use metrics and the link between performance and reimbursement, the focus of pharmacy practice

EXHIBIT 18.4
Metrics Found in the 2017 Medicare Part D Star Ratings System

Measure ID	Measure Name	Part D Summary	MA-PD Overall
D01	Call Center – Foreign Language Interpreter and TTY Availability	1.5	1.5
D02	Appeals Auto–Forward	1.5	1.5
D03	Appeals Upheld	1.5	1.5
D04	Complaints about the Drug Plan	1.5	1.5
D05	Members Choosing to Leave the Plan	1.5	1.5
D06	Beneficiary Access and Performance Problems	1.5	1.5
D07	Drug Plan Quality Improvement	5	5
D08	Rating of Drug Plan	1.5	1.5
D09	Getting Needed Prescription Drugs	1.5	1.5
D10	MPF Price Accuracy	1	1
D11	High Risk Medication	3	3
D12	Medication Adherence for Diabetes Medications	3	3
D13	Medication Adherence for Hypertension (RAS antagonists)	3	3
D14	Medication Adherence for Cholesterol (Statins)	3	3
D15	MTM Program Completion Rate for CMR	1	1

Source: Data from CMS (2018c).

is shifting to include not only the number of prescriptions dispensed but also performance and improvement in the quality of patient care.

Pharmacists are among the most accessible of all healthcare professionals. Research indicates that some patient groups visit a pharmacy as many as 35 times per year, or more, which can equate to 1.5 to 10 times more visits than they have with their primary care provider (Community Care of North Carolina 2018; Tsuyuki et al. 2018). As a result, pharmacists are uniquely positioned to develop strong, personal relationships with the patients they serve. A strong pharmacist–patient relationship allows pharmacists to individually optimize medication regimens for their patients, leading to improved care. Furthermore, because of the frequency of pharmacy visits, pharmacists often have a better understanding of the social determinants affecting the patient's life, enabling them to further tailor medication regimens to fit individual lifestyles, thereby increasing adherence and decreasing drug–drug and drug–food interactions (Benjamin 2016; Vest et al. 2017).

Historically, pharmacists have primarily served a dispensing role; however, given their extensive training and the evolving nature of the field, pharmacists today are performing an increasing number of patient care services, including medication therapy management (MTM). The American Pharmacists Association (APhA) defines MTM as "a service or group of services that optimize therapeutic outcomes for individual patients," potentially including "medication therapy reviews, pharmacotherapy consults, anticoagulation management, immunizations, health and wellness programs and many other clinical services" (APhA 2018). By providing these unique services, pharmacists are well positioned to improve healthcare quality via the safe and effective use of medication.

MTM does not simply focus on an individual medication product; rather, it encompasses the assessment, evaluation, and management of the patient's complete medication therapy regimen (McGivney et al. 2007). It involves a multifaceted approach of reviewing medications, identifying and remedying medication-related problems, providing disease-state management and self-management education, addressing medication adherence issues, and considering preventive health strategies. The goal of MTM is to optimize medication use for improved patient care. Pharmacist-delivered MTM services have potential to improve both economic and clinical outcomes, especially for older adults taking multiple medications for chronic disease management (Ai et al. 2014)

Given their extensive medication knowledge and close patient relationships, pharmacists provide a unique opportunity to optimize quality performance measures. They can work directly with patients to increase adherence through tools such as medication synchronization and refill reminders. They can also reduce medication safety risks by communicating with patients and providers to remove medications from a regimen or to switch to more appropriate ones. Further, pharmacists (and plans) have access to performance-tracking tools that display quality measure data, which can help ensure optimal patient care, support quality improvement efforts, and enable benchmarking with other organizations in the region.

A variety of performance-tracking tools are available to suit the needs of the vendor. One example is the Electronic Quality Improvement Platform for Plans and Pharmacies (EQuIPP), provided by Pharmacy Quality Solutions (PQS), a joint venture between PQA and Premier. EQuIPP is the first national pharmacy quality measurement, benchmark, and reporting platform for pharmacies and health plans (EQuIPP 2018; PQS 2018). It consistently and reliably connects stakeholders to quality information, which allows for rapid movement from measurement to improvement (see exhibit 18.5).

Performance-tracking dashboards present information to enable users to readily and proactively identify areas for improvement. In a dashboard such as the one in exhibit 18.6, a pharmacy (or plan) can distinguish areas of success from the areas where improvement is needed. Pharmacies can also view information for the total number of patients in the population and drill down to the patient level to identify groups of patients for which certain initiatives will be most effective. In addition, dashboards often offer pharmacies and plans the ability to compare their performance with those of other pharmacies and plans. Overall, tracking tools help pharmacists improve performance, effect change for value-based care, and serve as key collaborators in the drive to five stars (see exhibit 18.7) (EQuIPP 2018).

EXHIBIT 18.5
How PQS Provides Performance Information to Plans and Pharmacies

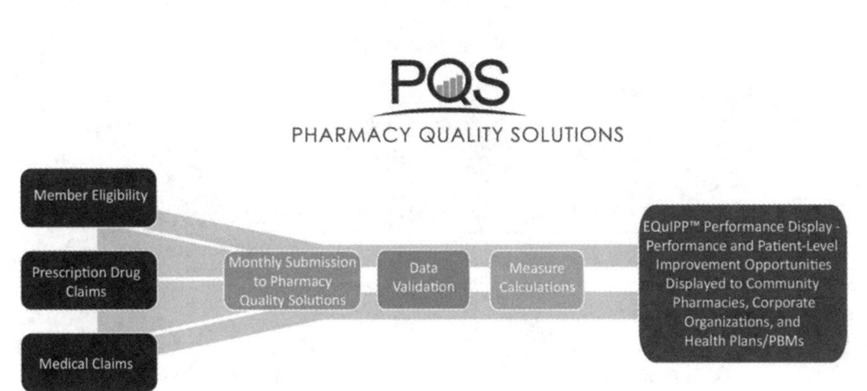
PQS
PHARMACY QUALITY SOLUTIONS
Member Eligibility
Prescription Drug Claims
Medical Claims
Monthly Submission to Pharmacy Quality Solutions
Data Validation
Measure Calculations
EQuIPP™ Performance Display - Performance and Patient-Level Improvement Opportunities Displayed to Community Pharmacies, Corporate Organizations, and Health Plans/PBMs

Source: Used with permission from Pharmacy Quality Solutions.

EXHIBIT 18.6
Example of a Tracking Tool Report Dashboard

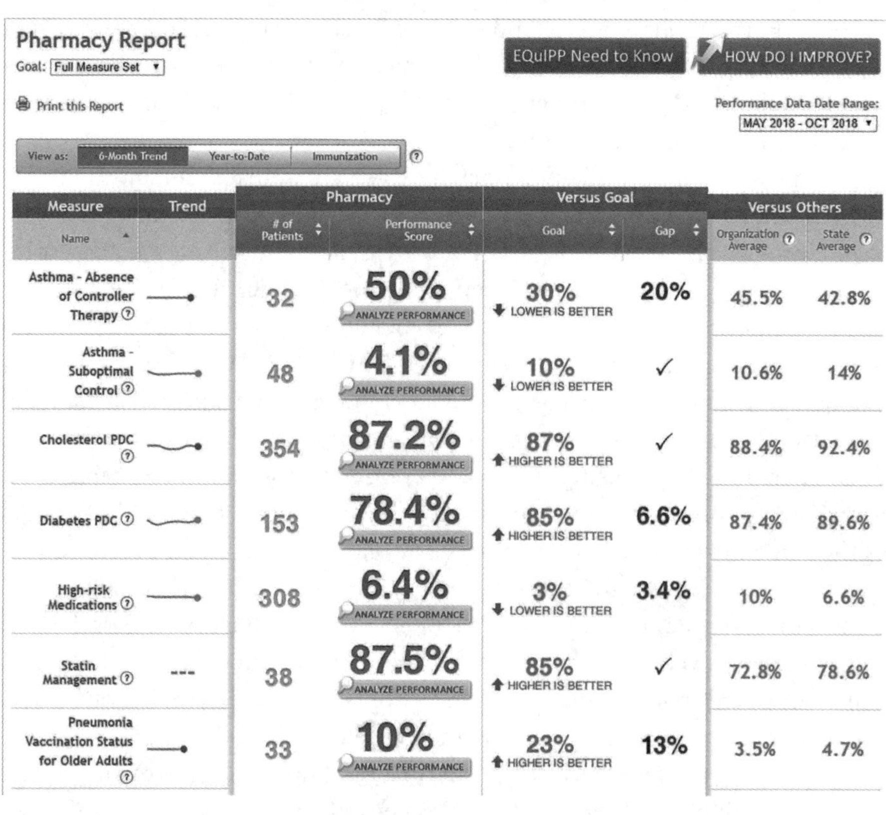

Pharmacy Report

Goal: Full Measure Set

EQuIPP Need to Know | HOW DO I IMPROVE?

Print this Report

Performance Data Date Range: MAY 2018 - OCT 2018

View as: 6-Month Trend | Year-to-Date | Immunization

Measure	Trend	Pharmacy		Versus Goal		Versus Others	
Name		# of Patients	Performance Score	Goal	Gap	Organization Average	State Average
Asthma - Absence of Controller Therapy		32	50% ANALYZE PERFORMANCE	30% LOWER IS BETTER	20%	45.5%	42.8%
Asthma - Suboptimal Control		48	4.1% ANALYZE PERFORMANCE	10% LOWER IS BETTER	✓	10.6%	14%
Cholesterol PDC		354	87.2% ANALYZE PERFORMANCE	87% HIGHER IS BETTER	✓	88.4%	92.4%
Diabetes PDC		153	78.4% ANALYZE PERFORMANCE	85% HIGHER IS BETTER	6.6%	87.4%	89.6%
High-risk Medications		308	6.4% ANALYZE PERFORMANCE	3% LOWER IS BETTER	3.4%	10%	6.6%
Statin Management	---	38	87.5% ANALYZE PERFORMANCE	85% HIGHER IS BETTER	✓	72.8%	78.6%
Pneumonia Vaccination Status for Older Adults		33	10% ANALYZE PERFORMANCE	23% HIGHER IS BETTER	13%	3.5%	4.7%

Source: Used with permission from Pharmacy Quality Solutions.

EXHIBIT 18.7
How Can Pharmacists Work Collaboratively with the Healthcare Team to Reach the Drive to Five Stars?

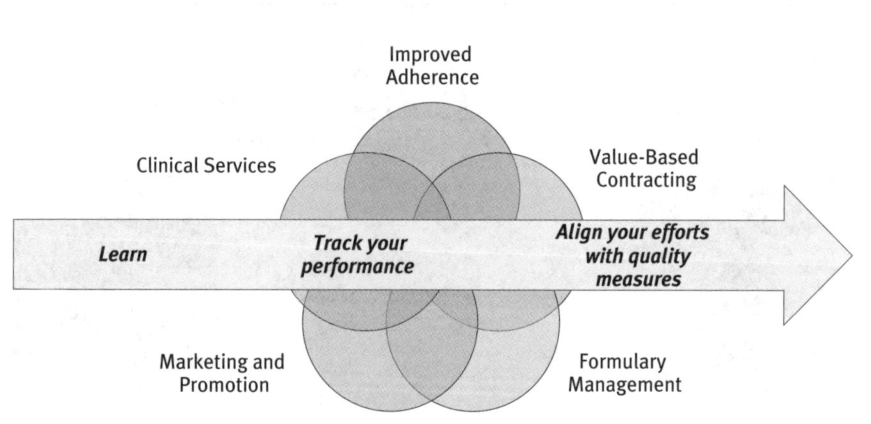

Source: Used with permission from Pharmacy Quality Alliance.

Emerging Trends: Pharmacist Engagement in a Value-Based Healthcare System

The US healthcare system has undergone a tremendous transformation over the past decade. New payment models, regulatory developments, clinical advances, digital and information technologies, and workforce trends have created a landscape of rapid change across just about every area of healthcare. Several emerging trends and innovative solutions specifically target appropriate medication use and safety.

The medication performance metrics used in many quality improvement programs help to monitor and inform medication use quality. At the same time, new payment arrangements—such as value-based insurance design and risk-sharing agreements—help to optimize the use of high-value drug therapies. The increased generation of comparative effectiveness research and patient-centered outcomes research further advance value-based care. Finally, present within all of these trends are new team-based models of care in which the pharmacist and MTM play significant roles in driving health outcomes. The following sections will discuss these emerging trends—and their potential for improving value-based care—in greater detail.

Enhanced Medication Therapy Management

In addition to using PQA's medication adherence measures, CMS has also implemented PQA's MTM completion rate measure, mandating all MTM programs to perform a comprehensive medication review for eligible Medicare beneficiaries (CMS 2018d). In 2003, the Medicare Prescription Drug, Improvement, and Modernization Act (MMA) amended the Social Security Act to provide Medicare Part D, a voluntary prescription drug coverage program for Medicare beneficiaries (GovTrack.us 2017). The MMA also established an MTM program to ensure that covered prescription drugs provided to beneficiaries under Part D are appropriately used to optimize therapeutic outcomes. Under this program, Medicare Part D plans are required to incorporate MTM into their benefit structure.

To foster innovation within MTM programs and to further expand the role of pharmacists in Medicare Part D MTM, CMS launched a new Enhanced MTM test model in 2017 (CMS 2018d). Over a five-year period, the model will test whether high-quality medication management can save the federal government money and provide seniors with better health. The goal of the test model will be to leverage MTM to identify ways to

- reduce medication problems and errors;
- improve medication adherence;
- increase patient education about the prescription drugs they take; and
- improve communications between prescribers, pharmacists, caregivers, and patients.

This new model should enable insurance plans to design creative MTM programs and leverage key services to improve outcomes and reduce resource utilization (i.e., hospitalizations, emergency department visits). To accomplish these goals, the pharmacist will be an integral stakeholder. With their clinical expertise at the intersection of regular patient interaction, pharmacists are uniquely positioned to set these improvements in motion.

Value-Based Insurance Design and Risk-Sharing Agreements

Risk-sharing agreements—sometimes called *value-based contracts* or *outcomes-based contracts*—are another innovative mechanism that health plans are using to improve medication-use quality while simultaneously controlling spend. A risk-sharing agreement brings together two key stakeholders—healthcare payers and biopharmaceutical manufacturers—to deliver medicines to patients.

Under risk-sharing agreements, medication reimbursement is linked to a drug's effectiveness and/or the frequency with which it is used. The payer does not simply cover all prescriptions at a single price. Rather, the initial price remains in place only if a specified percentage of patients achieves the agreed-upon target outcome. If the outcome threshold is not met, the manufacturer refunds some of the original price to the payer. When new drug products become available to the market, their high prices can be difficult to accommodate in the budgets of public and private payers, as well as patients. Therefore, risk-sharing agreements have attracted significant interest.

For example, in 2015, the Novartis drug Entresto (sacubitril/valsartan) was introduced to treat congestive heart failure. Evidence from a clinical trial showed that Entresto led to a 20 percent relative risk reduction in death or hospitalization. In 2016, Novartis disclosed that it had established separate deals with multiple private health plans to provide additional rebates if a higher level of hospitalizations occurred among their patients taking Entresto (*Managed Healthcare Executive* 2016).

Several other outcomes-based contracts have the potential to shift spending toward more effective treatments. However, these arrangements generally can only use outcomes that can be measured using claims data. Despite advances in technology, using electronic health records to access outcomes data and convert them into an analyzable form for use within these contracts remains difficult. Additionally, these value-based contracts apply only to a limited subset of drugs and, in many cases, are tied to surrogate measures that do not directly reflect outcomes that matter to patients (e.g., they reflect hospitalizations as opposed to quality of life). Nevertheless, the testing of these risk-sharing agreements in various populations (e.g., Medicare, Medicaid) could serve as an important first step in determining whether they have true improvement potential for the value of medication use.

Comparative Effectiveness Research / Patient-Centered Outcomes Research

Another aspect of the value agenda in US healthcare is the promotion and use of medical research—termed *comparative effectiveness research* (CER)—to support informed decision making by physicians and patients. According to the IOM, CER is "the generation and synthesis of evidence that compares the benefits and harms of alternative methods to prevent, diagnose, treat and monitor a clinical condition, or to improve the delivery of care" (Sox and Greenfield 2009, 203). The purpose of CER is to inform patients, clinicians, purchasers, and policymakers about which interventions are most effective for improving healthcare at the individual and population levels.

The key element of CER is the evaluation of an intervention in the "real world," which requires the use of key data sets (e.g., administrative claims, patient registries) to compare the outcomes of several effective interventions in a population that is representative of daily care. The large number of patients in these data sets enables researchers to study subgroups and identify key predictors of response to a specific intervention. Thus, the word *effectiveness* in CER refers to how well something works when it is implemented in a realistic setting (Gordis 2009); the term contrasts with *efficacy*, which refers to how the intervention works under ideal conditions. What works for patients in some closely monitored and controlled clinical trials might not work as well under "real world" conditions. Therefore, CER takes a more realistic and generalizable perspective to identify what works for patients.

We can take CER a step further by including the patient community within the research. *Patient-centered outcomes research* (PCOR) is an emergent approach that aims to help people and their caregivers communicate and make informed healthcare decisions by allowing patients' voices to be heard when assessing the value of healthcare options. The Patient-Centered Outcomes Research Institute (PCORI) was authorized by Congress in 2010 to support studies that advance patient-centered CER relevant to healthcare decisions confronting patients and their caregivers. Since the founding of PCORI, patient-centered outcomes have been more consistently incorporated into clinical research (PCORI 2017).

As more therapies become available to consumers to treat diseases, CER/PCOR aims to provide better information that will result in improved health outcomes and more effective use of resources. However, CER/PCOR is not by any means a silver bullet; it is simply another important cog in a larger mechanism for promoting better healthcare practices.

Conclusion

Medication use quality is an essential component of overall healthcare quality in the United States. As US healthcare continues to shift toward a value-based system, with performance increasingly tied to reimbursement and/or punitive action, accountability and performance measurement have become major areas of focus. Given their clinical expertise and direct interactions with patients, pharmacists are uniquely poised to have a strong, positive impact on performance measures related to medication use. Pharmacists are active in many current quality improvement programs, and their involvement will be essential for the success of the various value-based initiatives that continue to emerge. In the years ahead, pharmacists will be increasingly called upon to collaborate with healthcare teams to meet performance expectations to improve the overall quality of healthcare in the United States.

Study Question

1. This chapter—along with several others in this textbook—has discussed the shift from volume to value in healthcare and the importance of performance measurement to ensure accountability. How might the measurement burden affect our healthcare system, and what can be done to prevent or minimize this burden, particularly with regard to medication use?

Interactive Exercise

Think about the broad array of issues that healthcare providers face daily, and review the six healthcare priorities that are highlighted by the National Quality Strategy (available at www.ahrq.gov/workingforquality/about/index.html). For each of the NQS priorities, write a list of issues that need stronger marketplace and/or regulatory solutions to effect change in a positive way for the patients you serve. Using AHRQ's (2017b) NQS Toolkit (available at www.ahrq.gov/workingforquality/nqs-tools/alignment-toolkit.html), think about what kinds of organizational approaches might best address these concerns. Use the NQS Quality Strategy Template, which includes an Alignment Table, to begin defining actions to address the priorities, and choose one of the nine levers that best apply to the organization's actions.

The six NQS priorities—and a high-level description of related pharmacist opportunities—are presented here (AHRQ 2017b):

1. **Making care safer by reducing harm caused in the delivery of care**
   Pharmacist opportunity: How do we identify and/or reduce the high prescribing of opioid medications in persons without cancer, which could potentially lead to inappropriate or unsafe levels of opioid use?
2. **Ensuring that each person and family is engaged as partners in their care**
   Pharmacist opportunity: As states begin to allow for pharmacists to prescribe and/or dispense Plan B medications, what is the role of those pharmacists in ensuring that all partners are engaged in the care of the person seeking the medication?
3. **Promoting effective communication and coordination of care**
   Pharmacist opportunity: Coordination of care can be a challenge for many pharmacists as they try to reconcile patients' medications postdischarge. Effective coordination of a patient's medications postdischarge can help prevent hospital readmissions.
4. **Promoting the most effective prevention and treatment practices for the leading causes of mortality, starting with cardiovascular disease**
   Pharmacist opportunity: Raising adult immunization rates and assessing for gaps related to the Advisory Committee on Immunization Practices guidelines are two ways that pharmacists can lead effective prevention practices in their communities.
5. **Working with communities to promote wide use of best practices to enable healthy living**
   Pharmacist opportunity: Many pharmacists host seminars in the community, are active in health fairs, hold immunization clinics, and participate in other activities that promote healthy living.
6. **Making quality care more affordable for individuals, families, employers, and governments by developing and spreading new healthcare delivery models**
   Pharmacist opportunity: Many pharmacists work with patients and caregivers to find lower-cost medications or to find patient-assistance programs.

References

Agency for Healthcare Research and Quality (AHRQ). 2017a. "About the National Quality Strategy." Accessed December 17. www.ahrq.gov/workingforquality/about/index.html.

———. 2017b. "National Quality Strategy Toolkit." Published August. www.ahrq.gov/workingforquality/nqs-tools/alignment-toolkit.html.

Ai, A. L., H. Carretta, L. M. Beitsch, L. Watson, J. Munn, and S. Mehriary. 2014. "Medication Therapy Management Programs: Promises and Pitfalls." *Journal of Managed Care and Specialty Pharmacy* 20 (12): 1162–82.

American Pharmacists Association (APhA). 2018. "APhA MTM Central." Accessed December 7. http://pharmacistsprovidecare.com/mtm.

Aspden, P., J. A. Wolcott, J. L. Bootman, and L. R. Cronenwett (eds.). 2007. *Preventing Medication Errors.* Washington, DC: National Academies Press.

Benjamin, G. C. 2016. "Ensuring Population Health: An Important Role for Pharmacy." *American Journal of Pharmaceutical Education* 80 (2): 19.

Blumenthal, D., E. Malphrus, and J. M. McGinnis (eds.). 2015. *Vital Signs: Core Metrics for Health and Health Care Progress.* Institute of Medicine. Accessed December 1, 2017. www.nap.edu/catalog/19402/vital-signs-core-metrics-for-health-and-health-care-progress.

Bonner, L. 2016. "As Pay for Performance Grows, Health Plans Work with Pharmacies." *Pharmacy Today* 22 (3): 50–53.

Branigin, W., and N. C. Aizenman. 2010. "Obama Bypasses Senate by Appointing Medicare Chief." *Washington Post.* Published July 7. www.washingtonpost.com/wp-dyn/content/article/2010/07/07/AR2010070700394.html.

Burwell, S. M. 2015. "Setting Value-Based Payment Goals—HHS Efforts to Improve U.S. Health Care." *New England Journal of Medicine* 372: 897–99.

Centers for Medicare & Medicaid Services (CMS). 2018a. "CMS Measures Inventory." Updated March 27. www.cms.gov/Medicare/Quality-Initiatives-Patient-Assessment-Instruments/QualityMeasures/CMS-Measures-Inventory.html.

———. 2018b. "National Health Expenditure Data—Historical." Accessed December 7. www.cms.gov/Research-Statistics-Data-and-Systems/Statistics-Trends-and-Reports/NationalHealthExpendData/NationalHealthAccountsHistorical.html.

———. 2018c. "Part C and D Performance Data." Accessed February 2. www.cms.gov/Medicare/Prescription-Drug-Coverage/PrescriptionDrugCovGenIn/PerformanceData.html.

———. 2018d. "Part D Enhanced Medication Therapy Management Model." Updated December 4. https://innovation.cms.gov/initiatives/enhancedmtm/.

———. 2016a. "Introduction to the Consistent Poor Performer Notice." Published October. www.cms.gov/Medicare/Eligibility-and-Enrollment/MedicarePresDrugEligEnrol/Downloads/October-11627-combined.pdf.

———. 2016b. "Medicare 2017 Part C & D Star Rating Technical Notes." Updated August 3. www.cms.gov/Medicare/Prescription-Drug-Coverage/PrescriptionDrugCovGenIn/Downloads/2017_Technical_Notes_preview_1_2016_08_03.pdf.

———. 2016c. "2017 Star Ratings." Published October 12. www.cms.gov/newsroom/fact-sheets/2017-star-ratings.

Community Care of North Carolina. 2018. "Community Pharmacy Enhanced Services Network." Accessed December 7. www.communitycarenc.org/population-management/pharmacy/community-pharmacy-enhanced-services-network-cpesn/.

Donabedian, A. 1988. "The Quality of Care: How Can It Be Assessed?" *JAMA* 260 (12): 1743–48.

Electronic Quality Improvement Platform for Plans and Pharmacies (EQuIPP). 2018. "Learn About EQuIPP." Accessed January 3. www.equipp.org/default.aspx.

Gordis, L. (ed.). 2009. *Epidemiology*, 4th ed. Philadelphia, PA: Elsevier/Saunders.

GovTrack.us. 2017. "H.R. 1 (108th): Medicare Prescription Drug, Improvement, and Modernization Act of 2003." Accessed December 10. www.govtrack.us/congress/bills/108/hr1.

Institute for Healthcare Improvement (IHI). 2017. "The IHI Triple Aim." Accessed December 19. www.ihi.org/Engage/Initiatives/TripleAim/Pages/default.aspx.

IQVIA Institute for Human Data Science. 2017. "Medicines Use and Spending in the U.S.: A Review of 2016 and Outlook to 2021." Published May 4. www.iqvia.com/institute/reports/medicines-use-and-spending-in-the-us-a-review-of-2016.

Kaiser Family Foundation. 2017. "Medicare Advantage." Published October 10. www.kff.org/medicare/fact-sheet/medicare-advantage/.

Kohn, L. T., J. M. Corrigan, and M. S. Donaldson (eds.). 2000. *To Err Is Human: Building a Safer Health System*. Washington, DC: National Academies Press.

Managed Healthcare Executive. 2016. "Novartis Signs on to Value-Based Pricing for Entresto." Published May 4. www.managedhealthcareexecutive.com/benefit-design-and-pricing/novartis-signs-value-based-pricing-entresto.

McGivney, M. S., S. M. Meyer, W. Duncan-Hewitt, D. L. Hall, J. V. Goode, and R. B. Smith. 2007. "Medication Therapy Management: Its Relationship to Patient Counseling, Disease Management, and Pharmaceutical Care." *Journal of the American Pharmacists Association* 47 (5): 620–28.

National Center for Health Statistics. 2017. "Therapeutic Drug Use." Centers for Disease Control and Prevention. Updated May 3. www.cdc.gov/nchs/fastats/drug-use-therapeutic.htm.

Patient-Centered Outcomes Research Institute (PCORI). 2017. "Vision & Mission." Accessed December 19. www.pcori.org/vision-mission.

Pharmacy Quality Alliance (PQA). 2017a. "About." Accessed December 4. http://pqaalliance.org/about/default.asp.

———. 2017b. "PQA Measures Used by CMS in the Star Ratings." Accessed December 4. https://pqaalliance.org/measures/cms.asp.

Pharmacy Quality Solutions (PQS). 2018. "About Pharmacy Quality Solutions." Accessed January 3. www.pharmacyquality.com/about.

Shrank, W. H., M. E. Porter, S. H. Jain, and N. K. Choudhry. 2009. "A Blueprint for Pharmacy Benefit Managers to Increase Value." *American Journal of Managed Care* 15 (2): 87–93.

Sox, H. C., and S. Greenfield. 2009. "Comparative Effectiveness Research: A Report from the Institute of Medicine." *Annals of Internal Medicine* 151 (3): 203–5.

Tsyuki, R. T., N. P. Beahm, H. Okada, and Y. N. Al Hamarneh. 2018. "Pharmacists as Accessible Primary Health Care Providers: Review of the Evidence." *Canadian Pharmacists Journal* 151 (1): 4–5.

Vest, J. R., S. J. Grannis, D. P. Haut, P. K. Halverson, and N. Menachemi. 2017. "Using Structured and Unstructured Data to Identify Patients' Need for Services that Address the Social Determinants of Health." *International Journal of Medical Informatics* 107: 101–6.

CHAPTER

19

POPULATION HEALTH SAFETY AND QUALITY

Keith Kosel

To say that much has been written on the topic of population health safety and quality would be misleading; in fact, just the opposite is true. There exists only scant scientific literature—only a small number of white papers and peer-reviewed journal articles—examining safety and quality with a population health focus. The fact that so little has been written on the subject only magnifies the need for the healthcare field, its leaders, and clinical and social practitioners to devote their time and energies to clarifying this important issue.

Overview: Where We Stand Today

According to a widely held definition, *population health* refers to "the health outcomes of a group of individuals, including the distribution of such outcomes within the group," with attention to the determinants that give rise to those outcomes and the policies and interventions that affect those determinants (Kindig 2007, 143). Note that we do not see any explicit mention here of quality or patient safety. One could argue that both of these elements are implied within the definition, but even so, we are still left wondering just where exactly safety and quality fit into the concept of population health.

Exhibit 19.1 provides a conceptual framework for our current understanding of population health and the key factors that arise from the definition. It highlights the idea that the operational definition of *population health* consists of three pivotal pieces of information: (1) the policies and interventions that

EXHIBIT 19.1 Conceptual Framework for Our Current Understanding of Population Health

Drivers	Outputs
Health outcomes and their distribution within a population	Morbidity, mortality, quality of life
Health determinants that influence the outcomes	Medical care, genetics, socioeconomic status
Policies and interventions that affect the determinants	Social, environmental, and individual

affect (2) the determinants of health, which in turn drive (3) health outcomes within a group of individuals. As we discuss population health safety and quality, keep these three key elements in mind, as much of what we know or believe we know centers around them.

A quick look at the recent history of population health can help us better understand the challenge of describing what constitutes population health safety and quality. Although today we speak about population health as a core element of the care continuum, one step removed from ambulatory care, not all that long ago the concept of population health was foreign to many hospital administrators, physicians, and payer organizations. Only over the past half-dozen years or so has discussion of the role and relevance of population health become mainstream, thanks to pioneers in the field such as David Kindig and David Nash—both of whom have furthered our understanding of the concept and raised awareness of how population health fits within today's notion of the care continuum.

As payment approaches were redesigned away from fee-for-service models to incorporate greater degrees of provider financial risk, a natural evolution began to take place, elevating the discussion of populations and what it would take to (1) identify, (2) assess, (3) segment/stratify, (4) deliver services for, and (5) effectively measure them. No longer were populations and the social determinants that affected them topics for the uninformed; rather, providers and payers began to see how addressing "upstream" social and physical determinants of health—things like food, housing, domestic violence, and air quality—could effectively reduce the mismanagement of medications and the overuse of healthcare services such as emergency department (ED) visits. This shift in focus would demonstrate potential to lower utilization, lower healthcare expenditures, and increase the satisfaction of patients and families.

McGinnis, Russo, and Knickman (2002) described the determinants of health as being 40 percent behavioral, 30 percent genetic, 20 percent environmental, and 10 percent related to medical care. Soon, many people began to understand that optimizing the health of a population was a complex undertaking made up of disparate elements, each contributing to the final outcome. This new thinking about the determinants of health and the ways they affect the health of populations meant that our ideas about what constituted safe, high-quality care—ideas that had developed primarily around an inpatient medical model—needed to change, and change they did.

As clinical leaders and administrators were becoming more comfortable with the concept of population health, a natural question emerged: How do we define a population? A great deal of time and effort has been devoted to establishing what we mean when we use the word *population*. For some, it refers to the employees of a business who are covered under that particular business's employee benefit plan. For others, it includes all the insured lives of a Medicare Advantage plan or similar health plan. For still others, a population encompasses all the individuals living within a designated community with defined geographic boundaries. Clearly, the way we define a population depends on how wide a net we choose to cast over a group of individuals or a specific geographical locale. Fortunately, the question of how to define a population has no wrong answer—only a need to be clear about how narrow or expansive our definition is.

At the same time that the concept of population health was becoming more mainstream, the healthcare field was witnessing a parallel evolution in how it viewed patient safety and quality. In 2000, the landmark *To Err Is Human* report by the Institute of Medicine (IOM) shocked the industry and the general public with the assertion that between 44,000 and 98,000 Americans die each year because of medical errors, misdiagnoses, or avoidable injuries while under treatment (Kohn, Corrigan, and Donaldson 2000). The report raised serious concerns and sparked a movement of patient safety programs, research, and coalitions. Throughout the 2000s, quality improvement efforts in healthcare evolved, with a growing focus on coordination of care and the use of health information technology.

As these two industry trends—increased awareness of population health concepts and the growing safety and quality movement—evolved simultaneously, we naturally expected to see areas of meaningful interplay between the two concepts. Unfortunately, population health had to wait for several other major milestones to be achieved first.

The first of these milestones occurred in 2011, when the Centers for Medicare & Medicaid Services (CMS) launched its Partnership for Patients (PfP) initiative (CMS 2018a). The PfP campaign aimed to focus attention on patient safety by directing a group of 26 organizations, called Hospital Engagement Networks (HENs), to work with some 3,900 hospitals across the United States to reduce patient harms—specifically, hospital-acquired conditions and preventable readmissions. Participating HENs at the time of the program's launch included Premier, VHA Inc., the American Hospital Association–affiliated Health Research and Educational Trust, state hospital associations, and large healthcare systems such as Dignity Health and Ascension Health. With the PfP initiative, CMS encouraged acute care hospitals to focus on reducing ten conditions: falls; catheter-associated urinary tract infections (CAUTIs); adverse drug events; central line–associated bloodstream infections (CLABSIs); pressure ulcers; surgical site infections (SSIs); obstetrical adverse events, including early elective deliveries; ventilator-associated pneumonia (VAP); venous thromboembolism (VTE); and readmissions. From 2010 to 2013, incidents of patient harm decreased nationwide, from 144 per 1,000 discharges to 121, representing more than 50,000 lives saved and savings of more than $12 billion (Agency for Healthcare Research and Quality [AHRQ] 2015). Continuation of the program in subsequent years has resulted in further reductions, culminating in more than 87,000 lives saved, 2.1 million fewer instances of patient harm, and more than $20 billion in savings.

CMS continued to make progress in reducing patient harm within the acute care environment with HEN 2.0 (in 2014 and 2015) and the Hospital Improvement and Innovation Networks (HIIN 3.0). It then turned its attention to addressing quality in the ambulatory environment with its Transforming Clinical Practice Initiative (TCPI), launched in 2016. TCPI was designed to support 140,000 clinician practices in sharing, adapting, and further developing their comprehensive quality improvement strategies, with some 29 Practice Transformation Networks (PTNs) and 10 Support and Alignment Networks (SANs). Together, the PTNs and SANs were able to engage clinicians in practice redesign, making care safer by eliminating inappropriate care (e.g., unnecessary diagnostic tests, questionable therapies, unnecessary ED visits) while improving the overall quality of care in the ambulatory environment. Improvements sought to expand access; engage patients, families, and their caregivers; and address healthcare equity. Between the PfP and TCPI, CMS was working its way across the care continuum, thereby reducing patient harm and improving quality.

The next major chapter in CMS's attempt to address quality and safety across the care continuum had to wait until 2017, when its Accountable Health Communities (AHC) initiative launched (CMS 2018b). The initiative was developed based on a three-track model of Awareness, Assistance, Alignment, though it was later scaled back to just two parts: Assistance and Alignment. The AHC initiative was CMS's first systematic attempt to address the health-related social determinants that studies had shown to be conclusively linked to higher readmission rates and a host of morbidities. It marked the first time that a major payer organization (CMS) was driving the healthcare field to focus on safety and quality across the entire care continuum (i.e., in acute, ambulatory, and community settings). With this push, population health safety and quality now took center stage.

Safety and Quality in Various Populations

Employee Populations

Businesses that sponsor and pay for their employees' health insurance—whether they are large, for-profit enterprises such as Boeing and Intel or healthcare systems such as Mayo Clinic or Providence Health Services—are becoming increasingly concerned about the health of their workforce and the quality of care their employees receive. Such concerns are driven in large part by the negative impact that poor-quality care has on workers' productivity, attendance, and healthcare costs.

Managing the health of defined populations, such as employee groups, poses challenges different from those encountered when dealing with larger insured or noninsured populations. For small group populations, such as a health system's employees, healthcare safety and quality efforts focus on designing and promoting wellness and disease management programs tailored to the employees' unique situation and to various employee segments (e.g., active/retiree, hourly/salaried). These programs customize employee benefits to require or encourage the use of the hospital's own facilities, including physicians, pharmacies, and other affiliated resources. Typically, these types of population groups adopt some of the tactics that have proved effective for organizations seeking to manage costs and improve quality—for instance, high-deductible plans, narrow networks, centers of excellence, and health spending accounts. Leadership in these types of organizations emphasizes the tracking of health improvement results and disease outcomes to allow for midcourse corrections if necessary. The organizations recognize the importance of tailoring programs to the various needs of multiple tiers of workers and incorporating appropriate incentives and/or penalties to further drive desired behaviors and outcomes.

At the same time, an array of innovative benefit plan structures have gained popularity across many industries as ways to encourage healthy behaviors, improve the health of the employee population, and reduce costs. Most of these structures include a strong financial mechanism to effect positive change. For example, many organizations use differential cost sharing—that is, having lower deductibles and copays for employees who use domestic resources or requiring employees to pay more of the cost for low-value, high-cost procedures (Towers Watson 2012).

Health Plan Populations

Recognizing that social and physical determinants have a substantial impact on health outcomes and health status, many managed health plans have sought to help enrollees address their broader needs, from food to housing to dealing with multiple chronic conditions. For instance, CareSource, Ohio's largest Medicaid managed care plan, launched a statewide case management strategy that employed 60 patient navigators who visited the homes of more than 8,000 high-risk enrollees, many with diabetes, to better understand the challenges the enrollees faced. After an initial assessment, the plan realized that addressing food insecurity needed to be a top priority, so it partnered with a local community organization to create a portable, diabetic-friendly food bank that not only provided nutritious food but also helped educate patients in proper food selection and preparation (Heiman and Artiga 2015).

Commercial Medicaid and Medicare Advantage plans have also worked to develop programs to reflect the cultural and ethnic needs of members. Such programs emphasize preventive care, community and member health education, case management, and disease management tracking, and they incorporate sophisticated technology to help analyze and coordinate services. Managed care plans, especially Medicare and Medicaid plans, have taken the lead in addressing disparities of care through the use of voluntary or, in some cases, mandatory guidelines. For example, state Medicaid programs are required by CMS to provide race, ethnicity, and language data on enrollees (Nerenz 2005). Medicare Advantage plans operate under similar requirements to conduct periodic quality improvement projects in the areas of culturally competent care and linguistic services. Other commercial carriers, such as Aetna, Cigna, UnitedHealth Group, and Kaiser Permanente, have also undertaken large-scale, data-driven efforts to address health disparities.

What Should Safety and Quality Look Like in a Community?

As noted earlier in the chapter, one of the ways a population can be defined is as a community of residents, all contained within given geographical boundaries. When looking at communities as representative populations, we typically consider them in terms of three key elements: (1) their health status, (2) their level of health equity, and (3) their social and physical determinants of health and disease.

Health Status

The health status of individual communities, states, and the nation has been the subject of assessment for many years. Over that time, the number and types of focus areas have changed dramatically, as the culture and demographic make-up of populations have shifted. As we continue to focus on the health status of communities, we can measure their progress against standards developed by various agencies within the Department of Health and Human Services (HHS).

Healthy People 2020, a program within HHS, provides a comprehensive set of ten-year national goals and objectives for improving the health of all Americans (US Office of Disease Prevention and Health Promotion 2018). The program contains 42 topic areas with more than 1,200 objectives. A select set of 26 objectives, called Leading Health Indicators (LHIs), communicates high-priority health issues and highlights actions that can be taken to address them. The indicators can be used to assess the health of the nation; facilitate collaboration across sectors; and motivate action at the national, state, and community levels. Exhibit 19.2 lists the 12 topics around which the 26 LHIs were developed.

Progress toward the Healthy People 2020 targets has generally been encouraging. According to the program's midcourse review in 2014, 16 of the 26 LHIs had either met their target or shown improvement (US Office

EXHIBIT 19.2
Topics of Leading Health Indicators for Healthy People 2020

Access to Health Services	Nutrition, Physical Activity & Obesity
Clinical Preventative Services	Oral Health
Environmental Quality	Reproductive and Sexual Health
Injury and Violence	Social Determinants
Maternal, Infant & Child Health	Substance Abuse
Mental Health	Tobacco Use

Source: US Office of Disease Prevention and Health Promotion (2018).

of Disease Prevention and Health Promotion 2014). Among the notable successes to date are that

- fewer adults are smoking cigarettes,
- fewer children are being exposed to secondhand smoke,
- more adults are meeting physical activity targets, and
- fewer adolescents are using illicit drugs.

Health Equity

Until recently, the aim of achieving equity in care received only minimal attention in the quality arena. However, persistent disparities in care raise concerns about the overall quality of healthcare provided to a community and may have substantial implications for overall healthcare expenditures. If subpopulations are receiving suboptimal care or care that does not meet a healthcare system's standards, then the system must identify the deficiencies and remedy them; otherwise, it cannot claim to deliver superior quality and safety. The elimination of any observed disparities in care must be synergistically integrated within the healthcare system's quality strategy.

Issues related to health equity have a major impact on individuals in "minority" populations, people of low socioeconomic standing, and members of other vulnerable populations. Data suggest that African Americans, Hispanic Americans, and Native Americans have a higher burden of chronic disease, complications, substance use disorders, and disabilities than other groups do, yet they have lower healthcare expenditures and receive fewer healthcare services (particularly for high-end procedures, such as catheterization). Members of racial and ethnic minority groups tend to enter the healthcare system at more advanced stages of their disease, have higher rates of rehospitalization, and are more likely to be hospitalized for preventable conditions (e.g., diabetes, hypertension) (Davis, Liu, and Gibbons 2003). Furthermore, African Americans have nearly twice the rate of premature birth as the white population does (Heiman and Artiga 2015), leading to a greater need for neonatal intensive care.

Inequities in the healthcare system, especially those relating to underuse of recommended or necessary services, result in the use of more costly services at a later stage of illness, poorer outcomes, and lost productivity. Hence, they have health and social costs that extend beyond the individuals or specific population groups directly affected.

Addressing disparities and ensuring health equity present opportunities for systems to reduce unnecessary expenditures and improve the quality of care. Health equity also positively affects organizations' bottom line. As in any business, satisfaction with healthcare is a function of perceived quality, the competency of the professionals who are providing services (i.e., clinicians), and the degree of personal respect shown during interactions (i.e., during patient visits). High patient satisfaction is correlated with compliance with prescribed treatments, adherence to mutually agreed-upon goals, and reduced likelihood of hospital utilization. Conversely, poor public perception of a health system's quality can have a deleterious impact on community relations and the system's ability to hold market share.

Racial and ethnic disparities related to health outcomes are not limited to low-income, uninsured, or government-insured groups. They are also observed among privately insured patients, and they persist when socioeconomic and other determinants (e.g., age, gender, insurance status) are accounted for (Mayberry, Mili, and Ofili 2000). These findings indicate that socioeconomic status, insurance coverage, health status, disease severity, and patient preferences do not completely explain the disparities in health outcomes. Interpersonal factors (e.g., culture, patient–provider communication, provider bias, intentional and unintentional racism) may offer a partial explanation. However, system-level characteristics (e.g., care coordination, inefficiencies, lack of evidence-based clinical decisions, uncertainty in clinical decisions) may prove to offer the best explanation for such disparities—and also the best opportunities for achieving equity in healthcare access, use, and outcomes.

The nature of disparities is complicated by the fact that race and ethnicity are correlated with demographic factors such as economic status, insurance coverage, care-seeking behavior, and preexisting conditions. Despite these complex interrelationships, evidence indicates that health inequity can be reduced or eliminated in healthcare systems, such as the Department of Defense and the Veterans Health Administration, that provide universal access and comprehensive services regardless of an individual's race or ethnicity.

People may disagree on the specific strategies to eliminate inequities in healthcare, but most agree that a comprehensive, multidimensional strategy is needed to address the problem. The collection of accurate race, ethnicity, and language data (often called REAL data) is a prerequisite for a comprehensive strategy to initiate clinical and social interventions to improve quality of care and promote health equity for all. In addition, the development of alliances with local community and faith-based organizations and local health departments is increasingly recognized as an essential element in improving access to care. Research has shown that partnerships between community organizations and local health departments can be effective for "the elimination of significant disparities in breast cancer and cervical cancer screening rates between Whites and African Americans and a substantial reduction in disparities in breast cancer screening rates between Whites and Hispanics" (Mayberry et al. 2006, 107).

Healthcare organizations often build formal and informal relationships with local community groups through participation in community screenings, health fairs, health awareness campaigns, speaker bureaus, and community forums. As healthcare institutions around the country become more actively engaged with their communities, they develop into pivotal resources—improving access and quality; enhancing ongoing community-based activities; and addressing other aspects of population health safety, quality, and equity.

Another approach for enhancing health equity focuses on creating a culturally competent, or culturally sensitive, healthcare system—one capable of delivering the highest quality and safest care available to every patient regardless of race, ethnicity, social class, culture, ability to pay, or language proficiency. Cultural competence is an important element of healthcare quality. It means that an organization has the capacity to function effectively within the context of cultural beliefs, behaviors, values, needs, and social norms of patients and the patients' communities of origin, affiliation, or residence (Anderson et al. 2003). An early indication of cultural competence is the extent to which ethnic and cultural characteristics and norms are incorporated into the design, delivery, and evaluation of healthcare interventions.

Cultural competence and its effects on population health quality have attracted considerable interest among healthcare providers, public health services, policymakers, and academics, particularly in light of the growing racial and ethnic diversity of the US population and the desire of healthcare professionals to address the needs of vulnerable residents and underserved groups. However, despite widespread agreement on the need for culturally competent care interventions, the adoption of cultural competence into mainstream thinking about healthcare has been slowed by confusion, debate, measurement challenges, and a lack of consensus on the term's definition.

Nevertheless, cultural competence is emerging as a strategy not only for eliminating inequities but also for improving safety and quality in population health (Betancourt et al. 2005). Generally speaking, a culturally competent healthcare system would have the following components:

- Interpreter services, to improve communication between people who speak different languages
- Recruitment and retention efforts, to employ a culturally diverse clinical staff that reflects the community being served

- Training that helps educate staff on effective communication methods and increase cultural awareness
- Community workers, to serve as liaisons to the community and serve as mediators and endorsers of the health system
- Health promotion that incorporates culturally specific and sensitive messages to encourage healthy behaviors that decrease risk
- Administrative and organizational accommodations (including physical environments) that enhance sensitivity to the unique languages and cultures of the people being served

Finally, a culturally competent healthcare system also improves communication between providers and patients, families, and other caretakers and recognizes that ethnicity and culture influence health beliefs, perception of health and disease, care-seeking behaviors, and overall use of healthcare services. Inappropriate treatment and referral practices and negative provider attitudes and stereotypes—whether conscious or unconscious—must be eliminated so that the quality and safety of the population's care can be enhanced.

Social and Physical Determinants

A focus on racial and ethnic disparities does not preclude the need to pay attention to other personal, social, and physical characteristics that are known to be related to healthcare access, use, and health outcomes. We know that health starts in our homes, schools, workplaces, and communities and that taking care of ourselves by eating well, staying active, and getting the recommended immunizations all influence our health and that of our communities. Our health is also influenced by access to social and economic opportunities, the quality of our schools, the safety of our workplaces, and the nature of our social interactions. The conditions in which we live explain, in part, why some people are healthier than others and why Americans in general are not as healthy as they could be.

Although overall spending on social services and healthcare in the United States is comparable to that of other Western countries, the United States disproportionately spends less on social services and more on healthcare (Heiman and Artiga 2015). Increasing access to healthcare and transforming the healthcare delivery system are important, but research clearly indicates that improving population health and achieving health equity will require broader approaches that address myriad social, economic, and environmental factors.

Social and physical determinants of health are conditions in people's environments—the settings in which people are born, live, work, play, worship, and so on—that affect health, functioning, and quality of life in various ways. Examples of social determinants include the following:

- Safe housing and local food markets
- Access to educational, economic, and job opportunities
- Access to healthcare services
- Access to transportation
- Public safety
- Social support
- Language/literacy
- Residential segregation
- Social norms and attitudes

The following are examples of physical determinants:

- The natural environment, such as green space (trees and grass) and weather
- The built environment, such as buildings, sidewalks, roads, and bike lanes
- Work sites, schools, and recreational settings
- Physical barriers, especially for people with disabilities
- Exposure to toxic substances and other physical hazards

For population health purposes, the social, economic, and physical conditions in the various environments of people's lives (e.g., schools, churches, workplaces, and neighborhoods) can be collectively referred to as "place."

People's environments significantly affect their patterns of social engagement and sense of security and well-being, and resources that enhance quality of life can have a significant influence on population health outcomes. Examples of such resources include safe and affordable housing, access to education, public safety, availability of healthy foods, and environments devoid of life-threatening toxins. Understanding the relationship between how population groups experience "place" and the impact of "place" on health is fundamental to explaining the role of social and physical determinants on the health of communities (Swift 2002).

Through a meta-analysis of nearly 50 studies, researchers found that social factors such as education, social support, racial segregation, and poverty accounted for more than a third of all deaths in the United States (Heiman and Artiga 2015). Researchers also found that the likelihood of premature death increases as income decreases and that lower education levels are directly correlated with lower income, a higher likelihood of smoking, and a shorter life expectancy. Children born to parents who have not completed high school are more likely to live in environments that pose barriers to good health—for instance, neighborhoods that are unsafe, have exposed garbage or litter, and have substandard or dilapidated housing and vandalism.

A growing number of initiatives have emerged to address these social, economic, and physical determinants of health and to develop integrated solutions within the context of healthcare delivery system reform. In particular, a number of efforts to link healthcare to broader social needs have been included in commercial and Medicaid delivery and payment initiatives. The place-based approach used in Camden, New Jersey, provides a useful example.

The population of Camden had historically experienced a high poverty rate and poor access to care, with a high share of ED and hospital admissions for preventable conditions that could have been treated by a primary care provider. Furthermore, the population was having difficulty accessing behavioral health and social services because resources were in short supply. In response to these issues, the Camden Coalition created a citywide care management system to help connect high utilizers of hospital ED services with primary care providers (Heiman and Artiga 2015). The care management system included medical and behavioral health providers and a social worker who interacted with patients in the community to help identify and address their medical and social needs. Results have shown that patients managed through the initiative have had decreased ED and hospital utilization and improved management of health conditions. The initiative has also been successful in connecting patients to primary care following a hospital discharge.

As the relationship between neighborhoods and health status continues to be better understood, zip code has proved to be a strong predictor of a person's health. Recognizing the powerful impact of neighborhoods and housing, many people have begun focusing on how Medicaid can be used to support housing for vulnerable and underserved populations. In 2015, CMS released information about the circumstances under which Medicaid would pay for certain housing-related activities, with the aim of supporting states in community integration efforts. Most of these opportunities stem from various waivers contained in the Affordable Care Act of 2010. According to the CMS guidelines, Medicaid funds cannot be used to pay for room and board, but funds can support a range of housing-related activities, including referral, support services, and case management services that help connect and retain individuals with stable housing. Some states have gone further. In Texas, a major project is under way, with the help of Medicaid waivers, to direct funding to provide services for individuals in supportive housing and for people experiencing homelessness and mental illness (Heiman and Artiga 2015).

By establishing policies that positively affect social, economic, and physical conditions and that support changes in individual behavior, we can improve the general health and welfare of the population; in so doing, we can bring about lower utilization of inappropriate healthcare services and a better experience for patients and their families.

One of the primary challenges involved in addressing population health safety and quality—particularly as it relates to the social and physical determinants of health within a community—is the difficulty of connecting healthcare providers with community-based service delivery organizations (CBOs). For far too long, providers have lacked actionable information on the availability of local support services (e.g., food banks, homeless shelters, transportation providers). Even when community resource directories have been available—and up to date—providers have often had little or no way of making a connection with them.

In 2014, Parkland's Center for Clinical Innovation (PCCI)—a nonprofit off-shoot of Parkland Health and Hospital System in Dallas, Texas—launched a new initiative to address this issue. PCCI is a cutting-edge research and analytics organization focused on integrating data science with clinical best practices to improve care for indigent, vulnerable, and underserved populations. Recognizing the need for a population health framework to link clinical delivery sites with CBOs, PCCI developed a cloud-based Information Exchange Portal (IEP) to enhance the care coordination function between the two ecosystems (Cohen 2017). The system allows care managers to make referrals directly to hundreds of CBOs within the Dallas metropolitan area and receive information back from these CBOs when patients arrive for their referral appointments. For instance, in the case of a diabetic patient living within food-restricted areas, or food deserts, the IEP and local support staff can help guide the patient in selecting nutritious foods; post reminders for follow-up visits; and help counsel the patient on good nutrition, exercise, and other health-promoting behaviors.

Early results from the PCCI project have indicated dramatic improvement among patients with diabetes, hypertension, and food insecurities in terms of reduced ED visits, increased ambulatory appointments kept, and better medication management. At the same time, patients have reported that they feel more cared for, more a part of the decision-making process, and better able to navigate the complex healthcare system. PCCI's work and the IEP that supports it have now been expanded to support a contract with CMS pertaining to its Accountable Health Communities initiative. Further work is planned to help link the IEP to local school health programs working to reduce pediatric asthma, as well as to local criminal justice systems trying to manage the cross-traffic affecting various social institutions within the community.

Who Should Be Responsible for Population Safety and Quality?

The way that safety and quality are ultimately positioned within our concept of population health as it evolves will be the result of a dynamic interplay between two key stakeholder groups: (1) healthcare providers (including individual clinicians, the organizations with which they are affiliated, and nontraditional/ancillary providers) and the patients they care for and (2) public health agencies at the federal, state, and local levels.

Healthcare Providers

Traditional healthcare providers are the stakeholder group that has been tasked with delivering safety and quality in both the acute care and ambulatory care environments. Thus, logically, we can expect them to assume much of the responsibility for defining, delivering, and evaluating safety and quality in a future population health model. Physicians, nurses, care managers, and other clinical providers will play an important role in shaping how safety and quality are addressed not only through the technical expertise they display but also through the relationships they establish with their patients.

Much has been written about patient activation and patient engagement and the role those concepts play in strengthening the provider–patient relationship and affecting the management of patient care, the utilization of services, and ultimately the success or failure of a care plan. A population health model, by necessity, involves a high degree of interaction, communication, and trust—an authentic partnership between healthcare providers and patients and their families or caregivers. This partnership serves as the foundation for shared decision making with regard to the direction and intensity of the care plan and the roles and responsibilities each partner will assume.

In a population health model, the provider–patient relationship will be strengthened by the inclusion in the partnership of community health workers, care navigators, and patient advocates. These nontraditional lay providers will assume a critical role in linking the healthcare team and the patient to resources and services within the community and helping navigate the complexity that surrounds most chronic care today. As liaisons between the patient, the provider, and the community, they will support the continuity and coordination of care, helping patients make and keep appointments and adhere to treatment plans and medication regimens. Community health workers can also contribute to various activities related to health promotion, disease prevention, and patient education and support. Finally, because they are familiar with the particular communities in which the patients reside, these individuals can help traditional healthcare providers to better understand community norms, cultural challenges, and the availability of local resources.

Public Health Agencies

Historically, health and healthcare have been addressed through a combination of personal healthcare (often called "medical care") and public health systems. The personal healthcare system primarily provides curative services (e.g., treating illnesses and injuries) to individuals, with relatively little attention paid to prevention. The public health system, on the other hand, emphasizes prevention through population-based health promotion—those public services and interventions aimed at protecting entire populations from illness and injury.

The primary providers of public health services are government public health service agencies, such as the Centers for Disease Control and Prevention (CDC) at the federal level, as well as state, county, and municipal health departments. These agencies are responsible for ensuring individual, community, and environmental health by building partnerships and providing or coordinating adequate services to communities. In many instances, public health agencies have also sought to address the healthcare service needs of vulnerable and at-risk groups. Public health agencies meet their obligations to their communities in a variety of ways, such as by fostering policy-guided community initiatives to promote health or improve health conditions, directing the provision of services in the community or the home, and advancing community education. Another role of public health agencies involves regulating sources of risk and promoting health and safety practices—for instance, licensing restaurants and health facilities and regulating water and air quality.

Public health interventions focus on the health needs of the entire population or specific subgroups within the population. In contrast, personal healthcare providers have, until recently, had little incentive to consider population-based services, many of which have been unfunded. Even with the increased attention to the provision of preventive services by managed care organizations such as Medicare or Medicaid plans, the preventive services provided are often limited to those with immediate or short-range payoffs. Populations most at risk for increased morbidity and mortality may be the least likely to receive preventive services, whether because of financial or nonfinancial barriers. Public health agencies seek to address these issues through outreach, education, transportation, translation services, and culturally sensitive service provision.

Whereas personal healthcare might heal injuries, alleviate disorders, and treat diseases, public health programs can prevent the onset and spread of disease by addressing risk factors such as smoking, obesity, air quality, and drug use. Nonetheless, the vast bulk of spending on healthcare in the United States is focused on the private, personal healthcare sector, while public health programs receive just a small (and decreasing) portion of expenditures. This approach results in a society that is not provided with all the public health services necessary to maintain the public's health (Public Health Service 1994). If we are to optimize safety and healthcare quality within our community populations, the nature of all future health-promoting activities and their funding mechanisms must be altered to focus more on disease prevention and health awareness (i.e., risk-reduction activities) and less on private-sector personal healthcare services.

Since the early 2000s, a collaborative approach known as Health in All Policies (HiAP) has sought to improve health by incorporating health considerations into decision making across multiple sectors and policy areas (Rudolph et al. 2013). The approach engages diverse partners and stakeholder groups to work together to promote sustainable health and simultaneously advance other goals, such as promoting employment and economic stability. HiAP seeks to ensure that decision making across sectors within the healthcare industry is informed about the health, equity, safety, and quality consequences of policy decisions made in nonhealth sectors. Policies and practices in areas as diverse as education and early childhood development, community development, and transportation all affect the health and quality of care delivered to the population.

HiAP is being promoted and implemented at the federal level, by state and local governments, and by various community-based organizations. National and local funders are also shifting their focus to support broader policies and practices that promote opportunities for improved health. The Robert Wood Johnson Foundation, for instance, underwent a major reorientation aligned with its goal to look beyond traditional models of healthcare to improve population health. The foundation seeks to change the way the nation thinks about health by focusing on collective impact and cross-sector collaboration on issues ranging from early childhood education to food insecurity (Heiman and Artiga 2015).

Although an expanded and more central role for public health agencies is key to advancing the quality of health and healthcare within community populations, the role of private-sector personal health service delivery organizations (i.e., medical care) should not be diminished. In fact, much of the advancement taking place today in artificial intelligence, predictive modeling, and decision support technology can markedly improve the quality and safety of care delivered within community populations. Although the curative aspects of medical care will always remain a key focus, advancements in technology are helping to identify at-risk individuals earlier and to connect those individuals with appropriate clinical workflows to optimize care.

Work being done at Health Partners in Minneapolis, Minnesota, for example, seeks to help individuals identify and address risk factors that contribute to heart disease. Through sophisticated data algorithms and predictive models, individuals are able to see the impact that addressing one or more cardiovascular risk factors can have on reducing the likelihood of a heart attack or stroke (O'Connor 2017). Similar work is being done at Parkland Community Health Plan in Dallas, Texas, with the use of cutting-edge decision support tools to serve at-risk pediatric asthma populations.

These and other private-sector initiatives have sought to build outward from the traditional curative core of medical care by identifying at-risk individuals earlier and then engaging them in care delivery models that focus on evidence-based leading practices, patient engagement, and resource optimization to improve the health of individuals and communities.

Ideally, activities in the public health and personal healthcare systems should be more closely integrated and coordinated than they are today. Rapid changes in the organization and delivery of medical care—specifically, the growth of for-profit medical care, managed care health plans, and precision medicine—affect access for vulnerable populations, the health outcomes of the general public, and the activities and abilities of local public health agencies. Going forward, public health agencies will have a critical new role to play with regard to these changes. They should be tasked with ensuring that healthcare providers have the capacity to care for all populations within the community; monitoring, evaluating, and improving quality; and understanding the relationship between the clinical and social services delivered and the impact on the health of the population.

Reflecting the expanded role expected of state and local public health agencies in ensuring the quality of health for community populations, many US policymakers have discussed transitioning healthcare funding, in the form of block grants, from the federal government to individual states. Although a number of hurdles stand in the way of successful implementation of this type of model, the discussions reinforce important ideas—namely, that all health and healthcare are local and that engaging local public health entities along with the resident health systems, clinicians, and community-based organizations makes intuitive sense to foster better population health. The short case studies that accompany this section illustrate how traditional medical providers can work with public health agencies to bring about meaningful improvement in the health and well-being of the communities they serve.

Case Study: Hearts Beat Back: The Heart of New Ulm Project

Hearts Beat Back, the population health arm of the Minneapolis Heart Institute Foundation (MHIF), began in 2009 as a partnership with Allina Health, the New Ulm Medical Center, and several local public health departments (Heart Beats Back 2018). The program set out to reduce the incidence of heart attacks over a ten-year period by focusing on preventing cardiovascular disease, rather than on treating the disease after it occurs.

The medical organizations participating in the project provided registry data, screening protocols, and the identification of high-risk patients,

(continued)

and the collaborating public health departments conducted phone/mail surveys and generated supporting data to aid in community screenings. The public health departments also engaged in an extensive social marketing campaign to raise awareness of cardiovascular risk factors and preventive strategies to mitigate these risks. After just two years, the project was able to demonstrate statistically significant improvements in lifestyle behaviors (e.g., smoking cessation, health nutrition, stress reduction). At five years postimplementation, the project showed significant improvement in key clinical indicators such as blood pressure and lipid levels.

Case Study: Boston Community Asthma Initiative

Launched in 2005 and still ongoing, the Boston Community Asthma Initiative represents a partnership between Boston Children's Hospital, state and city public health agencies, and a host of local community organizations, including the YMCA, Boys and Girls Clubs, and Boston Public Schools. Its goal is to improve health outcomes and reduce disparities among children with asthma.

To facilitate the improvement effort, Boston Children's Hospital provided financial and administrative support, while also using the hospital's real-time data system to identify children with the highest risk and greatest need. Participating public health agencies were responsible for conducting in-home visits that focused on medication reconciliation and disease management, in addition to inspecting the homes for pests and environmental triggers. By working together, the hospital, public health agencies, and various community organizations were able to achieve an 80 percent reduction in hospital admissions and a 58 percent decrease in ED visits, as of December 2016 (Boston Children's Hospital 2018).

The Role of Measurement in Driving Population Health Safety and Quality

Study after study has told us that focusing on healthcare safety and quality is fundamental to achieving better health outcomes while avoiding unnecessary costs. Although great strides have been made in the area of quality measurement within the acute care setting, and more recently in the ambulatory environment, much less has been written about how we should measure quality in the context of population health.

Many published articles have cited the existing publication of vital statistics and other measures associated with public health agencies, such as the rate of smoking among high school students or the morbidity and mortality associated with national health problems such as obesity or the opioid epidemic. Many have described approaches for measuring quality in commercial health plans or employer-sponsored plans, emphasizing the use of Healthcare Effectiveness Data and Information Set (HEDIS) measures. What is lacking in all these discussions, however, is the central element of what's most important when assessing quality for populations. We need to answer the question of how we harmonize our various measures and measurement strategies to eliminate duplication and to focus on what really matters.

The challenges facing quality measurement in population health are numerous. They include lack of alignment of key measures between public- and private-sector quality improvement efforts; issues regarding data transfer, such as merging data across different information technology platforms or across different organizations on the healthcare continuum; ensuring protection of sensitive patient data; and developing, endorsing, and implementing measures of value—that is, measures that include both quality and cost information (McClellan 2013). However, the most important obstacle to greater use and impact of quality measures in population health is the fact that, today, quality still plays a relatively minor role in those systems that finance population health initiatives.

Obtaining a meaningful picture of the overall quality of healthcare within a population, particularly at the patient level, is difficult when quality measures have to accompany dozens of specific services across the various provider types and locations. Although these specific aspects of care do matter, what really matters to most patients is how these specific services or aspects of care come together for their individual needs. Patients with a chronic disease such as diabetes or hypertension will likely be most concerned with answers to such questions as, "Am I using the right medications that minimize the chance of the disease progressing?" For other individuals in the population with risk factors for a chronic disease, the questions might center on whether they are receiving the support they need to make the necessary lifestyle changes to reduce the risk of the disease becoming manifest. These questions reflect multidimensional, complex, and highly personal issues that cannot be measured perfectly and that, in the end, depend on clinicians' ability to focus on the needs and goals of each individual patient. These challenges are multiplied a thousandfold when the focus changes from a hospital's intensive care unit to a community population within a large metropolitan area.

Addressing these challenges will require a clear commitment to establishing a quality measurement strategy for population health. Although the

National Quality Forum has endorsed hundreds of measures, many of which are included in Medicare's payment system, relatively few assess quality in populations and even fewer address outcomes of interest for patients and their families. Measurement of population health safety and quality will likely be facilitated by a growing set of case- and patient-level measures that are becoming available or that could soon transition into more widespread use (McClellan 2013).

For instance, instead of tracking body mass index screenings, a more effective and meaningful outcome-oriented measure for gauging quality of care within a population would be the percentage of individuals screened as obese who actually followed up on recommended actions as prescribed by their physician or care manager. An even broader measure that is being implemented in some healthcare organizations is a ten-year mortality predictor developed by Elliott Fischer and colleagues at Dartmouth Medical School and the University of Washington. The measure incorporates 12 major health and behavioral risk factors and can be used to counsel and engage patients, while also tracking risk reduction across the population (McClellan 2013).

These newer measures are geared toward improving the outcomes that matter to patients. Thus, they can be regarded as much more patient centered, and they begin moving us along the evolutionary pathway toward true patient-reported outcome measures (PROMs) addressing experience and functionality.

In the context of system-level quality improvement and the notion that improving quality concurrently reduces or eliminates inequities, the same measures used for quality improvement should be applied to initiatives aiming to reduce inequities. AHRQ uses identical quality measures—across the quality dimensions of patient safety, timeliness, effectiveness, and patient centeredness—in both its *National Healthcare Quality Report* and its *National Healthcare Disparities Report*. The use of identical measures for improving quality and concurrently eliminating healthcare inequities is based on previous guidance by IOM (Hurtado, Swift, and Corrigan 2001).

Healthcare organizations need a sound methodological approach to establish a balanced set of measures to assess quality, safety, and equity as they relate to population health. The measures should be selected based on importance (e.g., potential impact of health problems, policymakers' and consumers' concerns, the systems' capacity to address the problem), scientific soundness (e.g., scientific evidence for the measure, validity, reliability across population groups), and feasibility (e.g., amount and timeliness of data collection, cost of data collection, comparison across population groups). The measures should also be linked to the various perspectives and priorities articulated in the organization's mission and goals. Focused data collection and analysis of specific safety and quality problems identified in hospital, ED, and ambulatory practice settings, as well as the targeted interventions to address these problems, must complement this approach of measuring and reporting a core set of population health safety and quality indicators.

Some providers and collaborations across providers are moving forward with implementing population-focused patient registries and tracking systems with detailed quality assessments to take advantage of new value-based and risk-sharing models of reimbursement (McClellan 2013). The reasoning is that quality improvement initiatives that lead to optimizing the patient experience and outcomes within a population (e.g., a managed Medicaid health plan or a bundled-payment demonstration project) will result in greater financial support, which in turn will allow for more innovative care delivery initiatives to take place, thereby producing better outcomes and patient experiences.

Going Forward

Having examined the topic of population health safety and quality in the preceding pages, we are at last left with the need to plot our path forward—to continue the conversation about what safety and quality should look like in a population health world.

The greatest benefit for a population comes from a comprehensive view of the needs of that population and the improvements made to address those needs. The well-being of a population, as measured by the yardsticks of safety and quality, is best achieved by viewing the healthcare ecosystem as a whole and focusing policies on those changes that will have the greatest impact across that ecosystem. To that end, the landmark IOM report *Crossing the Quality Chasm: A New Health System for the 21st Century* lays out a clear vision for what a robust population health safety and quality road map should entail (IOM 2001, xi).

The IOM report asserts that healthcare safety and quality problems within a population exist because of limited infrastructure and outmoded care systems, which result in a cycle of suboptimal care being repeated throughout the many levels of care. The report calls for fundamental reform "to ensure that all Americans receive care that is safe, effective, patient centered, timely, efficient, and equitable" (IOM 2001). Those six aims can be further described as follows.

- *Safe*: Avoid harming patients with the care that is intended to help them.
- *Timely*: Reduce waiting times and delays for both those who receive care and those who give it.
- *Effective*: Provide evidence-based services to all who are likely to benefit and refrain from providing services to those not likely to benefit.
- *Efficient*: Avoid waste; use finite resources with prudence.

- *Equitable*: Provide care that does not vary in quality based on personal characteristics such as gender, ethnicity, age, or socioeconomic status.
- *Patient-centered*: Place the patient and the patient's family at the center of everything we do; be respectful and responsive to the patient's preferences, needs, and values.

Only through such a comprehensive approach, driven by data and established by policy, can we hope to deliver a healthcare ecosystem that optimizes safety and quality for all people all of the time.

Although major federal legislation has brought significant reform to the healthcare system, much remains to be done legislatively to arrive at a place that optimizes population health; engages patients; and effectively addresses the numerous social, physical, environmental, and economic determinants that are now known to contribute to a population's health. Many influential policy leaders—including Mike Leavitt, Donna Shalala, Tom Daschle, and Mark McClellan, among others—have argued that the most important thing that policymakers can do to improve patient safety and healthcare quality is to make changes in healthcare payments and benefits so that they can better support patient-centered care (McClellan 2013). Such changes should allow providers and other community-based organizations to deliver to individual patients the services they need, rather than just what is covered in a traditional fee-for-service payment environment.

In addition to the reform of healthcare financing and regulatory policy, we need to develop a better understanding of the dynamics of population health safety and quality and their impact on health disparities and patient experience. Such an understanding can be advanced through a research framework that addresses three critical areas:

1. *The individual*—examining factors such as individual health promotion, care-seeking behaviors, and the way the individual interacts with social networks related to health and disease processes
2. *The community*—seeking to clarify the engagement of community-based organizations and the ways they interact with the individual in terms of access, utilization of services, and outcomes of care
3. *The patient–clinician relationship*—focusing on the nature of the relationship between patient and clinician, especially its establishment, the communication and trust that underlies such a partnership, participation in shared decision making, and the impact of health literacy

A focus on these three dimensions will be essential for building a more cohesive and sustainable model for population health safety and quality.

Conclusion

The challenge of population health safety and quality does not lie solely in how we choose to define the concept, though competing definitions have certainly introduced a degree of ambiguity. Nor is it exclusively an issue of what and how we measure, or the divide that exists between private personal healthcare (i.e., medical care) and public health services. Rather, the challenge we face with understanding and optimizing the concept are multidimensional, extending across a variety of disciplines and stakeholder groups. Compared to safety and quality in the acute care or ambulatory environments, population health safety and quality reflect an amorphous, all-encompassing state—one that we are only just now recognizing and coming to terms with.

Stakeholders and industry leaders must push for the healthcare delivery and financing reforms needed to improve population safety and quality. By advocating for policy and legislative changes that foster better patient-centered care and support the hardworking professionals who make a difference in patients' lives every day, we can, in time, make progress on, or even resolve, the challenges outlined in this chapter.

Study Questions

1. Why is the concept of population health safety and quality relatively new to healthcare's lexicon of terms?
2. Describe the importance of health equity and socioeconomic determinants of health in developing a comprehensive definition of population health safety and quality.
3. In today's healthcare ecosystem, how do traditional medical care providers and public health agencies work together to bring about population health safety and quality?

References

Agency for Healthcare Research and Quality (AHRQ). 2015. "2013 Annual Hospital-Acquired Condition Rate and Estimates of Cost Savings and Deaths Averted from 2010 to 2013." Published October. www.ahrq.gov/sites/default/files/publications/files/hacrate2013_0.pdf.

Anderson, L. M., S. C. Scrimshaw, M. T. Fullilove, J. E. Fielding, and J. Normand. 2003. "Culturally Competent Healthcare Systems: A Systematic Review." *American Journal of Preventive Medicine* 24 (Suppl. 3): 68–79.

Betancourt, J. R., A. R. Green, J. E. Carrillo, and E. R. Park. 2005. "Cultural Competence and Health Care Disparities: Key Perspectives and Trends." *Health Affairs* 24 (2): 499–505.

Boston Children's Hospital. 2018. "Community Asthma Initiative." Accessed December 13. www.childrenshospital.org/centers-and-services/programs/a-_-e/community-asthma-initiative-program.

Centers for Medicare & Medicaid Services (CMS). 2018a. "About the Partnership for Patients." Accessed December 11. https://partnershipforpatients.cms.gov/about-the-partnership/aboutthepartnershipforpatients.html.

———. 2018b. "Accountable Health Communities Model." Updated October 23. https://innovation.cms.gov/initiatives/ahcm/.

Cohen, J. K. 2017. "How a Texas Innovation Hub Is Eliminating Socioeconomic Disparities in Health." *Becker's Hospital Review.* Published September 21. www.beckershospitalreview.com/population-health/how-a-texas-innovation-hub-is-eliminating-socioeconomic-health-disparities.html.

Davis, S. K., Y. Liu, and G. H. Gibbons. 2003. "Disparities in Trends in Hospitalization for Potentially Preventable Chronic Conditions Among African Americans During the 1990s: Implications and Benchmarks." *American Journal of Public Health* 93 (3): 447–55.

Hearts Beat Back. 2018. "Who We Are." Accessed December 13. http://heartsbeatback.org/about-us/who-we-are.

Heiman, H. J., and S. Artiga. 2015. "Beyond Health Care: The Role of Social Determinants in Promoting Health and Health Equity." Kaiser Family Foundation. Published November 5. http://files.kff.org/attachment/issue-brief-beyond-health-care-the-role-of-social-determinants-in-promoting-health-and-health-equity.

Hurtado, M. P., E. K. Swift, and J. M. Corrigan. 2001. *Envisioning the National Health Care Quality Report.* Washington, DC: National Academies Press.

Institute of Medicine (IOM). 2001. *Crossing the Quality Chasm: A New Health System for the 21st Century.* Washington, DC: National Academies Press.

Kindig, D. A. 2007. "Understanding Population Health Terminology." *Milbank Quarterly* 85 (1): 139–61.

Kohn, L. T., J. M. Corrigan, and M. S. Donaldson (eds.). 2000. *To Err Is Human: Building a Safer Health System.* Washington, DC: National Academies Press.

Mayberry, R. M., F. Mili, and E. Ofili. 2000. "Racial and Ethnic Differences in Access to Medical Care." *Medical Care Research and Review* 57 (Suppl. 1): 108–45.

Mayberry, R. M., D. A. Nicewander, H. Qin, and D. J. Ballard. 2006. "Improving Quality and Reducing Inequities: A Challenge in Achieving Best Care." *Baylor University Medical Center Proceedings* 19 (2): 103–18.

McClellan, M. B. 2013. "Improving Health Care Quality: The Path Forward." Brookings Institute. Published June 26. www.brookings.edu/testimonies/improving-health-care-quality-the-path-forward/.

McGinnis, J. M., P. G. Russo, and J. R. Knickman. 2002. "The Case for More Active Policy Attention to Health Promotion." *Health Affairs* 21 (2): 83.

Nerenz, D. R. 2005. "Health Care Organizations' Use of Race/Ethnicity Data to Address Quality Disparities." *Health Affairs* 24 (2): 409–16.

O'Connor, P. 2017. "Point-of-Care Prioritized Clinical Decision Support Reduces Cardiovascular Risk in Adults with Elevated Cardiovascular Risks: A Randomized Trial." Invited abstract, 10th Annual Conference on the Science of Dissemination and Implementation in Health, Academy Health, Arlington, VA, December 4–6.

Public Health Service. 1994. *For a Healthy Nation: Returns on Investment in Public Health.* Washington, DC: US Department of Health and Human Services.

Rudolph, L., J. Caplan, K. Ben-Moshe, and L. Dillon. 2013. *Health in All Policies: A Guide for State and Local Governments.* Washington, DC, and Oakland, CA: American Public Health Association and Public Health Institute.

Swift, E. K. 2002. "Disparities in Health Care: Methods for Studying the Effects of Race, Ethnicity, and SES on Access, Use, and Quality of Health Care." Institute of Medicine. Revised March 7. www.nationalacademies.org/hmd/~/media/Files/Activity%20Files/Quality/NHDRGuidance/DisparitiesGornick.pdf.

Towers Watson. 2012. "Wellness Programs and In-House Care: How Hospitals Can Lower Employee Health Coverage Costs." Accessed December 11, 2018. www.towerswatson.com/~/media/Pdf/Services/hospitals/Hospital-wellness-programs.ashx.

US Office of Disease Prevention and Health Promotion. 2018. "Leading Health Indicators." Accessed December 12. www.healthypeople.gov/2020/Leading-Health-Indicators.

———. 2014. "Midcourse Review." Accessed December 12, 2018. www.healthypeople.gov/2020/data-search/midcourse-review/lhi.

INDEX

Note: Italicized page locators refer to tables and figures in exhibits.

AAFP. *See* American Academy of Family Physicians (AAFP)
AAP. *See* American Academy of Pediatrics (AAP)
abcdeSIM game, 222–23
Absenteeism, 449
Abstract conceptualization: in Kolb's cycle of learning, 219, *219*
ACA. *See* Affordable Care Act (ACA)
Academy for Emerging Leaders in Patient Safety (AELPS): curriculum for, 291–92; expansion of, 291; gaming and low-fidelity simulation in, 292, 294–95; program acceptance for, 292; as spin-off of Telluride Interdisciplinary Roundtables, 291; stories, narratives, and reflective practice in, 292, 293–94; unique aspects of, 292
Access to Better Care Act, 426
Accountability, 230; creating culture of, 186; performance measurement and, 458; safe systems and, 271; safety culture and, 264. *See also* Transparency
Accountable care organizations (ACOs), 59, 185, 376, 399, 403; ambulatory quality and safety and, 368, 370; analyzing variation and, 82; definition of, 368; development of, 54; measurement burden and, 406, 407; measures used in establishing quality performance standards for, in meeting shared savings, *369*; new applications of variation data and, 93; quality measures focus of, 461; quality metrics submitted by, 302
Accountable Health Communities (AHC) initiative (CMS), 478
Accreditation: healthcare quality improvement and, 366; medical home, 396; NCQA, 392–93, 402; quality measures and metrics and, 301
Accreditation Association for Ambulatory Health Care: medical home accreditation and certification program, 396
Accreditation Council for Graduate Medical Education (ACGME): Clinical Learning Environment Review (CLER) program, 286–88; Task Force on Quality Care and Professionalism, 286
Accuracy: of measure calculations, 408
ACE inhibitors: CHF patients and use of, 114
ACGME. *See* Accreditation Council for Graduate Medical Education (ACGME)
ACOs. *See* Accountable care organizations (ACOs)
ACP. *See* American College of Physicians (ACP)
ACS. *See* American College of Surgeons (ACS)
Action: health IT for, literature and discussion of, 192; health IT for: case study, 201–4
Actionable level: survey results reporting at, 118
Active experimentation: in Kolb's cycle of learning, 219, *219*

Activities of daily living (ADL) measure, 54
Acute care hospitals, 363; CMS PfP initiative and, 477
Acute myocardial infarction (AMI): aspirin and beta-blocker therapy for, 115; beta-blocker treatment for, 391–92; improved quality metrics and savings for patients with, 348
ADA. *See* American Diabetes Association (ADA)
Adherence: clinical nuance and, 418; clinical nuance in V-BID programs and, 419; health equity issues and, 482; higher-value care and, 445; pharmacist–patient relationships and, 464
Adjusted Risk Choice & Outcomes Legislative Assessment (ARCOLA) simulation model, 425
Administrative compensation, 60
Administrative data, 104, 124n2; cost-effectiveness and, 110–11
Administrative databases, 115–17; maintenance costs and, 117; reliability issues with, 117
Administrative data sources: advantageous use of, 116; examples of, 115–16
Administrators: STEEEP aims and, 13
Adult learning: implications of, on simulation training, 218–20
Advanced Alternative Payment Models (APMs), 176, 185, 371, 449
"Advanced medical home": history behind, 394–95. *See also* Patient-centered medical homes (PCMHs)
Adventist Health System, 264
Adverse drug events, 477; preventable, 457; transitions of care in ambulatory setting and, 373. *See also* Medication errors
Adverse events: hospital-related, diagnostic errors and, 9; prevalence of, 60; preventing, 258. *See also* Medical errors
Advisory Committee on Immunization Practices, 419
AELPS. *See* Academy for Emerging Leaders in Patient Safety (AELPS)
Aetna, 480
Affordable Care Act (ACA), 65, 176, 360, 458, 486; Hospital Readmissions Reduction Program and, 448; HVBP Program and, 88; marketplaces and, 402; Michigan's Medicaid expansion under, 428; NCQA accreditation requirements and, 392; passage of, 234, 367, 402; preventive health provisions of, 418; proliferation of ACOs and, 93; reporting of quality measures and, 184–85; solidified role of V-BID and, 419
African Americans: health equity issues and, 481
Agency for Health Care Policy and Research (AHCPR), 62
Agency for Healthcare Research and Quality (AHRQ), 41, 234, 257, 270, 338, 371, 392; founding of, 365; history behind, 62; identical quality measures used by, 494; metrics for quality measures, 341; *National Healthcare Disparities Report,* 494; *National Healthcare Quality Report,* 5, 7–8, 494; National Quality Strategy established by, 405; National Quality Strategy updates by, 458; patient safety in ambulatory setting report, 372; TeamSTEPPS and, 223
Aging population, polypharmacy and, 457
AHCPR. *See* Agency for Health Care Policy and Research (AHCPR)
AHIP. *See* America's Health Insurance Plans (AHIP)
AHRQ. *See* Agency for Healthcare Research and Quality (AHRQ)
Airline industry: deregulated, 65
Alerts: safe and effective clinical decisions and, 195; as subset of clinical decision support, 191, 205
Algorithmic diagnostic trees, 191
Algorithms: for just culture, 272

Alignment: of incentives, for ambulatory quality and safety, 375; of measures throughout healthcare system, 407–8
Alignment, creating around organizational quality strategy, 301–25; as critical leadership function, 301; leadership, measurement, and improvement, 308–17, 319–24; quality assurance, 305, *305,* 306; quality control, 305, *305,* 306–7; quality improvement, 305, *305,* 307–8; quality measures and metrics, 301–5
Alliance coalition (Wisconsin): QualityPath's innovative approach and, 442–43
Allina Health, 491
Alternative dispute resolution, 60
Alternative payment models (APMs): moving payment from fee-for-service models to, 405; value-based, MACRA and, 403–4
Amalberti, Rene, 263
Amazon: collaboration between Berkshire Hathaway, Chase, and, 361, 453
Ambulatory care, 56; definition of, 363; fragmented nature of, 372; traditional sites of, 363
Ambulatory Care Quality Alliance (AQA): creation of, 405
Ambulatory care settings, 363–64; challenges to delivery of safe care in, 372–74; diagnostic errors in, 373–74; medication safety concerns in, 373; referrals throughout, 373; regulation and, 364; test tracking in, 373; transitions of care in, 373; unique challenges related to, 364
Ambulatory quality improvement, 364–68, 370–71; accountable care organizations and, 368, *369,* 370; Affordable Care Act and, 367–68; compensation and aligning incentives in, 375; future challenges and keys to success in, 374–76; historical development of, 364–66; MACRA and shift from measuring process to measuring outcomes, 370–71; number and standardization of measures in, 375–76; pay for performance and expansion of, 366–67; role of primary care and subspecialty providers in, 374–75; transparency of data to other providers and the public, 376
Ambulatory safety, 359, 371–74; challenges in, 372–74; evolution of patient safety movement, 371–72; referral follow-up and, 382; strategies for, 374
Ambulatory surgery centers, 359, 363
American Academy of Family Physicians (AAFP), 405; "Future of Family Medicine" report, 395
American Academy of Pediatrics (AAP), 394, 395
American Association for Colleges of Nursing, 288
American Benefits Council, 453
American Board of Internal Medicine Foundation: Choosing Wisely campaign, 452
American Board of Internal Medicine (ABIM) Foundation, 430
American College of Cardiology: clinical practice guidelines, 92
American College of Physicians (ACP), 52, 394, 395, 405; Council of Subspecialty Societies, 397
American College of Surgeons (ACS), 51, 52, 58; National Surgical Quality Improvement Project, 238
American Diabetes Association (ADA), 112, 121, 122
American Heart Association: clinical practice guidelines, 92
American Heart Society, 226
American Hospital Association, 41, 52, 477
American Medical Association, 52, 63
American Osteopathic Association (AOA), 395
American Pharmacists Association (APhA): medication therapy management defined by, 464

American Recovery and Reinvestment Act (ARRA), 401
America's Health Insurance Plans (AHIP), 405, 406
AMI. *See* Acute myocardial infarction (AMI)
Analytic statistics, 105, 130, 156, 162
Anatomic models of human body, 215
Anderson, Odin, 52
Anesthesia, 50
Anesthesia Crisis Resource Management program, 218
Animals: practice of surgical skills on, 215
Antibiotics, 50, 63
Antibiotic stewardship programs, 372
Anticipation: in "Weick and Sutcliffe five," elements within, 264
AOA. *See* American Osteopathic Association (AOA)
API. *See* Associates in Process Improvement (API)
APMs. *See* Advanced Alternative Payment Models (APMs)
Apprenticeship model, in medical education, 216–17
AQA. *See* Ambulatory Care Quality Alliance (AQA)
ARCC mechanism (Healthcare Performance Improvement), 270
ARCOLA simulation model. *See* Adjusted Risk Choice & Outcomes Legislative Assessment (ARCOLA) simulation model
ARRA. *See* American Recovery and Reinvestment Act (ARRA)
Artificial intelligence, 490
Ascension Health, 477
Asheville Project (North Carolina), 441
Assignable (or special-cause) variation, 92, 94; definition and relevance to healthcare quality research/improvement, *76*
Associates in Process Improvement (API): model for improvement, 19, *19*
Association of American Medical Colleges, 279; Integrating Quality Leadership Group, 231
Attention: universal skill bundles and, 269
Attribution: analyzing variation and challenge of, 82–83
Augmented reality, 215
Autocorrelation: control charts and, 86
Automated dispensing units, 257
Automated systems: reliability, resilience, and, 261
AvaMed, 63
Avatars, 361
Average(s): avoid using indicators based on, 321–22; in control charts, 141; using median *vs.*, for run chart, 138–39
Averill, Rich, 55
Aviation industry: guidance document use and, 270; high reliability organizing and, 259; learning from, 280; safety culture and, 257

Back surgeries: appropriate use of MRIs and outcomes of, 62
Balanced Scorecard, The: Translating Strategy into Action (Kaplan and Norton), 303
"Balanced Scorecard, The: Measures That Drive Performance" (Kaplan and Norton), 303
Balanced scorecards, 321, 325n3; first use of term, 303; organizational strategy and, 304
Baldrige Award winners: transparency and, 324
Bar-code scanning, 257, 261
Bar graphs, 313
Barraclough, Bruce, 283
Barrows, Harold, 217
Bass, Eric B., 279
Batalden, Paul, 54
BayCare Health System (Florida): governing for quality in, 353–56
BayCare Physician Partners, 353

Baylor Scott & White Health (BSWH), case example, 91–92, *92*; inconsistent use of evidence-based HF therapies in observed hospitals within, 91; performance on "all indicated services" bundle measure for heart failure, 92, *92*
Baylor Scott & White Quality Alliance (BSWQA): patient-risk stratification process used by, 93, *93*; warranted variation and risk stratification conducted at contract population level, 94
Beane, Billy, 63, 64
Beecher, Henry, 51
Behavioral economics: consumer engagement and, 445
Behavior-shaping factors: reliability and, 260; safety, quality, and, 261
Benchmarks/benchmarking, 105; effective boards, quality of care, and, 333–34; examples of, for structure, process, and outcome measures, *16*; external benchmark data used to establish standards and targets, 323; goal of, 341; for patient and employee satisfaction, 316; performance information to pharmacies and, 465; physician's performance, 180; in quality dashboard report for the board, 342–43; reducing unwarranted variation in effective care and, 81
Berkshire Hathaway: collaboration between Amazon, Chase, and, 361, 453
Berwick, Donald, 59, 127, 458
Best practices: benchmarking of physician's performance and, 180; high reliability, improved quality, and, 266; for quality oversight, 339; researching and defining, AHRQ and, 365. *See also* Benchmarks/benchmarking
Better Care, Lower Cost Act of 2014, 420
Bipartisan Budget Act of 2018, 421
Black, Diane, 423, 426
Block grants, 491
Blue Cross Blue Shield of Michigan: medical home accreditation and certification program, 396
Blumenauer, Earl, 423, 426
Blunt-end factors: reliability and, 260
Board certification: provider profiles and, 175
Board of directors, 329; fiduciary duties of, 330; governance for quality and, 329
Board of trustees, 329; governance for quality and, 329
Boeing, 453, 478
Boston Children's Hospital, 492
Boston Community Asthma Initiative case study, 492
Boundarilessness: as high-impact leadership behavior, *309*
Bradley, Vernon, 258
Brainstorming, 155
Breast cancer screening rates: racial/ethnic disparities and, 483
Bridges to Excellence (BTE) program, 360, 451
British Medical Journal, 9
Brittleness: system resilience equation and, 261
Brook, Bob, 56
BTE program. *See* Bridges to Excellence (BTE) program
Bundle compliance data: control chart of baseline data, intervention, and completed transition, *161*; control chart of baseline data and first three months of intervention data, showing beneficial special cause, *161*; Pareto analysis, 155–59; Pareto analysis data as two-dimensional matrix, *158*; Pareto chart of bundle element noncompliances, 156, *156*; Pareto chart of bundle noncompliances by hospital, 156, *157*; Pareto matrix data with special causes highlighted,

158; relaxing the eight-in-a-row rule, 160; run chart of most recent baseline with five months of intervention data, *160*
Bundle element noncompliances: Pareto chart of, 156, *156*
Bureau of Labor Statistics, 254
Burnout: healthcare workforce and, 279; physicians, poor alignment and, 375

Cadaveric dissections, 215
Cadaveric models: procedural training and, 223
CAHPS measures: advent of, 234; framing of, 235; top-box rating, 235, *235,* 241
Camden, New Jersey: place-based healthcare approach in, 486
Camden Coalition, 486
Canadian Medical Association, 52
Cancer Care Quality Alliance, 405
"Can You Prove Anything With Statistics?" (Balestracci), 130
Capitation: HMO structure and, 365, 366
Cardiac angiographies: variation data on, 90
Cardiac surgery: surgical site infections metric for, 345
"Care bundles" use of, 154
Caregivers: bundles of universal skills for, 268–69
Care managers: population safety and quality and, 488
Care navigators: population health model and, 488
Care outcomes: research on board practices and, 333
Care protocols: standardizing, quality improvement and, 350
CareSource (Ohio), 479
Carper, Thomas R., 426
Case managers, 59
Case mix, 2, 54, 64
Case rates, 447
Case studies/case examples: Baylor Scott & White Health, 91–92, *92*; Boston Community Asthma Initiative, 492; Comprehensive Primary Care Plus, 379–80; difficulty of measuring quality of mental health and substance abuse services, 58–59; governance oversight of quality performance, *318,* 318–19; governing for quality, 353–56; Hearts Beat Back, 491–92; implementation of Connecticut's Health Enhancement Plan, 433–34; improving mortality from sepsis, *202,* 202–4, *203, 204*; Mr. Roberts and the US healthcare system, 33–37; new pay-for-performance contract, 380–81; preventing high-risk safety events through use of a hard-stop alert, 195–97; private practice in Pennsylvania Chronic Care Initiative, 377–79; reducing length of stay of orthopedic postoperative patients, 198–201, *199, 200*; referral follow-up and ambulatory safety, 382
Catalyst for Payment Reform (CPR), 444
Caterpillar charts, 83
Catheter-associated urinary tract infections (CAUTIs), 477; CUSP toolkit and, 43
Catheter-related bloodstream line infections, stopping at Johns Hopkins and hospitals across US, 38–43; average CLABSI rates per unit, *42*; CUSP program, 38–39, *39–40,* 41, 43; percentage of reporting units with CLABSI rate of 0/1,000 or less than 1/1,000 central line days, *42*
Catholic Healthcare Partners. *See* Mercy Health
CathPCI Registry: variation data in, 90
Cause analysis, 23–24; cause-and-effect/fishbone diagrams, 23–24, *24*; "five whys" exercise in, 23; skillful, 23
Cause-and-effect diagrams, 23–24, 154, *155*
CAUTIs. *See* Catheter-associated urinary tract infections (CAUTIs)
CBO. *See* Congressional Budget Office (CBO)

CBOs. *See* Community-based service delivery organizations (CBOs)
c-charts, 147
CCM. *See* Chronic Care Model (CCM)
Center for Medicare & Medicaid Innovation (CMMI), 402–3, 421; V-BID Model Test announced by, 420–21
Center for Transforming Healthcare, 257
Centers for Disease Control and Prevention (CDC), 489; Total Worker Health movement promoted by, 450
Centers for Medicare & Medicaid Services (CMS), 57, 103, 134, 174, 239, 312, 334, 363, 370, 404, 406, 423; Accountable Health Communities (AHC) initiative, 478, 487; ACOs defined by, 368; Berwick's administrative leadership at, 458; Comprehensive Primary Care Plus program, 379–80; data collection methods and, 243; Enhanced MTM test model, 467–68; expansion of V-BID Model, 421; Five-Star Quality Rating System for Medicare Advantage, 461; HCAHPS survey adopted by, 234; Health Care Payment Learning and Action Network, 405; Hospital-Acquired Condition (HAC) Reduction Program, 448; Hospital Compare website, 177, 184; Hospital Readmissions Reduction Program administered by, 88; Hospital VBP Program, 448; as largest public purchaser, 439; Medicare administered by, 447; Medicare's nonpayment of "never events," 447–48; medication therapy management completion rate measures, 360; metrics for quality measures, 341; Oncology Care Model, 181; Partnership for Patients (PfP) initiative, 477; Physician Compare performance scores, *177*; Physician Compare website, 172, 177, 184; Physician Quality Reporting System, 185, 367, 376; purchasing power of, 447; qualified clinical data registries recognized by, 172–73; quality and clinical indicators requirements, 303; quality measures defined by, 173; quality measures used by, 301, 302; Quality Payment Program, 176; ratings posted on consumer website of, 461; review set for heart attack, 322; Transforming Clinical Practice Initiative, 478; transition of eCQMs to CQL announced by, 408; Uniform Bill of, 124n2; value-based healthcare goals and, 460; Value-Based Purchasing (VBP) data set, 335; value-based purchasing programs, 447–49
Centers of excellence, 479
Central line–associated bloodstream infections (CLABSIs), 477; average rates, per unit, *42*; CUSP and elimination of, 38; percentage of reporting units with rate of 0/1,000 or less than 1/1,000 central line days, *42*; reductions in, 372
CEO. *See* Chief executive officer (CEO)
CER. *See* Comparative effectiveness research (CER)
Certification: in quality and safety fields, 296
Cervical cancer screening rates: racial/ethnic disparities and, 483
Cesarean rates: variation in, 75
CFO. *See* Chief financial officer (CFO)
CG-CAHPS. *See* Clinician and Groups CAHPS (CG-CAHPS)
Chalk, Mady, 58, 59
Change management model, 267
Charleston Community Memorial Hospital, 330
Chart audits, 282
Charts. *See* Control charts; Flowcharts; I-charts; Run charts
Chase: collaboration between Berkshire Hathaway, Amazon, and, 361, 453
Checklist and protocol use: universal skill bundles and, 270
Checklist interventions, 372
Checklist Manifesto, The (Gawande), 30
Checklists, 29–30, 260

CHF. *See* Congestive heart failure (CHF)
Chief executive officer (CEO): quality, role of the board, and, 331–32
Chief financial officer (CFO): quality/cost linkage and, 348
Chief medical officer (CMO): quality, role of the board, and, 332
Chief quality officer, 332
Children's Health Insurance Program (CHIP), 402, 403
Choosing Wisely campaign, 360, 430, 452
Chronic Care Model (CCM): development and elements of, 394
Chronic disease/health conditions: HDHP enrollees with, 417; quality measurement in population health and, 493
Chronic Disease Management Act of 2018, 426
Chronic obstructive pulmonary disease (COPD): fiscal implications of MA V-BID programs and, 420, 421
Cigna, 480
CINs. *See* Clinically integrated networks (CINs)
CLABSIs. *See* Central line–associated bloodstream infections (CLABSIs)
Claims-based data, 57, 64
Claims-based metrics: medical records-based outcomes metrics *vs.*, 57
Claims databases, 120
Cleary, Paul, 61
Cleveland Clinic, 247
Clinical decision support: alerts as subset of, 191, 205
Clinical guidelines: decreasing unwarranted variation and, 81
Clinical indicators: capturing six domains of healthcare quality with, 87; evolving approaches to, 322
Clinical-level measures: costliness of measurement burden, 407
Clinically integrated networks (CINs), 103, 399, 406, 407
Clinical nuance: cost sharing and, 417–18; implementing in value-based insurance design, 418–19; low-value care issues and, 431; out-of-pocket costs for Medicare beneficiaries and, 423; value-based insurance design and tenets of, 441
Clinical outcomes, 174
Clinical outcomes score: VBP program and calculation of, 336
Clinical quality: current curricular work in, 286–98; early curricular work in, 281–86; reviewing, 312
Clinical quality domain: for data collected for quality measurements, 107, 110
Clinical Quality Language (CQL): trial-use, Health Level Seven (HL7) standard for, 408
Clinical quality measures: classification of, 174; development and validation of, 174
Clinical reporting (CR) system: in categories of data: case example, 107; clinical dashboard for total knee replacement, *109*; clinical dashboards for high-volume, high-cost medical conditions, and surgical procedures, *108*; optimal use of, 123–24; producing, 108; validation of common measures from, 117
Clinical trial statistics: statistics for improvement *vs.*, 128
Clinical variation, 2–3; unexplained, 175. *See also* Variation
Clinician and Groups CAHPS (CG-CAHPS), 234, 237
Clinicians: STEEEP aims and, 11–12
Clostridium difficile infections, hospital-onset, reductions in, 372
CMMI. *See* Center for Medicare & Medicaid Innovation (CMMI)
CMO. *See* Chief medical officer (CMO)
CMS. *See* Centers for Medicare & Medicaid Services (CMS)
CMS Innovation Center, 367

Cochrane Database of Systematic Reviews, 60
Codman, Ernest A., 2, 51, 52, 174
Cognitive debiasing field, 269
Cohen, Jordan, 279
Coinsurance: consumer cost sharing and, 416, *416*; definition of, 445; funding of healthcare system through, 439; high-cost services and, 431. *See also* Copayments; Deductibles; Premiums
Collective mindfulness principle, 262
College for Value-Based Purchasing of Health Benefits, 440
Colonoscopies: reference pricing and, 445–46
Colorado: family medicine resident curriculum in, 297–98
Color coding: color-coded indicators for data report formats, 313; color-coded quality performance, sample scorecard for a hospital board, 317, *317*; in quality dashboard report for the board, 342
Colorectal cancer (CRC) screening: clinically nuanced cost-sharing approach to, 418
Combination systems: reliability, resilience, and, 261
Comcast, 453
Command and control: high reliability organizations and, 262–63
Committee on the Costs of Medical Care, 59
Common cause limits: standard deviations and, 143
Common cause range: underestimating breadth of, 150
Common cause strategy: stratification, 152–59; Pareto analysis, 155–59; vague projects have some vague issues, 153–55
Common cause (or systemic) variation, 105, 135, 139, 162, 163; common mistakes involving calculation of, 143–45; process summary using run and control chart analyses, 142. *See also* Random variation
Commonwealth Fund, 174; healthcare spending study, 415; value-based purchasing strategies identified by, 440
Communication: safety culture and, 264; universal skill bundles and, 269; workforce safety cultures and, 263
Community-based service delivery organizations (CBOs), 487
Community health workers, 59; population health model, 488
Comparative effectiveness research (CER), 81, 361; definition and purpose of, 469
Compensation: impact of, on ambulatory quality and safety, 375
Complication rates, 57
Composite clinical indicators: using for processes, 322
Comprehensive Accreditation for Hospitals (TJC): Standard LD.01.03.01 of, 357n2
Comprehensive Anesthesia Simulation Environment, 216
Comprehensive Primary Care Plus (CPC+) model: case study, 379–80; primary care physicians and, 374
Comprehensive Unit-Based Safety Program (CUSP): addressing other hospital-acquired infections with, 43; creation of, 38; flowchart, *39–40*; implementing in hospitals across US, Spain, and England, 41; steps in implementation of, 38–39; success of, 41
Computed tomography (CT) scans: reference pricing and, 445
Concerned, uncomfortable, stop (CUS), 270
Concrete experience: in Kolb's cycle of learning, 219, *219*
Congestive heart failure (CHF): ACE inhibitors and, 114; Entresto and treatment for, 468; fiscal implications

of MA V-BID programs and, 420, *421*
Congressional Budget Office (CBO): offset estimate, high-value health plans, 424–25
Connecticut Health Enhancement Program (HEP), 419; implementation of, 433–34; value-based insurance design example, 428–29
Consumer Assessment of Healthcare Providers and Systems (CAHPS) survey, 366, 392
Consumer cost sharing, 360; clinical value and, 433; Connecticut Health Enhancement Program, 428; Healthy Michigan and, 428; increasing, 416–17; Medicaid and constraints on, 427; theoretical motivation for, 417; TRICARE usage and, 427
Consumerism, 2
Consumer reviews, online, 247–49
Consumers: behavioral economics and engagement of, 445; empowerment of, 49, 63, 65; increasing management role of, 60; STEEEP aims and, 13
Containment: in "Weick and Sutcliffe five," elements within, 264
Continuous flow: in Lean, 20
"Continuous Improvement as an Ideal in Health Care" (Berwick), 127
Continuous Quality Improvement (CQI), 282, 308
Contract strategy: quality goals and, 462, *463*
Control chart analysis: process summary conclusions, 142
Control chart for individual values. *See* I-charts
Control charts, 28, 105, 313; appropriate, according to data type and distribution, 85, *86*; averages used in, 141; correct, of diabetes guideline compliance data, 145, *146*; creating, 141; of diabetes guideline compliance data generated by typical statistical software, *145*; incorrect, of diabetes guideline compliance data using overall average and standard deviation, 144, *144*; inventor of, 143; pioneering use of, 50; statistical process control and, 84, 85; as very powerful tool, 139–47; of year-end review performance data, *142*
"Controlling Variation in Health Care: A Consultation from Walter Shewhart" (Berwick), 127
Co-occurrences, health IT and: co-occurrence codes in descending order, *192*
Cook, Richard, 260
"Cookbook medicine," 184
Copayments: Connecticut Health Enhancement Program, 428; consumer cost sharing and, 416, *416*; definition of, 445; employee populations and, 479; funding of healthcare system through, 439; Healthy Michigan and, 428; TRICARE program, 427; value-based design, 441. *See also* Coinsurance; Deductibles; Premiums
COPD. *See* Chronic obstructive pulmonary disease (COPD)
COPIC insurance company, 291
Core Quality Measure Collaborative: sets of measures produced by, 406
Coronary artery bypass grafts, 63
Cost sharing: employee populations and, 479; payments by type, distribution of (2004-2014), *416*. *See also* Consumer cost sharing
"Count Data: Easy as 1-2-3? Hardly" (Balestracci), 151
Countermeasures, 28
CPR. *See* Catalyst for Payment Reform (CPR)
CQI. *See* Continuous Quality Improvement (CQI)
CQL. *See* Clinical Quality Language (CQL)
Creating High-Quality Results and Outcomes Necessary to Improve

Chronic (CHRONIC) Care Act of 2017, 421, 423
Credentialing: board's quality oversight duties and, 346–47; provider profiles and, 175
Credit card industry: healthcare industry and, 189
Crew resource management (CRM), 106, 217, 223
Crimean War, 51
Crisis management training: simulation and, 217
Critical strategies: clear and measurable, 321
Critical thinking, 162; quality improvement and, 128; universal skill bundles and, 269
CRM. *See* Crew resource management (CRM)
Crossing the Quality Chasm (IOM), 1, 5, 7, 9, 11, 33, 172, 232, 233, 315, 365, 495
C-section rates: reducing, recommended actions for employers, 451–52
CT scans. *See* Computed tomography (CT) scans
Cultural competence: health equity and, 361, 483–84
Culture: behavior-shaping factors and, 260–61; intersection of leadership and, 229–32; of quality and safety, building, 352–53, 356
Culture transformation models: fundamental principles of, 266–67
Curricular work in clinical quality and patient safety, current, 286–98; Academy for Emerging Leaders in Patient Safety: Telluride experience, 291–95; ACGME Clinical Learning Environment Review Program, 286–88; family medicine resident curriculum in Colorado, 297–98; graduate-level educational programs in quality improvement and patient safety, 295–96; IHI Open School, 288–90, *289*; Quality and Safety Education for Nurses, 288; quality reports for residents at Thomas Jefferson University, 297; resident engagement in quality improvement at Detroit Medical Center, 297
Curricular work in clinical quality and patient safety, early, 281–86; Lucian Leape Institute, 284–86; Telluride experience, 282–83; *WHO Patient Safety Curriculum Guide for Medical Schools,* 283–84
CUS. *See* Concerned, uncomfortable, stop (CUS)
CUSP. *See* Comprehensive Unit-Based Safety Program (CUSP)
Customized health IT solutions: prevention and, 191
CVS/Aetna merger, 361

Dallas County hospitals: forest plot showing variation in 30-day risk-standardized heart failure mortality in Medicare patients in, *80*; funnel plot showing variation in 30-day risk-standardized heart failure mortality in Medicare patients in, *81*
Dana-Farber Cancer Institute, 256
Darling, Dorrence, II, 330, 331
Darling v. Charleston Community Memorial Hospital, 330, 356–57n1
Dartmouth Atlas of Health Care, 3, 50, 54, 75, 77
Dartmouth Medical School, 494
Daschle, Tom, 496
Dashboards, 231, 304, 324; description of, 173; formats for organizing, 312–13; overseeing quality in multiple-board health systems and, 345; performance-tracking, pharmacies and, 465, *466*; of quality aims tracked by board, *318*; quality dashboard report for the board, 342–44, *343–44*; results *vs.* activities focus and system of, 323; scorecards *vs.,* 304, 305; strategic, 321; in a strategic leadership system, 311–12; of strategic measures, 314; Strategic Quality and Safety Plan sample, *349*; using

organizational performance dimensions to align efforts with, 321. *See also* Scorecards
Data: administrative, 115–17; "dirty," 113; good, need for, 127; looking at horizontally, 138
Data, sources for quality improvement, 113–23; administrative databases, 115–17; essential objectives for, steps in, 113; functional status surveys, 119; health plan databases, 119–22; in-home and wearable technology, 123; medical record review (retrospective), 113–14; patient experience surveys, 117–19; patient (specialty-specific) registries, 122–23; prospective data collection, 114–15
Data analysis of patient experience, advances in, 244–45
Data analytics companies, 408
Data categories: case example, 107–10; clinical dashboard for total knee replacement, *109*; clinical dashboards for high-volume, high-cost medical conditions, and surgical procedures, *108*; clinical reporting (CR) system, 107–8
Data collection, 104, 107–23; categories of data: a case example, 107–10; challenges with, in healthcare, 85–86; focused, balanced set of quality measures and, 494; inpatient *vs.* outpatient data, 112; overview, 107; patient experience, advances in, 243–44; physician profiles and, 181; "point-of-care," 244; prospective, 110, 114–15; retrospective, 113; stockpiling, "just in case," 111–12; time and cost involved in, 110–11
Data collection and analysis, 23, 27–28; run charts and control charts in, 27–28, *28*; SMART aims in, 27
Data quality: patient experience, advances in, 243–44
Data report formats: types of, 313
"Data Torturing" (Mills), 130
Data warehouses, 119
Deaths: caused by human error, prevalence of, 254; medical errors and, 9, 254, 477
Debriefing: simulation and, 215, 220, 221
"Decision fatigue," 445
Decision support technology, 490
Decision Tree for Determining the Culpability of Unsafe Acts (Reason), 272
Deductibles: Connecticut Health Enhancement Program and elimination of, 428; consumer cost sharing and, 416, *416*; employee populations and, 479; funding of healthcare system through, 439; for high-deductible health plans, 423; increase in, 416–17; value-based design, 441. *See also* Coinsurance; Copayments; Premiums
Defects: Deming on, 50
Defense healthcare reform: use of V-BID in, 427
Dekker, Sidney, 271
Deming, W. Edwards, 2, 25, 50, 52, 55, 62, 135, 143, 303; PDSA cycle, 18, 19; on reducing variation, 130; seven deadly diseases of management, 64; System of Profound Knowledge, 308
Democrats: Affordable Care Act passed by, 402; MACRA and, 403
Density: in network diagrams, 192, *193, 194*
Department of Veterans Affairs, 103
Dependent variable: defining, case mix and, 54
Depression: healthcare workforce and, 279
Descriptive statistics, 105, 129
Determinants of health: new thinking about, 476. *See also* Physical determinants of health; Social determinants of health
Detroit Medical Center: resident engagement in quality improvement at, 297

Diabetes disease-management project: diabetes provider report, *120–21,* 121–22; inpatient data *vs.* outpatient data and, 112
Diabetes guideline compliance data, 137–38; applying the run chart rules in, 137; contrasting with use of trend lines, 137–38; control chart of, generated by typical statistical software, 145, *145*; correct control chart of, *146*; diabetes guideline compliance data with fitted trend line, 137, *138*; goal trap and, 146–47; incorrect control chart of, using overall average and standard deviation, 144, *144*; with most recent stable history identified, *154*; proper summary of, 145–46; run chart of diabetes guideline compliance data, *137*
Diabetes mellitus (DM): clinical nuance and eye examinations for people with, 418; fiscal implications of MA V-BID programs and, 420, *421*
Diabetes Recognition Program (NCQA), 394
Diablo Canyon Power Plant, 262
Diagnosis-related groups (DRGs), 447; development of, 55; implementation, important effects of, 56
Diagnostic errors: in ambulatory care settings, 373–74; definition of, 373; prevalence of, 9
Dialysis, 63
Dignity Health, 477
Dingell, Debbie, 423
"Dirty data," 113
Disease management programs: for employee populations, 479
Disparities in healthcare: health equity issues and, 481–84; health plan populations and, 480; poor quality and, 49; quality goals and alleviation of, 8; systemic factors related to, 482
DM. *See* Diabetes mellitus (DM)
DMAIC (define, measure, analyze, improve, and control), 21, 32
Donabedian, Avedis, 2, 14, 53, 54, 64, 174, 258, 364, 460
DRGs. *See* Diagnosis-related groups (DRGs)
"Drive to five": quality bonus payments and, 462; reaching, pharmacist–healthcare team collaboration and, 465, *466*; strategies to improve health plan improvement and, 462, *462*
Drug alerts, 195
Duke University Hospital: costs related to quality measures at, 302; HCAHPS survey questions example, 238–39
Duty of care: board of directors and, 330
Duty of obedience: board of directors and, 330
Dysfunction in care delivery: patient needs and, *243*; preventing, 242

Economic outcomes, 174
eCQM testing method, 408
Eddy, David, 281
Edington, Dee, 446
Education: health status and, 485
Education for healthcare quality and safety, 279–98; current curricular work in clinical quality and patient safety, 286–98; early curricular work in clinical quality and patient safety, 281–86; overview of, 280–81
Effective care, 2, 10, 232, 361; implications of unwarranted variation within, 78; population health safety and quality and, 495; quality improvement and, 7; quality measures and, 173
Effectiveness: AHRQ use of identical measures and quality dimension of, 494; organizational performance and, 315; organizational scorecard creation and potential measures for, 317; of quality improvement programs, maximizing, 376; in STEEEP framework, 10

Efficacy: comparative effectiveness research and, 469
Efficiency: organizational performance and, 315; organizational scorecard creation and potential measures for, 317; of quality improvement programs, maximizing, 376; resource focus, high reliability, and, 266; in STEEEP framework, 10–11
Efficient care, 2, 10, 232, 361; population health safety and quality and, 495; quality improvement and, 7; quality measures and, 173–74
EHR-generated documentation: primary goal of, 407
Eight-in-a-row rule: relaxing, 160
80/20 rule, 154, 163
Electronic health records (EHRs), 103, 181, 231, 257, 366, 468
Electronic Health Records (EHR) Incentive Program, 176, 185, 401, 404
Electronic medical records, 57, 58, 60, 64, 341
Electronic Quality Improvement Platform for Plans and Pharmacies (EQuIPP), 465
eMeasure Certification program (NCQA), 408
Emergency departments (EDs): freestanding, 359, 363; overuse of, 476
Emergent properties: reliability and, 260–62
Emerging trends, 359–61
Employee Benefits Research Institute, 446, 453
Employee populations: safety and quality in, 478–79
Employee satisfaction: benchmarks for, 316
Employer-focused VBP programs, examples of: Bridges to Excellence, 451; Choosing Wisely campaign, 452; Leapfrog Group and Leapfrog VBP platform, 450–51; Purchaser Value Network, 451–52
Employer-provided health insurance, 176–77, 439, 449
Employers: direct and indirect medical costs and, 449; self-funded *vs.* fully insured, 449; zero trend strategies for, 446
Employers as value-based purchasers, 449–52
Employment support: mental health and substance abuse services and, 59
Endogenous forces: unwarranted variation and, 79
Entresto, 468
Enumerative statistics, 105, 129–30, 155–56, 162
EQuIPP. *See* Electronic Quality Improvement Platform for Plans and Pharmacies (EQuIPP)
Equitable care, 2, 11, 232, 361; population health safety and quality and, 496; quality improvement and, 7; quality measures and, 174
Equity: organizational performance and, 315; organizational scorecard creation and potential measures for, 317; in STEEEP framework, 11
ERR. *See* Excess readmission ratio (ERR)
Error trapping: reliability improvement and, 270, *271*
e-surveys: response rates with, 243–44
"Evaluating the Quality of Medical Care" (Donabedian), 54, 364
Evaluation and decision making, 23, 24–25; Pareto chart and, 25; scatter diagrams and, 24, *25*
Evaluative measures: importance of, 236
Evidence-based medicine, 16; definition of, 62; quality management, impact of politics, and, 62–63
Evidence-based practice: safety culture and, 264
Excess readmission ratio (ERR), 448
Exclusive provider organizations (EPOs): NCQA accreditation and, 392

Executive leadership: changes in, 276
Exogenous forces: unwarranted variation and, 79–80
Expert Consensus Working Group, 283
Explicit chart review, 51
External failure: learning systems geared toward, 273
External success: learning systems geared toward, 273
Eye examinations: clinically nuanced cost-sharing approach to, 418

Faces of Medical Error, The: From Tears to Transparency (film series), 293
Faculty physicians, 217
Failure mode and effects analysis (FMEA): mistake proofing and, 27; in situ simulations and, 218
Falk, I. S., 52
Falls, 253, 308
Family physicians: successful population health strategy and, 374
"Faulty Systems, Not Faulty People" (Leape), 152
Feasibility: cost of data collection and reporting and, 125n6
Federal poverty level (FPL): Healthy Michigan and, 428; Medicaid eligibility and, 402
Fee-for-service payment models/system, 365; calls for phasing out, 443; moving payment to alternative payment models, 405; shift away from, 183, 476; transition to value-based payment system, 176, 302, 330, 347, 458
Ferguson, Tom, 65
Fetter, Bob, 55
Fidelity: simulation and, 214
Fiduciary duties: board-related, 330, 356
Finance: linking quality and, 347–48
Financial incentives, 367; consumer behavior and, 445; for high-quality care, 365; Hospital VBP Program and, 367–68; performance improvement infrastructures and, 363–64; provider profiles and, 185–86; quality metrics incorporated into, 176; "three-legged stool" of quality management and, 49
Financial performance: data collected for quality measurements and, 107, 110
"Find-a-doctor" websites, 248, 249
"First, do no harm" *(primum non nocere)*, 256
Fiscal indicators: capturing six domains of healthcare quality with, 87
Fischer, Elliott, 54, 494
Fishbone diagrams, 23–24, *24,* 154
Fitbits, 361
5 Million Lives Campaign, 257
5S program, steps in, 30–31
"Five Alive" program, 226
Five-in-a-row rule, 160
"Five whys" exercise, 23
Flexner, Abraham, 51
Flight simulators, in aviation industry, 215–16
Flowcharts: Comprehensive Unit-Based Safety Program, *39–40*; example of, *26*; quality improvement and, 26
FMEA. *See* Failure mode and effects analysis (FMEA)
Food deserts, 487
Forest plots: analyzing variation data with, 83; showing variation in 30-day risk-standardized heart failure mortality in Medicare patients for Dallas County hospitals, *80,* 84
"Form follows function" concept: healthcare quality and, 17
Formulary management: "drive to five" and, 462, *462*
For-profit organizations: performance scorecard development for, 315–16
"Four Data Processes, Eight Questions" (Balestracci), 155
Fourth Generation Management (Joiner), 141
FPL. *See* Federal poverty level (FPL)
Frames: simulation learners and, 215

Front line engagement: as high-impact leadership behavior, *309*
Functional status: data collected for quality measurements and, 107, 110
Functional status surveys, 119
Funnel plots: analyzing variation data with, 84; showing variation in 30-day risk-standardized heart failure mortality in Medicare patients for Dallas County hospitals, *81,* 84

Gaba, David, 216
Gainesville Anesthesia Simulator, 216
Galen, 103
Gaming: in AELPS programs, 292, 294–95
Gawande, Atul, 30
GDP. *See* Gross domestic product (GDP)
General Electric (GE), 20, 453
General internists: successful population health strategy and, 374
Georgetown University: graduate-level programs in quality and safety, 296
Gingrich, Newt, 63, 64
Gittelsohn, Alan, 54
Glover, J. Allison, 75
Glucometers, 123
Goal trap: diabetes guideline compliance data and, 146–47
Goldwater, Barry, 53
Good, Michael, 216
Google, 249
Google Glass, 215
Gordon, Michael, 216
Governance: definition of, 329
Governance for quality, 329–56; best practices for quality oversight, 339; board–hospital management relationship and, 331–32; case example, 353–56; as ethical and legal obligation, 329–31; fiduciary duties and responsibility for, 330, 356; in multiple-board health systems, 345; need and reasons for, 329–30, 331; research connecting board practices with quality, 332–36, 338
Governance function measures, 313, *313*
Governance Institute, The (TGI), 229, 232, 335, 338; best practices for quality oversight, 339; quality survey of not-for-profit hospitals and health systems, 334
Governing boards: engaging in development of organizational performance measures, 319; organizational performance assessment and, 311
Governing board's quality oversight duties, 340–48, 350; credentialing, 346–47; ensuring clinician engagement and leadership to promote quality, 348, 350; ensuring quality and patient safety, 340; framework for board's leadership of quality, 340, *340*; going beyond measuring to dig deeper, 344–46; linking quality and finance, 347–48; measuring quality and setting performance targets, 340–46; quality dashboard report and, 342–44, *343–44*
Governing body: organizational scorecard use and, 316
Graduate-level educational programs: in quality improvement and patient safety, 295–96
Great Recession of 2009, 401
Greenfield, Shelly, 56, 58
Gross domestic product (GDP): healthcare spending as percentage of, 49, 176, 415
Groundedness: in network diagrams, 192, *193, 194*
Group Health Research Institute: MacColl Center for Health Care Innovation, 394
Group practice model of care, 52, 59
Grundy, Paul, 395

Haldol: Parkinson's disease patients and, 196; stop-order results: number of attempts in ordering of, for Parkinson's patients, *197*
Hannan, Ed, 57, 58

Happiness, quality of life and, 52
Hard-stop alerts, 205; preventing high-risk safety events through use of, 195–97
Harm: definition of, 253. *See also* Patient harm
Harvard Business Review, 303
Harvard Malpractice Study, 60
Harvey, cardiology patient simulator, 216
HCAHPS surveys: experience measures in, 342
HCPLAN. *See* Health Care Payment Learning and Action Network (HCPLAN)
HDHPs. *See* High-deductible health plans (HDHPs)
Health: determinants of, new thinking about, 476; physical determinants of, 479, 484–87; social determinants of, 361, 479, 484–87
Health Affairs, 429
Healthcare: dimensions of performance in, 314–15; elements of complete safety management system for, 255; as high-risk industry, 280; politics of, 2; rising costs of, 371
Healthcare, volume-to-value shift in, 457–63; "drive to five" and, *462*, 462–63; National Quality Strategy as a road map, 457–58, *459*; performance measurement and, 458, *460*, 460–61
Healthcare Bluebook website, 66n7
Healthcare delivery process: stories and narratives in, 293
Healthcare delivery system(s): correct care for, 256; human factors and, 275; QC measures collected throughout, 306
Healthcare Effectiveness Data and Information Set (HEDIS), 174, 303, 360, 366, 390, 409, 442, 493; Audit Committee, 391; health plans and reporting requirements, 391; measures, domains of care encompassed by, 391; retirement of measures in curation of, 391–92; retrospective medical record review and, 114
Healthcare expenditures: wasteful, low-value care and, 429. *See also* Healthcare spending
Health Care Financing Administration, 57, 174. *See also* Centers for Medicare & Medicaid Services (CMS)
Healthcare financing policy: reform of, 496
Healthcare industry: credit card industry and, 189
Healthcare leadership system: elements in, 311, *311*
Healthcare organizations: critical dimensions of performance in, *314*
Healthcare outcomes: nonhealthcare factors and, 52
Health Care Payment Learning and Action Network (HCPLAN): Alternative Payment Model (APM) Framework typology, 443–44; "big dot" measures as defined by, 408; CMS and creation of, 405
Healthcare Performance Improvement, 270; timeline of safety science and high reliability organizing, 257–58, *258*
Healthcare providers: population safety and quality and, 488. *See also* Nurses; Physicians
Healthcare quality: foundation of, 1–3; as a novel concept, 389; politics of, 404
Healthcare Quality and Safety Act: passage of, 371
Healthcare safety and quality leader: role of, 261
Healthcare spending: consumer cost sharing and slowing growth of, 416–17; as percentage of GDP, 49, 176, 415; serious fiscal challenges related to, 426; total, in United States, 457
Healthcare systems: applying variation to quality improvement, examples of, 90–91; board oversight of quality in, 329, 330; culturally competent,

483–84; four levels of, 7, *8*; profit motive and, 49
Health Enhancement Plan (Connecticut), 419
Health Enhancement Research Organization (HERO), 453
Health equity, 361; enhancing, approaches to, 483; safety and quality in a community and, 481–84
Healthgrades, 112, 185
Health in All Policies (HiAP), 489–90
Health information exchanges, 408
Health information technology, improving care delivery through: action: case study 3, 202–4; identification: case study 2, 198–201; prevention: case study 1, 195–97
Health information technology, in healthcare quality and safety, 189–92, 195; action, literature and discussion of, 192; co-occurrence codes in descending order, *192*; co-occurrences, 192; identification, literature and discussion of, 191–92; improving reliability of healthcare quality and safety, *190*; network diagram—action, *193*; network diagram—identification, *194*; network diagram—outcomes, *193*; network diagram—prevention, *194*; overview of the literature, 205–9; prevention, literature and discussion of, 191; resource planning and, 205
Health Information Technology for Economic and Clinical Health (HITECH) Act, 401–2; Title XII of, 401
Health information technology interventions: common, examples of, 205
Health insurance: early efforts in providing, 52; employer-sponsored, 176–77, 439, 449; value-based purchasing and, 176
Health insurance exchanges: Affordable Care Act and, 402
Health Insurance Portability and Accountability Act (HIPAA), 124n3
Health Level Seven (HL7) standard: for trial-use Clinical Quality Language, 408
Health maintenance organizations (HMOs), 59; cost-management capabilities of, 389; development of, 365; enrollment in, 389; NCQA accreditation and, 392; population health and success of, 366; premiums for, 425
HealthNEXT: central philosophy of, 446; "pressure points" identified by, 447
Health Partners (Minneapolis), 490
Health plan accreditation (HPA): by National Committee for Quality Assurance, 392–93
Health plan databases, 104; limitations of, 122; population health management and, 119–22
Health plan populations, 479–80
Health reform: solidified role of V-BID and, 419
Health reform, new era of (2009–2017), 400–404; Affordable Care Act, 402; Center for Medicare & Medicaid Innovation, 402–3; future of policy and politics of healthcare quality, 404; HITECH Act, 401–2; Medicare Access and CHIP Reauthorization Act of 2015, 403–4
Health Research and Educational Trust (HRET), 59, 416, 477; On the CUSP: Stop BSI program, 41, 43
Health Resources and Services Administration: preventive care and screenings supported by, 419
Health safety environmental (HSE) programs: workforce safety cultures and, 263
Health savings accounts (HSAs), 402; "triple tax advantage" with, 423
Health savings accounts–high-deductible health plans (HSA-HDHPs): enrollment growth in, 423; IRS guidelines for, 423, 424, 425–26; removing regulatory barriers for expanding

options for, and increasing uptake, 425–26
Health spending accounts, employee populations and, 479
Health status: measurement of, 54; safety and quality in a community and, 480–81
Health system board quality committee: responsibilities of, 351
"Health systems": transition to, 359
Health Transformation Alliance (HTA), 453
Healthy Michigan, 428
Healthy People 2020, 361; topics of Leading Health Indicators for, 480, *481*
Heart failure (HF) mortality/morbidity: reducing, treatment modalities for, 91
Hearts Beat Back case study, 491–92
Heart/Stroke Recognition Program (NCQA): Physician Practice Connections (PPC) program, 394
HEDIS. *See* Healthcare Effectiveness Data and Information Set (HEDIS)
Helmreich, Robert, 280
HENs. *See* Hospital Engagement Networks (HENs)
HEN 2.0, 478
HERO. *See* Health Enhancement Research Organization (HERO)
Heuristic evaluation, 274, *275*
Hewlett-Packard, 20
HFE. *See* Human factors engineering (HFE)
HHCAHPS. *See* Home Health CAHPS (HHCAHPS)
HHS. *See* US Department of Health and Human Services (HHS)
HiAP. *See* Health in All Policies (HiAP)
Hibbard, Judith, 61, 445
High-deductible health plans (HDHPs), 360, 479; changes to, 423–26; Choosing Wisely campaign and, 452; enrollment in, 416, 417. *See also* Health savings accounts–high-deductible health plans (HSA-HDHPs)
Higher-value care: engaging consumers in seeking, 445–46
Higher-value health plans: selectively contracting with, 442–43
High-fidelity simulation, 214, 226
High-impact leadership behaviors, *309*
High-Impact Leadership Framework (IHI), 308, *309*, 310, *310*
"High-Impact Leadership: Improve Care, Improve the Health of Populations, and Reduce Costs" (IHI), 308
High-performing organizations: transparency and, 324
High reliability: creating in practice, 266–71; important topics in, 271–75; leader bundles for, 267; learning systems and, 273; starting points with, 270, *271*; sustaining cultures of, 276
High reliability chassis, *265*, 265–66
High reliability organizations: descriptive theories of, 262–65
High reliability organizing (HRO): emergence of, as field related to safety culture, 258; knowledge for improvement and, *259*, 259–60; timeline of, 257–58, *258*; zero preventable harm and, 265
High-risk medications (HRMs), 462
High-value health plans (HVHPs), 360; potential impact of, 424–25; projected uptake in employer market, 425, *425*
High-value services: promoting use of, 441
HIPAA. *See* Health Insurance Portability and Accountability Act (HIPAA)
Hippocrates, 103
Hippocratic Oath, 256
Hispanic Americans: health equity issues and, 481
Histograms, 30
HMOs. *See* Health maintenance organizations (HMOs)
Hollnagel, Erik, 258
Home Health CAHPS (HHCAHPS), 234

Homelessness, 486
Hospital-Acquired Condition (HAC) Reduction Program, 448
Hospital-acquired infections, 477
Hospital-centric paradigm: transforming, 359
Hospital Compare, 302
Hospital complication measures: developing first, 57
Hospital Consumer Assessment of Healthcare Providers and Systems (HCAHPS), 230, 234, 238, 241, 301, 448
Hospital Engagement Networks (HENs), 477
Hospital Improvement and Innovation Networks (HIIN 3.0), 478
Hospital management: quality and relationship between board and, 331–32
Hospital mortality: quality improvement and, 307–8
Hospital performance: engaging hospital boards in improving, 333
Hospital Quality Alliance, 405
Hospital quality departments: voluminous reports generated by, 312
Hospital Readmissions Reduction Program (HRRP), 88, 448; variation-based strategy used by, 89
Hospitals: acute care, 363, 477; benchmarking themselves against "the best," 341; board oversight of quality in, 329, 330; high- *vs.* low-performing, differences in board activities of, 335; linking quality and finance in, 347–48; mergers of, 64; modern, Nightingale and, 51; patient safety movement and, 371–72; total case injury rate for, 254; TPS, and calculation of value-based incentive percentage, 88–89
Hospital Safety Grade, 450
Hospital Survey of Patient Safety (HSOPS), 257
Hospital Value-Based Purchasing (HVBP) program, 88, 89, 367–68, 448
Housing: Medicaid and activities related to, 486; mental health and substance abuse services and, 59
Howard, Donna M., 279
HRET. *See* Health Research and Educational Trust (HRET)
HRMs. *See* High-risk medications (HRMs)
HRO. *See* High reliability organizing (HRO)
HRRP. *See* Hospital Readmissions Reduction Program (HRRP)
HSA-HDHPs. *See* Health savings accounts–high-deductible health plans (HSA-HDHPs)
HSAs. *See* Health savings accounts (HSAs)
HSOPS. *See* Hospital Survey of Patient Safety (HSOPS)
HTA. *See* Health Transformation Alliance (HTA)
Huddles, 267
Hudson, Patrick, 258, 263
Human-centered design, 17, 21–22; design process steps, 22; healthcare setting applications, 21–22
Human errors: number of patient deaths caused by, 254. *See also* Medical errors
Human factors engineering (HFE), 21, 274
Human factors integration, 274, *275*; process for, 275
Human factors methods: summary of, *275*
Humanistic outcomes, 174
Human patient simulators, 214
HVBP program. *See* Hospital Value-Based Purchasing (HVBP) program
HVHPs. *See* High-value health plans (HVHPs)
Hybrid simulations, 223
Hysterectomies: practice pattern variation in, 51

Iatrogenic injury, 253
IBI. *See* Integrated Benefits Institute (IBI)

IBM, 396
I-charts, 105, 141; correct control chart of diabetes guideline compliance data, *146*; of Press Ganey "top box" data, *149*; questions related to, 147–48; of "top box" scores' percentile rankings, *149*; as your "Swiss army knife," 147–48, 150
Idea creation, 23, 28, *29*
Identification: health IT for: case study 2, 197–201
Identification of quality and safety issues: health IT for, literature and discussion of, 191–92
Iezzoni, Lisa, 57
IHC. *See* Intermountain Healthcare (IHC)
IHI. *See* Institute for Healthcare Improvement (IHI)
IHI high-impact leadership: improve care, improve population health, and reduce costs, *309*
Immunizations: Affordable Care Act and, 419; alerts for, 195
"Impending Collapse of Primary Care Medicine and Its Implications for the State of the Nation's Health Care, The" (ACP), 394–95
Improvement: patient experience measurement and goal of, 240; three bodies of knowledge for, 258–60, *259*
Improvement statistics: function of, 128; process-oriented thinking as context for, 128–30
Improving Diagnosis in Health Care (National Academies of Sciences, Engineering, and Medicine), 5, 9, 373
Incentives: aligning, ambulatory quality and safety and, 375. *See also* Financial incentives
Incident reporting, 60
Indemnity insurance model, 389
Independent practice associations (IPAs), 390
Industrial quality measurement and management: leaders in field of, 50
Information technology (IT), 105–6. *See also* Health information technology
In-home technology, 123
Injuries: healthcare workplace-related, 254–55; iatrogenic, 253
Inpatient data: outpatient data *vs.*, 112
Inpatient Prospective Payment System (IPPS), 55, 56, 88
Inputs: process and sources of, 129
In situ simulations: for mock codes, advantages of, 225
Institute for Healthcare Improvement (IHI), 19, 32, 257, 281, 338; on board's fiduciary responsibility, 331; founding of, 59, 66n1; High-Impact Leadership Framework, 308, *309*, 310, *310*; "High-Impact Leadership: Improve Care, Improve the Health of Populations, and Reduce Costs," 308; Open School, 288–90, *289*; reliability of healthcare cycle, 190; Triple Aim, 171, 189, 307, *307*, 308, 375, 403, 405, 458
Institute for Safe Medication Practices (ISMP), 257
Institute of Medicine (IOM), 390; on comparative effectiveness research, 469; *Crossing the Quality Chasm: A New Health System for the 21st Century*, 1, 5, 7, 9, 11, 33, 172, 232, 233, 315, 365, 495; *To Err Is Human: Building a Safer Health System*, 1, 5, 6–7, 9, 33, 60, 233, 254, 256, 279, 280, 298, 365, 371, 450, 457, 477; establishment of, 365; *Preventing Medication Errors*, 457; quality indicators for capturing six domains of healthcare quality defined by, 87; "The Urgent Need to Improve Health Care Quality," 5–6; use of identical measures guidance by, 494; "Vital Signs: Core Metrics for Health and Health Care Progress," 404. *See also* National Academy of Medicine (NAM)
Instrumental activities of daily living (IADL) measure, 54

Insulin, 50, 63
Integrated Benefits Institute (IBI), 453
Intel, 453, 478
Intermountain Healthcare (IHC): variation data used at, 90–91
Internal failure: learning systems geared toward, 273
Internal Revenue Code: safe harbor expansion and, 426
Internal success: learning systems geared toward, 273
International Classification of Diseases, 124n3
International Society for Quality in Health Care (ISQUA), 282
IOM. *See* Institute of Medicine (IOM)
IPAs. *See* Independent practice associations (IPAs)
IPPS. *See* Inpatient Prospective Payment System (IPPS)
Ishikawa diagrams, 23–24, 154
ISMP. *See* Institute for Safe Medication Practices (ISMP)
ISQUA. *See* International Society for Quality in Health Care (ISQUA)
IT. *See* Information technology (IT)

James, John, 254
Jefferson Center for Character Education, 269
Jefferson College of Population Health, 60
John A. Hartford Foundation, 59
Johns Hopkins University Medical Center, 256; Department of Behavioral Sciences at, 52; Quality and Safety Research Group, 38; stopping catheter-related bloodstream line infections at, 38–43
Johnson, Lyndon B., 53, 59
Joiner, Brian, 141
Joint Commission, The (TJC), 287, 301, 303, 323, 331, 338; core measures, 112, 114, 124n1; formation of, 52; medical home accreditation and certification program, 396; metrics for quality measures, 341; safety practices and standards, 257; sentinel events and, 253, 273; Standard LD.01.03.01 of *Comprehensive Accreditation for Hospitals*, 357n2
"Joint Principles of the Patient-Centered Medical Home" (ACP), 396
Juran, Joseph M., 2, 25, 50, 130, 143, 153, 154, 306
"Juran on Quality Improvement" video series, 157
"Juran Trilogy," 306
Just culture, 230, 267, 268; algorithms for, 272; development of concept for, 271; effectiveness of, 273; safety culture and, 264; safety management system for, 272
Just Culture (Dekker), 271
Just Culture Algorithm from Outcome Engenuity (Marx), 272
Just Culture Community, 271

Kaiser Family Foundation (KFF), 59, 416, 417
Kaiser Permanente, 269, 365, 480
Kaiser Permanente Center for Health Research, 59
Kaiser Permanente Community Benefit, 290
Kaiser Permanente Medical Group: history behind, 52
Kaizen blitz/event, 31–32
Kaplan, Robert S., 303, 304, 313, 321, 325n3
Katz, Sidney, 54
Keeler, Emmett, 58
Keller, Robert, 54
Kennedy, Ted, 65
Kern, David E., 279
Kerr, Robert, 53
Kerr-Mills Act, 53
Kerry, John, 63, 64
Key performance indicators (KPIs), 306
KFF. *See* Kaiser Family Foundation (KFF)
Khuri, Shukri, 57, 58
Kidney Care Quality Alliance, 405
Kindig, David, 476

King, Josie, 256
King, Willie, 256
Knowledge, skills, and attitudes (KSA), 260
Knowledge transfer and spread techniques, 23, 31–33; *kaizen* blitz/event, 31–32; rapid-cycle testing and pilots, *32,* 32–33
Kolb, Ben, 6
Kolb, David: cycle of learning, 219, *219*
KPIs. *See* Key performance indicators (KPIs)
KSA. *See* Knowledge, skills, and attitudes (KSA)

LaPorte, Todd, 262
Latent safety threats (LSTs): exposing, simulation and, 225
Leader behaviors/tools: for leader safety or high reliability bundles, 267–68
Leadership: function measures, 313, *313*; intersection of culture and, 229–32; safety culture, 264; system of, 311, *311*
Leading Health Indicators (LHIs): topics of, for Healthy People 2020, 480, *481*
League tables: misinterpreting, 83
Lean, 2, 127, 308, 352, 353, 364; 5S program, steps in, 30–31; goal of and steps in methodology, 20; history behind, 19–20; operational excellence and, 259; value stream mapping in, 26, 32
Lean thinking: *kaizen* as central concept in, 31
Leapfrog Group, 302; aims of, 124n4; founding of, 450; Hospital Survey, 114, 450; patient safety measures, 112; value-based purchasing platform, 360
Learning: game-based, 294–95; Kolb's cycle of, 219, *219*
Learning boards, 268
Learning environment: safety culture and, 264
Learning systems: for safety and high reliability, 273
Leavitt, Mike, 496
Legacy systems, 116
Lehman, Betsy, 6, 256
Lehman, Tony, 58
Lembcke, Paul, 51
Lessons-learned (or operating experience) programs, 273
Levine, Sol, 52, 58
Levodopa: Parkinson's disease and treatment with, 196
LHIs. *See* Leading Health Indicators (LHIs)
Liaison Committee for Graduate Medical Education. *See* Accreditation Council for Graduate Medical Education (ACGME)
Libuser, Carolyn, 262
Licensure: of physicians, 51
Link, Edwin Albert, 216
Linn, Larry, 61
LLI. *See* Lucian Leape Institute (LLI)
Local learning systems, leading, 268
Local public health agencies: expanded role of, 491
Loma Linda Hospital, 262
Lorig, Kate, 61, 65
Lovelace Health System: Episode of Care Disease Management Program and, 125n9; point-of-service patient experience surveys, 118
Low-fidelity simulation, 214, 226; in AELPS programs, 292, 294–95
Low Performing Icon (LPI): low-performing Medicare plans and, 462
Low-value services and care, 433; discouraging use of, 441; identifying and reducing, 429–31; provider- and patient-facing methods of reducing, *430*; risks related to, 429; role of value-based insurance design in, 431–32
LPI. *See* Low Performing Icon (LPI)
LSTs. *See* Latent safety threats (LSTs)
Lucian Leape Institute (LLI), 231, 284–86

MA. *See* Medicare Advantage (MA)
MacArthur Foundation, 290
MACRA. *See* Medicare Access and CHIP Reauthorization Act (MACRA)
Magnetic resonance imaging (MRI) scans: evidence-based guidelines, 62; reference pricing and, 445
Main Line Health (Philadelphia), 229
Managed care: Medicaid and, 461
Managed care organizations (MCOs), 56; NCQA accreditation and, 392
Managed care plans: health plan populations and, 479
Management function measures, 313, *313*
Managing the Unexpected (Weick and Sutcliffe), 263–64
Manufacturing industry: safety culture and, 257
MAPs. *See* Multiple Measurement Advisory Panels (MAPs)
Marx, David, 271, 272
Massachusetts Institute of Technology (MIT), 19, 248
Mastery training: safety through, 220–21
Maternal Child Health Bureau (MCHB), 394
Maternity-related services: recommended actions for employers, 451
Mayo Clinic, 247, 478
McClellan, Mark, 496
McClinton, Mary, 257
MCHB. *See* Maternal Child Health Bureau (MCHB)
McLellan, Tom, 58, 59
McLeod Health (Florence, SC): quality improvement philosophy at, 308
McMorris Rodgers, Cathy, 423
MCOs. *See* Managed care organizations (MCOs)
Meaningful Use, 401. *See also* Electronic Health Records (EHR) Incentive Program
Measurement: dealing with burden of, 406–7; role of, in improving healthcare quality and safety, 439. *See also* Metrics; Performance measures/performance measurement; Quality measures/quality measurement
Measurement, quality of care: best of, 15; metrics and benchmarks, *16*, 16–17; outcome, 15; process, 14–15; structure, 14
Measure specifications, 174
MEC. *See* Medical executive committee (MEC)
Median: in run chart, 132, 133, 134, 136; using for a run chart, *vs.* using average, 138–39
Medicaid, 2, 49, 54, 439; ACA and expanded eligibility for, 402; Adult and Pediatric Core Set of Measures, 461; enactment of, 50, 53; federal poverty level and eligibility for, 402; health plan populations and, 479, 480; housing-related activities and, 486; increased enrollment in, 401; meaningful use of EHRs and, 401; measurement burden and, 406; NCQA accreditation requirements and, 392; new quality management/measurement research institutions since passage of, 59–60; quality measure development since passage of, 53–54; reporting of audited HEDIS data to state and, 391; risk-sharing agreements and, 469; section 1115 waiver, 360, 401; state reforms, 360; value-based insurance design and, 427–28
Medical auditing, 51
Medical education, 231; reforming, challenges in, 280–81, 298. *See also* Medical schools
Medical errors, 6; achieving dramatic reduction in, 341; in ambulatory care settings, 372; disclosing, 60; lack of patient safety culture and, 38; as leading cause of death, 9, 254, 477; "never events," 447–48; patient safety movement and, 371; scope of, 9; severity of, 1

Medical executive committee (MEC): physician credentialing and, 346, 347
Medical Expenditure Panel Survey, 237
Medical home model, 379. *See also* Patient-centered medical homes (PCMHs)
Medical home "neighborhood": NCQA's vision for and extension of, 397–98
Medical malpractice: quality measures focusing on, 60
Medical Outcomes Study, 58; 12-Item Short Form Health Survey developed by, 325n5
Medical record review: retrospective, 113–14; time and cost involved in, 110
Medical records–based outcomes metrics: claims-based metrics *vs.*, 57
Medical schools: Flexner and reform of, 51; safety issues and curriculum development in, 1, 5, 6–7, 9, 33, 60, 233, 254, 256, 279, 280
Medical simulation: definition of, 213
Medical sociology, 52
Medicare, 2, 49, 54, 185, 439; administration of, 447; consumer cost sharing and, 417; enactment of, 50, 53; health plan populations and, 480; Hospital Compare, 302; Hospital Value-Based Purchasing (HVBP) program, 88, 302; low-value services and, 429; meaningful use of EHRs and, 401; medical home demonstration project, 395; metrics in 2017 Part D star ratings system, 463, *463*; new quality management/measurement research institutions since passage of, 59–60; Nursing Home Compare, 302; Part B, 367; Part D, 361, 461, 467; patient experience incentive, 245–46; prescription drug benefit, 401; Prospective Payment System, 447; quality indicators in Shared Savings Program, 341–42; quality measure development since passage of, 53–54; "refreshing" of process-of-care measures by, 89; repeal of sustainable growth rate formula for physician payment, 176; risk-sharing agreements and, 469; value-based healthcare goals and, 460; value-based purchasing programs, 447–49; V-BID principles and, 420
Medicare Access and CHIP Reauthorization Act (MACRA), 105, 176, 302, 360, 379, 403–4, 449; participation in NCQA PCSP program and, 399; passage of, 325n1, 403; Quality Payment Program, 185, 371, 449; quality reporting requirements, 404; shift from measuring process to measuring outcomes and, 370–71
Medicare Advantage (MA), 360, 420–23; actuarial analysis of value-based insurance design programs, by condition and stakeholder, *421*; health plan populations and, 479, 480; incorporation of V-BID principles into, 420; increased cost sharing with, 417; measurement burden and, 406; NCQA accreditation requirements and, 392; PQA metrics within CMS Five-Star Quality Rating System for, 461; Prescription Drug plans, 461; quality and performance measures, 370; star ratings for health plans, 302; states eligible for value-based insurance design model test, year 2, *422*; value-based insurance design model test plans and conditions, year 1, *422*; V-BID model test, 420–21, 423
Medicare Payment Advisory Commission (MEDPAC), 420
Medicare Prescription Drug, Improvement, and Modernization Act (MMA), 467
Medicare severity DRGs (MS-DRGs), 57, 88
Medicare Shared Savings Program, 181

Medication errors, 253, 308; drug alerts and decrease in, 195; preventable, 457

Medication reconciliation programs, 372

Medication reimbursement: under risk-sharing agreements, 468

Medication safety concerns/risks, 51; in ambulatory setting, 373; pharmacists and reduction in, 464–65

Medication synchronization, 464

Medication therapy management (MTM): enhanced, 467–68; goal of, 464

Medication use quality, 457–70; comparative effectiveness research and, 469; "drive to five": high-stakes implications and, *462,* 462–63; enhanced medication therapy management, 467–68; National Quality Strategy as a road map, 457–58, *459*; overall healthcare quality and, 470; patient-centered outcomes research and, 469; performance measurement and, 458, 460–61; pharmacist as medication use expert, 463–65, *466*; types of quality measures, with examples for, *460*; value-based insurance design, risk-sharing agreements, and, 468–69; volume-to-value shift in healthcare, 457–63

MedInsight Waste Calculator, 452

MEDPAC. *See* Medicare Payment Advisory Commission (MEDPAC)

Mental health and substance abuse (MHSA) services: difficulty in measuring, 58–59

Mercy Health, 229

Mergers: hospital, 64

Merit-Based Incentive Payment System (MIPS), 105, 176, 325, 375, 449; domains for payment in, 371; "Improvement Activities" category of, 399; performance categories of, 185

Methicillin-resistant *Staphylococcus aureus* (MRSA) bacteremia: hospital-onset, reductions in, 372

Metrics: definition of, 16; derivation of, change in, 16; examples of, for structure, process, and outcome measures, *16*; medication-related, 458, 463; Pharmacy Quality Alliance, 461

MHIF. *See* Minneapolis Heart Institute Foundation (MHIF)

MHSA services. *See* Mental health and substance abuse (MHSA) services

Michigan hospitals: CUSP and dramatic decreases in CLABSI rates in, 41

Military defense industry: learning from, 280

Millennial generation: technological literacy of, 294

Miller, George: Pyramid of Assessment, 220, *220*

Mills, Ron, 55

Mills, Wilbur, 53

Minneapolis Heart Institute Foundation (MHIF), 491

Minority populations: health equity and, 481–84

MIPS. *See* Merit-Based Incentive Payment System (MIPS)

Mission: linking quality measures to, 494

Mistake proofing (or *poka yoke*): goal of, 27

Misuse, quality defects and, 1, 6

MIT. *See* Massachusetts Institute of Technology (MIT)

MMA. *See* Medicare Prescription Drug, Improvement, and Modernization Act (MMA)

Mock codes: simulation and, 225–26

Model for improvement (API), 17, 19, *19*

Mortality rates, 57, 174

Motorola, 20

Moving range (MR), 143; calculations for performance data, *140,* 140–41

MRI scans. *See* Magnetic resonance imaging (MRI) scans

Mr. Roberts and the US healthcare system (case study), 33–37; communication deficits and lack of a team

approach, 34–35; knowledge-based care, 36–37; mismatch between supply and demand, 36; nonphysician/nonhospital care, 37; removing question mark from patient–provider interactions, 35–36
MS-DRGs. *See* Medicare severity DRGs (MS-DRGs)
MTM. *See* Medication therapy management (MTM)
Multimodality systems: data collection and, 243
Multiple-board health systems: overseeing quality in, 345
Multiple Measurement Advisory Panels (MAPs), 391
Musson, David, 280

Narratives: in AELPS programs, 292, 293–94
Narrow networks, 479
Nash, David, 476
National Academies of Sciences, Engineering, and Medicine: *Improving Diagnosis in Health Care,* 5, 9
National Academy of Medicine (NAM), 62, 390, 457; *Improving Diagnosis in Health Care,* 373; safety defined by, 253. *See also* Institute of Medicine (IOM)
National Alliance of Healthcare Purchaser Coalitions, 453; eValue8 tool, 442
National Association for Healthcare Quality: Certified Professional in Healthcare Quality (CPHQ) certification, 296
National Business Group on Health, 453
National Center for Vital Statistics, 57
National Commission on Physician Payment Reform, 443
National Committee for Quality Assurance (NCQA), 174, 177, 180, 303, 360, 389, 401, 402, 409, 442; ACA and demand for accreditation services of, 402; accreditation status by product line determined by, 393; accreditation status levels, 393; Committee on Performance Measurement (CPM), 391; defining and measuring quality, 390–92; development of, 390–93; develops/launches Patient-Centered Specialty Practice, 397–99, *398*; eMeasure Certification program, 408; founding of, 366, 390; future of quality measurement and, 404; future of recognition programs, 399–400; health plan accreditation and, 392–93; Health Plan Report Card, star ratings, 393; HEDIS Compliance Audit, parts within, 391; launches PCMH program, 396–97, *398*; Oncology Medical Home program, 398; participation and scope of recognition programs, 398; Patient-Centered Connected Care, 398, *398*; PCSP recognition program, 375; Physician Practice Connections (PPC) program, 394, 396; physician profiling and, 184; practice-level focus of, 393–400; Quality Compass database, 391; recognition programs and patient-centered care, *398*; recognition programs developed by, 394; rise in overall revenue for, 403; role of, 389–409; SIM grants and, 403; *Standards and Guidelines for the Accreditation of Health Plans,* 392; Standards Committee categories, 393; 2017 standards for PCMH program, 400, *400*
National Defense Authorization Act (NDAA): for Fiscal Year 2018, V-BID principles and, 427
National Healthcare Disparities Report (AHRQ), 8, 494
National Healthcare Quality Report (AHRQ), 5, 7–8, 494
National Health Interview Survey, 416
National Health Service (UK): Incident Decision Tree, 272
National Heart, Lung, and Blood Institute, 391

National League for Nurses, 288
National Patient Safety Foundation (NPSF), 257, 284; Certified Professional in Patient Safety (CPPS) certification, 296
National Patient Safety Goals, 257
National Quality Forum (NQF), 151, 174, 257, 406, 494; establishment of, 367; HCAHPS survey approved by, 234; metrics for quality measures, 341; mission of, 124n5; National Voluntary Consensus Standards for Hospital Care, 114; "never events" list, 448; Quality Positioning System, 375
National quality improvement efforts: applying variation, examples of, 88–90
National Quality Strategy (NQS): establishment and aims of, 405; three aims, six priorities, nine levers in, *459*; updates of, 458
National Registry of Myocardial Infarction, 117
National Strategy for Quality Improvement in Health Care. *See* National Quality Strategy (NQS)
Native Americans: health equity issues and, 481
NCQA. *See* National Committee for Quality Assurance (NCQA)
NDAA. *See* National Defense Authorization Act (NDAA)
Neave, Henry, 129
Nelson, Eugene, 54, 58
Netherlands: ensured consistency of healthcare system in, 77
Network maps: co-occurrences and, 192
Network of Regional Health Initiatives (NRHI), 453
"Never events": dealing with, 151–52; examples of, 447–48
New England Journal of Medicine, 399
Newhouse, Joe, 56
New Ulm Medical Center (Minnesota), 491
NICU conference poster session, 150–51; typical displays of incident data, *151*
NICU infection rate example: dangers of applying vague strategies and, 153–54; run chart of, *152*
Nightingale, Florence, 51
Nixon, Richard, 59
Nolan, Tom, 19
North American Spine Society, 62, 63
Northwestern University, 248, 295
Norton, David P., 303, 304, 314, 321, 325n3
Not-for-profit organizations: performance scorecard development for, 316
Not-for-profit physician groups: board oversight of, 329
Novartis, 468
NPSF. *See* National Patient Safety Foundation (NPSF)
NQF. *See* National Quality Forum (NQF)
NQS. *See* National Quality Strategy (NQS)
NRC Health, 229
NRHI. *See* Network of Regional Health Initiatives (NRHI)
Nuclear power industry: guidance document use and, 270; high reliability organizing and, 259; learning from, 280; safety culture and, 257
Numerical goals: arbitrary, 163
Nurses: mock codes, in situ simulation, and, 226; population safety and quality and, 488
Nursing education: transformation of, 288
Nursing Home Compare, 302
Nursing Home Quality Initiative, 405
Nursing homes, 56

Obama, Barack, 401, 404, 458
"Obamacare." *See* Affordable Care Act (ACA)
Obesity epidemic, 493
Obesity screening, 494
Objective structured clinical examination (OSCE), 215
Obstetrical adverse events, 477

Obstfeld, David, 262
Occupational safety: ill health issues and, 450
Office of the National Coordinator of Health Information Technology (ONC), 401; Health IT Certification Program's testing of EHR systems, 408
"Off to the Milky Way" (Balestracci), 141
Ohno, Taiichi, 20
O'Kane, Margaret E. "Peggy," 390, 408
ONC. *See* Office of the National Coordinator of Health Information Technology (ONC)
Oncology Medical Home program (NCQA), 398
100,000 Lives Campaign, 257
100 percent appropriate care: culture of safety and high reliability and, 276
Online consumer reviews, 247–49
On the CUSP: Stop BSI program: implementation of, 41; iterations of, 43; success of, 41, 43
Open School (IHI), 288–90, *289*; eight knowledge domains, 289; founding of, 290; success of, 290; three pillars of, 288, *289*
Operational Excellence (OpEx): knowledge for improvement and, 259, *259*
Opioid epidemic, 239, 493
Optum, 361
Organizational accident, 258
Organizational attitudes: workforce safety cultures and, 263
Organizational behavior: workforce safety cultures and, 263
Organizational performance: six IOM aims and, 315
Organizational performance measures: strategic measures and, 314
Organizational scorecards: creating, 315–17, *317*
Orthopedic postoperative patients, reducing length of stay of, 198–201; four-pronged approach for, 198; LOS for patients with a primary ICU orthopedic admission diagnosis, before and after improvement, *200*; Pareto chart showing ICU admission by diagnosis, *199*; statistical process control chart showing LOS for patients with a primary ICU orthopedic admission diagnosis, *200*
OSCE. *See* Objective structured clinical examination (OSCE)
Outcome indicators: using for results, 322–23
Outcome measures: subclassification of, 174
Outcomes, 259; evaluation of care based on, 2; MACRA and shift to measurement of, 370–71; metrics and benchmarks for, examples, *16*; quality measures for medication use quality and, 460, *460*; quality of care measurement and, 15
Outcomes-based contracts, 468
Outcome variation: definition and relevance to healthcare quality research/improvement, *76*
Out-of-pocket costs: ACA and elimination of, for preventive services, 419; increased burden of, 417; low-value care and, 429; for Medicare beneficiaries, clinical nuance and, 423; value-based insurance design, 441
Out-of-pocket maximums: rising, for HSA-HDHPs, 423–24
Out-of-pocket payments: funding of healthcare system through, 439
Outpatient data: inpatient data *vs.*, 112
Overuse, quality defects and, 1, 6

Pacific Business Group on Health (PBGH), 451
Pacific Gas and Electric, 262
Pareto, Vilfredo, 25
Pareto analysis, 155–59
Pareto analysis data: as a two-dimensional matrix, *158*
Pareto charts, 25, 30, 156; development of, 25; of guideline noncompliances compared by bundle element, *156*;

of guideline noncompliances tallied by hospital, 156, *157*; showing frequency with which causes contribute to error, *26*
Pareto matrix, 157–59, 160
Pareto matrix data: with special causes highlighted, *158*
Pareto principle, 154, 163
Parkinson's disease: hard-stop alerts and patients with, 196; stop-order results: number of attempts to order Haldol for, *197*
Parkland Community Health Plan (Texas), 490
Parkland Health and Hospital System (Texas), 487
Parkland's Center for Clinical Innovation (Texas): cloud-based Information Exchange Portal developed by, 487
Park Nicolett (Minneapolis): quality improvement philosophy at, 308
Partnership for Patients (PfP) initiative (CMS), 477
Patient, physician, and staff satisfaction domain: data collected for quality measurements and, 107
Patient activation measure, 61
Patient advocates: population health model, 488
Patient care quality: characteristics of quality-focused board actions and, 334
Patient-centered care, 2, 11, 232, 241, 361; population health safety and quality and, 496; quality improvement and, 7; quality measures and, 174; segmentation and, 244
Patient-Centered Connected Care (NCQA), 398, *398*
Patient-centered culture: safety culture and, 264
"Patient-Centered Medical Home Neighbor, The: The Interface of the Patient-Centered Medical Home with Specialty/Subspecialty Practices" (ACP), 397
Patient-centered medical homes (PCMHs), 54, 360, 376, 377; Affordable Care Act and, 367; benefits of, 366–67; history of, 394–95; improved patient safety and, 374; joint principles of, 395–96; primary care physicians and, 374
Patient centeredness: 2, 494; high reliability coupled with, 266; organizational performance and, 315; organizational scorecard creation and potential measures for, 317
Patient-centered outcomes research (PCOR), 361, 469
Patient-Centered Outcomes Research Institute (PCORI), 367, 469
Patient-Centered Specialty Practice (PCSP), 366, 375, *398*; NCQA and launch of, 397
Patient confidence measure, 61
Patient-derived outcomes measures: three-legged stool and, 61
Patient empowerment measure, 61
Patient engagement: provider-patient relationship and, 488
Patient experience, 233–49; data collected for quality measurements and, 107, 110; "deconstructing" notion of suffering in, 242; emergence of, 233–36; key drivers of overall rating in the inpatient setting, *247*; online posting of comments and ratings, 247–49; replacement of term "patient satisfaction" with, 235; transparency and, 247–49
Patient experience data: conceptual issues, 237–39; concerns about, 236–41; data issues, 239–41; reviewing, 312; using to improve, 245–49
Patient experience measurement and reporting, improving, 241–45; advances in data analysis, 244–45; advances in data quality and collection, 243–44; measuring what matters to patients, 241–43

Patient experience of care score: VBP program and calculation of, 336
Patient experience surveys, 117–19, 230; administering, 118–19; conducting via telephone, 119; point-of-service, 118
Patient harm: categories of, *254*; reducing, CMS PfP initiative and, 477–78
Patient harm index, 307
Patient needs: examples of, within the inpatient setting, *243*
Patient outcomes: board practices with significantly positive correlations with, 334–35
Patient Protection and Affordable Care Act. *See* Affordable Care Act (ACA)
Patient registries, 104; advantages of, 122; common conditions in, 122; specialty-specific, 122–23; versatility of, 123
Patient-reported outcome measures (PROMs), 494
Patient reports, 60–61
Patients: STEEEP aims and, 12
Patient safety: AHRQ use of identical measures and quality dimension of, 494; current curricular work in, 286–98; early curricular work in, 281–86; ensuring, board's quality oversight and, 340; human factors engineering and, 274; physician credentialing and, 346; workforce safety and, 255
Patient safety culture: medical errors and lack of, 38
Patient safety indicators: gap between tracking *vs.* improvement, 312
Patient safety movement: evolution of, 371–72
Patient safety organizations (PSOs): learning systems and, 273
Patient safety simulations: educational frameworks applied to, 218–21
Patient satisfaction: benchmarks for, 316
Patient satisfaction measurements: early, 233
Patient satisfaction metric, 61
Patient satisfaction scores, 307
Patient surveys: functional status surveys, 119; patient experience surveys, 117–19
Payers: physician profiling and, 172; STEEEP aims and, 12–13
Pay-for-performance contract: new, 380–81
Pay-for-performance pharmacy networks, 463
Pay-for-performance programs, 370; attribution and questions about effectiveness of, 83; expansion of quality improvement through, 366–67; provider profiles and, 175
Pay-for-reporting program, PQRS as, 367
Payment reform: pursuing, 443–44
PBGH. *See* Pacific Business Group on Health (PBGH)
p-charts, 147; of Press Ganey "top box" data, *149*
PCMHs. *See* Patient-centered medical homes (PCMHs)
PCOR. *See* Patient-centered outcomes research (PCOR)
PCORI. *See* Patient-Centered Outcomes Research Institute (PCORI)
PCSPs. *See* Patient-centered specialty practices (PCSPs)
PDSA cycle. *See* Plan-Do-Study-Act (PDSA) cycle
Pediatricians: successful population health strategy and, 374
Peer Review Organizations (PROs), 53
Penalties: Hospital Readmissions Reduction Program, 89; for hospitals with high excess readmission rates, 448; inpatient and ambulatory quality measures and, 367
Pennsylvania Chronic Care Initiative (CCI): private practice in, 377–79
People-only systems: reliability, resilience, and, 261
Percentage p-chart, 148

"Perfectly designed" concept: dealing with "never events" and, 152
Performance data: moving range calculations for, *140,* 140–41; year-end review, 130–32, *131, 133*
Performance in healthcare, dimensions of, 314–15
Performance measures/performance measurement: changing, being prepared for, 320; develop clear understanding of intended use of, 319; developing composite indicators for high-volume, high-profile conditions, 322–23; engage governing board in development of, 319; focus on results, not on activities, 323–24; ideal cycle time for, 315; integrating to achieve a balanced view, 320–21; leadership system changes and, 323; provider profiles and, 175; quality improvement efforts and, 458, 460; quality indicators and, 185–86; transparency and, 324; using performance scorecard to evaluate organizational/leadership performance, 319–20
Performance scorecards: changing, being prepared for, 320; organization's governance system and, 319–20; sample, for hospital board, 317, *317*
Performance targets: setting, board's quality oversight and, 340–46
Performance-tracking tools: pharmacies and, 465, *466*
Performance variation, 92; definition and relevance to healthcare quality research/improvement, *76*
Perinatal Quality Collaborative of North Carolina, 43
Personal diagnostic testing devices, 361
Personal healthcare: public health programs *vs.,* 488–89
Personalized medicine, 184, 361
Person centeredness: as high-impact leadership behavior, *309*
Pew Research Center, 248
Pharmaceutical Manufacturers Association, 63
Pharmacist engagement in value-based healthcare system, 467–69; comparative effectiveness research and, 469; enhanced medication therapy management, 467–68; patient-centered outcomes research and, 469; value-based insurance design and risk-sharing agreements, 468–69
Pharmacists: collaborating with healthcare team to reach drive to five stars, 465, *466*; medication-related metrics and, 458; medication therapy management and, 464; as medication use experts, 463–65; quality improvement programs and, 470; role of, in Medicare Part D MTM, 467
Pharmacy networks: quality goals and, 463
Pharmacy Quality Alliance (PQA), 405, 465; medication-use metrics, 463; MTM completion rate measure, 467; quality measures development and, 461
Pharmacy Quality Solutions (PQS): provision of performance information to plans and pharmacies, 465, *465*
Pharmacy visits: frequency of, 464
Physical determinants of health, 484–87; examples of, 485; health plan populations and, 479
Physician conflict-of-interest policies, 347
Physician credentialing: board's quality oversight duties and, 346–47
Physician Practice Connections—Patient-Centered Medical Home (PPC-PCMH): launch of, 396
Physician practices: hospital acquisition of, 65
Physician profiles/profiling, 105; background and terminology related to, 171; challenges related to, 183–85; in a changing healthcare landscape, 185–86; choosing measures for, 181; data collection and, 181; data

interpretation and, 182; dissemination of findings, 182–83; examples of, 177; functions of, 171; keys to success with, 183; quality measures and, 174; use of, in healthcare organizations, 176–77. *See also* Provider registries
Physician Quality Reporting System (PQRS), 176, 367, 404
Physicians: benchmarking performance of, 180; changing financial incentives for, 365; licensure of, 51; online consumer reviews and, 248–49; population safety and quality and, 488; primary care, 374–75; role in improving quality, 174–75; variation in demand and, 79
Physician Voluntary Reporting Program, 405. *See also* Physicians Quality Reporting System
Pilots: conducting, 32–33
Pilot Schools Learning Collaborative, 288
Pitney Bowes, 419
"Place": social and physical determinants of health and, 485
Placebo effect, 51
Plan design: taking value-based insurance design approach to, 441
Plan-Do-Study-Act (PDSA) cycle, 2, 17, 18–19, 32, 380, 381; Comprehensive Unit-Based Safety Program, *40*; rapid-cycle testing and, 32
"Point-of-care" data collection, 244
Point-of-service (POS) plans: NCQA accreditation and, 392
Poka yoke (mistake proofing), goal of, 27
Politics: of healthcare, 2; quality management, evidence-based medicine and impact of, 62–63; quality management and engagement in, 65
Polypharmacy, 457
Population: defining, 476–77
Population-based management: ambulatory setting and, 364
Population-Based Payment Work Group: within CMS's HCPLAN, 405
Population health, 361; challenges facing quality measurement in, 493; current understanding of, conceptual framework, *475,* 475–76; definition of, 475; pivotal information in operational definition of, 475–76; recent history of, 476; success of HMOs and, 366; supporting through wellness, disease prevention, and disease management, 446–47; variation data being applied for, examples of, 93–94
Population health management: health plan databases and, 119–22
Population health model: provider–patient relationship and, 488
Population health safety and quality, 475–97; case studies, 491–92; employee populations, 478–79; facing challenge of, 497; healthcare providers and, 488; health plan populations, 479–80; IOM's six aims and, 495–96; moving forward with, 495–96; overview of, 475–78; public health agencies and, 488–91; responsibility for, 487–91; role of measurement in driving, 492–95; understanding dynamics of, research framework for, 496
Population health safety and quality, in communities, 480–87; health equity and, 481–84; health status and, 480–81; social and physical determinants of health and, 484–87
Positive autocorrelation, 86–87
POS plans. *See* Point-of-service (POS) plans
Poverty: health status and, 485
PPC-PCMH. *See* Physician Practice Connections—Patient-Centered Medical Home (PPC-PCMH)
PPOs. *See* Preferred provider organizations (PPOs)
PQA. *See* Pharmacy Quality Alliance (PQA)
PQRS. *See* Physician Quality Reporting System (PQRS)

PQS. *See* Pharmacy Quality Solutions (PQS)
Practice Transformation Networks (PTNs), 478
Prebrief: simulation and, 221
Precision medicine: value-based insurance design and, 432–33
Pre-deductible coverage: high-value health plans, 424–25; lack of, health savings accounts and, 424
Prediction science, 64
Predictive modeling, 490
Preference-sensitive care: implications of unwarranted variation within, 78; unwarranted variation identified in, 81–82
Preferred pharmacy networks, 463
Preferred prescription drugs: improving health plan performance and, 462, *462*
Preferred provider organizations (PPOs), 59; NCQA accreditation and, 392; premiums for, 425
Premature births: African Americans and, 481
Premier, 465, 477
Premiums: Connecticut Health Enhancement Program, 428, 434; for employer-sponsored health insurance, 449; funding of healthcare system through, 439; Healthy Michigan and, 428; for high-deductible health plans, 423; for high-value health plans, 424, 425. *See also* Coinsurance; Copayments; Deductibles
Prescription drug costs: healthcare spending total and, 457
Prescription drug coverage: for Medicare beneficiaries, 467
Prescription drugs: initial V-BID programs and, 419; preferred, 462, *462*; refill reminders, 464
Prescription drug use: high rate of, in US, 457
Presenteeism, 449
"Present-on-admission" flag: implementing on insurance claims forms, 57
Press Ganey, 236; patient satisfaction survey and feedback process, 148, 235; "top box" data, p-chart and I-chart of, *149*
Pressure ulcers, 253, 477
Preventing Medication Errors (IOM), 457
Prevention: health IT for, literature and discussion of, 191; health IT for: case study 1, 195–97
Preventive care services: Affordable Care Act and, 419; in HSA-HDHPs, 424
PricewaterhouseCoopers V-BID survey, 419
Primary care offices, 363
Primary care physicians: demand for, 374–75; successful population health strategy and, 374
Primary care providers: ambulatory quality and safety and role of, 374–75
Private health insurance plans: ambulatory quality programs and, 370; value-based payment programs and, 302
Private insurers: value-based purchasing and, 176
Private purchasers, 439
Private-sector personal health service delivery organizations: role of, 490
Problem reporting culture: just culture and approach to, 273–74
Process analysis, 23, 25–27; failure mode and effects analysis / mistake proofing, 27; flowcharts in, 25–26, *26*
Process auditing: high reliability organizations and, 262
Process behavior charts, 141
Process(es): aspects of, quality of care measurement and, 14–15; evaluation of care based on, 2; MACRA and shift from measurement of, to measuring outcomes, 370–71; metrics and benchmarks for, examples, *16*; quality measures for medication use quality and, 460, *460*; sources of inputs for, 129

Process improvement: behavior-shaping factors and, 261
Process maps, 25–26, *26*
Process measures, 174
Process-of-care (POC) score: VBP program and calculation of, 335
Process-oriented thinking, 139, 162; benefits of, 138; as context for improvement statistics, 128–30; never events and, 152
Process variation: control chart and determining presence of, 139; definition and relevance to healthcare quality research/improvement, *76*
Professional Standard Review Organizations (PSROs), 53
Profile development, 105
Profit motive, 49
Progressive discipline, 267
Project Cypress, 408
Project planning and implementation, 23, 28–31; checklists, 29–30; 5S program, 30–31; stakeholder analysis, 28–29; 2 × 2 matrix, 30, *30*
PROMs. *See* Patient-reported outcome measures (PROMs)
PROs. *See* Peer Review Organizations (PROs)
Prospective data collection, 114–15; advantages of, 115; methods for, 114–15; time and cost involved in, 110
Prospective payment case mix systems: adjusting for severity, 56–57
Prospective payment systems: development and implementation of, 56; introduction of, 447
Providence Health Services, 478
Provider registries, 105; background and terminology related to, 172–74; in a changing healthcare landscape, 185–86; function of, 171; use of, in healthcare organizations, 175. *See also* Physician profiles/profiling
Providers: bundles of universal skills for, 268–69
Provost, Lloyd, 19
PSOs. *See* Patient safety organizations (PSOs)
PSROs. *See* Professional Standard Review Organizations (PSROs)
PTNs. *See* Practice Transformation Networks (PTNs)
Public health agencies: population safety and quality and, 488–91
Public health programs: personal healthcare *vs.*, 488–89
Public purchasers, 439
Purchasers: definition of, 439
Purchaser Value Network (PVN), 360; establishment of, 451; Maternity Care Toolkit, 451
Pyramid of Assessment (Miller), 220, *220*

QA. *See* Quality assurance (QA)
QBPs. *See* Quality bonus payments (QBPs)
QC. *See* Quality control (QC)
QDM. *See* Quality Data Model (QDM)
QI. *See* Quality improvement (QI)
QPP. *See* Quality Payment Program (QPP)
QSEN Expert Panel: competency areas outlined by, 288
QSEN Forum, 288
QSEN project. *See* Quality and Safety Education for Nurses (QSEN) project
Qualified clinical data registries, 172–73
Quality: building culture of, 352–53, 356; collecting information on, 440–41; defining/measuring, NCQA's rebirth and, 390–92; definition of, 390; growing focus on, 5–9; important elements of, 2; knowledge for improvement and, 259, *259*; linking finance and, 347–48; public reporting of, 174; six aims of, 2; transformation of the healthcare system and, 1. *See also* Governance for quality
Quality Alliance Steering Committee, 405
Quality and Safety Education for Nurses (QSEN) project, 288

Quality assurance (QA), 305, 308; characteristics of, *305*; description of, 306
Quality bonus payments (QBPs): "drive to five" and, 462; Medicare Advantage plans and, 461
Quality committee, board-level, 350–52; meeting frequency, 350; need for, 350; recruiting for, 352; responsibilities of, 351–52
Quality Compass database (NCQA), 391
Quality control (QC), 305, *305*, 306–7, 308; characteristics of, *305*; description of, 306; in "Juran Trilogy," 306
Quality dashboard reports: for the board, 342–44, *343*; regular review of, 341
Quality data: gathering and reporting, 341
Quality Data Model (QDM): updates to, 408
Quality defects: categories of, 6
Quality degradation monitoring: high reliability organizations and, 262
Quality healthcare: national debate over, 390
Quality improvement (QI), 305, *305*, 307–8; applying evidence of unwarranted variation to, 80–82; characteristics of, *305*; description of, 307; in "Juran Trilogy," 306; physician's role in, 174–75
Quality improvement committees: data collection for physician profiles and, 181; data interpretation for physician profiles and, 182; dissemination of findings on physician profiles and, 182; physician profile measure and, 181; successful physician profiling systems and, 183
Quality improvement initiatives: relative strength of, framework for, *29*
Quality improvement models, 17–22; API model for improvement, 17, 19, *19*; basic format of, 17; human-centered design, 17, 21–22; Lean, or Toyota Production System, 17, 19–20; Plan-Do-Study-Act (PDSA) cycle, 17, 18–19; quality improvement tools *vs.*, 22–23; Six Sigma, 17, 20–21
Quality improvement tools, 22–33; categories of, 23; cause analysis, 23–24; data collection and analysis, 23, 27–28; evaluation and decision making, 23, 24–25; idea creation, 23, 28; knowledge transfer and spread techniques, 23, 31–33; process analysis, 23, 25–27; project planning and implementation, 23, 28–31; quality improvement models *vs.*, 22–23
Quality indicators: variability in, 87
Quality landscape: evolving trends in, 64–65
Quality landscape, historical context of, 49–65; Medicare, Medicaid, and subsequent developments, 53–63; new outcomes metrics and future of quality measurement/management, 63–65; overview, 49–50; quality measurement/management prior to 1965, 50–53
Quality measurement and management: consumer information and, 60–62; evidence-based medicine and impact of politics, 62–63; following passage of Medicare and Medicaid, 53–54; medical malpractice and, 60; new outcomes metrics and future of, 63–65; new research institutions since passage of Medicare and Medicaid, 59–60; prior to 1965, 50–53
Quality-measurement sets: commonly used, 303
Quality measures/quality measurement: assessing healthcare performance across the US, 404–8; background and terminology, 303–5; categories of, 364; clinical, 174; CMS definition of, 173; collection and publication of, 302; creating balanced set of, 494; dealing with burden of, 406–7; development of, entities

involved with, 461; explosion in, across healthcare, 301; getting to meaningful measures, 407–8; High-Impact Leadership Framework (IHI) and, 310; history behind, 174; number and standardization of, 375–76; organizing by category, 312–13; role of, in driving population health safety and quality, 492–95. *See also* Dashboards; Scorecards
Quality metrics: explosion in, across healthcare, 301; High-Impact Leadership Framework (IHI) and, 310; submitted by ACOs, 302
Quality of care: evaluations of, measures for, 2; healthcare organizations' mission and, 330
Quality of life, happiness and, 52
Quality outcomes measures: improvements in, 64
Quality Payment Program (QPP): creation of, 371; establishment of, for Medicare-participating clinicians, 449; MACRA and creation of, 325
Quality planning: in "Juran Trilogy," 306
Quality rating systems: evolution of, 458

Race and ethnicity: equity in health services delivery and, 11
Racial and ethnic disparities, 361; health equity issues and, 481–84
Racial segregation: health status and, 485
Radar charts, 313, 320
RAND, 16
RAND Health Insurance Study (HIS), 56, 58
Random (or common-cause) variation, 94; definition and relevance to healthcare quality research/improvement, *76*
Rapid-cycle testing (or rapid-cycle improvement): description of, 32; example of, *32*
Readmissions: delineating preventable, 57; "excess," HRRP and, 89; preventable, 477; reducing likelihood of, 364
Reagan, Ronald, 55
REAL data, 482
Reason, James, 258, 260, 271, 272
Reference pricing: employer adoption of, 446; services subjected to, 445
Referrals: ambulatory safety and follow-up for, 382; throughout ambulatory care system, 373
Reflection-in-action process: simulation and, 221
Reflection-on-action process: simulation and, 221
Reflective observation: in Kolb's cycle of learning, 219, *219*
Reflective practice: in AELPS programs, 292, 293–94
Registry(ies): definition of, 172; forms of, 173
Regulatory policy: reform of, 496
Rehabilitation care, 56
Reimbursement: tiered structures of, 197
Relentless focus: as high-impact leadership behavior, *309*
Reliability: as an emergent property, 260–62; definition of, 230, 255; repeatability *vs.*, 255; safety and, 230, 260
Reliability of healthcare: IHI and three-part cycle of, 190; improving, *190*; quality and safety, improving, *190*
Reliability science, 341
Reliable care: definition of, 256
Repeatability: reliability *vs.*, 255
Report cards: limitations of, 185; provider profiles and, 175; reducing unwarranted variation in effective care and, 81
Republicans: MACRA and, 403; US healthcare policy and, 400–401
Residency, 217
Resident physicians, 217
Resilience engineering, 258; aims and goals of, 261–62, 273
Resilient systems, 261

Resource focus: high reliability coupled with, 266
Resource planning: organizational culture and, 205
Resusci-Anne manikin (Laerdal), 216
Resuscitation: "Five Alive" program and, 226
Retail clinics, 359, 363
Retrospective data collection, 113
Revenue sharing: ACO model and, 368
Reward systems: high reliability organizations and, 262
Rickover, Hyman G., 276
"Right Chart or Right Action?" (Balestracci), 147
Risk adjustment, 2, 64
Risk awareness: high reliability organizations and, 262
Risk-based contracts/contracting, 103; measurement burden and, 406
Risk-sharing agreements: value-based insurance design and, 468–69
Roberts, Karlene, 258, 262, 263
Robert Wood Johnson Foundation (RWJF), 59, 288, 390, 490
Robust Process Improvement (RPI), 308
Rochlin, Gene, 262
Roemer, Milton, 52
Romano, Patrick, 57
Romney, Mitt, 401
Root cause analysis, 163, 261, 273, 282; hindsight and, 153; overuse and poor execution of, 152; real meaning of, 152–53
Rosenfeld, Leonard, 51
Rounding, reinforcing safe practices through, 267
Rounding to influence (RTI), 268
RPI. *See* Robust Process Improvement (RPI)
RTI. *See* Rounding to influence (RTI)
Run: definition of, 136
Run chart analysis: process summary conclusions, 142
Run chart rules: applying, 137; did a process shift occur?: run chart rule # 2, 136; trend rule: run chart rule #1, 136
Run charts, 27, *28,* 105, 313, 320; of diabetes guideline compliance data, *137*; median in, 132, 133, 134, 136; of most recent baseline with five months of intervention data, *160*; of NICU infection rate, *152*; plotting data over time with, 132–34; time-ordered plot of year-end review performance data, *133*; using median *vs.* average for, 138–39; of year-end review performance data, *133*; of year-end review performance data with first postintervention point added, *134*
RWJF. *See* Robert Wood Johnson Foundation (RWJF)
Rx Foundation, 290

Safar, Peter, 216
Safe care, 2, 10, 232, 361; population health safety and quality and, 495; quality improvement and, 7; quality measures and, 173
"Safe harbor" services: bipartisan support for expansion of, 426; in HSA-HDHPs, 424
Safety: ambulatory, 371–74; building culture of, 352–53, 356; creating in practice, 266–71; definition of, 253; important topics in, 271–75; leader bundles for, 267; learning systems and, 273; organizational performance and, 315; organizational scorecard creation and potential measures for, 316; reasons for caring about, 265–66; reliability and, 230, 260; standardized care protocols and, 350; in STEEEP framework, 10
Safety and quality movement: growth of, 477
Safety culture(s): characteristics of, 263; domains or subcultures of, 264; goal of, 273; high reliability organizing field and, 258; starting points with, 270, *271*; sustaining, 276

Safety moments, 267–68
Safety movement: modern, history of, 256–60
Safety science, 267; definition of, 255; timeline of, 257–58, *258*; zero preventable harm and, 265
Sammer, Christine, 264
Sample sizes: in academic (enumerative) statistics, 155–56; patient experience data and, 239, 240
SANs. *See* Support and Alignment Networks (SANs)
SBAR. *See* Situation-background-assessment-request (SBAR)
Scanners: patient experience surveys and, 118
Scatter diagrams: demonstrating two data sets, *25*; function of, 24
Scorecards, 184, 231, 304–5, 324; balanced, 303, 304, 321, 325n3; comparison of HbA1c screening rates by provider, *179*; dashboards *vs.*, 304, 305; description of, 173; examples of, 177–78; organizational, creating, 315–17, *317*; performance, 319–20; performance, for a hospital board, 317, *317*; physician profile, pay for performance (through third quarter), *178*; practice profile template, *179*; practice profile with cost and patient visit data, *180*; results *vs.* activities focus and system of, 323; in a strategic leadership system, 311–12; useful, understandable formats for, 320; using organizational performance dimensions to align efforts with, 321; using to evaluate organizational and leadership performance, 319–20. *See also* Dashboards
Segmentation, 246; patient-centered care and, 244
Seiketsu (standardize): in 5S program, 31
Seiri (sort): in 5S program, 31
Seiso (shine): in 5S program, 31
Seiton (straighten): in 5S program, 31
Senior leadership: organizational scorecard use and, 316
Seniors' Medication Copayment Reduction Act of 2009, 420
Sentinel events: definition of, 253
Sepsis, 308; key interventions for, 201; morbidity and mortality related to, 201
Sepsis, improving mortality from, 202–4; percent sepsis mortality, before and after improvement implementation, *203*; percent sepsis mortality over 24-month period, *202*; time to antibiotic administration before and after improvement, *204*
Sepulveda, Martin, 395
Serious safety events (SSEs), 316
Service indicators: capturing six domains of healthcare quality with, 87
Service outcomes measures: quality of care and, 342
SF-12 health surveys, 317
Shalala, Donna, 496
Shapiro, Sam, 51, 64
Shared decision making: positive impact of, 61
Sharp-End Model, 260
Shell Oil Company, 258; Hearts and Minds campaign, 263
Sheps, Cecil, 51
Sheps, Mindel, 51
Sherbourne, Cathy, 60
Shewhart, Walter A., 2, 18, 20, 50, 143
Shingo, Shigeo, 27
Shitsuke (sustain): in 5S program, 31
Short-Form Health Survey (SF-36), 56
Sia, Calvin, 394
Simulation, 106; benefits of, 218, 221–22; clinical environment for, 218; debriefing and, 215, 220, 221; evolution and history of, 215–16; hybrid, 223; integration into educational programming, 216–18; making the case for, 221–22; mode of delivery and, 214–15; as a pedagogy, 213; procedural training and clinical skills for, 222–23; realism of, 214; in situ simulation, 218; terminology, 213–15; virtual reality and interacting with, 215

Simulation center: physical workplace *vs.*, 218
Simulation in patient safety landscape, 221–26; making the case for simulation, 221–22; mock codes, 225–26; procedural training and clinical skills, 222–23; systems errors and latent threats, 225; TeamSTEPPS, 223–25
Simulation-mediated education, 213
Simulation training: adult learning and its implications on, 218–20
Situation-background-assessment-request (SBAR), 269
Six Sigma, 2, 17, 20–21, 127, 352, 353, 364; central concepts of, 20; DMAIC and, 21
Skinner, Jonathan, 54
SMART (specific, measurable, achievable, relevant, and time bound) aims, 27
Smart infusion pumps, 257
Smith, G. Richard, 58
SNOMED project. *See* Systematized Nomenclature of Medicine (SNOMED) project
Social determinants of health, 361, 484–87; examples of, 484–85; health plan populations and, 479
Social Security Act: Title XIX of, 53; Title XVIII of, 53
Social Security Amendments of 1983, 55
Sociotechnical systems: definition of, 255; examination of, high reliability organizing and, 262; relationships within, 275
Soft sciences of medicine, 281
Soft-stop alerts, 195, 205
Sower, Kevin, 302
Speaking up for safety: universal skill bundles and, 270
Special causes, 135, 138, 139, 162; deeply hidden, Pareto matrix and, 157; goal trap, diabetes guideline compliance data, and, 147; hidden, sequence for understanding and exposing, 161–62; highlighted, Pareto matrix data with, *158*; indications of, 139–40
Special causes, rules for determining, 135–36; run chart rule # 1: trend rule, 136; run chart rule # 2: did a process shift occur?, 136
Special cause strategy: process summary using run and control chart analyses, 142
Special cause (or unique) variation, *76,* 105, 162. *See also* Assignable variation
Specialty offices, 363
Spread models: effective, characteristics of, 32
Spreadsheet graphs, 320
SPs. *See* Standardized patients (SPs)
SSEs. *See* Serious safety events (SSEs)
SSIs. *See* Surgical site infections (SSIs)
Stakeholder analysis, 28–29
Stakeholders: board's fiduciary duties and, 330; categories of, 29; physician profiling and, 184; population safety and quality and, 497
Stakeholders, STEEEP aims and, 11–13; administrators, 13; clinicians, 11–12; commonality among, 13; patients, 12; payers, 12–13; society/public/consumers, 13
Standard deviations: what common cause limits represent in terms of, 143
Standardization: reliability improvement and, 270, *271*
Standardized patients (SPs): simulation and, 217
Standards and Guidelines for the Accreditation of Health Plans (NCQA), 392
Stanford Chronic Disease Self-Management Program, 61
STAR technique. *See* Stop-think-act-review (STAR) technique
State employee health plans, 360; value-based insurance design and, 427, 428
State health reform: value-based insurance design and, 427–28

State Innovation Model (SIM) grants program, 403
State public health agencies: expanded role of, 491
Statistical process control (SPC): limitations of, 84–85
Statistical tools for quality improvement, 127–63; cause-and-effect diagram, 154, *155*; c-charts, 147; control chart, 139–47, *140, 142, 144, 145, 146, 161*; I-chart, 147–48, *149,* 150; Pareto analysis, 155–59, *158*; Pareto chart, 156, *156, 157*; Pareto matrix, 157–58, *158*; p-charts, 147; run chart, 132–39, *133, 134, 160*; u-charts, 147
Statistics: analytic, 130, 156, 162; descriptive, 129; enumerative, 129–30, 155–56, 162; for improvement, clinical trial statistics *vs.,* 128; role of, in quality improvement, 162; types of, 105, 129–30
STEEEP focus areas: quality improvement and, 7
STEEEP framework, 10–11, 232; effectiveness, 10, 232; efficiency, 10–11, 232; equity, 11, 232; patient centeredness, 11, 232; safety, 10, 232; timeliness, 10, 232
Steinwachs, Don, 58
Stockpiling "just in case": fulfilling requirements "just in time" *vs.,* 111
"Stoplight" color scheme: performance indicators and, 325n4
Stop loss insurance, 449
Stop-think-act-review (STAR) technique, 269
Stories: in AELPS programs, 292, 293–94
Story of Lewis Blackman, The (film), 293
Story of Michael Skolnik, The (film), 293
Strang, Carly, 290
Strategic dashboards, 321
Strategic leadership system: dashboards and scorecards in, 311–12
Strategic measures: organizational performance measures and, 314; transparency and, 324
Strategic Quality and Safety Plan Dashboard, sample, *349*
Stratification: common cause strategy, 153–59; Pareto analysis, 155–59; vague projects have some vague issues, 153–55
Strengthening Medicare Advantage Through Innovation and Transparency for Seniors Act of 2015, 420
Stroke patients: thrombolytic therapy for, 115
Structure: evaluation of care based on, 2; metrics and benchmarks for, examples, *16*; quality measures for medication use quality and, 460, *460*; quality of care measurement and, 14
Structure measures, 174
Structure/process/outcomes triad framework: for assessing quality measures, *460,* 460–61
Subsidiary board quality committee: responsibilities of, 351–52
Subsidies: Affordable Care Act, 402
Subspecialty providers: ambulatory quality and safety and role of, 374–75
Suffering: patient experience and, 242
Suicide: healthcare workforce and prevalence of, 279
Supply-sensitive care: elimination of overuse and unwarranted variation in, 82; implications of unwarranted variation within, 78
Support and Alignment Networks (SANs), 478
Supreme Court of Illinois, 331
Surgical site infections (SSIs), 372, 477
Sustainable Growth Rate formula: repeal of, 325
Sustainable improvement: defining, 33
Sutcliffe, Kathleen, 258, 262, 263, 267, 268
Switzerland: healthcare spending as percentage of GDP in, 415
Systematic reviews, 16
Systematized Nomenclature of Medicine (SNOMED) project, 124n3

System errors: determining, 255–56; exposing, simulation and, 225
System-level quality improvement: newer measures for, 494
System reliability: determining, 255–56
System reliability equation, 255
System resilience equation, 261
Systems thinking, 282

Tampering, 135, 145, 163
Target behaviors: culture transformation models and, 266, 267
Tarlov, Al, 58
Task trainers: in simulation, 214
Tax Relief and Health Care Act of 2006, 367, 395
TCPI. *See* Transforming Clinical Practice Initiative (TCPI)
TeamSTEPPS: safety concerns and, 270; simulation and, 223–25
Teamwork: safety culture, 264; safety outcomes and quality of, 223
Technical Measurement Advisory Panel (TMAP), 391
Technology: wearable, 123. *See also* Health information technology; Information technology
Technology and process solutions: reliability improvement and, 270, *271*
Teeter-totter game, 295, *296*
Telluride, Colorado: roundtables in, educational themes and, 282–83
Test tracking: in ambulatory setting, 373; maximizing safety of, 374
Texas: housing and Medicaid waivers project in, 486
TGI. *See* Governance Institute, The (TGI)
ThedaCare (Wisconsin): quality improvement philosophy, 308
Third-party payers: STEEEP aims and, 12–13
Thomas, Patricia A., 279
Thomas Jefferson University: level-3 recognition in PCSP program, 398; quality reports for residents at, 297; School of Population Health, 295
Thompson, John, 55
Thrombolytic therapy: for stroke patients, 115
Thune, John, 426
Tiered networks, 445
Tiered reimbursement structures, 197
Timeliness: AHRQ use of identical measures and quality dimension of, 494; organizational performance and, 315; organizational scorecard creation and potential measures for, 317; in STEEEP framework, 10
Timely care, 2, 10, 232, 361; population health safety and quality and, 495; quality improvement and, 7; quality measures and, 174
Time series models, 87
TMAP. *See* Technical Measurement Advisory Panel (TMAP)
To Err Is Human (IOM), 1, 5, 6–7, 9, 33, 60, 233, 254, 256, 279, 280, 298, 365, 371, 450, 457, 477
Tonsillectomies: Glover's study on, in England and Wales, 75, 77; practice pattern variation in, 51
Total composite score: VBP program and calculation of, 336
Total knee replacement: clinical dashboard for, *109*; improving patients' functional status with, 110
Total Performance Score (TPS): Medicare's "achievement" and "benchmark" thresholds and, 88; value-based incentive percentage calculated with, 88–89
Total Worker Health movement, 450
Toyota Motor Corporation, 20
Toyota Production System (TPS), 17, 20, 259, 308
Transforming Clinical Practice Initiative (TCPI), 478
Transitions of care: in ambulatory setting, 373
Transparency: ambulatory measures and, 376; fostering, 440–41; as high-impact leadership behavior, 308, *309*; high-performing organizations and,

324; patient experience and, 247–49; regulatory reporting requirements and, 302; safety culture and, 264. *See also* Accountability
Trend line, fitted: diabetes guideline compliance data with, 137, *138*
Trend thinking: limitations of, 138
TRICARE, 360; Pharmacy Benefits Program, 427; value-based insurance design and, 426–27
Triple Aim (IHI), 171, 189, 307, *307,* 308, 375, 405; ACA and achievement of, 403; as basis for National Quality Strategy, 458
Trump, Donald, 404, 421
Turnover rates: ill health issues and, 450
12-Item Short Form Health Survey (SF-12), development of, 325n5
2 × 2 matrix, 30, *30*

u-charts, 147
Uncontrolled variation: Deming on, 50
Underserved populations: linking community-based services and healthcare providers with, 487
Underuse, quality defects and, 1, 6
Unhealthy Politics (Patashnik, Gerber, and Dowling), 62, 63
Unified Medical Language System, 124n3
Uniform Hospital Discharge Data Set, 124n2, 125n7
Uninsured population: ACA and decrease in, 402; quality management and measurement and, 65; rate of, early 21st century, 401
United Airlines, 270
UnitedHealthcare, 396
UnitedHealth Group, 480
United States: dynamic healthcare landscape in, 363; lack of universal insurance coverage in, 50; spending on social services and healthcare in, 484; total healthcare spending in, 457; uneven healthcare quality in, 174–75, 189, 233, 415, 429; variability in supply of healthcare services in, 77
"Units of accountability": definition of, 244; modern medicine and, 245
"Units of improvement": definition of, 244; modern medicine and, 245
Universal insurance coverage: lack of, in US, 50
Universal skill bundles: for caregivers and providers, 268–69
University Community Hospital of Tampa, 256
University of California (Berkeley), 262
University of Illinois (Chicago), 282; Full Disclosure and Transparency Program, 298; online master of science in patient safety leadership program, 295
University of Michigan: Center for Value-Based Insurance Design, 441
University of Utah Health System: online patient comments and ratings, key findings on, 247, 248–49
University of Washington, 494
Unmet Needs: Teaching Physicians to Provide Safe Patient Care (Lucian Leape Institute): recommendations in, 284–86
Unwarranted variation: applying evidence of, to quality improvement, 80–82; effects of, 3, 77; sources of, in medical practice, 78–80; three categories of care and implications of within each, 77–78; warranted variation *vs.*, 77, 94–95
URAC: medical home accreditation and certification program, 396
Urgent care centers, 359, 363
"Urgent Need to Improve Health Care Quality, The" (IOM), 5–6
Usability evaluation, 274, *275*
US Army Air Corps, 216
US Department of Defense, 223, 482
US Department of Education: 2010 National Education Technology Plan, 294
US Department of Health and Human Services (HHS), 480; National Quality Strategy updates and, 458; Office

for Health Maintenance Organizations, 390
US National Center for Health Statistics: 2016 National Health Interview Survey, 416
US Preventive Services Taskforce: colorectal cancer screening recommendations, 418; value-based insurance designs guidelines and, 419
USS Carl Vinson, 262
US Senate Committee on Armed Services, 427
Utilization: clinical nuance and, 418; rates, comparing in practice variation studies, 80–81

Validity: of measure calculations, 408
Value: defining, in healthcare, 347, 439
Value-based care, 403; proliferation of physician profiles and, 183
Value-based contracts, 468
Value-based healthcare system: transition from volume-driven healthcare system to, 415
Value-based healthcare system, pharmacist engagement in, 467–69; comparative effectiveness research, 469; enhanced medication therapy management, 467–68; patient-centered outcomes research, 469; value-based insurance design and risk-sharing agreements, 468–69
Value-based insurance design (V-BID), 360, 415–34; Affordable Care Act and, 419–20; applied example: Connecticut Health Enhancement Program, 428–29, 433–34; bipartisan support for, 420; definition of, 441; future of, 429–33; high-deductible health plans and, 423–26; identifying and reducing low-value care, 429–31; implementing clinical nuance in, 418–19; Medicare Advantage and, 420–21, *422,* 423; precision medicine and, 432–33; putting innovation into action, 419–29; risk-sharing agreements and, 468–69; role of, in low-value care, 431–32; state health reform and, 427–28; TRICARE and, 426–27
Value-based marketplace: driving toward, 453
Value-based payment models, 302, 347
Value-Based Payment Modifier, 176, 185
Value-based payments, 176, 330
Value-based purchasing (VBP), 176–77, 185; beginning of, 57–58; importance of quality considerations in funding healthcare system and, 439–53; patient satisfaction and, 61; public-purchaser: CMS and Medicare, 447–49
Value-Based Purchasing (VBP) data set (CMS): process-of-care and clinical outcomes scores from, 335–36
Value-based purchasing programs, 105, 376
Value-based purchasing scores: higher, board practices associated with, *336–38*
Value-based purchasing strategies, overview of, 440; collecting information on quality and fostering transparency, 440–41; engaging consumers in seeking higher-value care, 445–46; pursuing payment reform, 443–44; selectively contracting with higher-value health plans and providers, 442–43; supporting population health, 446–47; taking a value-based design approach to plan design, 441
Value-driven system: transition from volume-based system to, 458
Value stream mapping, 26, 32
VAP. *See* Ventilator-associated pneumonia (VAP)
Variation: across healthcare providers, recognizing, 441; common cause (or systemic), 105, 162, 163; common causes *vs.* special causes of, 134–39; decision making in face of, 132; as

enemy of quality, 127; reducing, Deming on, 130; special cause (or unique), 105, 162
Variation data: applied for population health, examples of, 93–94; tools for analyzing, 83–87; using to drive healthcare quality initiatives, 87–91, 93–94
Variation in medical practice, 75, 77–82, 365; analyzing, 82–87; assignable, *76*, 92, 94; challenge of attribution and, 82–83; determining value of, 77; forest plot of variation in 30-day risk-standardized heart failure mortality in Medicare patients in Dallas County hospitals, *80*; funnel plot showing variation in 30-day risk-standardized heart failure mortality in Medicare patients in Dallas County hospitals, *81*; healthcare systems applying to quality improvement, examples of, 90–91; important procedural characteristics of, 77; minimizing or eliminating, 77, 94; national quality improvement efforts applying, examples of, 88–90; outcome, *76*; patterns, geography of, 54; performance, *76*, 92; process, *76*; random, *76*, 94; successful management of, 94–95; terminology of, *76*; warranted *vs.* unwarranted, 77
Variation in physician practice, board and reduction in, 348
V-BID. *See* Value-based insurance design (V-BID)
V-BID for Better Care Act of 2017, 423
VBID Health, 452
Venous thromboembolism (VTE), 477
Ventilator-associated pneumonia (VAP), 477
Verma, Seema, 406
Veterans Health Administration, 482
VHA Inc., 477
Virginia Mason, 257; quality improvement philosophy at, 308
Virtual reality: simulation and, 215
"Vital Deming Lessons STILL Not Learned" (Balestracci), 132
"Vital Signs: Core Metrics for Health and Health Care Progress" (IOM), 404
Vital statistics, 493
Voltaire, 320
Volume-driven healthcare system: transition to value-based healthcare system, 415
Volume-to-value shift in healthcare, 457–63; clinical nuance, 417–18; consumer cost sharing, 416–17; "drive to five" and, *462*, 462–63; implementing clinical nuance in V-BID, 418–19; key concepts in, 416–19; National Quality Strategy as a roadmap, 457–58, *459*; performance measurement and, 458, *460*, 460–61
VTE. *See* Venous thromboembolism (VTE)

Wagner, Ed, 394
Walmart, 453
Walton, Merilyn, 283
Ward, Lawrence: perspective on NCQA Patient-Centered Specialty Practice program, 399
Ware, John, 56, 58, 60, 119
Warranted variation: BSWQA strategy and creation of, 94; unwarranted variation *vs.*, 77, 94–95
Washington Health Alliance, 452
Wasson, John, 54, 61
Waste: types of, 20
Wasteful care, 10–11
Waste (or *muda*) removal: Lean and, 20
Wearable technology, 123
Weick, Karl, 258, 262, 263, 267, 268
Wellness Council of America, 453
Wellness programs: for employee populations, 479
Wennberg, John, 54, 77
Westrum, Ronald, 258, 263
Wheeler, Donald, 141

White, Kerr, 52
WHO Patient Safety Curriculum Guide for Medical Schools, 283–84; *Teacher's Guide* component, 284
Woods, David, 260
Work-based clinics, 359, 363
Worker compensation claims, 255
Workforce populations: safety and quality in, 478–79
Workforce safety: healthcare quality and, 254–55; patient safety and, 255
Workforce safety cultures: successful, characteristics of, 263
Working behavior: workforce safety cultures and, 263
Workplace culture: reviewing, 312
World Health Organization (WHO), 283; health system performance rankings, 175

Yale School of Management, 55
Year-end review performance data, 130–32, *131, 133*; control chart of, *142*
Yelp, 185
YMCA diabetes program: Medicare reimbursement and, 61

Zero harm to patients: reliable care and, 256
Zero preventable harm: culture of safety and high reliability and, 276; safety science, high reliability organizing, and, 265
Zero Trends (Edington), 446
Zip code: as predictor of health, 486
Zoo lions scenario: clinical trial findings and, 128; types of statistics applied to, 129–30

ABOUT THE EDITORS

David B. Nash, MD, was named the founding dean of the Jefferson College of Population Health in 2008, capping nearly three decades on the faculty of Thomas Jefferson University in Philadelphia. He is also the Dr. Raymond C. and Doris N. Grandon Professor of Health Policy. Dr. Nash is a board-certified internist who is internationally recognized for his work in public accountability for outcomes, physician leadership development, and quality-of-care improvement.

Dr. Nash has repeatedly been named to *Modern Healthcare*'s list of "Most Powerful People in Healthcare," and his national activities cover a wide scope. He is a principal faculty member for quality-of-care programming for the American Association for Physician Leadership (AAPL) in Tampa, Florida. He also serves on the National Quality Forum Task Force on Improving Population Health and the John M. Eisenberg Award Committee for The Joint Commission. He is a founding member of the Association of American Medical Colleges Integrating Quality (AAMC-IQ) Steering Committee, the group charged with infusing the tenets of quality and safety into medical education. Dr. Nash was recently appointed to the board of the Pharmaceutical Quality Alliance in Washington, DC. He also has governance responsibilities for various organizations in the public and private sectors.

Dr. Nash has received many awards in recognition of his achievements. He earned the top recognition award from the Academy of Managed Care Pharmacy in 1995, received the *Philadelphia Business Journal* Healthcare Heroes Award in 1997, and was named an honorary distinguished fellow of the American College of Physician Executives (now the AAPL) in 1998. In 2006, he received the Elliot Stone Award for leadership in public accountability for health data from the National Association of Health Data Organizations. The Wharton School honored Dr. Nash in 2009 with the Wharton Healthcare Alumni Achievement Award and in 2012 with the Joseph Wharton Social Impact Award. Also in 2012, he received the *Philadelphia Business Journal* award for innovation in medical education.

Dr. Nash's work is well known through his many publications, public appearances, "Nash on the Road" blog, and online column in *MedPage Today*. He has authored more than 100 peer-reviewed articles and edited 23 books, including *Connecting with the New Healthcare Consumer* (Jones & Bartlett

Learning, 2001); *The Quality Solution* (Jones & Bartlett Learning, 2005); *Demand Better!* (Second River Healthcare Press, 2011); and, most recently, *Population Health: Creating a Culture of Wellness*, second edition (Jones & Bartlett Learning, 2016). He was also the inaugural deputy editor of *Annals of Internal Medicine* (1984–1989). Currently, Dr. Nash is editor-in-chief of the *American Journal of Medical Quality, Population Health Management, P&T* (pharmacy and therapeutics), and *American Health and Drug Benefits.*

Dr. Nash received his BA in economics (Phi Beta Kappa) from Vassar College, his MD from the University of Rochester School of Medicine and Dentistry, and his MBA in health administration (with honors) from the Wharton School at the University of Pennsylvania. While at Penn, he was a former Robert Wood Johnson Foundation Clinical Scholar and medical director of a nine-physician faculty group practice in general internal medicine. He has received three honorary doctorates, from Salus University, Geisinger Commonwealth School of Medicine, and the University of Rochester.

Maulik S. Joshi, DrPH, is the chief operating officer and executive vice president of integrated care delivery at the Anne Arundel Health System (AAHS) in Annapolis, Maryland. At AAHS, Dr. Joshi oversees health system operations and, with a team of more than 4,000 employees, leads the integration of care delivery across the continuum, including acute, ambulatory, post-acute, and ancillary care through owned, affiliated, and joint venture arrangements.

Previously, Dr. Joshi was at the American Hospital Association in Chicago, where he served as associate executive vice president and president of the Health Research and Educational Trust. He has served as senior adviser at the Agency for Healthcare Research and Quality and as president and CEO of the Delmarva Foundation, where he received the 2005 US Senate Productivity Award. He has also served as vice president at the Institute for Healthcare Improvement, as senior director of quality for the University of Pennsylvania Health System, and as executive vice president for The HMO Group.

Dr. Joshi has served on the board of trustees for Anne Arundel Medical Center, the Board Quality and Patient Safety Committee for Mercy Health System, the Health Outcomes Committee for Advocate Health Care, and the board of governors of the National Patient Safety Foundation. He has also been treasurer of the board of trustees for the Center for Advancing Health. Dr. Joshi was editor-in-chief for the *Journal for Healthcare Quality.*

Dr. Joshi received his DrPH and MHSA from the University of Michigan and his BS in mathematics from Lafayette College. He authored *Healthcare Transformation: A Guide for the Hospital Board Member* (CRC Press and AHA Press, 2009) and *Leading Healthcare Transformation: A Primer for Clinical Leaders* (CRC Press, 2015). He is an adjunct faculty member at the University of Michigan School of Public Health in the Department of Health Management and Policy.

Elizabeth R. Ransom, MD, is the executive vice president and clinical leader for the eight-hospital north zone of Texas Health Resources (THR). She and the operations leader are jointly responsible for strategy, operations, finance, hospital management and leadership, and physician and board relations for the region, with revenues of more than $2 billion. She focuses on collaborating with clinical partners, communities, employers, schools, religious organizations, physicians, and clinicians to create healthier lives for North Texans. Her work continues THR's efforts to round out continuum-of-care capabilities and evolve into a fully integrated system of health that excels in physician-directed population health management.

Previously, Dr. Ransom served as chief quality officer at Texas Health Harris Methodist Hospital Southwest Fort Worth, where she was responsible for the quality improvement and safety program, as well as oversight of medical staff affairs, pharmacy, patient safety and risk management, laboratory services, case management, and the environment of care. She also worked with the Texas Health Research & Education Institute on a strategic feasibility assessment of a coordinated graduate medical education initiative for THR.

Prior to joining THR, Dr. Ransom was the vice chair and chair-elect of the board of governors of the Henry Ford Medical Group. Additionally, she was the residency program director for the Department of Otolaryngology–Head and Neck Surgery and chair of the credentials committee of the Henry Ford Health System.

Dr. Ransom received her BSc in microbiology and immunology from McGill University in Montreal and her MD from Wayne State University School of Medicine in Detroit, Michigan. She completed her residency in otolaryngology–head and neck surgery at Henry Ford Hospital and was a senior staff physician there.

Scott B. Ransom, DO, FACHE, is a partner in the Health Industries Advisory at the PricewaterhouseCoopers Strategy& consulting team. He serves as a consultant to health systems, academic medical centers, universities, insurance companies, private equity firms, and other leading institutions on issues related to strategy-enabled transformation, physician engagement, organizational redesign, turnarounds and restructuring, mergers and acquisitions, clinical and research operations, quality, and medical education. He has served more than 100 health systems and academic medical centers, including eight of the top ten as ranked by *U.S. News & World Report.*

Dr. Ransom has more than 25 years of operations, clinical, and leadership experience, including appointments as president and CEO of the University of North Texas Health Science Center. He served previously as a hospital vice president for medical affairs and then as senior vice president and chief quality officer at the Detroit Medical Center / Wayne State University. Dr. Ransom has been a faculty member of three universities, including the University of Michigan in Ann Arbor, where he was a tenured professor in obstetrics, gynecology, and health management and policy and director of the program for health improvement and leadership development. He has conducted research supported by the National Institutes of Health and National Science Foundation and has authored more than 150 publications, including ten books, on topics related to healthcare management, quality, and women's health. He has delivered more than 4,000 babies and completed more than 10,000 surgeries as a practicing obstetrician.

Dr. Ransom is a Fellow of the American College of Healthcare Executives, the American College of Surgeons, and the American Congress of Obstetricians and Gynecologists. He is a Distinguished Fellow and past president of the American College of Physician Executives (now the American Association for Physician Leadership). He is board certified by the American Board of Obstetrics and Gynecology, the American Board of Medical Management, and the Certifying Commission in Medical Management.

Dr. Ransom received his MPH in clinical effectiveness from the Harvard University School of Public Health, his MBA from the University of Michigan Ross School of Business, and his medical degree from the Kansas City University of Medicine and Biosciences. He earned an undergraduate degree in chemistry at Pacific Lutheran University and is a graduate of the US Marine Corps Officer Candidates School.

ABOUT THE CONTRIBUTORS

Bracken Babula, MD, is a clinical assistant professor at Thomas Jefferson University in Philadelphia. He studied at Weill Cornell Medical College in New York City and completed his internal medicine / primary care residency at Beth Israel Deaconess Medical Center in Boston. He currently practices as a board-certified internist with Jefferson Internal Medicine Associates and works in quality improvement as an associate quality officer for the Department of Medicine.

Davis Balestracci is well known for delivering his message of "data sanity" with a passionate, provocative, challenging, yet humorous and down-to-earth public speaking style. He began his career with 3M in the mid-1980s and received several awards for his teaching and innovative uses of statistical methods. Since 1992, he has devoted his efforts primarily to healthcare, and he was a regular presenter at the Institute for Healthcare Improvement annual forum for 21 consecutive years. His book *Data Sanity: A Quantum Leap to Unprecedented Results* provides a unique synthesis of W. Edwards Deming's teachings into an improvement-based leadership philosophy designed to transform organizations to cultures of excellence. Balestracci holds a BS degree in chemical engineering and an MS degree in statistics.

David J. Ballard, MD, PhD, is chief quality officer of Baylor Scott & White Health (BSWH), the largest nonprofit healthcare system in Texas, which includes 49 hospitals, more than 1,000 patient care sites, 6,000 affiliated and/or employed physicians, more than 44,000 employees, and the Scott & White Health Plan. He also serves as president of the BSWH STEEEP Global Institute, which has a mission of providing performance improvement solutions to healthcare organizations throughout the world. A board-certified internist, Dr. Ballard trained at the Mayo Graduate School of Medicine following completion of degrees in chemistry, economics, epidemiology, and medicine at the University of North Carolina (UNC). At UNC, he was a Morehead Scholar, North Carolina Fellow, and junior-year Phi Beta Kappa inductee. Dr. Ballard received the AcademyHealth New Investigator Award in 1995, the Distinguished Alumnus Award of the UNC School of Medicine in 2008, and the 2012 *Health Services Research* John M. Eisenberg Article-of-the-Year Award. His books *Achieving*

STEEEP Health Care and *The Guide to Achieving STEEEP Health Care* both received the Shingo Research Award for their contributions to operational excellence. Dr. Ballard was named in 2015, 2016, and 2017 by *Becker's Hospital Review* as one of "50 Experts Leading the Field of Patient Safety."

Michael S. Barr, MD, is a board-certified internist and executive vice president for the Quality Measurement and Research Group at the National Committee for Quality Assurance (NCQA). His portfolio at NCQA includes performance measurement development; research; management of NCQA's contracts and grants portfolio; and contributions to strategic initiatives, public policy, and educational programs.

Bettina Berman, RN, is the associate director for ambulatory performance improvement at the Jefferson College of Population Health, where she is responsible for the development, implementation, and evaluation of quality initiatives for the Jefferson Clinically Integrated Network. Her background includes extensive experience in inpatient and outpatient quality management, including the implementation of value-based strategies. She has authored peer-reviewed papers on quality management and coauthored book chapters on ambulatory quality measurement.

Scott E. Buchalter, MD, is a professor of medicine in the Division of Pulmonary and Critical Care Medicine at the University of Alabama at Birmingham (UAB) School of Medicine. In addition to his clinical duties, he serves as the quality education officer for UAB Medicine and as the medical director for healthcare quality and safety within the UAB School of Health Professions. A graduate of the School of Medicine, he completed his residency and fellowship training at UAB. His many clinical and medical staff leadership responsibilities have led to his strong interest and leadership in the field of quality improvement and patient safety.

John Byrnes, MD, is a nationally recognized expert in healthcare quality and safety. He has more than 25 years of experience leading, designing, and implementing quality and safety programs throughout the United States and Europe. During his 11-year tenure as chief quality officer at Spectrum Health in Grand Rapids, Michigan, the organization received more than 100 quality awards and was ranked three times as one of the nation's top 15 health systems. Dr. Byrnes is chief medical officer for the Adventist Health Northern California region.

Craig Clapper, PE, is a founding partner of Healthcare Performance Improvement (HPI) and a partner in Press Ganey Strategic Consulting. Clapper has

30 years of experience improving reliability in nuclear power, transportation, manufacturing, and healthcare. He specializes in cause analysis, reliability improvement, and safety culture improvements. He has led safety culture transformation engagements for Duke Energy, the US Department of Energy, ABB, Westinghouse, Framatome ANP, Sentara Healthcare, and Sharp HealthCare. Prior to becoming a partner in Press Ganey consulting, Clapper was the chief knowledge officer of HPI, the chief operating officer of HPI, the chief operating officer of Performance Improvement International, systems engineering manager for Hope Creek Nuclear Generating Station, and systems engineering manager for Palo Verde Nuclear Generation Station.

Laura Cranston, RPh, serves as the executive director of the Pharmacy Quality Alliance, a multistakeholder membership-based organization that develops medication use measures and works with organizations (including health plans, pharmacy benefit managers, community pharmacy organizations, and employers) to encourage the uptake and implementation of meaningful medication use measures in the marketplace.

Briget da Graca, JD, is a senior medical writer with the Center for Clinical Effectiveness at Baylor Scott & White Health (BSWH) in Dallas, Texas, and a clinical assistant professor of health services research with the Robbins Institute for Health Care Policy and Leadership at Baylor University in Waco, Texas. She holds degrees in biochemistry and science and technology journalism from Texas A&M University, and in 2012 she received her JD *summa cum laude* from the Southern Methodist Dedman School of Law. She has worked with health services researchers within BSWH for more than ten years, examining a variety of topics related to the effectiveness and efficiency of care. In 2012 she received the *Health Services Research* John M. Eisenberg Article-of-the-Year Award, and in 2015 she was a Presidential Scholar for the AcademyHealth Institute on Advocacy and Public Policy.

Sue S. Feldman, RN, PhD, is associate professor and director of graduate programs in health informatics in the School of Health Professions at the University of Alabama at Birmingham. She also has a dual appointment in the School of Medicine. Dr. Feldman has been published in a variety of top-tier peer-reviewed journals and conference proceedings and has served as program chair for several national forums. Dr. Feldman has a master's degree in education and a PhD in education and in information systems and technology from Claremont Graduate University.

A. Mark Fendrick, MD, is a professor of internal medicine in the School of Medicine and a professor of health management and policy in the School of

Public Health at the University of Michigan. He received a bachelor's degree in economics and chemistry from the University of Pennsylvania and a medical degree from Harvard Medical School. Dr. Fendrick conceptualized and coined the term "value-based insurance design" (V-BID) and currently directs the V-BID Center at the University of Michigan, the leading advocate for development, implementation, and evaluation of innovative health benefit plans.

Hannah M. Fish, PharmD, at the time of this writing, was associate director for education and communications for the Pharmacy Quality Alliance (PQA). In that role, she was responsible for leading a broad range of activities focused on guiding PQA's communications strategy, consistently articulating the organization's mission, and ensuring that PQA was viewed as the primary source, disseminator, and conduit of medication use quality information for outside stakeholders and members. In addition, she led special projects to drive organizational awareness, improve educational engagement, and advance patient care, including the development of immunization-related performance measures.

Neil Goldfarb is president and CEO of the Greater Philadelphia Business Coalition on Health (GPBCH), an employer-led nonprofit organization with the mission of developing best practices for maintaining a healthy workforce and ensuring that healthcare is safe, high-quality, accessible, and affordable. GPBCH, established in 2012, represents more than 1.5 million covered lives nationally. Mr. Goldfarb brings more than 30 years of healthcare research and management experience to his coalition leadership position.

Norbert Goldfield, MD, is CEO of Ask Nurses and Doctors, a bipartisan venture, incorporated in April 2018, that supports competitive congressional candidates who have practical plans for universal health coverage for all Americans. Dr. Goldfield is also founder and CEO of Healing Across the Divides, which focuses on peace building through health in the Israeli–Palestinian conflict. Prior to February 2018, Dr. Goldfield worked for 30 years as medical director for a private healthcare research group, developing tools linking payment for healthcare services to improved quality of healthcare outcomes. Dr. Goldfield edits a peer-reviewed medical journal, the *Journal of Ambulatory Care Management*; has published more than 50 books and articles; and is a practicing internist.

Anne J. Gunderson, GNP, EdD, is professor of medicine and associate dean for innovation in clinical education at Georgetown University, where she created and directs the Executive Master's in Clinical Quality, Safety, and Leadership program. She is also assistant vice president of quality and safety education for MedStar Health, a ten-hospital system. She has spent the past 17 years in medical education, has authored more than 20 manuscripts and a book, and has secured funding from multiple national agencies.

Marianthi N. Hatzigeorgiou is an administrative fellow at Anne Arundel Medical Center. She received her master of health services administration degree from the University of Michigan. Prior to receiving her master's, she worked at Park View Health Systems of Fort Wayne, Indiana, designing and launching integrated care clinics.

Leslie W. Hayes, MD, is the associate quality education officer for University of Alabama at Birmingham (UAB) Medicine. She is also an associate professor of pediatrics in the UAB School of Medicine, Division of Pediatric Critical Care, and serves as the associate medical director of UAB Healthcare Quality and Safety Programs in the School of Health Professions. She is certified by the American Board of Pediatrics Subboard of Pediatric Critical Care Medicine. Dr. Hayes is a graduate of The Ohio State University School of Medicine, and she completed her combined internal medicine and pediatrics internship and residency at UAB. She is a Six Sigma Black Belt with extensive experience working with healthcare systems on quality improvement and patient safety initiatives.

Richard Jacoby, MD, is a clinical associate professor in the Jefferson College of Population Health. He is director of ambulatory quality performance improvement for Jefferson University Physicians, a large multispecialty clinical practice.

Rebecca C. Jaffe, MD, received her medical degree from the Perelman School of Medicine at the University of Pennsylvania, and she completed her residency training in internal medicine at the University of Pennsylvania Health System. She is board certified in internal medicine and a clinical assistant professor of medicine in the Division of Hospital Medicine at Thomas Jefferson University Hospital (TJUH). Dr. Jaffe serves as TJUH's first assistant patient safety officer and associate designated institutional official for quality and safety education, acting as a liaison between graduate medical education and the institution's infrastructure for patient safety and quality improvement. Dr. Jaffe has been recognized for her teaching, receiving in 2014 the Jefferson University Alpha Omega Alpha Volunteer Clinical Faculty Award, the Leon A. Peris Memorial Award for Excellence in Teaching and Superior Patient Care, and the Internal Medicine Teaching Attending of the Year for Humanism in Medicine.

Keith Kosel, PhD, is vice president of strategic enterprise relationships at the Parkland Center for Clinical Innovation (PCCI), a leading nonprofit research and innovation affiliate of Parkland Health & Hospital System in Dallas, Texas. Dr. Kosel has responsibility for introducing innovative solutions and advisory services and managing engagements to help clients address pressing needs in the areas of population health, quality and safety, and patient engagement. Before coming to PCCI, Dr. Kosel was senior vice president of government affairs at Vizient Inc., where he procured and oversaw all of Vizient's government grants and contracts as well as member advocacy via the organization's Washington, DC, office.

Hyunjoo Lee, MD, is a medical education fellow and clinical instructor in the Department of Emergency Medicine at Thomas Jefferson University in Philadelphia. Born and raised in New York, she left to pursue her undergraduate studies at Swarthmore College in Pennsylvania, where she received a BA in biology. She returned to New York and researched B-cell biology and chronic lymphocytic leukemia, before heading back to school to obtain her MD from Stony Brook University School of Medicine. She completed her emergency medicine residency at Mount Sinai Beth Israel in New York City.

Thomas H. Lee, MD, is chief medical officer for Press Ganey, Inc. He is a practicing internist and cardiologist at Brigham and Women's Hospital and a professor (part time) at Harvard Medical School. He is a member of the board of directors of Geisinger Health System, the Panel of Health Advisors of the Congressional Budget Office, and the editorial board of the *New England Journal of Medicine.*

David Mayer, MD, is vice president of quality and safety for MedStar Health. He is responsible for overseeing the infrastructure for clinical quality and its operational efficiency for MedStar and each of its entities. Dr. Mayer also founded and has led the annual Telluride International Patient Safety Roundtable and Patient Safety Educational Summer Camps for health science students and resident physicians over the past 13 years.

Frank Micciche is the vice president of public policy and communications for the National Committee for Quality Assurance. He has worked in the area of state and federal health policy for more than two decades, including four years as the director of the Commonwealth of Massachusetts's Washington, DC, office, where he advised Governor Mitt Romney on intergovernmental issues, including healthcare reform. Micciche holds a master's degree in public policy from the John F. Kennedy School of Government at Harvard University, as well as a bachelor's degree in political science from Tufts University.

Deirdre E. Mylod, PhD, is the executive director of the Institute for Innovation and senior vice president of research and analytics at Press Ganey Associates. She is the architect of Press Ganey's Suffering Framework, which reframes the view of the patient experience as a means to understand unmet patient needs and reduce patient suffering. She holds a PhD in psychology from the University of Notre Dame.

Mel L. Nelson, PharmD, is the director of research and academic affairs at the Pharmacy Quality Alliance (PQA). In this role, she is responsible for the advancement and coordination of PQA's research portfolio. She also directs PQA's student and postgraduate programs, to support PQA's commitment to educating the next generation of healthcare quality leaders. Prior to her work for PQA, Dr. Nelson spent several years as a research assistant at the University of Arizona College of Pharmacy, with a focus on investigating healthcare quality improvement, health professions education, and health outcomes.

David Nicewander received his master's degree in biostatistics from the School of Public Health of the University of Illinois at Chicago. His more than 20 years of experience in healthcare analytics and research include five years as a statistician with the Centers for Medicare & Medicaid Services, where he was involved in national quality improvement projects targeting Medicare beneficiaries. He currently serves as director of analytics at Baylor Scott & White Health in Dallas, Texas, where he oversees analytic support provided to performance improvement and clinical effectiveness initiatives.

Susan Lynne Oesterle is the program manager for the University of Michigan Center for Value-Based Insurance Design (V-BID), a public policy center and the leading advocate for development, implementation, and evaluation of innovative health benefit plans. In this role, she manages and coordinates all aspects of the V-BID Center's activities. Oesterle holds degrees in business and education from Eastern Michigan University, which prepared her surprisingly well for work in the public policy realm.

Dimitrios Papanagnou, MD, is the vice chair for education in the Department of Emergency Medicine at Thomas Jefferson University, the assistant dean for faculty development in the Sidney Kimmel Medical College of Thomas Jefferson University, and the director for the In Situ Simulation Program at Thomas Jefferson University Hospitals.

Kathryn C. Peisert is managing editor of The Governance Institute. She oversees The Governance Institute's library of publications in print and online, video programs, webinars, e-learning courses, and customized board education curriculum. She also develops the overall education agenda and programs for Governance Institute conferences. She has authored or coauthored articles in *Health Affairs*, the *Journal of Health & Life Sciences Law*, *Prescriptions* *for Excellence in Health Care*, and *Healthcare Executive*, as well as numerous articles, case studies, and research reports for The Governance Institute. She has a bachelor's degree in communications from the University of California, Los Angeles, and a master's degree from Boston University.

Matthew K. Pickering, PharmD, serves as the associate director of research and quality strategies at the Pharmacy Quality Alliance (PQA). In this role, he identifies needed studies to further validate the impact of PQA's measures on improving patient care, reducing overall healthcare spending, and filling recognized gaps in performance measurement. Dr. Pickering is also responsible for coordinating PQA research and demonstration project portfolios. He works closely with the PQA research team to implement high-quality, responsive, and timely activities that support PQA research functions and internal operations.

Rhea E. Powell, MD, is an assistant professor of medicine at Thomas Jefferson University in Philadelphia. She is a practicing primary care physician in internal medicine and a health services researcher interested in how the organization can support the delivery of quality care and improve health.

Michael D. Pugh has more than 30 years of CEO experience in hospitals, healthcare systems, managed care organizations, and consulting and healthcare technology companies. He is an internationally known adviser and consultant to healthcare providers, payers, trade associations, technology companies, and government organizations. He is an adjunct professor in the University of Colorado Denver Business School Health Administration Program, an instructor in the Mount Sinai Medical School Health Care Leadership Program, and a senior faculty member for the Institute for Healthcare Improvement. Pugh holds a BS and an MPH in healthcare administration from Tulane University in New Orleans, Louisiana, and is the author of multiple articles and book chapters on quality and governance.

Margaret F. Shope received her bachelor of science degree in interdisciplinary physics from the University of Michigan in 2018. She is a research assistant at the University of Michigan Center for Value-Based Insurance Design and plans to pursue a combined degree in medicine and public health.

Brett D. Stauffer, MD, is a practicing hospitalist and vice president associate chief quality officer for Baylor Scott & White Health (BSWH) in Dallas, Texas. He has led a variety of BSWH efforts focused on quality measurement and improvement, including standardization of quality reporting for the system, electronic order sets, and development of other clinical decision support tools. Dr. Stauffer's research has focused on the care of patients with chronic disease, including the improvement of care transitions for patients with heart failure to prevent readmission. He attended medical school at the University of Medicine and Dentistry of New Jersey (New Jersey Medical School) and trained in internal medicine at Parkland/UT Southwestern in Dallas. Following his residency, Dr. Stauffer was an assistant professor at UT Southwestern and part of the strategic planning office for Parkland hospital. He completed a Robert Wood Johnson Clinical Scholars Fellowship at Yale University from 2006 to 2008 and, since graduating, has held various leadership positions within BSWH.

Lawrence Ward, MD, is the vice chair for clinical practice and quality and associate professor of medicine in the Department of Medicine at the Sidney Kimmel Medical College of Thomas Jefferson University. He is also the medical director, primary care and population health, for Jefferson University Physicians. In these roles, he develops innovative practice designs and leads efforts on quality improvement, value-based care, population health, and pay for performance.

Alexis Wickersham, MD, is a hospitalist at Thomas Jefferson University Hospital and a clinical instructor of internal medicine at the Sidney Kimmel Medical College. Prior to joining Jefferson in 2016, she completed her residency training at the University of Iowa Hospitals and Clinics and served as the chief resident in quality and safety through the Iowa City Veterans Administration Medical Center. She enjoys teaching and mentoring students and residents in quality improvement and patient safety and is active in resident curricular design.